second edition

# Philosophies and Theories

## for Advanced Nursing Practice

*Edited by*

Janie B. Butts, PhD, RN
Professor
College of Nursing
The University of Southern Mississippi
Hattiesburg, Mississippi

Karen L. Rich, PhD, RN
Associate Professor
College of Nursing
The University of Southern Mississippi
Long Beach, Mississippi

JONES & BARTLETT
LEARNING

*World Headquarters*
Jones & Bartlett Learning
5 Wall Street
Burlington, MA 01803
978-443-5000
info@jblearning.com
www.jblearning.com

Jones & Bartlett Learning books and products are available through most bookstores and online booksellers. To contact Jones & Bartlett Learning directly, call 800-832-0034, fax 978-443-8000, or visit our website, www.jblearning.com.

**Production Credits**
Executive Publisher: William Brottmiller
Senior Editor: Amanda Martin
Associate Acquisitions Editor: Teresa Reilly
Editorial Assistant: Rebecca Myrick
Production Editor: Keith Henry
Senior Marketing Manager: Jennifer Stiles

VP, Manufacturing and Inventory Control: Therese Connell
Composition: Aptara®, Inc.
Photo Research and Permissions Coordinator: Joseph Veiga
Cover Design: Michael O'Donnell
Cover Image: © kwest/ShutterStock, Inc.
Printing and Binding: Edwards Brothers Malloy
Cover Printing: Edwards Brothers Malloy

**Library of Congress Cataloging-in-Publication Data**
Philosophies and theories for advanced nursing practice / [edited by] Janie B. Butts, Karen L. Rich.—2e.
    p. ; cm.
    Includes bibliographical references and index.
    ISBN 978-1-284-04134-7 (pbk.)
    I. Butts, Janie B., editor of compilation. II. Rich, Karen L., editor of compilation.
    [DNLM: 1. Nursing Theory. 2. Advanced Practice Nursing. 3. Evidence-Based Nursing. 4. Models, Nursing. WY 86]
    RT84.5
    610.7301—dc23
                                                                2013042019

6048

Printed in the United States of America
17 16 15 14    10 9 8 7 6 5 4 3 2

# TABLE OF CONTENTS

**CHAPTER 23**    **The Praxis Theory of Suffering    559**

**Part 5**    **Tools for Integrating and Disseminating Knowledge in Advanced Nursing Practice    591**

**CHAPTER 24**    **Theory Testing and Theory Evaluation    593**

*Philosophies and Theories for Advanced Nursing Practice,* by Janie B. Butts and Karen L. Rich (editors), is an essential resource for advanced practice nurses and for students in graduate nursing programs, both DNP and master's-level programs. The authors who contributed to this text are distinguished nursing and interdisciplinary scholars with expertise in theory.

## Arrangement of the Book

There are 25 chapters that are presented in 5 parts:
- Part 1: Foundations of Nursing Science
- Part 2: The Structure and Function of Theory
- Part 3: Interdisciplinary Philosophies and Theories
- Part 4: Select Nursing Models and Theories
- Part 5: Tools for Integrating and Disseminating Knowledge in Advanced Nursing Practice

The chapters in Parts 1 and 2 provide the foundation for philosophy of science, the development of nursing knowledge, and theory. Advanced practice nurses and nursing students can use Parts 1 and 2 as sequential building blocks for the information in Part 5—theory evaluation, testing, and integrating, translating, and disseminating evidence-based findings from research to practice.

Part 3 focuses on a selection of interdisciplinary philosophies and theories relevant for advanced practice. Part 4 is a focus on select conceptual models, grand theories, and middle-range theories of nursing. Conceptual nursing models and grand nursing theories both bring advanced practice nurses a certain reality of conceptual arrangements, theoretical variables, and propositions used for deriving middle-range theory. Middle-range nursing theories derived from conceptual models and grand theories of nursing translate theory and research findings directly into practice.

## Acknowledgments

We would like to thank the Jones & Bartlett Learning staff, editors, and administrators for their diligent work and their support given to us. We also thank our colleagues who enthusiastically shared their expertise with us. Without their contributions, we could not have this book. For these reasons, we extend to you a big thank you!

*Janie B. Butts and Karen L. Rich*

**Janie B. Butts, PhD, RN,** The University of Southern Mississippi, College of Nursing, Hattiesburg, Mississippi

Janie B. Butts is Professor at The University of Southern Mississippi College of Nursing in Hattiesburg, Mississippi, and teaches classroom and online nursing courses at the doctoral, master's, and baccalaureate levels. Courses include ethics, advanced theory, advanced practice issues, professional development, research, and professional nursing practice. Dr. Butts was elected to serve beginning in 2008 in the capacity of Consultant Editor for *Nursing Ethics* journal, an international journal with headquarters located in England. Current specific research interests include death and dying ethical issues. Dr. Butts' journal articles and book chapters include topics on ethics, her research, theory, education, professional issues, and home care ethics, and she reviews for top nursing journals and book companies. Dr. Butts' doctoral degree is from the University of Alabama at Birmingham with an emphasis in nursing education and nursing science, and her master's degree is from the University of Mississippi at the Medical Center, Jackson, with an emphasis in adult health nursing and nursing management.

**Karen L. Rich, PhD, RN,** The University of Southern Mississippi, College of Nursing, Long Beach, Mississippi

Karen L. Rich is an Associate Professor at The University of Southern Mississippi College of Nursing in Long Beach, Mississippi, where she teaches public health nursing, ethics, and professional development. Dr. Rich's doctoral degree in nursing with an emphasis in ethics is from The University of Southern Mississippi. She has a master's in public health nursing from Louisiana State University and a post-master's in psychiatric–mental health nursing, nurse practitioner emphasis, from The University of Southern Mississippi. Dr. Rich serves as a Consultant Editor for the international *Nursing Ethics* journal. She serves on the ethics committees of a large county hospital in Gulfport, Mississippi, and a private hospital in Biloxi, Mississippi. Dr. Rich has written a number of articles and book chapters about ethics and philosophy. Her special interests are communitarian ethics, virtue ethics, ethics in public health, Eastern philosophy and ethics, and critical thinking in nursing.

# CONTRIBUTORS

**Patsy Anderson, DNS, RN**
Associate Professor
DNP Assistant Coordinator,
  College of Nursing
The University of Southern Mississippi
Gulf Coast Campus
Long Beach, Mississippi

**Sandra Bishop, DNS, RN**
Assistant Professor
Academics Coordinator,
  College of Nursing
The University of Southern Mississippi
Gulf Coast Campus
Long Beach, Mississippi

**Margaret M. Braungart, PhD**
Professor Emeritus, Psychology
Center for Bioethics and Humanities
SUNY Upstate Medical University
Syracuse, New York

**Richard G. Braungart, PhD**
Professor Emeritus, Sociology
Maxwell School
Syracuse University
Syracuse, New York

**Lora E. Burke, PhD, MPH, RN**
Professor, School of Nursing
  and Graduate School of
  Public Health, Department
  of Epidemiology
University of Pittsburgh
Pittsburgh, Pennsylvania

**Janie B. Butts, PhD, RN**
Professor
PhD Assistant Coordinator,
  College of Nursing
The University of Southern Mississippi
Hattiesburg, Mississippi

**Peggy L. Chinn, PhD, RN, FAAN**
Professor Emerita
School of Nursing
University of Connecticut
Storrs, Connecticut

**Lisa Astalos Chism, DNP, APRN, BC**
Nurse Practitioner
Department of Internal Medicine
Beaumont Hospitals
Woodhaven, Michigan

**Joanne R. Duffy, PhD, RN, FAAN**
Professor
Department of Environments
  for Health
Indiana University-Purdue
  University Indianapolis
Indianapolis, Indiana

**Joan C. Engebretson, DrPH, RN,
  AHN-BC**
Professor
The University of Texas Health
  Science Center at Houston
Houston, Texas

**Jacqueline Fawcett, PhD, FAAN**
Professor
College of Nursing and
    Health Sciences
University of Massachusetts,
    Boston
Boston, Massachusetts

**Karen Glanz, PhD, MPH**
Faculty
Rollins School of Public Health
Emory University
Atlanta, Georgia

**Yolanda M. Gonzalez, DNS, MSN**
Nursing Faculty
Universidad de Panama
Panama, Republic of Panama

**Patricia Goodson, PhD**
Professor, Department of Health &
    Kinesiology
Texas A&M University
College Station, Texas

**Sherry Hartman, DrPH, RN**
Professor Emeritus of Nursing
The University of Southern
    Mississippi
Hattiesburg, Mississippi

**Joanne V. Hickey, PhD, RN,
    ACNP-BC, FAAN, FCCM**
Professor, Patricia L. Starck
    Professor of Nursing
Director, Doctor of Nursing
    Practice Program
University of Texas at Houston,
    School of Nursing
Houston, Texas

**Violet M. Malinski, PhD, RN**
Associate Professor
Hunter-Bellevue School of Nursing
New York, New York

**Kathleen Masters, DNS, RN**
Associate Professor
Associate Director, College of Nursing
The University of Southern
    Mississippi
Hattiesburg, Mississippi

**María Elisa Moreno-Fergusson,
    MSN, RN**
Nursing Faculty
Universidad de La Sabana
Bogotá, Columbia

**Janice M. Morse, PhD, RN, FAAN**
Professor
College of Nursing
University of Utah
Salt Lake City, Utah

**Sandra Nelson, PhD, APRN-BC**
Associate Professor
Psychiatric Mental Health Nursing
Eastern Michigan University
Ypsilanti, Michigan

**E. Carol Polifroni, EdD, CNE,
    NEA-BC, RN**
Associate Professor
School of Nursing
University of Connecticut
Storrs, Connecticut

**Larry Purnell, PhD, RN, FAAN**
Professor
Department of Nursing
The University of Delaware
Newark, Delaware

**Karen L. Rich, PhD, RN**
Associate Professor, College of Nursing
The University of Southern Mississippi
Gulf Coast Campus
Long Beach, Mississippi

**Barbara K. Rimer, DrPH**
Dean and Alumni Distinguished
Professor
UNC Gillings School of Global Public
Health
Chapel Hill, North Carolina

**Beth L. Rodgers, PhD, RN, FAAN**
Professor
College of Nursing
University of Wisconsin, Milwaukee
Milwaukee, Wisconsin

**Mary W. Stewart, PhD, RN**
Associate Professor
School of Nursing
University of Mississippi
    Medical Center
Jackson, Mississippi

**Rosemarie Tong, PhD**
Director
Distinguished Professor of
    Healthcare Ethics
Center for Professional and
    Applied Sciences
Department of Philosophy
University of North Carolina,
    Charlotte
Charlotte, North Carolina

**Steven J. Vanderheiden, PhD**
Assistant Professor of Political
    Science
Department of Political Science
University of Colorado at Boulder
Boulder, Colorado

**Martha V. Whetsell, PhD,
    RN, ARNP**
Faculty
Department of Nursing CUNY
Lehman College
Bronx, New York

# PART 1

# Foundations of Nursing Science

# Philosophy of Science: An Introduction

*E. Carol Polifroni*

## Introduction

A philosophy of science is a perspective—a lens, a way one views the world, and, in the case of advanced practice nurses, the viewpoint the nurse acts from in every encounter with a patient, family, or group. A person's philosophy of science creates the frame on a picture—a message that becomes a paradigm and a point of reference. Each individual's philosophy of science will permit some things to be seen and cause others to be blocked. It allows people to be open to some thoughts and potentially keeps them closed to others. A philosophy will deem some ideas correct, others inconsistent, and some simply wrong. While philosophy of science is not meant to be viewed as a black or white proposition, it does provide perspectives that include some ideas and thoughts and, therefore, it must necessarily exclude others. The important key is to ensure that the ideas and thoughts within a given philosophy remain consistent with one another, rather than being in opposition.

Discussions of science, philosophy, and philosophy of science could all fill books unto themselves. This chapter introduces readers to these topics. It is constructed in the form of a survey and is designed to launch inquiry in myriad ways. The purpose is to encourage nurses to think in ways that they may not yet have discovered and to examine their assumptions and actions in their role as advanced practice nurses. If nurses leave this chapter without questioning their assumptions, the author has not done her job! One must appreciate the personal assumptions used in everyday professional life. Nurses, for example, must question their assumptions and reaffirm (appreciate and understand) what it is that they believe.

# Science

Before the concept of a philosophy of science is examined in greater depth and particular philosophies of science are specifically explored, it is important to begin by developing an appreciation of the meaning of the terms *science* and *philosophy*. Science, which comes from the Latin word *scientia*, meaning "knowledge," traditionally refers to both processes and the outcomes of processes, such as general laws and observations. General laws are the laws of nature that guide physical life, such as the laws of gravity, energy, and motion. Generators of science use these laws in a systematic way to create a body of knowledge about a specific topic. The culmination of using the scientific method (systematic process) provides a set of data (evidence) supported by propositions about an area of study (Boyd, Gasper, & Trout, 1991).

## Natural Hard Sciences

As an outcome, science is a body of knowledge. Physics, mathematics, and chemistry are three examples of scientific disciplines composed of unique bodies of knowledge. These sciences are often classified as *natural sciences* because they employ the general laws of nature and begin with the physical notion of the world. These natural sciences (which are also sometimes referred to as the *physical sciences*) are also known as *pure sciences*. "Pure," in this context, means a unique body of knowledge. A pure science is independent of others; it is able to stand alone, and it may be developed and furthered for the abstract cause of the knowledge itself. Pure science is not pursued for its utility or value.

Natural and pure sciences are based on the assumption that reality is objective, rather than subjective. As a result of this objectivity, natural science is consistent—in other words, it is reproducible and reliable. Natural science further encompasses the assumption that human beings have the capacity to be accurate in their objectivity.

Natural scientists believe that explanations (obtained using the method described later in this chapter) are present within the natural or real world. As a consequence, explanations are reasonable, constant and consistent, accurate, objective, discoverable, and understandable. Owing to its basis in objectivity, natural science is predicated on the belief that there is an external world structure independent of self that is grounded in reliability.

Natural physical sciences are referred to as *hard science*. In recent years, quantum physicists have begun to integrate the role of the observer into their discipline, which is still categorized as a hard science. This conundrum will be addressed as part of the discussion of complexity science found at the end of this chapter.

Examples of the physical sciences present in health care include the biophysical and biochemical processes related to diabetes, cardiovascular disease, and cancer. Using the physical sciences in health care involves assuming a disease focus, rather than a person focus. The science is about diagnosis, treatment, and outcomes of treatment. It is about side effects and it is about pathology.

## Soft Applied Sciences

Sociology, psychology, and anthropology are three examples of applied sciences. *Applied sciences* have their own unique body of knowledge, albeit a different one than is found in the natural sciences category. They are known as applied sciences because the focus is on the application of related knowledge, usually to meet some human need (and not to generate knowledge for the sake of knowledge). Additionally, the word "applied" is used to convey the understanding that, in the development of their own knowledge, applied scientists use the knowledge from the pure sciences. Sociologists, who study people and behavior, rely on and use the natural sciences and their inherent assumptions to further their work. Thus sociology is an applied science. Mathematicians and physicists do not use psychology or sociology to add knowledge to their scientific disciplines, because mathematics and physics are pure sciences, whereas psychology and sociology are applied sciences.

Although applied scientists use what they deem accurate and appropriate from the natural sciences, they do not subscribe to the rigid belief of objectivity and reliability. In applied science, the focus is on human beings and the utility of the science to them and for them. Consequently, objectivity, observation, and reproducibility are diminished or perhaps not present at all. Therefore, the applied sciences are sometimes referred to as *soft science*.

Inherent in the distinction between hard and soft science are certain assumptions and beliefs. Hard scientists assume objectivity, whereas soft scientists do not. Hard scientists operate from a belief in an external world structure independent of self, whereas soft scientists do not. The hard sciences are grounded in a worldview based on reliability and consistency as contrasted with the soft sciences, which allow for individuality and originality. These distinctions are not minor semantics, but rather indicators of major differences in philosophy and perspective.

Examples of using soft applied sciences in health care can be found in social work, the work of a psychotherapist, and the examination of healthcare disparities between people of color, those of wealth, and fragile elders. Some state practice acts define nursing as specialized knowledge integrating both physical and social sciences. In these instances, the acts combine the concepts of hard, soft, pure, and applied sciences.

## Human Science

In addition to the categories of science discussed previously, human science is an important type of science. Few scholars would choose to classify human science as either hard or soft, but rather might prefer to classify it as something totally different. *Human science* is not a new term. It was introduced by Dilthey in the late 1800s (Ermarth, 1978). As a German philosopher, Dilthey was concerned about the focus on objectivity and value-free science, which left the person out of the process. He expressed concern about a science and a subsequent knowledge base that did not include the everyday lived reality of individuals. Along the way, Dilthey created the discipline of human science, which captures human beings and their experiences as the source for knowledge.

With this understanding of human science, the scientist becomes as much a part of the experience as does the participant. This view is in direct opposition to the neutral or value-free experience of the physical scientist, whose life is irrelevant to his or her work. Thus the nature and focus of the science and the process and role of the scientist are different when the subject area is viewed as a human science. In the physical sciences, the scientist and the subject are not one. In the applied sciences, the science and the scientist are not necessarily one. In contrast, in human science, they are one; they cannot be separated from each other.

Is nursing a human science? Is the work of the advanced practice nurse inextricably interwoven with the population served? When nurses speak of patients and families in one breath, is this a function of a human science view or of something else? For nursing to be a human science, nurses must recognize themselves as scientists. The work they do in the provision of care to individuals, families, and communities may be viewed from a lens of science that is simultaneously physical (hard), applied (soft), and human.

## Scientific Method for the Physical Sciences (Traditional)

As an approach or a method, traditional physical science uses a process of linear steps to solve a problem. Most nurses are familiar with the term *scientific method*, but few appreciate the assumptions inherent within the method itself. An assumption is a notion or fact that one takes for granted as true and right. The scientific method is based on the assumptions that observation is universal, that laws of nature guide every action, and that the outcome of an experiment will be useful in predicting and, therefore, controlling the object of the experiment. Being *universal*, as the term is used in relation to the scientific method and science, means that all essences are the same and that individuality does not apply. The laws of nature are those that are connected to the physical world structure independent of human consciousness, such as the laws of thermodynamics and gravity. Control through prediction is the ultimate aim of the scientific method. Control occurs through the accurate and reproducible prediction of events.

The scientific method is more than a linear process to conduct an experiment. Although hard scientists would say that it is value neutral, the scientific method is an interwoven and value-laden approach to the solution to a problem. Objectivity is a key factor that is used to validate the scientific method, yet what the scientist considers to be part of the process is a value-laden decision, regardless of whether objectivity is used later. Arguments about science being value neutral versus value laden color the aims of the two categories of science: pure and applied.

## Aim of Science

The pure hard sciences have a single aim of knowledge development for the sake of knowledge development and the search for truth. To the hard scientist, a single truth exists that can be discovered once human beings have the physical capacity to make the necessary discovery. This "single truth" approach is based on a belief that an objective world exists independent of human consciousness. Traditional science aims to describe and explain this external world structure. Another aim of the physical pure sciences is to control phenomena through an empirical approach to scientific inquiry. Control is achieved as a result of the accurate prediction of universal descriptions of outcomes. When it is known, the world can be controlled.

The aim of the applied sciences, by comparison, is the application of knowledge for a specific purpose, thereby yielding utility. Applied science is not focused on generating knowledge for the sake of having knowledge, but rather for the development of applications that can better a situation, improve a process, or change the way that situations are viewed.

In human science, the aims focus on individuals, families, and communities. Aims of human science may be to improve quality of life, ensure dignified beginnings and ends to life, uncover meaning in everyday life, and highlight the roles of individuals within this examination. The aims of human science may be simply stated as *to know and understand what works for people to maximize their ability to be fully functioning individuals, families, and communities at whatever level they are able to function.*

## Scientific Methods in Human Science

Human science requires different methods. While the scientific method may be applied in the abstract, the end for the human scientist is greater than the sum of the parts. Thus varied methods are needed. In human science, the scientists and the subject (content area) being studied are treated as parts of the same whole. Therefore, the methods used can be neither linear nor constant. Instead, the methods need to be dynamic, while still meeting the same expectation of rigor found in the hard sciences. Rigor—a notion usually associated with randomized control studies, reliability, and validity in the hard sciences—is not the goal in human science. Rather, contextual consistency, purpose sampling within the population experiencing the essence to be described, validity of questions, a detailed audit trail of data collection and data analysis, and a return to the participants for validation of the message sent and received are emphasized.

# Criteria for Science

An important distinction to address is the difference between science and non-science. This discussion has been going on for centuries. Some scholars may look at human science as nonscience. Pseudoscience—comprising theories that are presented as scientific but not proven with the scientific method or supported by data—is the bane of existence for the hard physical scientist, even though it clearly has popular appeal. Therefore, it is important for the hard physical sciences to demarcate themselves from pseudoscience and, perhaps, applied and human sciences. Five criteria are used for this purpose: (1) intersubjective testability, (2) reliability, (3) definiteness and precision, (4) coherence, and (5) comprehensiveness and scope (Feigl, 1988).

## Intersubjective Testability

Intersubjective testability is based on a belief in the value of corroboration and on the idea that two people who view the same entity in the same manner should obtain the same results; if this criterion is met, the method is objective. Using the word "objective" as a synonym for intersubjectivity means that "the belief is not based on hallucination or deception and it is not a state of mind but truly exists . . . the belief is neither private nor unique. It can be and must be verified . . . and be empirically tested" (Polifroni & Welch, 1999, pp. 3–4).

## Reliability

Reliability, the second criterion, means that researchers achieve the same result time and again when the circumstances of their study have not changed. If findings demonstrate reliability, then the same outcomes are achieved with repeated tests, thereby confirming the beliefs and premises set forth by the scientist. Reliability is the basis for prediction and subsequent control.

## Definiteness and Precision

Definiteness and precision, which collectively constitute the third criterion, are words used to convey exactness and rigid adherence to objectivity. Precision is not about approximation, but rather exactness; it is about specifics, not generalities. If experimentation meets the criterion of definiteness and precision, creating the same circumstances for repeated experimentation leads to a reasonable expectation that the same results will be achieved. Definiteness and precision are not about inclusion of the researcher or fluidity of ideas; indeed, they focus on the opposite goal.

## Coherence

Coherence or systematic character, the fourth criterion, addresses connectedness and wholeness. How do the parts relate to one another to form a unique body of knowledge? The connectedness (the sense of a whole with integrated parts, not disparate ideas) is the coherence required in science that is not necessarily present in pseudoscience. It is important to distinguish the wholeness of coherence from holism in human science. In coherence, the focus is on the parts and their relation to one another. In contrast, holism in human science focuses on the whole from the outset, not the parts.

## Comprehensiveness and Scope

The fifth criterion, comprehensiveness and scope, encompasses the ability of the science to be used for something other than its intended purpose. Comprehensiveness and scope define applications beyond than the basis of the planned study and achieving the expected outcome through appropriate utilization. "The thrust of this criterion is the maximum explanatory power of the science and its related theories. . . . a science is not a science if it does not explain and address events and related concerns beyond the issue under study at the present time" (Polifroni & Welch, 1999, p. 4).

# Questions for the Practitioner

The five criteria—intersubjective testability, reliability, definiteness and precision, coherence, and comprehensiveness and scope—serve to separate science and pseudoscience, as well as common sense. It is important for advanced practice nurses to ask, "Is nursing a science?" Is nursing work that of pure science or applied science? Is the care provided to patients, families, and communities done for the purpose of prediction and control? Are there universals within patient care provision? Is there an external world independent of human consciousness that colors the care delivered? Does nursing as a science satisfy the five demarcation criteria? Is nursing practice objective?

# Philosophy

Whereas science is about knowledge, the term *philosophy* (originally from the Greek word *philosophia*) means "love of wisdom." Enjoyment of the thought process, the notion of thinking for the sake of thinking (how often have you said, "If I only had time to think . . ."), the examination of ideas, and the search for truth are all part of philosophy. Philosophy also involves a search for meaning; it represents a perspective, and it is a set of beliefs. Philosophy, like science, is both a process and an outcome. The process of philosophy is the critical inquiry and examination of meaning and the method one undertakes when beliefs are examined, ideas are proposed, and assumptions are challenged.

---

### Box 1-1  Questions for Advanced Practice Nurses

1. Is nursing a science?
2. Does your practice "fit" with the five criteria of a science?
3. How do you use universals in your care and make the care individualized?

---

Philosophy encompasses more than rhetoric; it is the guide by which situations are approached, the viewpoint used to see what is before one, and the method by which one searches for truth, as well as an understanding of what truth is. Philosophy is contextually grounded; it relies on the present but is embedded in the historical past. Philosophy is dynamic, it evolves, and it is subtle while simultaneously being overt.

Philosophy captures the essence of a human being, such as the essence of what it means to be a provider in a caring profession. The deliberate use of the word "caring" here indicates a philosophical belief based on the author's experience, gender, and role as a scientist. Philosophy is more than just a belief—it is the *application* of that belief to situations known and unknown. Philosophy is epistemology *and* ontology, the knowledge of and the belief about something. Epistemology is the study of knowing, of determining what knowledge is and how that knowledge is relevant and related to extant knowledge. Ontology is the study of being and of meaning.

All schools of philosophical thought cannot possibly be explored in a single chapter. One way to undertake a large survey of philosophical thought is to examine the various perspectives in terms of two major schools of philosophical thought: analytical and continental. Analytical philosophers originally were those primarily located outside of Europe, whereas advocates of continental philosophy originally emanated from Europe. While the two schools are often discussed in opposition to each other, their discordant viewpoints are actually simply a matter of the philosophers using a different lens, differing approaches, and differing subjects. Analytical philosophy is wedded to objectivity and reproducibility, whereas continental philosophy is about essence and experience.

*Continental philosophy* is grounded in the viewpoint that the phenomena of interest are deeply embedded in the human experience. *Analytical philosophy*, by comparison, focuses more on the use of the process of logic and rational discourse than on the subject itself. Analytical philosophies include positivism, empiricism, instrumentalism, pragmatism, and rationalism, whereas continental philosophies include phenomenology, hermeneutics, critical social theory, feminism, structuralism, post-structuralism, and postmodernism. Some of these views will be discussed later in this chapter.

## Box 1–2 Essential Terminology in Philosophy

| | | |
|---|---|---|
| Analytical philosophy | Epistemology | Phenomenology |
| Antirealism | Essence | Positivism |
| A priori | Experience | Post-structuralism |
| Chaos | Hermeneutics | Pragmatism |
| Complexity science | Idealism | Priori |
| Continental philosophy | Logical positivism | Realism |
| Empiricism | Ontology | Truth |

# Philosophy of Science

Philosophy of science exists at the intersection of philosophy and science—where the two meet to form a new perspective that aims to examine the body of knowledge *and* the approaches to the study of the body of knowledge. Philosophy of science in nursing is an "examination of nursing concepts, theories, laws and aims as they relate to nursing practice. Through such an understanding and deliberate thought, praxis evolves" (Polifroni & Welch, 1999, p. 5). Praxis is the planned, deliberate, and thoughtful creation of a plan of action to achieve a set goal. Philosophy of science in nursing explores the meaning of truth, the meaning of evidence, and the meaning of life through praxis.

It is nurses' responsibility to view science from a multitude of perspectives: as nurse scientist; as care provider; and from the perspective of the patient, family, and society. Each perspective potentially offers a different lens for examining the same concept. Each lens brings certain assumptions to the forefront that color both the lens and the object of review.

Analytical philosophers, who are often physical scientists, examine the nature of truth using a lens of objectivity, linear thinking, and rationality. Continental philosophers explore the meaning and nature of truth from an individual lens focusing on the experience of truth from the perspective of the person (including the perspective of the scientist), which leads to some subjectivity in the results. These two lenses or perspectives require practitioners to examine their own perspective of truth and ask, "Is there only one truth? Does truth reside in the external world structure independent of human consciousness, or is truth found within the individual and highly contextual? Is there more than one truth? Is truth even a relevant subject for discourse, or should the focus of practice be on the outcomes of treatment modalities?" The answers to these questions enable providers to become comfortable with the assumptions and underpinnings of the various philosophical perspectives.

# How Do We Know?

Answering the question "How do we know?" is key to helping anyone understand philosophy of science. This question can be pondered by considering where knowledge and knowing originate. A first thought is that people know because of tradition: Experiences that happened yesterday color and shape what is known about today. Tradition often shapes experiences into a repetitive pattern of behavior. Authorities also inform what is known. An authority may be a person, a role, or an institution. A police officer is an authority; a college professor is an authority; an institution of higher learning is an authority, as is a church. In addition, doctrine can shape what is known. Without evidence or in the face of contradictory evidence, those who believe in and practice a religion profess it as their knowing. Reason, without regard for religion or tradition, is yet another realm of knowing. Reason may lead to a path that contradicts religion or tradition; thus individuals must decide what to believe.

Common sense is a form of knowing also: People know that they become wet when it rains and, therefore, they should seek shelter. If people do not eat, they know that they will become hungry and should find food. These are two examples of common sense.

Finally, there is science as a way of knowing (*to know = science*). Science is knowledge derived from methods that may be linear or complex (chaotic) depending on the view and approach. Science could be physical science, social science, human science, or nursing science. Science is how people know, regardless of the type of science.

## Analytical Philosophy of Science

The analytical and continental categories are merely one way to examine philosophical schools of thought. Other options include using received and perceived views (Suppe, 1977), a historical timeline, a context of major events in history, and many others. Choosing the analytical and continental categories as criteria implies nothing more than a framework choice for examination. It is important to note that continental philosophers analyze and analytical philosophers examine applications.

The analytical perspective is closely associated with positivism and, more specifically, with logical positivism. Given that a significant amount of what can be read about philosophy today is contrary to logical positivism, it is important to understand that base. Logical positivism is a school of thought that originated in the early 20th century under the aegis of the Vienna School in Austria. That geographic location, while on the European continent, does not mean that the analytical perspective is necessarily associated with continental philosophy, however.

Logical positivism actually began earlier than the 20th century, with Comte's (1788–1857) view of positivism. Comte, the father of positivism, asserted that human history progresses from the theological to the metaphysical to the positivistic. By the last term, he asserted the *positive* role that the universal laws of nature provided. Following in Comte's footsteps, Kolakowski (as cited in MacKenzie, 1977) suggested four characteristic rules of positivism: (1) phenomenalism, (2) nominalism, (3) the denial of cognitive value in value judgments and normative statements, and (4) the essential unity of the scientific method.

The major tenants of logical positivism, consistent with the use of an analytical approach to problem solving, require a rigid adherence to the scientific method (deductive nomological approach), a belief in cause and effect, a solid underpinning of replicability, and an unwavering belief in an external world structure that remains independent of self. It is the final point that provides the platform for the cause and effect relationship and the needed objectivity divorced from humans and subjectivity.

The noted philosophers Carnap, Feigl (demarcation criteria), Hempel and Oppenheim (1948), and Popper (2002) developed logical positivism with an aim to affirm the external world structure, solidify a reliance on the inherent laws of nature, and promote the deductive method of analysis to achieve a problem's solution. These logical positivists believed in the verifiability principle—the belief that a statement is meaningful only if it is proven true or false through the means of experience (experiment). They suggested that there is a logical structure of scientific theories, probability is meaningful in science (as opposed to possibility), science is a deductive experience, and the sources of knowledge are twofold (logical reasoning and empirical experience).

A large amount of literature in the nursing field has criticized logical positivism as being too rigid, too deductive, and lacking an appreciation or recognition of the human experience. To overcome these objections, logical positivism eventually segued into empiricism. Empiricism, which relies on the scientific method for the production of truth, held to tenets similar to those underlying logical positivism, except that the empiricist required actual experience. The logical positivist accepted the external world structure, whereas the empiricist, while neither accepting nor dismissing the existence of the external world's structure, required that science be generated through the senses of experience. Empiricism is what is commonly called science in today's world.

Over time, both empiricism and logical positivism were incorporated into the received view described by Suppe (1977). The received view of science states that a theory is either right or wrong, that mature or developed theories must be formalized, that a theory must be axiomized (taken apart into propositions and independently tested), that all sciences should be patterned after physics, and that there is a clear separation between theoretical and empirical understandings.

The received view is strongly supportive of the prominence and dominance of physical sciences. It is based on the search for truth, wherein a single truth is desired and possible to identify. Put simply, empirical (scientific) methods lead the knower to *the* answer.

This view of empiricism, which is embedded in analytical philosophy, is commonly known as traditional science. It is how most people are taught in elementary and high schools throughout the United States. Learning physical science by having opportunities to experience through observation is the gold standard of science, knowledge, and truth. Prediction, using descriptive laws and understanding initial conditions, is the purpose of science for scientists who advocate a received view. Such value-free science relies on a single universal scientific method. The received view is sometimes known as *realism*.

## Continental Philosophy of Science

Whereas the analytical philosophy of science focuses on the search for a single truth through a scientific process of controlled experimentation, the continental philosophy of science is concerned with the connection of an idea to the world around the idea and its historical context. Continental philosophy is not about theories or truths, but rather about the relationships between people, ideas, meaning, and their historical connectedness.

Georg Hegel, Wilhelm Dilthey, Pierre Duhem, Paul Thagard, Philip Kitcher (2001), Edmund Husserl, and Martin Heidegger (1962) all have written from the continental philosophy of science perspective. Their works focus on the applied sciences of sociology and psychology, the historical approach and context, the understanding of power (Foucault, 1976), and the lived experience of the subject and scientist (philosopher).

Human science is the domain of the continental philosophy of science. As described earlier, human science deals with persons and their connectedness to the world in which they live and the lived experiences of their life. Continental philosophers examine this lived experience in the past as well as the present. Using continental philosophy requires an examination of historical context as much as it does what is happening in the present time. Continental philosophers of science believe not in cause and effect, but rather in connectedness and the often used proverb "Past is prologue."

Phenomenology is an example of a philosophy that emanates from the continental philosophy of science perspective. In phenomenology, as in philosophy, value is placed on universal experiences. Husserl (1990), a continental philosopher, believed that while human experience is personal, the essence of it is universal. For example, the essence of grief is strikingly similar whether one is grieving the loss of a limb, a loved one, a home, or a pet. For Husserl, phenomenology entails a focus on examining phenomena that appear in the consciousness of the subjects. It is about personal experience; from an examination of such experience, the essences of the phenomena are drawn.

Hermeneutics is another continental philosophy. As a philosophy, hermeneutics deals with the interpretation and understanding of a message that is being delivered. The name of this school of thought derives from Hermes, the messenger of the Greek gods. Hermeneutics is characterized by the assumptions that people are social and dialogical beings; that culture, language, skills, and experiences create shared understandings; that there is a continual circle of connectedness and understanding; that understanding precedes interpretation; and that the interpreter and the interpreted are seen as one. In hermeneutics, meaning and understanding are identified as the aims of the philosophical inquiry.

Post-structuralism, another philosophy that falls under the broad rubric of continental philosophy, speaks to the premise that the study of structures (above and below the surface of relationships and contexts) must be viewed as a cultural phenomenon. As a result, the analysis is open to a variety of interpretations and likely misinterpretations. Post-structuralism conveys the message that both the object and its context for creation, development, and evaluation must be studied. This view is similar to that taken by all the continental philosophies, which are based on a contextual grounding for analysis. The assumptions of post-structuralism are typically that the meaning of a message is based on the perception of the receiver and that the person who conveys the message is not necessarily significant in terms of the message itself. For example, this view would suggest that an advanced practice nurse is not the important component in the delivery of a message; rather, what is important is what the patient hears and interprets the message to be. This approach serves to equalize the imbalance of power between healthcare providers and patients noted in the healthcare field today.

Although the three varieties of continental philosophy described in this section certainly demonstrate some differences, all revolve around context, meaning, and the knowing subject of the discourse or action. Collectively, continental philosophies may also be called the *perceived view, antirealism,* or *idealism.* These terms are meant to intrigue the reader and encourage further exploration, because the space limitations here do not permit an adequate discussion of them.

## Perceived View

Suppe (1977) examined the perceived view with a different lens. As with the view evinced by the continental philosophers, who engaged the notion of human science and the human experience in the search for truth and knowing, the perceived view is more fluid and dynamic than the received view. Within the perceived view, theories are neither right nor wrong. This position stands in stark contrast to the verification approach of the received view.

In the perceived view, observation leads to the generation of theory, which in turn is value laden. Both the received and perceived views rely on observation, but the meaning of this term and the process by which observation is achieved differ for the two views. Observation for the received, analytical philosopher is precise, detailed, physical, objective, and inherently value neutral or value free. For people subscribing to the perceived view, observation involves the use of the senses and the mind. Observation is accurate but is not reliant on precision; it is both physical and mental. Observation is detailed but not necessarily measurable, and it is subjective. Therefore, observation from the perceived view perspective is inherently subjective. What one chooses to observe is as much a part of the process as is the observation itself.

The received view supports the beliefs that progression in science leads to a deeper understanding and that this understanding leads to theories for examination. Perceived view proponents believe in using different kinds of theories and many methods to obtain truth, although some do not seek truth at all, only understanding. Whereas following the tenets of the received view requires use of the scientific method, exploration, and experimentation, proponents of the perceived view use varied approaches to science and seeking truth, such as phenomenology, grounded theory, case method, and hermeneutics. Received view scientists use the quantitative method in their pursuit of science, whereas perceived view scientists use methods appropriate to the question asked, which may be either quantitative, qualitative, or mixed methods.

> ## Box 1–3  What Image Emerges?
>
> | | | | |
> |---|---|---|---|
> | Work-up | Industry | Control | Emergent |
> | Diagnose | Engineer | Check | Self-organize |
> | Fine-tune | Design | Evolve | Diversity |
> | Prescribe | Operate | Adapt | Ecology |

## Chaos and Complexity Science

Contemporary philosophers of science synthesize the work of both the analytical and continental philosophers into a new and emerging philosophy of science. The emerging philosophy incorporates chaos and complexity science, which is closely aligned with quantum physics. Truth, the domain of the analytical scientists and philosophers, and understanding, the realm of the continental philosophers and scientists, come together in a different and dynamic way in chaos and complexity science. Complex adaptive, dynamic systems (organic or inorganic) are connected to environments and are influenced by what has come before and what will come after; these systems are irreducibly whole.

Complexity science and a view of complex adaptive systems with the language of fluidity and dynamicism push the scientist to look at things differently. Is there a real difference—not just a semantic difference—between the images conjured up by the terms "fine-tune" and "emergent" or "work-up" and "evolve"?

Bohm (1980) stated that the "universe is no longer seen as a machine, made up of objects, but rather pictured as one indivisible whole whose parts are essentially interrelated and can only be understood as patterns of a cosmic process" (p. 29). The assumptions about complex adaptive systems are many, and they include the characteristics of embeddedness (meaning patterns that can be traced backward and forward), distributed control (an equalization of power bases), nonlinearity, multidirectionality, emergence in the dynamic diversity of subjects and objects, a simultaneous coexistence of order and disorder, and outcomes that are inherently unpredictable. This perspective stands in direct contrast to the notion of traditional science, which aims to explain and predict in order to control.

## Question the Assumptions

There is more to philosophy of science than what is presented here. Whole schools of thought have not been addressed. Throughout the chapter, several underlying questions have colored all else: What are the assumptions of each nurse's philosophy of science? Do nurses aim to diagnose and treat illness, or to diagnose

---

### Box 1–4  Provider Questions

1. What is my view of truth?
2. Are there multiple truths?
3. What if my patient and I do not agree on the truth or the view of truth?
4. Is the lived experience important?
5. Is the lived experience more important than lab values and blood gases?
6. How do I justify/juggle evidence-based practice guidelines and individuality?

---

and treat human responses? Do nurses aim to control through prescription, or do they aim to understand and co-create meaning and action? Is there a single way to resolve a problem, or are different views and approaches permissible? Is one's praxis dynamic and wedded to a guideline, a critical path, or a set of standing orders? What do nurses need to be the best practitioners that they can be? What do patients, families, and communities need? Finally, each nurse is encouraged to ask, "Am I the nurse that I want to be?"

## Discussion Questions

1. What are the assumptions that color/shape my approach to care?

2. Describe the revolution needed within health care to address the major issues facing us today.

## References

Bohm, D. (1980). *Wholeness and the implicate order*. London, UK: Routledge.

Boyd, R., Gasper, P., & Trout, J. D. (Eds.). (1991). *The philosophy of science*. Cambridge, MA: Blackwell.

Ermarth, M. (1978). *Wilhelm Dilthey: The critique of historical reason*. Chicago, IL: University of Chicago Press.

Feigl, H. (1988). The scientific outlook: Naturalism and humanism. In E. D. Klemke, R. Hollinger, & A. D. Kline (Eds.), *Philosophy of science* (pp. 427–437). Buffalo, NY: Prometheus Books.

Foucault, M. (1976). *The will to know*. Paris, France: Gallimard.

Heidegger, M. (1962). *Being and time* (J. Macquarrie & E. Robinson, trans.). New York, NY: Harper & Row.

Hempel, C., & Oppenheim, P. (1948). Studies in the logic of explanation. *Philosophy of Science, 15*, 135–175.

Husserl, E. (1990). *The idea of phenomenology* (W. Altson & G. Nakhnikian, trans.). Boston, MA: Kluwer Academic.

Kitcher, P. (2001). *Science, truth, and democracy*. Oxford, UK: Oxford University Press.

MacKenzie, B. D. (1977). *Behaviourism and the limits of scientific method.* London, UK: Routledge & Paul.

Polifroni, E. C., & Welch, M. (1999). *Perspective on philosophy of science in nursing: An historical and contemporary anthology.* Philadelphia, PA: Lippincott.

Popper, K. (2002) [1959]. *The logic of scientific discovery* (2nd English ed.). New York, NY: Routledge.

Suppe, F. (1977). *The structure of scientific theories.* Chicago, IL: University of Illinois Press.

CHAPTER

# The Evolution of Nursing Science

*Beth L. Rodgers*

---

## Introduction

In discussions of nursing, images that commonly come to mind are those of the nurse performing certain acts such as listening to blood pressure sounds, changing a dressing for a wound, assisting someone with ambulation, giving medication, or starting an intravenous line. Undoubtedly people who have been registered nurses for some time recall their early days in school and the tremendous anticipation of performing the first immunization or urinary catheterization, or the excitement the first time an intravenous catheter was inserted smoothly and successfully.

Nurses who have been engaged in the broad professional role of the registered nurse recognize that there is a great deal more to nursing than the performance of those skills. Nonetheless, when talking about nursing, discussion often turns quite easily to a focus on what nurses *do*—the skills, tasks, and functions that are associated with the actions and behaviors of nurses. Much less common is an emphasis on what nurses *know*—the knowledge base that underlies the performance of those acts—as well as the many more things that nurses do beyond obvious physical functions. No doubt it is much easier to describe the mechanics of listening to breath sounds than it is to describe the detailed thinking that goes into formulating a holistic portrayal of an individual patient for whom those breath sounds are only a small part of his or her scenario.

Nurses engage in a variety of actions that are far subtler than those involving the common skills that are directly observable. For example, they form important working relationships with patients to help them achieve their health and wellness goals; they counsel, educate, guide, facilitate, assess, plan, relate, evaluate, and engage with people as individuals or in groups or communities on a variety of levels consistent with a holistic approach to health concerns and health promotion. Nurses also engage in activities such as arranging for referrals, managing various stages of care, and facilitating access to necessary resources. This list is in no way exhaustive, but it provides some indication of the tremendous number of cognitive activities associated with nursing—activities that, because they lack implements or other tangible equipment, may be recognized less readily by the public. Perhaps even more significant, nurses also are less quick to describe these activities, possibly because of the difficulty associated with articulating the specific thought processes that are essential for effective and appropriate care. Many nurses seem to give themselves less credit than is warranted for the cognitive capabilities and knowledge that go into nursing. When asked why they reacted to a situation in a particular way or what prompted them to intervene, it is not uncommon to hear the nurse say, "I just knew," referring to a gut feeling or intuition as the basis for significant action.

These responses on the part of nurses fail to give credit to the vast amount of knowledge that nurses carry with them every day. It is not the tasks and skills that nurses perform that make them such an indispensable part of health care, but rather what they "know." The knowledge of nurses not only lies at the root of competent and effective care, but it also provides the foundation that makes nurses such important contributors to broader decision making and planning. When nurses argue that they should be involved in committees, on boards, or in other influential positions, and when they discuss why certain concerns or problems clearly could benefit from nursing involvement, it is the knowledge of nurses that makes these arguments so meaningful. Although nurses often find themselves in a position of needing, or at least wanting, to articulate what is unique about their particular level of preparation, discussion of the knowledge base of nursing can be a challenging undertaking. It is much easier to describe what nurses do than what they know.

## The Impact of the Doctor of Nursing Practice Degree

As nurses have achieved higher levels of education (particularly doctoral degrees), the need to understand the knowledge base of the discipline has become even more imperative. Nurses with doctoral-level education are likely to be perceived as leaders both in the discipline and in the broader community and they should be prepared and willing to assume roles as leaders in a number of contexts. They often are confronted with both the opportunity and the need to explain what constitutes nursing at that level. No doubt this need will persist and, it most likely will be greatly expanded as more nurses with Doctor of Nursing Practice (DNP) degrees work within a variety of settings. Not only does the DNP constitute an advanced degree, which surely will grab the interest of the public (whose familiarity with nursing is most likely limited to personal experience with hospital or clinic nurses), but it also is a new degree that carries with it credentials and titles that are not known to the broader public, and perhaps also not well understood within nursing.

At the same time, nurses with the DNP degree are in an important position to serve as leaders in the continuing articulation of the discipline, as well as contributors on multiple levels to the development of the knowledge base for nursing.

All of these factors create a tremendous need for nurses at all levels of preparation to articulate with clarity the nature of nursing knowledge and what nurses are capable of contributing to health in all realms—individual, family, local, community, and global. DNP-prepared nurses have particular responsibility for taking leadership to represent the discipline and profession of nursing well and to identify and discuss the particular expertise and advanced knowledge of the DNP-prepared nurse. In addition, nurses with the DNP degree are prepared and often placed in important positions as essential collaborators in research and innovations that add to the knowledge base of nursing as it continues to develop as a discipline.

## Science and Knowledge

Without an understanding of the overall discipline, including the knowledge that underlies the thoughts and actions of the nurse, both practice and research can become isolated, individualistic, situational endeavors. Science is the general term used to refer to the knowledge base of a discipline that has been developed rigorously and systematically. The idea of "science" has an interesting history, however, and science was not always the dominant term used to refer to credible knowledge. As evidenced by the writings of Aristotle, for example, and in the work of many others continuing into the 19th century, the terms *science* and *knowledge* were used almost interchangeably for much of recorded history. It is only in modern times that science has been recognized as a rather specialized form of knowledge, replete with specific methodologies and means to evaluate credibility. In exploring the underpinnings of nursing work, especially those elements that provide nurses with valuable and trustworthy information as a foundation for practice, it is helpful to look at not just science but the broader realm of nursing knowledge.

The discipline of nursing includes components other than just the knowledge base. Disciplines also involve a human component in that judgments are made about what is acceptable science and what are current priorities. This component necessarily involves the expression of the values embodied in the discipline in regard to what is needed for knowledge development. The human component, what Toulmin (1972) referred to as the "profession," works with and develops the knowledge base of the discipline and develops mechanisms for the sharing of ideas through debate and dialog, both oral and in the form of publications. Organizations within the discipline provide leadership, whether through societies that have bestowed honors upon esteemed nurses, research organizations that promote the conduct of research and dissemination of results, or specialty organizations that shape practice. Those organizations also have important roles in the ongoing development of nursing as a discipline. Discussion of the science of nursing, or the knowledge base, cannot be carried out without recognition of the context that exists for that knowledge in the discipline. In addition, this nursing context exists within a larger societal context that includes expectations for nurses, as well as standards for what is considered to be knowledge or science, and especially "good" science.

It is easy to identify examples of how knowledge has changed, sometimes rapidly, and just as often in radical ways. Recent discoveries related to genetics are stimulating revolutionary developments in treatment as well as renewed efforts at prevention as that genetic knowledge evolves. Dietary guidelines are evolving as awareness develops that blood lipid profiles are not inextricably linked to dietary intake of fats, with new information being in substantial opposition to prevailing ideology about nutrition and illness. Awareness of the effect of environmental conditions and artificial substances on health and the development of health problems has raised questions in areas that were not given much consideration in the prior germ theory–oriented approach to medicine, questions ranging from food production to vaccination guidelines. In such a context of ever-changing science, often accompanied by competing values and priorities, significant challenges are presented for nurses who provide not only "best practice" in whatever realm they work, but who also must defend those practices in the face of changing knowledge.

It is clear that context has considerable influence on the discipline of nursing and the development of the corresponding knowledge base. Because of that influence, it is reasonable to look at the evolution of nursing knowledge using a chronological approach; in fact, many aspects of context are associated with historical events and timing. One limitation associated with such a chronology is that it gives the impression that change is linear. That would be quite a naïve view, however. Science is inextricably tied to human behavior and attitudes; given that science is a human enterprise, and multiple stakeholders and influences exist, the development and change of knowledge over time is far from linear. In contrast, the movement of knowledge often involves multiple and simultaneously existing and competing areas of focus influenced by diverse philosophical systems and sets of values.

Nonetheless, early ideas do provide the impetus for later ideas; societal needs and expectations at one period of time eventually lead to other sets of ideas. As such, there is continuity in the progression of ideas, and that continuity provides a useful framework for studying the history of ideas about nursing science. It is important to keep in mind that changes in ideas and emphasis must be considered as an evolutionary process and not necessarily a progression. Progression implies movement toward some specified point or goal, such that it is possible to say that nursing knowledge or science is getting closer to whatever that goal might be. Because of the fluidity of the context of nursing, as well as the context of the greater society, that endpoint or goal must be amenable to change as well. Although the evaluation of progress in regard to knowledge is a difficult task, nurses can say with certainty and, perhaps, with pride that there have been incredible improvements in educational preparation, in leadership and organization within the discipline, and in the ability to address the changing needs of the people who are the beneficiaries of nursing care.

This element of continuity also needs to be examined from the standpoint of ideas about nursing. Nursing, in various forms, has existed, depending on how it is defined, since the beginning of time. Nursing also exists in a global context in spite of the variation that might exist from one setting to the next, even within general geographic regions. It is tempting sometimes to avoid defining nursing, or making clear statements about what nursing "is" because of this variation. However, there are some things that enable all of these disparate situations to be thought of as nursing. In spite of all the differences, there are some things that hold nursing together as a distinct type of knowledge and work; some essence persists across time and contexts and makes it proper to call these things nursing. Leaders and scholars in nursing have the obligation to be able to discuss nursing with others who may have different perceptions of nursing and be able to articulate to others the nature of nursing and the incredible contributions to human health that can be made by those who are registered nurses.

## Nursing As a Discipline

In spite of the tremendous contributions of nurses to meeting the healthcare needs of individuals, groups, and populations, and in spite of the pervasiveness of nursing throughout much of history, it can be difficult to delineate clearly what constitutes nursing as a discipline. Problems articulating the nature of the knowledge base of nursing can give the impression that there is not a specific, unique, substance of knowledge or science that underlies the practice of nurses. Such claims might seem absurd to any nurse who has been carrying out acts of nursing for an entire career. While it should be self-evident that nurses cannot act without some base of knowledge—otherwise, their actions would be totally without reason—significant challenges have arisen as they have tried to articulate precisely what constitutes that knowledge base.

This desire to define the knowledge base of nursing has been enhanced by some authors who have argued that it is essential for nursing's continued viability to distinguish its knowledge base from that of other disciplines (Feldman, 1981; Smith & McCarthy, 2010; Visintainer, 1986). While such concerns are not voiced in nursing as frequently today as they were a few decades ago, lingering questions persist about precisely what exemplifies nursing and what reflects or represents some other field of knowledge or inquiry.

To respond to these concerns, unique languages have been created in the form of nursing diagnoses and other taxonomies; research has been conducted rather extensively on intuition and critical thinking, two modes of thinking that are often thought to play a prominent role in nursing. Nurses have focused on the art of nursing and the realm of aesthetics as means other than science to capture the essence of nursing knowledge. These and more themes evident in the evolution of nursing science reflect the ongoing quest by nurse scholars to answer questions about the nature of nursing and, especially, the knowledge base or science that constitutes the discipline.

# The Education of Nurses

As noted previously, concern has been expressed in nursing literature, especially during the period of the late 1960s through the late 1980s, about the apparent lack of a unique knowledge base for the discipline. At other times, critics noted a failure to articulate what makes up that unique knowledge. No doubt the history of the development of nursing supports concerns about the existence of a distinct, unique knowledge base in the discipline. Education for nurses has been referred to historically as training, a term that was particularly relevant during the apprentice-type model of early nursing preparation. In spite of Florence Nightingale's revolutionizing the preparation of nurses for her day, even well into the 20th century a substantial portion of the preparation of nurses occurred through on-the-job apprenticeships.

Nurses educated as recently as the 1970s (and sometimes even more recently) may still refer to their preparation as training rather than as education. While these semantics might seem like a minor point, terminology can be quite powerful in terms of its capability to convey unintended messages, as well as those desired by the speaker or writer. The term *education* carries a different connotation than the term *training*; the latter is focused on the ability to perform certain actions, not on the knowledge and understanding that precede reasoned action. In addition to this distinction, the emphasis in early nursing training was placed on selecting the best candidates to be nurses based on personal characteristics that were presumed to be appropriate; the focus was not on the intellectual capacity or aptitude for gaining the knowledge needed to be an effective nurse. A review of conditions for nurse preparation in the early days of the discipline clearly reveals that fortitude and persistence were valued as characteristics essential to successful completion of these preparatory programs. At the same time, rules for nurses mandated subservient behaviors rather than critical thinking.

At the time that nurses began to receive formal education through actual involvement in classroom work and didactic presentations, much of the content of nursing programs was taught by physicians. Programs were associated with hospitals rather than colleges and universities, and the learning of the skills associated with nursing continued to occur primarily by actually doing the work of the nurse. Nursing was not associated closely with academic settings until 1909, when Richard Olding Beard successfully integrated the nursing program into the formal academic structure of the University of Minnesota. This program led to a 3-year diploma and was subsumed under the medical school, yet it was the first instance of nursing education as an official part of a university structure. Yale School of Nursing, which opened in 1924, was the first autonomous school of nursing with its own dean and budget (Kalisch & Kalisch, 1995).

Education at the graduate level developed slowly within the context of academic settings. Master's degrees were available in the early 1930s, yet by 1962 data revealed only 2,472 students pursued the master's degree in nursing; for the period 1961–1962, only 1,098 graduates were enrolled in master's degree programs (U.S. Public Health Service, 1963). Opportunities for doctoral-level education were severely limited in nursing, and nurses who wanted such preparation typically pursued their degrees in the discipline of education, rather than nursing per se. The first programs that enabled nurses to pursue doctoral degrees were established in schools of education at Teacher's College, Columbia University, and at New York University, both developed in the 1920s and 1930s.

As nursing evolved as a discipline, recognition of the need for nurses with doctoral-level preparation as researchers grew, yet there was almost no opportunity to obtain such education within the discipline of nursing. In 1962, the U.S. Public Health Service began the Nurse Scientist Program to support advanced education to prepare nurses as researchers. Because of the absence of doctoral programs in the discipline of nursing, nurses who pursued their education as a part of this program had no choice but to receive their education in other fields. As a result, they typically were socialized into those other disciplines, bringing the perspective of physiologists, sociologists, and educators to bear on their ideas about nursing.

Nurses with doctoral preparation in nursing and increased nursing research activity are fairly recent developments. The first doctoral nursing program was established at the University of Pittsburgh in 1954 and was limited to maternal–child health, with a Doctor of Nursing Science (DNS) program being established at Boston University 6 years later in 1960 (Kalisch & Kalisch, 1995). Because many universities did not support doctoral-level preparation in nursing, doctoral programs often had to offer a distinct degree, typically the DNS or DNSc. Journals devoted to nursing research did not emerge until the 1950s, with an additional surge of activity in this area occurring in the 1970s. It is only within the last 30 years or so that a preponderance of people teaching in programs that lead to a doctoral degree in nursing also have had their own doctoral-level preparation in nursing.

Awareness of this historical development in nursing helps to explain the nature of research that has been done and, similarly, the development of the discipline over the last several decades. It is only within the last two or three decades that the individuals conducting research within the field of nursing were likely to have been educated with degrees in nursing and socialized primarily as researchers and scholars in nursing. As a result, there has been an increase in research conducted by nurse investigators with a viewpoint that has been derived from and has reflected a nursing perspective toward the problems addressed by the research.

This brief glimpse into a significant aspect of the history of nursing education makes it easy to see why concerns about borrowed knowledge have had a prominent role in the evolution of nursing as a discipline. This lack of clarity in regard to a unique knowledge base for nursing was compounded by prevailing ideas about the nature of disciplines. Prominent nurse scholars in the 1960s through the late 1970s brought to nursing ideas from education about the nature and structure of disciplines.

# Delineating the Discipline

Underlying all of this historical activity was a variety of theoretical thinking about knowledge in nursing, including nursing as a discipline, the role of theory in nursing, mechanisms for theory development, and, in more recent years, a broad interest in nursing science and its development. In the early stages, attention was focused on the delineation and development of nursing as a discipline, motivated to some extent by the need to demonstrate the unique aspects of nursing. Early efforts were focused particularly on knowledge development consistent with prevailing ideas about the way disciplines were structured. This focus on structure likely was a result of, at least in part, close connections between nursing and the discipline of education, and the structure of disciplines was an area of considerable theoretical interest and emphasis in education, particularly in the 1960s. The premise in the literature that promoted this focus in nursing was that the determination of the nature of nursing as a discipline, including its structure and boundaries, would provide direction for continuing development. Donaldson and Crowley (1978) pointed out the need for work on the discipline of nursing, indicating that such investigation would determine "the essence of nursing research and of the common elements and threads that give coherence to an identifiable body of knowledge" (p. 113).

Invoking ideas about borrowed versus unique knowledge, Donaldson and Crowley (1978) argued that much of the basis for nursing was "tacit rather than explicit" (p. 113), and they emphasized the need to ensure that nursing research was actually research in the discipline of nursing and not merely research that was conducted by nurses. Donaldson and Crowley described a *discipline* as "characterized by a unique perspective, a distinct way of viewing all phenomena, which ultimately defines the limits and nature of its inquiry" (p. 113). Developing nursing knowledge consistent with this idea of disciplinary structure would make it possible to demonstrate what knowledge was unique to nursing in contrast to knowledge that might be considered borrowed. Donaldson and Crowley's (1978) work was seen as providing some important direction for continuing knowledge to develop what ultimately could be seen as a distinct discipline of nursing.

As part of their work, Donaldson and Crowley (1978) used an approach to disciplines based on the writings of Schwab (1962) to provide guidance for development of the discipline. Schwab (1962) and others who worked in the area of disciplinary structure (Shermis, 1962) argued that disciplines comprised two components: a *substantive structure* and a *syntax*. The content of the discipline constitutes the substantive structure; it includes concepts, theories, and other knowledge, principles, and ideas that make up the knowledge base of the discipline of nursing. Research to develop the discipline, therefore, should focus on content according to this idea of the disciplinary structure. The syntax includes the methods used in inquiry, as well as means to evaluate the value, credibility, or usefulness of inquiry done in the discipline. A general perspective, or worldview, provides the context for the substantive structure and the syntax to be brought together as characteristic of the particular discipline. Overall, these authors argued for the importance of delineating a distinct discipline of nursing, ensuring that the substance of the discipline served as a guide for practice, and establishing clear connections between research, the development of the discipline, and nursing practice.

It is worth noting that the approach to disciplinary structure that was advocated in nursing was that of the natural sciences. While this strategy may seem appropriate, it is important to consider how nursing might have developed differently if an idea relative to social sciences or humanities had been employed. This placement of nursing within the ranks of natural sciences became evident again when the philosophy of science known as *logical positivism* began to influence nursing knowledge development beginning in the 1970s, such that greater use of references in the area of natural, rather than social, sciences (although such works existed within philosophy of science) continues to be found throughout the nursing literature.

## The Idea of a "Professional" Discipline

The focus on disciplines occupied the nursing knowledge literature for some time, providing a framework for discussion of the uniqueness of nursing. This discussion encompassed topics such as the differences between basic and applied sciences, with nursing being held out as distinct from the basic sciences through its focus on application (Donaldson & Crowley, 1978; Johnson, 1959). The notion of applied science as a key aspect of nursing was captured sometimes through the references to nursing as a *professional discipline*. Professional or practice disciplines were thought to have specific characteristics that set them apart from those without a clear practice component. Thus professional disciplines, such as nursing, were viewed as different from the academic disciplines. A unique characteristic of the professional discipline is the delivery of service of some sort by those engaging in practice.

It is easy to argue that all disciplines have individuals who carry out the work of the discipline, who teach its substance, and who contribute to its ongoing development. Anyone who applies the knowledge of a discipline is engaging in practice related to that knowledge. The mere existence of people who engage in practice is not sufficient to differentiate a field from other disciplines whose members lack such a component. Nurses have used the argument that nursing is a "practice discipline" or a "professional discipline" to delineate nursing from other disciplines and to rationalize certain constraints or other challenges that set nursing apart from more traditional disciplines. However, describing nursing as a practice discipline is misleading because all disciplines have individuals who apply the knowledge. Without such application, there would be no opportunity for testing, studying, enhancing, refining, or sharing the knowledge of the particular discipline. What is important in regard to nursing, however, is that there are social constraints, licensing requirements, and means of public oversight that create a special context for nursing. These aspects are critical to the development of nursing and do require important considerations about the process of knowledge development. These characteristics also translate into specific needs for the nursing knowledge base (Dickoff, James, & Wiedenbach, 1968a, 1968b). Merely referring to nursing as a practice discipline may not draw sufficient attention to these aspects that affect its development. In spite of these social and legal constraints, however, it may not be beneficial to the development of nursing to emphasize these differences. It is not self-evident that nursing as a discipline is sufficiently distinct from other disciplines in its organization and development, and a focus on similarities may bring greater progress to understanding and valuing nursing than a continuing emphasis on differences. Indeed, failure to recognize the academic basis for nursing practice and the need for ongoing knowledge development may have contributed to the slow acceptance of nursing and valuing of nursing knowledge within university and healthcare settings.

The idea of a discipline having a unique substance, as advanced by scholars in nursing during the 1970s and 1980s, contributed to concerns mentioned previously about whether knowledge can be borrowed. This idea of borrowing knowledge from one discipline to the next does not hold up to further scrutiny. First, for something to be borrowed, it must belong to someone, yet it is not reasonable to think of knowledge as the possession of any one person or group of people. Researchers in the field of psychology may have created much of what is known about stress or behavior change, for example, yet it is clear that there are important connections to physiology, medicine, nursing, and sociology, in addition to other disciplines. Similarly, the members of other disciplines use, expand, critique, revise, and refine what is known on an ongoing basis, often with minimal regard for the origin of the knowledge.

There is some legitimate reason to be concerned about the perspectives that are represented in existing knowledge. To that end, nursing's holistic viewpoint and focus on relationships and contexts could be overlooked if nurses are not involved in the generation of that knowledge. Looked at another way, knowledge developed within other disciplines could fail to address the problems that nurses confront and that are important to their work with their populations of interest. Borrowing and the viability of the discipline of nursing are not the concerns here; rather, there is a legitimate concern that knowledge be generated that addresses the epistemic (knowledge-oriented) needs of nurses.

The idea of borrowed versus unique knowledge may not have much utility or support at this time, yet the need to pay attention to the knowledge base of nursing still has considerable merit. Nurses need to have an understanding of their discipline, particularly nurses who are in positions to help shape that knowledge. Nurses with DNP-level preparation will be in roles that enable them to have a significant influence over which knowledge development activities are pursued, and they should be engaged as members of research teams to ensure that the knowledge generated addresses areas of need. Because of the advanced practice focus of DNP education, DNP-prepared nurses are especially likely to have meaningful interaction with the public—the recipients of care—and, therefore, are in important positions to influence public perceptions of nursing. Understanding the current status of the discipline, and particularly the evolution of nursing to the present day, helps to create an understanding of the discipline that can be shared with others, can guide continuing research, and can shape the individual nurse's own perception of the role of nursing and the area of practice.

The brief mention of nursing history previously points to the continuing emergence of nursing as a discipline with a body of what can be called nursing knowledge. While there are occasional references to nursing as being in an early stage of development, particularly in reference to other disciplines, such a characterization does not do justice to the long history that exists, especially in connection with religious orders or the military, of people providing essential health services to those in need. Human beings have always needed individuals to whom they could turn for support with health and illness situations, whether that support has taken the form of the recommended cures of the day or more long-term care. To the extent that certain humans were identified as being particularly adept at providing such care, nursing has existed. As early as the time of the Crusades (the 11th century CE), efforts were made to provide a means for placing the work of tending to ill individuals in the hands of those skilled at providing needed care. These early efforts served as a harbinger of nursing that would develop in a more formal sense in later centuries, making it clear that nursing care in some form has been available to people for an exceptionally long period of time. Although the nursing of centuries ago bears little resemblance to the nursing of modern times, it does support the idea that the practice of nursing is not new or embryonic—a characterization occasionally used to describe nursing's state of development. Contemporary nursing involves formal education with complex substantive content reflecting a variety of disciplines, yet integrated into an approach to health and illness situations that represents the special influence of nursing. Arriving at this point in nursing education and practice reflects centuries of ongoing development.

## The Emergence of Nursing Science

As emphasis increased on nursing as a discipline, there emerged a concomitant drive to develop what can be referred to as *nursing science*. This emphasis became the specific focus of theory development for nursing and was the primary consideration in the development of the discipline from the 1960s through the 1980s. This section and subsequent sections of this chapter describe the major traditions in epistemology that have influenced the development of theory and nursing science (see **Box 2–1**).

A review of nursing knowledge development over the latter half of the 20th century shows the steady and profound influence of logical positivism. Logical positivism produced a lasting impact on nursing knowledge development, with one particularly strong example of its influence being extensive theory development activities demonstrated from the late 1960s and into the 1990s. Nurses who received

Box 2-1  Epistemologies in Nursing Science Development

| Logical positivism | Phenomenological | Feminist |
|---|---|---|
| Historicism | philosophy | epistemology |
| Postmodernism | Hermeneutics | |

their doctoral-level education in fields other than nursing were influenced by the dominance of this ideology at the time, a factor that helped to ensure its translation to a nursing context. Logical positivism, in fact, was pervasive throughout all of the sciences and has had a lasting impact on broad societal ideas about science and what constitutes appropriate or acceptable scientific activity. Logical positivism no longer occupies the forefront of philosophical thought about science; in fact, Webster, Jacox, and Baldwin (1981) declared it dead in the early 1980s. It is questionable, however, whether any philosophical movement ever dies completely, and there can be no doubt that the influence of logical positivism persists and has had a major role in shaping current ideas about science.

Logical positivism placed great emphasis on the demarcation of science from other forms of knowledge. Science was characterized as developing in a cumulative and linear fashion, with successive studies building on prior research. This process was oriented toward continuously refining and building theory in the quest for parsimonious statements that accurately corresponded with reality. Science, in essence, was seen as a theory-building activity, with the ideal theoretical statements being those that were capable of expression using the rules of logic and mathematics. Theory formed the core of scientific activity, and investigations represented an attempt to further develop, refine, or verify existing theory. With this emphasis on theory, it is easy to see how a discipline that lacked specific theoretical statements and clearly delineated bodies of theory might have been hindered in its efforts to gain recognition as a scientific discipline. If science was a theory-building activity, then nurse scholars suggested that there must be a theoretical foundation for nursing knowledge and practice for the discipline to be considered a science.

## The Theory Movement in Nursing

Nurse scholars and leaders devoted considerable effort to identifying the core or essence of nursing, to constructing theoretical formulations that would reflect this core, and to promoting further inquiry, as well as theory-based nursing practice. Federal funding was provided during the 1960s to support a series of conferences on theory development. The first conference was held at Case Western Reserve University in 1968; the second was held at the University of Colorado in 1969. Papers and discussion at these conferences clearly revealed the focus on the science of nursing and the influence of the philosophy of logical positivism on such activities during this time. The theoretical activity that took place under this influence amply illustrates the impact of logical positivism and this philosophical movement in the evolution of nursing as a discipline. Early nursing theory development activities, reflected in the work of Orlando (1961), Rogers (1970), Roy (1970, 1971), and others, served as important milestones in the effort to develop a theoretical basis for nursing.

Developing status as a science required not only the identification or development of theory for nursing, but also the use of existing theory as a basis for research. Logical positivism, after all, required that scientific activity focus on development and further articulation of theory. Descriptive research—that is, inquiry intended to discover or document events or conditions—did not meet the criteria for science that were espoused by philosophers and the dominant thinking of the period. As a result of this emphasis, the literature of nursing during this time includes a number of articles and ongoing discussion about the necessary connection between theory, research, and practice, with Fawcett's "double helix" metaphor being a particularly poignant example of this focus (Fawcett, 1978, 1985). Writings related to the role of theory in science reflected the tenets of logical positivism; theory development was viewed as a very formal activity with a focus on axioms and propositions in the construction of theory. Reynolds' (1971) *A Primer in Theory Construction* is referenced frequently in the nursing literature of this era and shows the emphasis on the development of formal theory, the importance of concepts being defined in operational terms to show their means of empirical testing, and a focus on quantitative testing of hypotheses derived from the theories. Research with an emphasis on describing situations or phenomena was possibly of some value, but only to the extent that it provided baseline data for further theory development (Fawcett, 1978, p. 60).

Science that was developed according to the tenets of logical positivism represented what is sometimes referred to as *hard science,* yet nurse scholars and leaders in the area of knowledge development encountered considerable difficulty with this philosophy in that a significant amount of nursing was not amenable to this conception of science. In spite of the great strides that were made during this time in developing the scientific and theoretical foundations of nursing, some aspects of nursing just could not fit these specific criteria. Nursing had maintained a long history of being regarded as holistic, humanistic, and relational, with an emphasis on psychological and social aspects of health and wellness as much as physiological and biological aspects. Concepts such as dignity, empathy, presence, and caring could not be forced into the mold of logical positivism without tremendous difficulty and, as nurses readily recognized, without considerable disservice to those crucial aspects of the human condition.

The lack of fit between nursing and prevailing ideas about science left nurses with some difficult choices. One option was for nurses to strive to meet the criteria of science as defined by the logical positivist philosophers. This endeavor would, however, require forcing some elements of nursing knowledge to meet the requirements of the prevailing ideology. Needless to say, this option was akin to the "square peg and round hole" metaphor, and it is debatable whether some of the highly valued aspects of nursing could ever be recast in this fashion without significantly changing their nature.

As a second option, nurses could argue that some components of nursing fit the idea of science, maintaining the logical positivist idea of science, while acknowledging that other aspects did not fit this ideology. Those other aspects are referred to as art: The dogma of nursing as "an art and a science" (Rodgers, 1991) persists throughout the history of modern nursing thought.

As a third option, nurses could accept that the knowledge base of the discipline, in its totality, did not meet the requirements of logical positivism. Carper's (1975, 1978) widely cited work identifying patterns of knowing in nursing addressed some of these concerns, identifying the empirical knowing that is consistent with traditional ideas of science as only one of four types of knowing inherent in nursing. Personal knowing, aesthetic knowing, and ethics were the terms used to label other forms of knowing that she argued were essential in nursing. This schema went beyond the mere separation of knowledge into science and everything else (e.g., art), and emphasized the existence of numerous ways of knowing, all of which are essential to the work of nursing.

## The Importance of Evaluating Philosophical Ideology

The fact that nurses largely failed to raise questions about the legitimacy of logical positivism as a useful and acceptable definition of science regardless of discipline is notable. The challenge for nurses should not have been viewed as only the determination of how to adopt and follow a particular line of activity or thought. In the case of logical positivism, nurses could have argued—as some did—that this philosophical approach just was not an acceptable or legitimate approach for nursing. In fact, there are significant problems with this philosophy regardless of discipline, even for those that seem to be a more reasonable fit with this idea of traditional science.

Although logical positivism was not an appropriate view for the development of the discipline of nursing, looking only at whether this philosophy "fit" nursing (rather than evaluating its merits overall) has two strong detrimental effects. First, it sets nursing apart as different, and not necessarily in a good way, but in a way that indicates nursing cannot, or will not, conform to prevailing standards for science. Second, and particularly significant in the case of logical positivism, it fails to address the crucial question of the legitimacy of the philosophy. Without that challenge, a philosophical tradition can continue to be held as an ideal, and progress in disciplines can be evaluated relative to its major tenets regardless of whether a particular discipline accepts that view. Those who rejected logical positivism as a suitable guide for the development of nursing without assessing the philosophy's inherent value created a situation where nursing could easily be viewed as "different," or as a lesser science than others that appeared to follow prevailing standards. The situation that resulted from this rejection (perpetuated in the argument that nursing is an art and a science) is similar to criticisms that continue to be levied against qualitative research, in other words, that it is "soft" and fails to meet the criteria of real science.

Trends and paradigm shifts are always occurring, and the critical questions asked by nurses cannot be limited to whether to follow along as viewpoints shift. The most important questions that need to be asked by nurses in regard to the knowledge base involve two things. First, is the latest ideology sound, not just for nursing, but for any discipline? Second, does it enable progress in nursing? In other words, is it an ideology that will help nurse scholars and researchers to make sound moves toward achieving the goals of the discipline? Applying such questions to logical positivism reveals quite quickly that the answer is *no* in regard to both aspects. Indeed, the shortcomings of logical positivism led to its demise as the dominant ideology of science by the mid-1900s.

The ideal put forth by the philosophers of this genre, however, continues to influence expectations and desires in the creation of science in nursing and elsewhere, ideals that persisted long after logical positivism lost its favored status. Science continues to be seen by society at large, as well as in many of the academic disciplines, as a special or unique form of knowledge with greater credibility than other forms of knowledge. Expectations for widespread generalizability of results, for statistical significance as the measure of meaningful results, for theory development as a focus of scientific activity, and for objectivity and a value-free orientation to inquiry continue to shape both the conduct of research and the needs of the public and others who will apply the results of scientific endeavors.

Webster and colleagues (1981) clearly pointed out the effects of "undue adherence to the positions and ideas of the received view" and noted how that perspective "stilted the development of nursing theories" (p. 34). *Truth*, as a criterion for evaluating theory, particularly in the form of correspondence with facts, presented other problems in the logical positivist viewpoint. The correspondence theory requires that phenomena be objectified—that is, measured in some way that is precise, repeatable, rigorous, and, as is evident in any research methods text, a valid measure of the phenomenon being studied. As a result, the phenomenon is believed to be captured successfully through the collection of empirical data.

Although this goal of precision and high validity certainly is an admirable one, it ignores elements of phenomena that can be the source of important information but are not reducible to means of measurement. With this approach, grief, for example, could be understood only as "grief as measured by a score on the grief instrument" because that is the only means for assigning numbers to grief to quantify and validate its existence. An individual's description of grief, including its emotional impact, its effect on daily life, and feelings that often are expressed by people using metaphors rather than checklists or Likert scales, could not be included under the heading of scientific.

It is easy to see how social or psychological phenomena are particularly troublesome to study from the perspective of logical positivism, because these phenomena have strong personal or what might be called subjective components. Physiological phenomena, however, are not immune to these difficulties either. Consider, for example, hypertension, measured as the pressure of the blood against vessel walls, or diabetes control, measured with glucose or HgbA$_{1c}$ levels. While these clearly are meaningful measures of these physical phenomena, they do not provide a broad or holistic perspective on how these conditions affect individuals with these diagnoses or what it is like to live with and try to maintain control of these physiological challenges. There are many challenges with the logical positivist philosophy of science. For purposes here, the significant point is to note the barriers to progress in the discipline of nursing that were confronted as a result of the rise in popularity of logical positivism and a staunch adherence to empirical ways of knowing, particularly within the context of a discipline that derives a significant amount of its identity from a holistic approach to human beings. These challenges also led to difficulties with the adoption of logical positivism in other disciplines. In spite of these barriers, however, logical positivism had a profound and lasting role on shaping views of science through the 20th century and beyond. Specifically, the philosophy created expectations for science in both academic settings and society at large that continue to influence the evaluation of knowledge for its applicability and meaningfulness.

Before moving on to address the changes that have arisen since the logical positivist approach became prominent, it is appropriate to reiterate some important points. Methods and philosophy are linked inextricably: The choice of method that a nurse or any scientist takes in regard to knowledge development has strong philosophical underpinnings that need to be recognized as an inherent part of the science or knowledge development enterprise. These foundations are not always obvious, yet the philosophical position taken by a researcher can be determined by assessing the approach to inquiry that is taken. It also is possible to use similar strategies for inquiry in spite of different philosophical positions.

When a researcher measures some phenomenon, the researcher is indicating that it is possible and appropriate to measure the phenomenon of interest. Yet, one researcher using a quantitative instrument to measure a phenomenon may believe that those measurements reflect true and meaningful data, whereas another may believe that the results are meaningful, but only a piece of a complex human situation, and that the answer to the research question is just one of many possible answers. Logical positivism, for example, undoubtedly leads to a quantitative approach to science, but, conversely, not all quantitative science is necessarily based on logical positivism.

From a philosophical or disciplinary standpoint, it is important to look at assumptions about the nature of reality, truth, the goals and purpose of science, and the criteria that are used for differentiating good science as reflective of the philosophical viewpoint of the researcher or scientist. Those underpinnings are reflected in the methods used, but the methods essentially are tools, and they can be used with perspectives that have some perhaps subtle—but important—variations.

Failure to distinguish method from philosophical underpinnings can lead to wholesale rejection (or, conversely, blind adoption) of alternatives to knowledge development without appropriate thought being given to the choices that are being made. The responses of nurses to various trends as evidenced in the literature of nursing do not always capture this subtle yet important difference. Without that understanding, however, there is a tendency to abandon useful aspects of some approaches to knowledge development or to develop a bandwagon mentality when new trends emerge and either become popular or later are found to be insufficient to meet the needs of the discipline.

As noted earlier, the logical positivist approach to knowledge had significant limitations as a focus for the development of knowledge, especially within the narrower realm of scientific knowledge. As a philosophy of science, it not only presented challenges within the philosophy itself with regard to views of the nature of reality, truth, and the proper goal of science, but it was also created as a prescriptive view—in other words, a directive dictating how science should be done. In essence, logical positivism was not comprehensive in terms of how science actually was conducted. Prescriptive approaches can be of great value, of course; this point is clearly seen in health care where prescriptions for all sorts of things are intended to set people on a healthier and more productive path, just as a prescriptive view of science could have the same intention. This prescriptive focus likely added to the strength of its influence because it was put forth as a directive for how science should be carried out.

## The Search for a Nursing Paradigm

An obvious problem raised by this prescriptive focus was the fact that it ignored much of how science actually was carried out. An insider view of science would provide great insight into how science worked, not just on the level of particular methods but also in regard to the broader enterprise of science—an enterprise consisting not only of theories and ideas but also of scientists (the people who do the work of science) and the context in which their work takes place. Thomas Kuhn (1970, 1974) provided just such insight into not only the workings of science but the people who did that work. Because logical positivism was found to be lacking for nursing, Kuhn's views quickly gained the attention of nurses looking for a useful understanding of science.

One of the major shifts presented in Kuhn's writing was the change in the philosophy of science from a focus on product to a focus on process—in other words, the way in which science was done. Kuhn's view of science was organized around the idea that a central paradigm provided a focal point for activity in a discipline. The paradigm served as a disciplinary matrix and included the values and aims inherent in the major substantive content of the discipline. The work of scientists, according to Kuhn, was to articulate this paradigm. Progress, truth, and theory, among other aspects of science, were determined by viewing these developments from the perspective of the paradigm. This was a radically different approach to science than the view of the logical positivist, because it allowed judgments about science to be made relative to a viewpoint—in this case, the disciplinary matrix or paradigm—rather than in reference to an objective reality.

Although there were some limitations to this new perspective, nurses writing during this period gave a great deal of attention to Kuhn's views and argued for the relevance of this philosophical position for knowledge development in nursing. Kuhn's discussion of scientific revolutions and the term *paradigm,* derived from his work, became common features in discussions of nursing as a discipline and, especially, as a science. Writers in nursing during this period ultimately concluded that nursing had a *metaparadigm,* a broader worldview and conceptualization or important elements of the discipline, yet evidence of a paradigm as required by Kuhn was presented as lacking (Hardy, 1983; Kim, 1989). Kim (1989) identified a number of distinct paradigms that were used in nursing but acknowledged the lack of a single overriding paradigm that would characterize nursing as a discipline in accordance with Kuhn's position.

Interestingly, while logical positivism experienced a relatively long life in nursing, Kuhn's view was quite short-lived in comparison. Nurse leaders and theorists during this time had become more familiar with philosophy and philosophical principles through their advanced education. As a result, there may have been a greater level of sophistication employed in evaluating ideology such as that presented by Kuhn. Limitations of Kuhn's view were quite obvious in nursing and perhaps contributed to acceptance of this tradition being less widespread, as well as shorter in duration in nursing. Although the term paradigm still has a prominent place in discussions about science, Kuhn's view overall was supplanted rather quickly by the views of other historicists and the rise of postmodernism, which followed shortly after the popularity of his work faded.

It is important to acknowledge the work of other historicist philosophers and the connection of such ideas to the development of nursing science. Larry Laudan was another noted philosopher of the late 1970s and a historicist whose work received some attention from nurse scholars. Laudan's (1977) philosophy was particularly noteworthy because he provided a view of science that addressed both conceptual and empirical problems in the conduct of science and the determination of progress. In general, Laudan focused on science as a problem-solving activity and assigned some weight to both conceptual and empirical work. Relatively few nurse authors (articles such as Fry, 1995, and Tinkle & Beaton, 1983, are good examples) described positions in support of Laudan's viewpoint and the practicality of his approach for nursing, and his work, like that of Kuhn, received far less attention than did the positions advocated by the logical positivists. Two significant aspects of the time could have contributed to this lack of attention. First, there was a continuing dominance of logical positivism and its influence on views of science even as historicist viewpoints were being articulated; this entrenched view would not be supplanted easily. Second, the philosophy of postmodernism emerged, developing particularly in the social sciences and then gradually spilling over into a number of other fields. Postmodernism served as a direct counterpoint to the rigidity of logical positivism, its emphasis on foundationalism, and its adherence to a belief in objective reality. This perspective represented quite a radical departure from both positivism and historicism, although it overlooked what might be considered the more moderate or intermediate position presented by historicist philosophers.

## Conceptual Problems and Concept Development

The potential contributions of historicism to nursing knowledge development are evident when reviewing the emphasis placed on concepts during the 1970s and 1980s. Although concepts and conceptual problems received attention during this time, the focus was not totally consistent with a historicist or postmodern perspective; in fact, discussion of concepts during this time had a strong positivist orientation. Concepts were valued primarily as elements of theory or, to use a popular phrase in nursing, as the "building blocks of theory," and not in a broader philosophical sense as ways to reflect, describe, and navigate through existence. Nonetheless, at least some attention was being paid to concepts, an occurrence that stands out in the history of the development of nursing science and points to the significance of concepts within the knowledge base.

Catherine Norris (1982) gave conceptual activity an important emphasis with the publication of a detailed book on concept clarification in nursing. Walker and Avant (1983, 1988) drew on the work of John Wilson (1969) to bring a method of concept analysis to nursing. This method remains popular in nursing and has been used in the analysis or clarification of a wide range of concepts. The text by Walker and Avant (1983, 1988) that addressed a method of concept analysis actually was focused on strategies for theory development in nursing, consistent with that common focus during the time of its initial publication. Content included analysis, synthesis, and derivation in the three categories of concepts, statements, and theories, all discussed as strategies for theory development. Perhaps as a remnant of logical positivism, or perhaps merely as recognition of the role of theory in science, work continued to be focused on theory development through much of the 1990s.

More recent work emphasizing concepts in nursing has been focused on developing useful concepts and resolving conceptual problems without being limited to theory development as the only relevant context for such work. Numerous philosophers addressed the role of concepts in cognition and, to a lesser extent, in science, yet their work has not received much of a reception in nursing. Rodgers (1989) constructed a view of concepts that emphasized concept development, not merely analysis, with analysis being a component of a broader process to generate meaningful and useful concepts. This work was informed by philosophers such as Laudan (1977), Toulmin (1972), Price (1953), and others, and was oriented toward providing a solid foundation for conceptual work as part of the development of science and the discipline. Since that time, increased attention has been paid to concept development rather than merely to analysis, or to analysis as a strategy oriented more broadly to the development of useful and effective concepts (Rodgers, 2000a, 2000b; Rodgers & Knafl, 2000). In spite of this development, a great deal of conceptual work in nursing continues to follow the techniques described by Walker and Avant, being empirical in orientation and poorly linked to resolution of conceptual problems. Although sound philosophy and techniques for improving the conceptual base of nursing are readily available, this aspect of knowledge development is not well utilized in nursing. This is an unfortunate situation, because a number of the significant problems regarding nursing knowledge are conceptual in nature rather than empirical. Even for problems that are clinical in nature, clear and sound concepts are needed to ensure that empirical problems are articulated with clarity and relevant variables are understood, defined, and measured appropriately.

There is a need for additional work in concept development because many of the problems that are paramount in nursing are conceptual in nature and because methodological advances in concept development are not well integrated into nursing inquiry. In addition, concepts are important in delineating the identity and scope of the discipline. Consistent with the earlier effort to identify the essence of nursing, fundamental concepts were stipulated as constituting the core of nursing knowledge. Kim (1987), Flaskerud and Halloran (1980), and others identified nursing, person, health, and environment as the key concepts in nursing, with Flaskerud and Halloran referring to the centrality of these concepts as an important area of agreement in nursing. Other writings around this time were consistent with this focus, specifying that these concepts could provide a foundation for theory development in the discipline (Hardy, 1978; Johnson, 1968; Newman, 1972). As noted previously, although work conducted during the 1980s and 1990s reveals attention to the role of concepts in developing the knowledge base, a significant part of this effort, particularly in the early phases, was consistent with the positivist focus on theory development. More recently (Rodgers, 1989, 2000b), concepts have begun to take on a role as significant parts of knowledge outside of theory development. There is a continuing need for attention to concept development that goes beyond the basic level of analysis to modes of inquiry that result in better ways to conceptualize important phenomena in nursing (Rodgers, 2000a, 2000b). The analysis of concepts should not be seen as an endpoint to inquiry; instead, the results of any analysis should be tied to a continuing process of developing knowledge that addresses significant problems in the discipline.

## The Postmodern Turn

The historicist tradition (*historicism*) presented a stark contrast to the major tenets of logical positivism. Historicism provided an emphasis on problem solving as evidenced by the work of Laudan (1977), conceptual repertoires as discussed by Toulmin (1972), the notion of science as an enterprise with work conducted by people with their own values and perspectives, and a focus on science as a process rather than the product—all of which prompted questions about appropriate ways of doing and evaluating science. The historicist tradition offered substantial advantages over the rigid requirements placed on science by logical positivism. The potential contributions of historicist philosophy, however, received relatively scant attention in nursing. A review of the literature for nursing knowledge development and nursing science in the 1980s and 1990s reveals few works that address the work of historicist philosophers. This lack of attention likely is related to the development of yet another philosophical tradition, *postmodernism*, which garnered substantial attention in nursing shortly after the peak of historicism.

Postmodernism involves an emphasis on hermeneutics, narrative traditions and discourse, and philosophies of critical social theory and feminism. The emergence of this array of ideologies overshadowed discussions of historicism and quickly became a major focus of interest in nursing. Postmodernism, to many nurse authors at the time, seemed to closely approximate many of the values and purposes of nursing knowledge. This philosophical tradition was based on ideas of relativism, or viewpoints that truths existed on an individual level. This orientation was consistent with a longstanding emphasis in nursing on the whole person and the uniqueness of each individual. Nursing had developed around a focus on individualized care, and postmodernism was wholly consistent with that idea, not only allowing for but requiring recognition of uniqueness related to gender, culture, social status, and other characteristics inherent in the individual. Postmodernism also captured the idea that power differentials present in society are reflected in the healthcare system and interactions with care providers. In contrast to the idea that one single, central, fundamental overarching reality exists, with the purpose of science being to discover that reality, postmodernism was founded on uniqueness, diversity, power structures, and multiple realities as a result of human and social variation. This notion that there is not one single, central truth or story that is applicable to everyone is a defining feature of postmodernism and is referred to as the rejection of metanarrative, overarching narratives that are broadly generalizable.

Feminism, in particular, received a tremendous amount of attention, and it was not uncommon for authors to stipulate that feminism was a natural fit for nursing given that the majority of nurses were female. Feminism provided a clear example of postmodernism and was seen by many nurse leaders as exemplary of the postmodern emphasis on the uniqueness of each individual; the importance of individual realities with their gender, class, social, economic, and other influences; recognition of cultural relativism; and awareness of the role of power differentials in health care as in the rest of society. As a result, postmodernism garnered considerable attention as a good fit as a philosophical system for nursing knowledge development.

Postmodernism represented a radical departure from earlier philosophies dealing with science and knowledge. As a result of its emergence, new modes of inquiry and new methodologies began to receive attention in nursing. The emphasis on individual beliefs, cultural and social contexts, multiple realities, power differentials, and so on required the development of methods that were able to capture these aspects of existence through research. With such significant philosophical differences, it was clear that traditional scientific principles could not be applied to the study of human beings given their individual and social contexts. At the very least, a pluralistic approach to inquiry would be necessary, balancing the supposedly objective and quantifiable facets with the more personal and individual aspects of human beings. A more extreme form of ideology at the time held that reduction and quantification could be rejected in their entirety and replaced with more holistic traditions of inquiry. Techniques for deconstruction could be applied to language, as well as images, and reveal power differentials and biases implicit in communication. Similarly, narrative or text, including the idea that action constitutes a text as described by Ricoeur (1981, 1984), provided a means to identify precepts, values, hidden meanings, and other contextual elements of experience. During this time there was an increasing emphasis on language and communication, with the development of narrative modes of inquiry that focused on individual story rather than attempts to uncover any form of truth.

Qualitative research began to emerge as a viable option for inquiry in nursing and in other disciplines. Philosophical methods such as phenomenology and hermeneutics had existed for an extended period of time, with hermeneutics having a particularly long history dating back to the early study of biblical texts. In spite of this extensive history, however, these philosophical methods had not been compatible with traditional ideas of science. Acceptance of qualitative research grew slowly and continues to meet resistance in some disciplines and by some researchers even in nursing. Nonetheless, the rise of postmodern philosophy opened the door for, and subsequently fueled rapid growth in, qualitative methodologies to develop knowledge for the discipline. In fact, the popularity of qualitative research grew so quickly that it appeared at times to be a sort of bandwagon, drawing significant attention and support simply because it offered such a stark contrast to the method supported by the quantitative methods of logical positivism. The quality of studies was variable, and there was evidence of some confusion regarding the various specific methods, resulting in awkward piecemeal combinations of different, and sometimes incompatible, methodological traditions. This blending of perspectives and methods was referred to as "method slurring" by Baker, Wuest, and Stern (1992). Over time, an increasing number of publications dealt with aspects of quality in qualitative research, and the initial excitement about qualitative methods gradually evolved to leave a variety of distinct, clear, and highly rigorous approaches for the conduct and the evaluation of such forms of inquiry.

Postmodernism led to the emergence of a particular form of qualitative inquiry referred to as *interpretive approaches*. These approaches focus on experiences as people live them with all their individual interpretations and reactions; consistent with this view is the idea that actions represent values, and an emphasis on the primacy of dialog and language as means to share realities. As a result, actions, dialog, and language provide a mechanism for the investigator to gain a greater understanding of those unique realities. Hermeneutical, phenomeno-logical, narrative, and other interpretive approaches have been used to explore a variety of experiences of interest to nurses, including suffering (Steeves, Kahn, & Benoliel, 1990), race and attrition in nursing programs (Jordan, 1996), the care provider–patient relationship (Sundin, Jansson, & Norberg, 2002), and nurses in various roles such as nurse consultant (Walters, 1996).

The philosophy of postmodernism reflects another unique turn in ideas about the development of knowledge by raising significant questions about the presumption of objectivity in the conduct of science. In postmodernism, the separation of what is known from who is doing the knowing no longer exists; moreover, social elements not only have an effect on knowledge, but they also are viewed as an appropriate focus for inquiry. As noted previously, feminism and feminist epistemology gained considerable attention in relation to the growth of postmodernism. Postmodern philosophy makes it clear that social elements, such as class and gender, are important in regard to knowledge development and, in feminism, the specific emphasis is on gender.

Feminism exists in numerous forms, ranging from a moderate view that gender is important when looking at ways of interacting with the world to a more extreme version that holds gender to be the most important factor in interactions. In the extreme view, political action to counteract the dominant patriarchy is crucial to social progress (Harding, 1986, 1991). Some of the roots of feminism can be traced to historical events in which women were denied what are now considered to be basic social and civil rights.

Adding to this historical origin is a considerable body of research that was biased against women. Kohlberg's (1981) research on moral development, for example, was groundbreaking, but the stages of moral development that were identified, when used in research with female subjects, led to the conclusion that females functioned at a considerably lower level of moral development than their male counterparts. Subsequent research using a different frame of reference, such as the work conducted by Carol Gilligan (1982), revealed the gender bias inherent in Kohlberg's work. The differences between male subjects and females in regard to development was argued by Gilligan to be not a matter of more or less of something, or one group being more developed than the other, but rather an altogether different way of approaching ethical problem solving. Gilligan's work was foundational in supporting the idea that females have a different frame of reference and a different way of working through ethical problems than males. Such differences do not equate to higher or lower levels of moral development. Additional work in this area was carried out by Belenky, Clinchy, Goldberger, and Tarule (1986), who interviewed a group of 135 women; their study revealed that women interact with the world and have ways of knowing that appear to be substantially different from how men interact with and know the world.

The recognition of gender differences evident in research, along with the postmodern emphasis on individual realities rather than grand narratives, made it easy to see how feminism could be viewed as a philosophy with a good fit for nursing.

In addition, a number of noted scholars in nursing recognized the consistency between a feminist view and the professional status of nurses. History is replete with references to nurses as the handmaidens of the physician, and it is likely that most nurses have heard stories of nurses giving up their chairs or handing over patient charts to the physician whenever he was present (and, of course, in early years, physicians were *he* rather than *she,* as the discipline of medicine demonstrated a similar bias against women). From a political standpoint, then, feminism was seen as offering some potential benefit to a predominantly female profession such as nursing.

Feminist ideology, however, often results in assigning a gender orientation to knowledge, labeling some approaches as distinctly feminine. This can create awkwardness in regard to thinking of knowledge claims as having a particular gender and presenting some views as superior to others based on a gender orientation. Rather than offering a means to overcome problems with bias that are presumed to be present in science, this approach sometimes seems only to offer yet a different form of bias in knowledge development. Some authors have justified this development, arguing that the masculine, patriarchal orientation is so strong that it is necessary to promote an equally strong feminist orientation as a counterpoint to the male hegemony. Others see feminism as opening the door to more diversity in a broad scope of perspectives that can be considered. Chinn (1989) described nursing as emphasizing wholeness, with any singular perspective—masculine or feminine—being insufficient to accomplish this idea of wholeness in health. According to Chinn, nurses see the world through the lens of integration and wholeness. We cannot conceive of knowing sufficiently in any way nor can we rely on any one way of knowing that disregards another dimension of experience. We know we experience reality in a whole way.

It seems essential that myriad viewpoints be considered in the development of a view that meets the expectations of being holistic and values the uniqueness of individuals. As societies and cultures evolve, the viewpoints to be considered and included in knowledge development have evolved as well, a situation evident in the development of viewpoints based on voices of many unique groups including immigrants and gay, lesbian, and transgendered persons.

The relationship between nursing and feminism as a political movement has been a difficult one in many regards. Historically, men had positions of prominence in nursing because of the association of nursing with the military and with religious orders. In addition, women who in earlier times had worked to advance the professional status of nursing did not always see this work as connected to promoting the status of women in general. The American Nurses Association, for example, was not a supporter of women's right to vote in the early years of the organization. At the same time, as opportunities for women have expanded throughout recent history, there has been a tendency for women in traditionally female occupations to feel disenfranchised for choosing those occupations rather than new ones that have become available to them. The tensions surrounding nurses in relation to feminism as a political movement in nursing, therefore, emanated from both the feminist action side and the nursing professional side.

In spite of political tensions and debates regarding the merits of gender as a specific focus in knowledge development, feminism has had a significant role in the development of nursing knowledge. Leaders in this movement in nursing brought energy to workplace issues that affect both nursing practice and the nursing workforce. Awareness of bias in scientific research—particularly the historical exclusion of women from a large body of medical research—raised questions about the applicability and generalizability of scientific findings to the care of patients. Recognition of the role of gender and science and what Lather (1991) referred to as the failure of traditional science increased awareness of numerous factors in the development of nursing knowledge and the ways in which knowledge is applied in practice.

The postmodern movement, including feminism, led to considerable research in nursing dealing with cultural and unique individual factors and helped to illuminate on a much broader scale the spectrum of human health and illness as lived by real people in their natural social and cultural settings. Through developments consistent with this ideology, meaningful work has been used not only to understand but also to empower people in their interactions related to health and health care. Philosophies of the postmodern, critical social theory, and feminist traditions continue to evolve and stimulate new ideas for research methodology and criteria for evaluating the quality and range of application for research results.

Work remains, however, to explore ideas of postmodernism and the methodologies consistent with these ideas in a context of contemporary science. Prevailing notions of quality and what constitutes science still tend to be consistent with a positivist or logical positivist philosophy. To date, considerable effort has been devoted to articulating standards for evaluating the quality of inquiry in postmodern traditions (Guba & Lincoln, 1989; Hall & Stevens, 1991; Rolfe, 2006), and the rules associated with such work represent a vast departure from traditional notions of science. Reconciling these disparate viewpoints is important so that the merit of each viewpoint is appreciated and the potential usefulness understood. This is an area in which continuing work can develop a cohesive body of nursing knowledge and have that knowledge valued across an array of situations and contexts.

## Emerging Trends in Nursing Science

The prior examination of developments and trends in the evolution of nursing science provides a glimpse into the progress made in the discipline and attempts to provide a solid foundation for nursing knowledge. Numerous approaches to knowledge relevant to nursing practice have been entertained within the discipline; some were taken as prescriptions for nursing thought, whereas others offered what was considered a closer fit with nursing as it currently exists. While the variety of philosophical approaches and methodologies appears appealing simply because of the diversity of perspectives offered, the plethora of philosophies also places some demands on the nurse in an advanced practice role.

One option for dealing with the myriad approaches that can be appealing to any nurse is to adopt a pluralistic view, or something similar to an *anything goes* attitude. Each era in nursing history has contributed to the development of the discipline of nursing through expansion and articulation of the knowledge base and, concomitantly, a stronger identity for nursing. In addition, each viewpoint has some merits, just as each has limitations. So why not selectively apply pieces of these traditions, if not the whole tradition, when addressing a problem relevant to nursing? Noted Austrian philosopher Feyerabend (1975) specifically supported an approach allowing for maximum creativity and innovation in the process of knowledge development. Numerous authors in nursing have taken such a position as well, by suggesting that there should be a variety of methods and perspectives from which nurses can choose whatever is appropriate to guide their research or practice (Baker, Norton, Young, & Ward, 1998; Coward, 1990; Schultz, 1987).

Some important considerations must be addressed when adopting an approach such as pluralism, however. The primary issues are *philosophical congruency* and *incoherence* and *fit* with the values and ontological perspective of the discipline. Philosophical congruency and coherence are evident as concerns when looking at whether different perspectives in nursing are compatible with a philosophical basis. If nursing holds that the human being is holistic and cannot be viewed specifically in terms of parts, the viewpoints that are taken relative to knowledge development need to be consistent on that point. Given this example, positions based on the philosophy of logical positivism are incompatible with views based on postmodernism and critical social theory.

This example also points out the importance of ontological fit with nursing. In this case, the ontological view supports the position that human beings need to be considered on a holistic basis. The human being cannot be both holistic and reducible at the same time, and advocating this position would be inconsistent with nursing's expressed metaphysical position on the nature of the human being. Positions about truth, generalizability, the nature of reality, the nature of facts, the role of the investigator, and the role of ethics and values are fundamental considerations and intrinsic parts of the discipline. There is certainly a need for differing perspectives in the process of knowledge development, but whatever approaches are taken need to be consistent with the espoused values and worldview held by the discipline at large.

Such a position does not preclude a variety of approaches to developing the knowledge base for nursing. The discipline will benefit most, however, if the use of a variety of means of knowledge development relevant to nursing is based on a consistent philosophical viewpoint that supports such diversity. The purpose of nursing knowledge is to support the work of nurses and provide information critical to both the delivery of effective care and the continuing development of the discipline. These real and practical aims provide an organizing viewpoint for continuing knowledge relevance. Capturing this need for applicable knowledge is the philosophy of *pragmatism* or, a more contemporary variation, *neopragmatism*. The discipline of nursing has paid relatively little attention to this philosophy, although a few articles can be found that have addressed this topic. For example, Rodgers (2005, 2007) advocated a problem-solving approach based on the philosophies of Laudan (1977) and Toulmin (1972) as a way to justify multiple approaches to knowledge development and nursing while still maintaining some consistency and identity for the discipline.

From a philosophical standpoint, a focus on problem solving pertains specifically to epistemic problems in the discipline. The advanced practice nurse with a practice-focused doctoral degree is the ideal person to facilitate this process. The advanced practice nurse has clinical expertise and practical experience that enables the nurse to detect problems that need to be addressed. The DNP-prepared nurse also has sufficient knowledge of processes of inquiry, as well as an understanding of the discipline of nursing, both of which help to ensure that attempts to expand the knowledge base are properly conducted and are relevant to the discipline.

Other developments in nursing have helped to bring some focus and direction to knowledge development in the discipline. During the 1980s and 1990s, a series of conferences was held in the northeastern United States, alternately sponsored by schools of nursing at the University of Rhode Island and Boston College. These conferences served as a vital forum for discussion of ideas about science and knowledge development relevant to the discipline of nursing. After this period of sharing and development, it became apparent to the conference organizers that the next appropriate step would be the development of a consensus statement reflecting crucial areas of agreement about nursing as a discipline. The purpose of the Knowledge Consensus Conference in Boston in 1998 was for the 40 participants "to discuss and synthesize various perspectives on knowledge development related to (1) the nature of the human person, (2) the nature of nursing, (3) the role of nursing theory, and (4) the links of each of these understandings to nursing practice" (*Consensus Statement on Emerging Nursing Knowledge*, 1999, p. 1). The document that resulted from this effort, the *Consensus Statement on Emerging Nursing Knowledge,* served as an important event in the history of contemporary nursing and reflected the values and knowledge that were thought by participants to be essential to the discipline, as well as the practice, of nursing.

The consensus statement was an attempt to move beyond repeated discussion of the nature of nursing and the knowledge base and provide a foundation for continuing focused development of the discipline. What this manifesto provided was a statement of agreed-upon values and perspectives that could provide some cohesiveness among nurses, a reminder of the lens through which nurses see the world and the recipients of their care. A variety of philosophical traditions, modes of inquiry, and research methods may be used to solve epistemic problems in nursing. Keeping in mind the key assumptions and values embedded in the discipline allows plurality in approaches to knowledge development while still supporting a sense of unity in the discipline and the knowledge that underlies the work of nurses. The consensus statement was disseminated through a website, and there was an opportunity for sharing and continuing dialog.

# The Future of Nursing Knowledge Development

Predicting the future is an onerous—if not absurd—task. Current trends do lead to future developments, yet precisely how change occurs and which changes may take place along the way are difficult, if not impossible, to predict with accuracy. Preparing for the future in nursing science, then, is more a matter of perspective development than an anticipation of specific occurrences. The future of nursing knowledge development requires nurses to blend philosophical aspects with the emerging social trends and needs in the discipline. It also requires nurses with strong analytical skills to clearly identify problem areas where research is needed, promote awareness of trends within society, as well as within the discipline, and demonstrate the leadership and interpersonal skills to address the needs on all levels.

Along those lines, patterns that reveal potential significance for nursing involvement can be identified. Changes in philosophy, as well as in social context, call for new methods to address pressing issues in nursing. Recognition of the role of culture and social context require increasing development, application, and evaluation of methods effective at capturing those aspects of existence. These changes also require nurses who understand the philosophy and knowledge development enterprises well enough to be able to articulate the value of differing approaches to inquiry. Advanced practice nurses will provide a critical link in this process through their skill and understanding of both the knowledge development and scientific enterprises, as well as the realm of application in practice. Nursing science work without that critical link to practice is likely to fail in meeting the needs of nurses who apply that science on a daily basis. Nurses at levels prior to advanced practice need leadership and guidance from advanced practice nurses to offer a few problems suitable for inquiry, as well as to help evaluate and apply new information for evidence-based practice.

Promoting continuing progress in nursing in regard to knowledge development also requires nurses who recognize that the future is something to be constructed as well as anticipated. Perhaps what the future of nursing knowledge development needs most is nurses who have a vision of what nursing can be and who have a commitment and desire to help create that idealized future. Advanced practice nurses will continue to be an essential part of the process of developing the discipline of nursing.

One area in need of increased attention in nursing is that of theory development. Theory often is poorly understood in nursing, with a common misperception being that theory is limited to the work of the grand theorists such as Orem, Johnson, and others. Exposure to theory in nursing programs unfortunately has perpetuated a gross misunderstanding about the role of theory in the knowledge base and in support of the practice of nursing. Ideas of theory need to be expanded beyond these broad narratives about nursing and also beyond the axiomatic and propositional constructions supported by the logical positivists. Theory is merely organized knowledge—knowledge that is connected and structured in such a way as to be slightly abstract, rather than case dependent, and potentially relevant to a variety of situations. Theories exist that can be immensely beneficial to nurses dealing with a wide array of topics commonly encountered in practice. Rather than reject theory development, a position taken by nurses at the 2013 Campaign for Action summit (Future of Nursing: Campaign for Action, 2013), nurses need to recognize the value of theory in regard to providing some organization to knowledge and focus on theory that is meaningful and useful in practical application. Nurses also need to recognize that knowledge changes. Just as the history of philosophical views about knowledge has changed over time, knowledge itself can and must change. Nurses need to develop skills that enable thoughtful critique of knowledge, characteristics of flexibility, a spirit of creativity, and a willingness to evaluate and embrace changes in knowledge. Along with this approach, particularly critical for nurses in leadership positions such as those with DNP degrees, nurses need to recognize the vital connection between the knowledge base and the discipline of nursing and look beyond immediate practice implications to promote changes in the discipline and perception of nursing among the public, other health professionals, and nurses. All activities, whether administrative, clinical, or research oriented, should be undertaken with an understanding of the essential connections among the discipline, the knowledge base, and the practice of nursing.

## Summary

In this chapter the nonlinear evolution of nursing science was explored in regard to philosophical traditions in epistemology and philosophy of science, specifically logical positivism, historicism, postmodernism, phenomenological philosophy, hermeneutics, and feminist epistemology. Events in the development of nursing as a discipline were examined in light of philosophical change. Emerging trends were presented along with suggestions for continuing development appropriate to the role of the DNP nurse.

## Discussion Questions

1. Discuss significant historical trends that have shaped the development of nursing knowledge.

2. Which trends in philosophy have influenced the development of nursing science?

3. Describe the role of the DNP-prepared nurse in the development of nursing science.

# References

Baker, C., Norton, S., Young, P., & Ward, S. (1998). An exploration of methodological pluralism in nursing research. *Research in Nursing and Health, 21, 545–555.*

Baker, C., Wuest, J., & Stern, P. N. (1992). Method slurring: The grounded theory/phenomenology example. *Journal of Advanced Nursing, 17, 1355–1360.*

Belenky, M. F., Clinchy, B. M., Goldberger, N. R., & Tarule, J. M. (1986). *Women's ways of knowing: The development of self, voice, and mind.* New York, NY: Basic Books.

Carper, B. A. (1975). *Fundamental patterns of knowing in nursing.* Doctoral dissertation, Teachers College, Columbia University, New York. University Microfilms Cat # 76–7772.

Carper, B. A. (1978). Fundamental patterns of knowing in nursing. *Advances in Nursing Science, 1*(1), 13–23.

Chinn, P. L. (1989). Nursing patterns of knowing and feminist thought. *Nursing and Health Care, 10, 71–75.*

*Consensus statement on emerging nursing knowledge: A value-based position paper linking nursing knowledge and practice outcomes.* (1999). Nursing Knowledge Consensus Conference, Boston, MA. Retrieved from http://www.bc.edu/bc_org/avp/son/theorist/roy.pdf

Coward, D. D. (1990). Critical multiplism: A research strategy for nursing science. *Image: Journal of Nursing Scholarship, 22, 163–167.*

Dickoff, J., James, P., & Wiedenbach, E. (1968a). Theory in a practice discipline: Part I. Practice-oriented theory. *Nursing Research, 17, 415–435.*

Dickoff, J., James, P., & Wiedenbach, E. (1968b). Theory in a practice discipline: Part II. Practice-oriented theory. *Nursing Research, 17, 545–554.*

Donaldson, S. K., & Crowley, D. M. (1978). The discipline of nursing. *Nursing Outlook, 26*(2), 113–120.

Fawcett, J. (1978). The relationship between theory and research: A double helix. *Advances in Nursing Science, 1*(1), 49–62.

Fawcett, J. (1985). Theory: Basis for the study and practice of nursing education. *Journal of Nursing Education, 24, 226–229.*

Feldman, H. R. (1981). A science of nursing: To be or not to be? *Image: Journal of Nursing Scholarship, 13, 63–66.*

Feyerabend, P. K. (1975). *Against method.* London, UK: Humanities Press.

Flaskerud, J. H., & Halloran, E. J. (1980). Areas of agreement in nursing theory development. *Advances in Nursing Science, 3*(1), 1–7.

Fry, S. T. (1995). Science as problem solving. In A. Omery, C. E. Kasper, & G. G. Page (Eds.), *In search of nursing science* (pp. 72–80). Thousand Oaks, CA: Sage.

Future of Nursing: Campaign for Action. (2013). Top actions we must stop doing. Retrieved from http://campaignforaction.org/resource/top-actions-we-must-stop-doing

Gilligan, C. (1982). *In a different voice: Psychological theory and women's development.* Cambridge, MA: Harvard University Press.

Guba, E. G., & Lincoln, Y. S. (1989). *Fourth generation evaluation.* Newbury Park, CA: Sage.

Hall, J. M., & Stevens, P. E. (1991). Rigor in feminist research. *Advances in Nursing Science, 13*(3), 16–29.

Harding, S. (1986). *The science question in feminism.* Ithaca, NY: Cornell University.

Harding, S. (1991). *Whose science? Whose knowledge?* Ithaca, NY: Cornell University.

Hardy, M. E. (1978). Perspectives on nursing theory. *Advances in Nursing Science, 1*(1), 27–48.

Hardy, M. (1983). Metaparadigms and theory development. In N. L. Chaska (Ed.), *The nursing profession: A time to speak* (pp. 427–437). New York, NY: McGraw-Hill.

Johnson, D. E. (1959). The nature of a science of nursing. *Nursing Outlook, 7,* 291–294.

Johnson, D. E. (1968). Theory in nursing: Borrowed and unique. *Nursing Research, 17,* 206–209.

Jordan, J. D. (1996). Rethinking race and attrition in nursing programs: A hermeneutic inquiry. *Journal of Professional Nursing, 12,* 382–390.

Kalisch, P. A., & Kalisch, B. J. (1995). *The advance of American nursing*. Philadelphia, PA: Lippincott.

Kim, H. S. (1987). Structuring the nursing knowledge system: A typology of four domains. *Scholarly Inquiry for Nursing Practice, 1,* 111–114.

Kim, H. S. (1989). Theoretical thinking in nursing: Problems and prospects. *Recent Advances in Nursing, 24,* 106–122.

Kohlberg, L. (1981). *Essays on moral development*. San Francisco, CA: Harper & Row.

Kuhn, T. S. (1970/1962). *The structure of scientific revolutions* (2nd ed.). Chicago, IL: University of Chicago.

Kuhn, T. S. (1974). Second thoughts on paradigms. In F. Suppe (Ed.), *The structure of scientific theories* (pp. 459–482). Urbana, IL: University of Illinois.

Lather, P. (1991). *Getting smart: Feminist research and pedagogy with/in the postmodern*. New York, NY: Routledge.

Laudan, L. (1977). *Progress and its problems*. Berkeley, CA: University of California Press.

Newman, M. A. (1972). Nursing's theoretical evolution. *Nursing Outlook, 20,* 449–453.

Norris, C. M. (1982). *Concept clarification in nursing*. Rockville, MD: Aspen.

Orlando, I. (1961). *The dynamic nurse–patient relationship*. New York, NY: G. P. Putnam's Sons.

Price, H. H. (1953). *Thinking and experience*. London, UK: Hutchinson House.

Reynolds, P. D. (1971). *A primer in theory construction*. New York, NY: Bobbs-Merrill.

Ricoeur, P. (1981). *Hermeneutics and the human sciences* (J. B. Thompson, Ed. & Trans.). Cambridge, UK: Cambridge University Press.

Ricoeur, P. (1984). *Time and narrative* (2 vols.). (K. McLaughlin & D. Pellauer, Trans.). Chicago, IL: University of Chicago Press.

Rodgers, B. L. (1989). Concepts, analysis, and the development of knowledge: The evolutionary cycle. *Journal of Advanced Nursing, 14,* 330–335.

Rodgers, B. L. (1991). Deconstructing the dogma in nursing knowledge and practice. *Image: Journal of Nursing Scholarship, 23,* 177–181.

Rodgers, B. L. (2000a). Concept analysis: An evolutionary view. In B. L. Rodgers & K. A. Knafl (Eds.), *Concept development in nursing: Foundations, techniques, and applications* (pp. 77–102). Philadelphia, PA: Saunders.

Rodgers, B. L. (2000b). Philosophical foundations of concept development. In B. L. Rodgers & K. A. Knafl (Eds.), *Concept development in nursing: Foundations, techniques, and applications* (pp. 7–38). Philadelphia, PA: Saunders.

Rodgers, B. L. (2005). *Developing nursing knowledge: Philosophical traditions and influences*. Philadelphia, PA: Lippincott Williams & Wilkins.

Rodgers, B. L. (2007). Knowledge as problem solving. In C. Roy & D. A. Jones (Eds.), *Nursing knowledge development and clinical practice* (pp. 107–117). New York, NY: Springer.

Rodgers, B. L., & Knafl, K. A. (Eds.). (2000). *Concept development in nursing: Foundations, techniques, and applications.* Philadelphia, PA: Saunders.

Rogers, M. E. (1970). *An introduction to the theoretical basis of nursing.* Philadelphia, PA: F. A. Davis.

Rolfe, G. (2006). Judgments without rules: Towards a postmodern ironist concept of research validity. *Nursing Inquiry, 13*(1), 7–15.

Roy, C. (1970). Adaptation: A conceptual framework for nursing. *Nursing Outlook, 18*(3), 42–45.

Roy, C. (1971). Adaptation: A basis for nursing practice. *Nursing Outlook, 19,* 254–257.

Schultz, P. R. (1987). Toward holistic inquiry in nursing: A proposal for synthesis of patterns and methods. *Scholarly Inquiry for Nursing Practice: An International Journal, 1,* 135–146.

Schwab, J. (1962). The concept of the structure of a discipline. *Educational Record, 43,* 197–205.

Shermis, S. (1962). On becoming an intellectual discipline. *Phi Delta Kappan, 44,* 84–86.

Smith, M., & McCarthy, P. M. (2010). Disciplinary knowledge in nursing education: Going beyond the blueprints. *Nursing Outlook, 58,* 44–51.

Steeves, R. H., Kahn, D. L., & Benoliel, J. Q. (1990). Nurses' interpretation of the suffering of their patients. *Western Journal of Nursing Research, 12,* 715–729.

Sundin, K., Jansson, L., & Norberg, A. (2002). Understanding between care providers and patients with stroke and aphasia: A phenomenological hermeneutic inquiry. *Nursing Inquiry, 9,* 93–103.

Tinkle, M. B., & Beaton, J. L. (1983). Toward a new view of science: Implications for nursing research. *Advances in Nursing Science, 5*(2), 27–36.

Toulmin, S. (1972). *Human understanding.* Princeton, NJ: Princeton University Press.

U.S. Public Health Service. (1963). *Toward quality in nursing: Needs and goals.* Washington, DC: Government Printing Office.

Visintainer, M. A. (1986). The nature of knowledge and theory in nursing. *Image: Journal of Nursing Scholarship, 18,* 32–38.

Walker, L. O., & Avant, K. C. (1983). *Strategies for theory construction in nursing.* Norwalk, CT: Appleton & Lange.

Walker, L. O., & Avant, K. C. (1988). *Strategies for theory construction in nursing* (2nd ed.). Norwalk, CT: Appleton & Lange.

Walters, A. J. (1996). Being a clinical nurse consultant: A hermeneutic phenomenological reflection. *International Journal of Nursing Practice, 2*(1), 2–10.

Webster, G., Jacox, A., & Baldwin, B. (1981). Nursing theory and the ghost of the received view. In J. C. McCloskey & H. K. Grace (Eds.), *Current issues in nursing* (pp. 26–35). Boston, MA: Blackwell Scientific.

Wilson, J. (1969). *Thinking with concepts.* New York, NY: Cambridge University Press.

# The Essentials of the Doctor of Nursing Practice: A Philosophical Perspective

*Lisa Astalos Chism*

## Introduction

The Doctor of Nursing Practice (DNP) degree has been recommended by the American Association of Colleges of Nursing (AACN) as the terminal practice-focused degree in nursing (AACN, 2004). Since its inception, the DNP degree has been met with both support and criticism (Burman, Hart, & McCabe, 2005; Chase & Pruitt, 2006; Dracup & Bryan-Brown, 2005; Hathaway, Jacob, Stegbauer, Thompson, & Graff, 2006). Despite the controversy associated with this innovative degree, approximately 184 DNP programs exist, with over 100 more currently in development (AACN, 2012). Because of the recommendations of the AACN (2004), as well as the growth in programs devoted to awarding this degree, it is necessary that graduate nursing students understand the definition and competencies of the DNP degree.

This chapter provides a definition of the DNP degree. This definition may be more easily understood from a historical perspective of nursing education; therefore, the history of doctoral education in nursing leading up to the development of the DNP degree is reviewed. The AACN's *Essentials of Doctoral Education for Advanced Nursing Practice* defines the competencies of the DNP degree (AACN, 2006a) and is also discussed. *Essential I, Scientific Underpinnings for Practice,* is extensively explored, with particular attention being paid to philosophical inquiry regarding the nature of the discipline of nursing and nursing science. The chapter concludes with a description of this author's development of a middle-range theory to exemplify bridging theory with practice.

## Overview of the Doctor of Nursing Practice Degree

The DNP degree is defined as a practice-focused, terminal degree in nursing practice (AACN, 2004). Nursing practice is defined as follows:

> Any form of nursing intervention that influences healthcare outcomes for individuals or populations, including the direct care of individual patients, management of care for individuals and populations, administration of nursing and healthcare organizations, and the development and implementation of health policy. (AACN, 2004, p. 1)

Historically, nursing has been concerned with care of the individual. This more contemporary definition accurately describes care that focuses on the healthcare outcomes of populations from an organizational perspective, as well as nursing's impact on healthcare policy (Chism, 2013). These themes remain consistent throughout the competencies of DNP curricula as well and are reflected in *Essentials of Doctoral Education for Advanced Nursing Practice* (see **Table 3–1**).

It should be noted that the DNP degree differs from the traditional PhD in both focus and content (see **Table 3–2**). The DNP degree is a *practice-focused degree*, whereas the doctor of philosophy (PhD) is a *research-focused* degree. Both degrees share a common goal regarding a "scholarly approach to the discipline and commitment to the advancement of the profession" (AACN, 2006a, p. 3). However, the DNP degree emphasizes practice, while the PhD degree emphasizes theory and research methodology (AACN, 2004, 2006a). The DNP graduate is expected to demonstrate scholarly activity through a theory-driven research project, often termed a capstone project. This project may be guided by middle-range

**TABLE 3–1    AACN's *Essentials of Doctoral Education for Advanced Nursing Practice***

| | |
|---|---|
| Essential I | Scientific Underpinnings for Practice |
| Essential II | Organizational and Systems Leadership for Quality Improvement and Systems Thinking |
| Essential III | Clinical Scholarship and Analytical Methods for Evidenced-Based Practice |
| Essential IV | Information Systems/Technology and Patient Care Technology for the Improvement and Transformation of Health Care |
| Essential V | Healthcare Policy for Advocacy in Health Care |
| Essential VI | Interprofessional Collaboration for Improving Patient and Population Health Outcomes |
| Essential VII | Clinical Prevention and Population Health for Improving the Nation's Health |
| Essential VIII | Advanced Nursing Practice |

*Source:* American Association of Colleges of Nursing (AACN). (2006a). Essentials of doctoral education for advanced nursing practice. Reprinted by permission of American Association of Colleges of Nursing.

**TABLE 3-2    Key Differences Between DNP and PhD/DNS/DNSc Programs**

|  | DNP | PhD/DNS/DNSc |
|---|---|---|
| Program of study | **Objectives**<br>Prepare nurse specialists at the highest level of advanced practice | **Objectives**<br>Prepare nurse researchers |
|  | **Competencies**<br>Based on AACN essentials of the DNP degree | **Content**<br>Based on indicators of quality in research-focused doctoral programs in nursing (AACN, 2001) |
| Students | Commitment to a practice career | Commitment to a research career |
|  | Oriented toward improving outcomes of care | Oriented toward developing new knowledge |
| Program faculty | Practice doctorate and/or experience in the area in which teaching | Research doctorate in nursing or a related field |
|  | Leadership experience in the area of specialty practice | Leadership experience in the area of sustained research funding |
|  | High level of expertise in specialty practice congruent with the focus of the academic program | High level of expertise in research congruent with the focus of the academic program |
| Resources | Mentors/preceptors in leadership positions across a variety of practice settings | Mentors/preceptors in research settings |
|  | Access to diverse practice settings with appropriate resources for areas of practice | Access to research settings with appropriate resources |
|  | Access to financial aid | Access to dissertation support dollars |
|  | Access to information and patient care technology resources congruent with the areas of study | Access to information and research technology resources congruent with the program of research |

*(Continues)*

TABLE 3-2    **Key Differences Between DNP and PhD/DNS/DNSc Programs** (*Continued*)

| | DNP | PhD/DNS/DNSc |
|---|---|---|
| Program assessment and evaluation | **Program Outcome** Healthcare improvements and contributions via practice, policy change, and practice scholarship | **Program Outcome** Contributes to healthcare improvements via the development of new knowledge and other scholarly projects that provide the foundation for the advancement of nursing science |
| | Oversight by the institution's authorized bodies (i.e., graduate school) and regional accreditors Receives accreditation from a specialized nursing accreditor Graduates are eligible for the national certification exam | Oversight by the institution's authorized bodies (i.e., graduate school) and regional accreditors |

*Source:* AACN DNP Roadmap Taskforce Report, October 20, 2006 (b). Reprinted by permission of American Association of Colleges of Nursing.

nursing theory and demonstrate ways in which research affects practice. Middle-range nursing theory and the DNP degree are discussed later in this chapter.

## Historical Perspectives

Doctoral education in nursing has, indeed, evolved over the past 40 years. In the 1960s, nurses' choices for doctoral education included a PhD in the basic sciences such as biology, anatomy, or physiology or an education doctorate (EdD; Carpenter & Hudacek, 1996; Marriner-Tomey, 1990). As doctoral education in nursing evolved, more nursing-related doctoral degrees emerged.

The first nursing-related doctorate degree originated at Teacher's College, Columbia University, in 1924. This degree was an EdD that was designed to prepare nurses to teach at the college level. It was unique in that it was the first doctoral degree in nursing to emphasize both nursing education and the needs of the profession (Carpenter & Hudacek, 1996). Later, in 1934, the first PhD in nursing was offered at New York University, followed by introduction of a maternal–child nursing PhD program in the 1950s at the University of Pittsburgh (Carpenter & Hudacek, 1996). Importantly, the latter PhD program was the first to recognize the importance of clinical research for the development of the discipline of nursing (Carpenter & Hudacek, 1996). Throughout the United States, other PhDs continued to focus on sociological fields such as psychology, sociology, and anthropology. Actual nursing PhDs did not become popular until the 1970s (Grace, 1978).

According to Murphy (1981), doctoral education in nursing developed in three phases. The focus of these phases included nursing doctorates that emphasized the development of (1) functional specialists, (2) nurse scientists, and (3) doctorates that were "in and of nursing" (p. 646). The first phase, which emphasized the development of functional specialists, focused on preparing nurses as teachers or administrators. Throughout the second phase—the development of nurse scientists—relevant questions emerged that directly affected the third and final phase of nursing doctoral education:

- What is the essential nature of professional nursing?
- What is the substantive knowledge base of professional nursing?
- What kind of research is important for nursing? As a knowledge discipline? As a field of practice?
- How can the scientific base of nursing knowledge be identified and expanded? (p. 646)

These questions led to the development of nursing doctorates that were "in and of nursing" (p. 646), and they continue to influence nursing doctoral education today.

More recently, a fourth phase of doctoral education in nursing has evolved. This phase emphasizes nursing practice and initially began with the development of the Doctor of Nursing Science (DNS). The first DNS degree was developed at Boston University and "focused on the development of nursing theory for a practice discipline" (Marriner-Tomey, 1990, p. 135). The DNS was perceived as the first practice-focused doctorate. Cleland (1976) noted that the research doctorate should focus on contributions to nursing science and the practice doctorate should focus on expertise in clinical practice. Grace (1978) suggested that nurses be prepared as "social engineers," with attention being given to the clinical field (p. 26). Finally, Newman (1975) indicated that a practice doctorate would prepare nurses as "professional practitioners" for entry into practice (p. 705).

Although the DNS was developed to prepare nurses as practice experts, over time curricula in these programs began to resemble the PhD in nursing (AACN, 2006b; Apold, 2008; Marriner-Tomey, 1990). Given this development, the AACN has designated all DNS degrees as research-focused degrees (AACN, 2004). Hence, the challenge to develop a true practice doctorate remained.

Rozella Schlottfeldt pioneered the development of a Doctorate of Nursing (ND) degree in 1979 at Case Western Reserve University in Cleveland, Ohio. Schlottfeldt posited that nursing needed a practice doctorate to address several needs of nursing education:

- The need to reorient the existing system of health care toward services that enhance the health status of all people, while maintaining the existing services that focus primarily on detection and treatment of disease

- The need to reorient the nursing community in ways to hasten the emergence of nursing as a scholarly discipline and a fully autonomous practice profession
- The need to reorient nursing's approach to preparing professionals with a view toward promptly augmenting the cadre of competent, independent, accountable nursing practitioners (Schlottfeldt, 1978, p. 302)

Unfortunately, ND programs did not have the same popularity as DNS or PhD degrees. It was also noted that the curricula for these programs lacked the uniformity needed to establish their credibility as practice doctorate programs (Marion et al., 2003). Interestingly, the needs outlined by Schlottfeldt are reflected in the curricula of present DNP programs.

## Development of the Doctor of Nursing Practice

In 2002, a task force was formed by the AACN to evaluate the current status of practice doctorates in nursing. The task force was charged with developing recommendations for a practice doctorate in nursing, as well as proposing practice doctorate curriculum models. This work led to the development of the AACN's *Position Statement on the Practice Doctorate in Nursing,* which was published in 2004. The position statement recommended that the DNP degree become the terminal practice-focused degree for nursing by 2015 (AACN, 2004).

The University of Kentucky's School of Nursing was the first to admit students to this program in 2001. Dr. Carolyn Williams, President of AACN (2000–2002) and Dean Emeritus of the University of Kentucky's School of Nursing, was an early proponent of the practice doctorate in nursing and, along with others, helped to facilitate the development of the DNP degree. Currently, more than 184 DNP programs exist in the United States, with more than 100 in development (AACN, 2012).

## Doctor of Nursing Practice Competencies

In 2006, the AACN developed the *Essentials of Doctoral Education for Advanced Nursing Practice.* The *Essentials* "address the foundational competencies that are core to all advanced nursing practice roles" (AACN, 2006a, p. 8). Also in 2006, the National Organization of Nurse Practitioner Faculties developed the *Practice Doctorate Nurse Practitioner Entry-Level Competencies,* and in 2008, the National Association of Clinical Nurse Specialists developed the *Core Practice Doctorate Clinical Nurse Specialist Competencies.* Together, these documents provide the curriculum standards for all DNP programs. The following is a summary of the *Essentials of Doctoral Education for Advanced Nursing Practice.*

### Essential I: Scientific Underpinnings for Practice

*Essential I* describes the scientific foundations for nursing practice. These scientific foundations are derived from the natural and social sciences and may include human biology, physiology, and psychology. This foundation also includes nursing science, which adds to the discipline of nursing. Within the discipline of nursing, specific nursing middle-range theories that guide practice are also part of the foundation for nursing practice (AACN, 2006a). *Essential I* provides the scientific basis necessary for advanced nursing practice. Because of the importance of understanding the foundations for nursing practice, *Essential I* will be discussed in more depth later in this chapter.

## Essential II: Organizational and Systems Leadership for Quality Improvement and Systems Thinking

*Essential II* describes preparation in organizational and systems leadership that affects subsequent healthcare delivery and patient care outcomes. Preparation in this area provides DNP graduates with expertise in "assessing organizations, identifying systems' issues, and facilitating organization-wide changes in practice delivery" (AACN, 2006a, p. 10). The DNP graduate is prepared to assume roles in leadership at every level, from informal leadership in the clinical setting to more formal leadership at an executive level (Chism, 2013).

## Essential III: Clinical Scholarship and Analytical Methods for Evidence-Based Practice

*Essential III* describes competencies related to the evaluation, integration, translation, and application of evidence-based practice. DNP graduates are unique in that their practice perspective allows them to merge nursing science, practice, human needs, and human caring (AACN, 2006a). Additionally, because of their practice perspective, DNP graduates are well positioned to apply research to practice, as well as to ask pertinent questions related to practice (Chism, 2013). Potential roles related to *Essential III* include partnering with research colleges and participating in clinical research, evaluating and developing practice guidelines, critically evaluating existing literature to determine best practices, and designing and evaluating methodologies that improve patient care (AACN, 2006a).

## Essential IV: Information Systems/Technology and Patient Care Technology for the Improvement and Transformation of Health Care

*Essential IV* prepares the DNP graduate to use information technologies in ways that improve patient care outcomes. Additionally, DNP graduates develop expertise in information technologies to support leadership and clinical decision making. Examples of information technologies important for improvement of healthcare outcomes include web-based communications, online documentation, telemedicine, and data mining. DNP graduates may employ their expertise in information technologies when evaluating programs for online documentation or data from large systems or databases as part of a search for practice outcome patterns. Graduates may also use information technologies to communicate and evaluate the accuracy, timeliness, and appropriateness of healthcare consumer information (AACN, 2006a). Finally, DNP graduates have a role in attending to the ethical and legal issues related to information technologies (AACN, 2006a).

### Essential V: Healthcare Policy for Advocacy in Health Care

*Essential V* describes the importance of nurses' involvement in healthcare policy and advocacy. As leaders in the practice setting, it is imperative that DNP graduates understand the relationship between practice and policy. Such graduates may be called on to analyze health policies and proposals from multiple points of view; provide leadership in the development of healthcare policies on different levels; actively participate on committees, boards, or task forces; and act as advocates for the nursing profession through organizational leadership (AACN, 2006a).

### Essential VI: Interprofessional Collaboration for Improving Patient and Population Health Outcomes

*Essential VI* prepares the DNP graduate to understand the importance of interprofessional collaboration within a multitiered healthcare environment. Nurses frequently function as collaborators with members of other professions. This essential skill expands on the collaboration that naturally occurs among professionals by ensuring that DNP graduates will develop the expertise needed to assume leadership roles when collaborating with teams, as well as participate in the work of the team. Graduates must also be prepared to act as consultants during times of change (AACN, 2006a).

### Essential VII: Clinical Prevention and Population Health for Improving the Nation's Health

*Essential VII* prepares DNP graduates to "analyze epidemiological, biostatistical, occupational, and environmental data in the development, implementation, and evaluation of clinical prevention and population health" (AACN, 2006a, p. 15). Nursing has traditionally been involved in health promotion and risk reduction/illness prevention. The DNP graduate is prepared to assume roles that improve health promotion and reduce risk from an advanced nursing practice perspective.

### Essential VIII: Advanced Nursing Practice

*Essential VIII* describes the clinical specialization content from a specific domain of advanced nursing practice. Post-baccalaureate DNP degree programs "provide preparation within distinct specialties that require expertise, advanced nursing knowledge, and mastery in one area of nursing practice" (AACN, 2006a, p. 16). The DNP graduate is prepared to develop therapeutic relationships with patients and other healthcare professionals to improve patient outcomes, assess health and illness parameters, utilize advanced clinical decision-making skills and critical thinking, serve as mentor to others in the nursing profession, and educate patients (AACN, 2006a).

## Focus on *Essential I: Scientific Underpinnings for Practice*

The scientific underpinnings of practice provide the basis of knowledge for advanced nursing practice. These scientific underpinnings include sciences such as biology, physiology, psychology, ethics, and nursing. Although the basic sciences are often accepted as the basis of knowledge for nursing practice, the role of nursing science may not be as readily understood. Nursing science has expanded the discipline of nursing to include the development of middle-range nursing theories and concepts to guide practice (AACN, 2006b). Graduates of DNP programs have a pertinent role in the implementation of middle-range nursing theories to guide nursing practice. Hence, understanding the scientific underpinnings for nursing practice is essential for all DNP graduates.

## Basic Sciences

It is often accepted that advanced nursing practice borrows from the social and basic sciences—much as medicine does—to build a scientific basis for practice. These sciences frequently include biology, physiology, psychology, and ethics. According to Webber (2008), nurse practitioners "rely on medical research to support their practice because not enough advanced practice research and researchers exist" (p. 466). Concerns have been raised that advanced nursing practitioners "adopt the practice values of medicine rather than identifying and adopting knowledge, skills, values, meanings and experiences unique to this nursing specialty" (p. 466). This point may be well taken; however, without the basic understanding of disease, how will nursing develop an understanding of the human responses to disease? Gortner (1980) noted this paradox also and suggested that if nursing rejects the medical model, it rejects the body of knowledge that describes and explains the pathology that leads patients to nurses' care. Through development of an understanding of the fundamentals of the sciences that predict and explain disease processes, nursing can build a basis for understanding how best to care for those affected by disease. Donaldson and Crowley (1978) described professional disciplines such as nursing as "emerging *along with* rather than *from* academic disciplines" (p. 116).

## The Discipline of Nursing

A discipline is characterized by a "unique perspective, a distinct way of viewing all phenomena, which ultimately defines the limits and nature of its inquiry" (Donaldson & Crowley, 1978, p. 113). The discipline of nursing has been defined as the body of knowledge concerned with the following aspects of care:

- The principles and laws that govern all life processes, well-being, and optimal functioning of human beings, sick or well
- The patterning of human behavior in interaction with the environment in normal life events and critical life situations
- The processes by which positive changes in health status are effected
- The wholeness of health of human beings, recognizing that they are in continuous interaction with their environments (adapted from AACN, 2006a; Donaldson & Crowley, 1978; Fawcett, 2005; Gortner, 1980)

Nursing is concerned "with the whole human, with lifestyles and with health behavior" (Gortner, 1980, p. 181) and looks beyond the biological and physiological perspectives on disease. In doing so, nursing seeks to explain and predict responses to therapy, improvement in health status, and wellness (Gortner, 1980).

## Nursing Science

The definition of nursing science may be somewhat more difficult to elucidate. Nursing science has been described as both a body of theoretical knowledge and the methods of reproducible modes of inquiry (Gortner, 1980; Jacobs & Huether, 1978; Jacox, 1974). Gortner (1980) defined it as "the base of knowledge underlying human behavior and social interaction under normal and stressful conditions across the lifespan" (p. 180). Interestingly, Jacobs and Huether (1978) defined nursing science as "the process, and the result, of ordering and patterning the events and phenomena of concern to nursing" (p. 65). Thus nursing science may be understood as both the "methods of inquiry specific to the discipline of nursing—the process—as well as the outcomes of that inquiry—the result" (Jacobs & Huether, 1978, p. 65). Nursing research has been differentiated from nursing science as "the systematic inquiry into problems associated with illness, health, and care" (Gortner, 1980, p. 180).

## Nursing Theory

Nursing theory has been described as the product of nursing science (Jacobs & Huether, 1978; Kerlinger, 1973). Specifically, Jacobs and Huether (1978) described the dual purposes of nursing science as "to define common goals and guide the practice of nursing" (p. 64)—hence, the development of nursing theory. A *theory* is defined as a relationship between two or more concepts, whereas the term *concept* describes objects, properties, or events, and indicates the subject matter of the theory (Jacox, 1974). The concepts within a theory are related by propositions that describe the relationships between two or more concepts (Jacox, 1974). In essence, then, nursing theory attempts to describe, predict, or explain phenomena consistent with nursing's perspective (Donaldson & Crowley, 1978).

## Middle-Range Theory

Nursing's body of knowledge, or discipline, includes both grand and middle-range theories (Fawcett, 2005). Grand theories are more abstract and are broader in type, whereas middle-range theories are more concrete and are narrower in type (Fawcett, 2005). For this reason, middle-range theories are more applicable to clinical practice (Lenz, 1998). Further, clinicians may use middle-range theory "situationally," or to help "direct their assessment, decision-making, and nursing interventions when cued by a particular kind of situation rather than practicing consistently according to the tenets of a given theory" (Lenz, 1998, p. 63).

## Doctor of Nursing Practice Graduates and Nursing Theory

Nursing has traditionally struggled to close the theory–practice gap (i.e., the lack of use of theory in practice or the inability of nurses to use theory in practice; Kenney, 2006). Reasons for this shortcoming include lack of knowledge, understanding, belief, or applicability of nursing theory as a guide for practice (McKenna, 1997).

Further, the use of medical knowledge, especially in advanced practice nursing roles, has prevailed as a guide for nursing practice (Meleis, 1993).

Because of the limited, narrower, and more applicable scope of middle-range theories, the understanding and application of such theories may be vital to closing the theory–practice gap. As a practice discipline, when nursing theories prove useful in the real world and are "logical and consistent with other validated theories, they may provide a rationale for nursing actions that lead to predictable client outcomes" (Kenney, 2006, p. 297). For this reason, DNP graduates must have an understanding of middle-range theories, as well as the skills necessary to apply those theories in practice.

In a book chapter entitled "Expectations for Theory, Research, and Scholarship," Magnan (2013) suggested that it was more important for DNP students to acquire the skills needed to apply theory to practice than to simply be exposed to a number of middle-range theories. Further, Magnan noted that these skills should be "transferable" and apply to the application of other middle-range theories to practice (p. 110). To achieve this goal, DNP students will need to meet the following criteria:

- Have a foundation in the language of theory (e.g., concepts, relational statements)
- Learn how to distinguish modifiable from nonmodifiable predictors and understand the meaning they have for planning theory-based interventions
- Understand how to interpret the research literature to determine the level of empirical support for relationships between theoretical concepts (Magnan, 2013, pp. 110–111)

As experts in the application of theory, and specifically in middle-range theory, DNP graduates are well positioned to close the theory–practice gap (Magnan, 2013). Such nurses are practice experts who combine their clinical expertise with a doctoral-level understanding of nursing science and theory. This combination prepares the DNP graduate to clearly articulate for others the importance of theory in practice. DNP graduates are ideal role models to increase the use and understanding of theory-guided practice.

## Doctor of Nursing Practice Graduates and Use of Other Theories

*Essential I* of the AACN's *Essentials of Doctoral Education for Advanced Nursing Practice* clearly recommends that DNP graduates garner an understanding of the scientific underpinnings of nursing practice (AACN, 2006a). It is well understood that these scientific underpinnings include other sciences such as biology, physiology, psychology, and ethics. *Essential I* reaffirms the notion that DNP graduates must apply other middle-range theories to practice in an effort to provide patient-centered care. As Meleis (1997) noted, because nurses study many disciplines as a foundation for practice, nursing theory tends to reflect a broad range of perspectives and premises.

Donaldson and Crowley (1978) asserted that nursing is—importantly—a practice-oriented discipline. In a book chapter entitled "Nursing Science for Nursing Practice," Donaldson (1995) thoughtfully emphasized the point that nursing practice, as well as society's need for nursing services, has shaped the discipline of nursing. Because of nursing's interest in societal needs and desired patient outcomes, the discipline of nursing may include many theories, and the most appropriate theory selection will depend on the patient or societal situation. Donaldson (1995) described the nurse pragmatist as a nurse who will use the most pragmatic theory to accomplish the desired patient outcome. Further, nursing science will be a source of theory to the nurse pragmatist only if that theory "fits" the desired patient outcome (Donaldson, 1995).

DNP graduates, therefore, not only have a responsibility to exemplify the application of nursing theory to practice, but they must also be "nurse pragmatists" (Donaldson, 1995) and apply various theories from other sciences to practice. The role of the DNP graduate in theory evaluation and selection may well be one of the most valuable roles that such a person fills. Hence, DNP graduates become the knowledge appliers and exhibit expertise in evaluating, applying, and supporting theory-based interventions to ensure patient-centered care.

## Dilution of the Discipline of Nursing: Philosophical Considerations for Doctor of Nursing Practice Graduates

Although applying and integrating theories from various disciplines may add to the knowledge base considered to be part of the discipline of nursing, some practitioners have expressed concerns that this trend dilutes the discipline of nursing (Cody, 1996; McKenna, 1997). McKenna (1997) expressed concerns that combining other theories with nursing theories compromises the context of the original nursing concepts. Additionally, if theories are constantly borrowed and incorporated into the discipline, it may become difficult to differentiate nursing as its own discipline (Cody, 1996). Johnson (1968) pointedly discussed this dilemma, stating that if nursing "continues to observe behavior from the perspective of the sciences such as sociology and psychology, if we continue to study disease with the aim of elucidating etiologies, properties, or life cycles, . . . we may be serving the cause of science, but not necessarily the cause of nursing" (Johnson, 1968, pp. 207–208).

The dilemma ensues upon reviewing *Essential I* of the AACN's *Essentials* document. DNP graduates are frequently advanced practice nurses. Many people who fill advanced practice nursing roles identify very closely with a medical model and may be viewed as "junior doctors" (Meleis, 1993). According to Fawcett (1997), nurses are often unaware of their discrete knowledge and instead glean fragmented information from a medical model. Moreover, DNP graduates are expected to understand the scientific underpinnings of practice, including the basic sciences—sciences that are traditionally associated with the medical model. An interesting question then arises: How do DNP graduates understand and contribute to the discipline of nursing through application of knowledge if this knowledge base has been infused with theories borrowed from other disciplines, specifically the basic sciences?

This dilemma may be resolved by DNP graduates developing a good understanding of nursing as a profession, a science, and a discipline. Nursing is a practice profession whose science and body of knowledge depend on its perspective. Further, if this understanding is developed, DNP graduates will integrate the necessary knowledge from a nursing perspective, understanding what nursing is and what it is not. While the basis of knowledge may include knowledge borrowed from various sciences to explain and predict disease, nursing is concerned with the laws and principles that govern the life processes, well-being, and optimal functioning of human beings; the human behavioral responses to disease; and the processes by which positive health status is effected (Donaldson & Crowley, 1978). The ability to elucidate what defines nursing practice, while employing various "pragmatic" (Donaldson, 1995, p. 6) scientific underpinnings from a nursing perspective, may be what truly differentiates the DNP-prepared nurse.

## Summary

The AACN recommended that the DNP degree become the terminal practice-focused degree for nursing by 2015 (AACN, 2004). Adoption of this recommendation has implications for the advancement of nursing as a profession, a science, and a discipline. Expanding their understanding of the scientific underpinnings for practice is perhaps the most essential expectation for DNP graduates. Through the process of gaining this understanding, DNP graduates will garner expertise in the differentiation and application of nursing knowledge. Moreover, as the practice experts and knowledge appliers, DNP graduates will be in an ideal position to bridge the theory–practice gap, an enduring ambition of nursing.

## Exemplar

The following discussion is a case scenario in which this author developed, tested, and applied a nursing middle-range theory, thereby bridging theory and practice.

> During my doctoral study at Oakland University in Rochester, Michigan, Dr. Morris Magnan charged the advanced theory class with writing a middle-range theory paper. I had only recently been introduced to middle-range theory and was struggling to develop an understanding of nursing as a science and a discipline. However, applying middle-range theory to an actual patient scenario helped me to develop a broader understanding of nursing.
>
> Dr. Magnan and I were having a telephone meeting one evening to discuss which middle-range theory I would use for my theory paper.

My research interest was spiritual care in nursing. I was drawn to Olson's empathic process theory (Olson, 1995) as the theoretical guide for my ideas. Dr. Magnan urged me to describe in more detail why I believed that this middle-range theory applied to spiritual care in nursing.

I explained that I had recently cared for a patient whose son had attempted suicide and was now in an intensive care unit (ICU) clinging to life. My patient was struggling with what to pray for: death or healing. She was disturbed also by how she was approached by a rabbi in the ICU who whispered to her in Hebrew and touched her knee when he spoke to her. She related, "Just because I am Jewish, it doesn't mean that I speak Hebrew. And furthermore, I don't want anybody whispering to me and touching me. I will pray in my own way and on my own terms." I replied to my patient, "So, you felt that instead of the rabbi asking you how you pray, or what your spiritual need was, he assumed what you needed and made you even more anxious." She immediately relaxed in the chair and exclaimed, "Yes! That's exactly how I feel." Her body language clearly exhibited an openness to further spiritual discussion. I added, "Why don't you pray for peace?" She agreed: "Yes, that's what I will pray for—peace."

I will never forget the night I shared this story with Dr. Magnan. When I had finished, he replied, "Well, I believe you have a middle-range theory here."

With Dr. Magnan's guidance, we developed my ideas into Chism's middle-range theory of spiritual empathy (MTSE; Chism, 2007). The MTSE was deductively derived from Olson's empathic process theory (1995; middle-range theory) and Orlando's dynamic nursing process theory (1990; grand theory). The MTSE purports that nurses' spiritual care perspectives—that is, nurses' attitudes and beliefs about spiritual care (Taylor, 2002)—will influence nurses' expression of spiritual empathy—that is, the nurse's expression of verbal understanding of a patient's spiritual concern (Chism, 2007; Chism & Magnan, 2009; Olson, 1995). Expression of spiritual empathy will then increase the patient's perception of empathy—patients feeling that they are understood by nurses (Olson, 1995). Spiritual distress—impairments in a sense of connectedness to self and others, faith and belief system, sense of purpose, inner peace, and inner strength (Villagomeza, 2005)—will then decrease. The final concept, spiritual well-being—a sense of inner peace and contentment resulting from one's perceived sense of connection to self or others (Chism, 2007)—is purported to increase at this point.

One portion of the MTSE was tested as my capstone project: the relationship between nurses' spiritual care perspectives and their expressions of spiritual empathy. The MTSE has been presented in two poster presentations, and findings from the theory testing study have been published (Chism & Magnan, 2009).

The development and testing of the MTSE during doctoral study in a DNP program was somewhat industrious and not a customary expectation of a DNP research project. This rewarding experience not only challenged me to develop my scholarship, but it also exemplified the use of theory (specifically, middle-range theory) to guide practice. As a DNP graduate and advanced practice nurse, I have a responsibility to understand, from a nursing perspective, the scientific underpinnings of disease processes and the care of my patients. Moreover, the development and testing of the MTSE reinforced for me the idea that the discipline of nursing truly guides nursing practice.

## Acknowledgment

*I would like to acknowledge Dr. Morris Magnan for his expert guidance and mentorship throughout my doctoral study and beyond. He is an exemplary nurse, scholar, mentor, and friend who continues to inspire me every day.*

## References

American Association of Colleges of Nursing. (2001). Indicators of quality in research-focused doctoral programs in nursing: AACN position statement updated 2001. Retrieved from http://www.aacn.nche.edu/publications/position/quality-indicators

American Association of Colleges of Nursing. (2004). AACN position statement on the practice doctorate in nursing. Retrieved from http://www.aacn.nche.edu/publications/position/DNPpositionstatement.pdf

American Association of Colleges of Nursing. (2006a). Essentials of doctoral education for advanced nursing practice. Retrieved from http://www.aacn.nche.edu/publications/position/DNPEssentials.pdf

American Association of Colleges of Nursing. (2006b). Doctor of Nursing Practice Roadmap Taskforce report. Retrieved from http://www.aacn.nche.edu/dnp/roadmapreport.pdf

American Association of Colleges of Nursing. (2012). DNP program list. Retrieved from http://www.aacn.nche.edu/dnp/program-schools

Apold, S. (2008). The doctor of nursing practice: Looking back, moving forward. *Journal for Nurse Practitioners, 4*(2), 101–106.

Burman, M., Hart, A., & McCabe, S. (2005). Doctor of nursing practice: Opportunity amidst chaos. *American Journal of Critical Care, 14*(6), 463–464.

Carpenter, R., & Hudacek, S. (1996). *On doctoral education in nursing: The voice of the student.* New York, NY: National League for Nursing Press.

Chase, S., & Pruitt, R. (2006). The practice doctorate: Innovation or disruption? *Journal of Nursing Education, 45*(5), 155–161.

Chism, L. (2007). *Spiritual empathy: A model for spiritual well-being.* Unpublished doctoral paper. Oakland University, Rochester, MI.

Chism, L. (2013). *The doctor of nursing practice: A guidebook for role development and professional issues* (2nd ed.). Burlington, MA: Jones & Bartlett Learning.

Chism, L., & Magnan, M. H. (2009). The relationship between student nurses' spiritual care perspectives and their expressions of spiritual empathy. *Journal of Nursing Education, 48*(11), 597–604.

Cleland, V. (1976). Develop a doctoral program. *Nursing Outlook, 24,* 631–635.

Cody, W. K. (1996). Drowning in eclecticism. *Nursing Science Quarterly, 9*(3), 86–88.

Donaldson, S. K. (1995). Nursing science for nursing practice. In A. Omery, C. E. Kasper, & G. G. Page (Eds.), *In search of nursing science* (pp. 3–12). Thousand Oaks, CA: Sage.

Donaldson, S. K., & Crowley, D. M. (1978). The discipline of nursing. *Nursing Outlook, 26*(2), 113–120.

Dracup, K., & Bryan-Brown, C. (2005). Doctor of nursing practice: MRI or total body scan? *American Journal of Critical Care, 14*(4), 278–281.

Fawcett, J. (1997). Conceptual models of nursing, nursing theories, and nursing practice: Focus on the future. In M. R. Alligood & A. Marriner-Tomey (Eds.), *Nursing theory: Utilization and application* (pp. 211–221). St. Louis, MO: Mosby.

Fawcett, J. (2005). *Contemporary nursing knowledge: Analysis and evaluation of nursing models and theories* (2nd ed.). Philadelphia, PA: F. A. Davis.

Gortner, S. (1980). Nursing science in transition. *Nursing Research, 29,* 180–183.

Grace, H. (1978). The development of doctoral education in nursing: In historical perspective. *Journal of Nursing Education, 17*(4), 17–27.

Hathaway, D., Jacob, S., Stegbauer, C., Thompson, C., & Graff, C. (2006). The practice doctorate: Perspectives of early adopters. *Journal of Nursing Education, 45*(12), 487–496.

Jacobs, M. K., & Huether, S. E. (1978). Nursing science: The theory–practice linkage. *Advances in Nursing Science, 1*(1), 63–73.

Jacox, A. K. (1974). Theory construction in nursing. *Nursing Research, 23*(1), 4–13.

Johnson, D. E. (1968). Theory in nursing: Borrowed and unique. *Nursing Research, 17*(3), 206–209.

Kenney, J. W. (2006). Theory-based advanced nursing practice. In W. K. Cody (Ed.), *Philosophical and theoretical perspectives for advanced nursing practice* (pp. 295–310). Sudbury, MA: Jones and Bartlett.

Kerlinger, F. N. (1973). *Foundations of behavioral research* (2nd ed.). New York, NY: Holt Rinehart & Winston.

Lenz, E. R. (1998). The role of middle-range theory for nursing research and practice: Part 2. Nursing practice. *Nursing Leadership Forum, 3*(2), 62–66.

Magnan, M. (2013). Expectations for theory, research, and scholarship. In L. Chism (Ed.), *The doctor of nursing practice: A guidebook for role development and professional issues* (2nd ed., pp. 107–140). Burlington, MA: Jones & Bartlett Learning.

Marion, L., Viens, D., O'Sullivan, A., Crabtree, M. K., Fontana, S., & Price, M. (2003). The practice doctorate in nursing: Future or fringe. *Topics in Advanced Practice Nursing eJournal, 3*(2). Retrieved from http://www.medscape.com/viewarticle/453247_print

Marriner-Tomey, A. (1990). Historical development of doctoral programs from the Middle Ages to nursing education today. *Nursing and Health Care, 3*(11), 132–137. Washington, DC: National Academies Press.

McKenna, H. (1997). Applying theories in practice. In H. McKenna (Ed.), *Nursing theories and models* (pp. 158–189). New York, NY: Routledge.

Meleis, A. I. (1993). Nursing research and the Neuman model: Directions for the future. Panel discussion conducted at the Fourth Biennial International Neuman Systems Model Symposium, Rochester, NY.

Meleis, A. I. (1997). *Theoretical nursing: Development and progress* (3rd ed.). Philadelphia, PA: Lippincott.

Murphy, J. (1981). Doctoral education in, of, and for nursing: An historical analysis. *Nursing Outlook, 29*(11), 645–649.

National Association of Clinical Nurse Specialists. (2008). Clinical Nurse Specialist core competencies. Retrieved from http://www.nacns.org/docs/CNSCoreCompetenciesBroch.pdf

National Organization of Nurse Practitioner Faculties. (2006). Practice doctorate nurse practitioner entry-level competencies. Retrieved from http://www.nonpf.com/associations/10789/files/DNP%20NP%20competenciesApril2006.pdf

Newman, M. (1975). The professional doctorate in nursing: A position paper. *Nursing Outlook, 23*(11), 704–706.

Olson, J. (1995). Relationship between nurse-expressed empathy, patient-perceived empathy, and patient distress. *Image: Journal of Nursing Scholarship, 27*(4), 317–322.

Orlando, I. (1990). *The dynamic nurse–patient relationship*. New York, NY: National League for Nursing.

Schlottfeldt, R. (1978, May). The professional doctorate: Rationale and characteristics. *Nursing Outlook,* 302–311.

Taylor, E. (2002). *Spiritual care: Nursing theory, research, and practice*. Upper Saddle River, NJ: Prentice Hall.

Villagomeza, L. (2005). Spiritual distress in adult cancer patients. *Holistic Nursing Practice, 19*(6), 285–294.

Webber, P. B. (2008). The doctor of nursing practice degree and research: Are we making an epistemological mistake? *Journal of Nursing Education, 47*(10), 466–472.

# PART 2

# The Structure and Function of Theory

# Theory as Practice

*Patricia Goodson*

## Defining Theory

People have a hard time understanding precisely what a theory is, what exactly it can do to guide research, and how to know which theory to use. Difficulties often begin when attempting to define theory, because uncovering a simple explanation is difficult. Scholars' conceptualizations and explanations are often abstract, convoluted, and complex. Actually, the question "What is theory?" can be an unimaginative question: on the one hand, presupposing simplistic, reduced accounts of a seemingly rich phenomenon, and on the other hand, offering abstract, complicated, and unintelligible answers. The impulse is to fill in the blank in "Theory is _____" with a quick, concise, one-sentence description. However, such concise and short definitions may render theory meaningless, lifeless, confusing, and dry.

A friend of mine enjoys reminding me that "Theory is not rocket science; it's much more complicated than rocket science." If this holds true, then it does not seem logical to define theory as one single, simple entity. As I came to understand late in my studies, theory is multifaceted and amazingly complex. To reduce it to a one-dimensional phenomenon would come close to mutilation. Theory's beauty lies precisely in its dynamic and intricate complexity (Hoffmann, 2003). Brief definitions never do it justice. If simply asking "What is theory?" leads nowhere interesting, then it may be more productive to ask a different set of interconnected questions:

- What does theory do?
- What does theory—in action—look like?

- How can one recognize theory?
- What does theory do that is uniquely "theory-*ish*"?

This chapter, which is primarily approached from a health promotion perspective, focuses on the first two questions: "What does theory do?" and "When theory is doing its 'thing,' what does it look like?" Put in simple terms, theories have at least two faces or may be found in two different varieties: *commonsense theories* and *scientific theories*. These familiar categories are covered in this chapter.

## Commonsense Theories

Commonsense theories comprise explanations that people invoke on a daily basis to make sense of their lives. Suppose, in the past couple of weeks, Laura's behavior seems a little "off." She arrives late for team meetings and appears distant and broody when the team interacts. Laura is a graduate assistant and doctoral student. As her teacher, I do have a theory (or a proposed explanation) for Laura's behavior: Laura has been under considerable stress lately, taking her comprehensive exams, finalizing a manuscript to submit for publication, and teaching two freshman-level classes.

My theory is a commonsense theory because it represents a personal attempt to make meaning of a situation (a sense-making task), based on the information at hand. I may choose to test this theory of mine, for instance, by asking Laura if what I'm thinking is valid or by asking some of her colleagues about what is happening, but such testing will not go far. As soon as I understand what is going on or as soon as Laura's behavior returns to "normal," I will forget my little theory and the need to test it and will gladly move on to the next problem.

Another good example of a commonsense theory is conspiracy theory. People can certainly recognize a conspiracy theory when they see or hear about one. Such a theory tends to grab one's imagination. Conspiracy theories combine challenging questions with sometimes outlandish answers, attempting to explain why something happened. An example is President John F. Kennedy's assassination: Many explanations have been proposed to make sense of the bizarre events that ended the president's life. Among these explanations, a handful of conspiracy theories have emerged. These theories started by zeroing in on the questions that were dismissed or brushed aside by the mainstream official reports because they (the questions) were unthinkable, outrageous, or too far-fetched. The theory proposing that President Kennedy and Governor John Connally were not struck by a single bullet is only one example of the many conspiracy theories that sprang up after the event (Kurtz, 2006).

Frequently, unique perspectives or approaches are followed, and unusual solutions to difficult problems are sometimes found because of these conspiracy-type accounts. More often, conspiracy theories are unsupported by available evidence and, with time, become tales and myths that societies' members enjoy telling and retelling. Underlying both commonsense and conspiracy theories is a shared element: an attempt to make sense of reality, to explain events and circumstances so that humans can function in a world, in a reality, in a place furnished with meaning.

## Scientific Theories

From the outset, scientific theories look different from commonsense theories. Definitions of scientific theories are much more elaborate, contain more clearly outlined characteristics, and have better defined purposes when compared with definitions of commonsense theories. The following are examples of these definitions as they appear, specifically, in the social sciences. In the now classic textbook on health behavior theories, *Health Behavior and Health Education*, for instance, *theory* is defined as "a set of interrelated concepts, definitions, and propositions that present a *systematic* view of events or situations by specifying relations among variables, in order to *explain and predict* the events or situations" (Glanz, Rimer, & Viswanath, 2008, p. 26).

Another elaborate, yet a bit clearer, definition of social science theory was proposed by Denzin (1970):

> A theory is a set of propositions that furnish an explanation by means of a deductive system. *Theory is explanation.* Durkheim's theory of suicide in Spain conforms to the above specifications. . . . It states that: (1) In any social grouping, the suicide rate varies directly with the degree of individualism (egoism); (2) the degree of individualism varies with the incidence of Protestantism; (3) therefore, the suicide rate varies with the incidence of Protestantism; (4) the incidence of Protestantism in Spain is low; (5) therefore, the suicide rate in Spain is low. (p. 34, emphasis added)

Other definitions provide additional details regarding scientific theory's main elements:

> A theory is a set of interrelated universal statements, some of which are definitions and some of which are relationships assumed to be true, together with a syntax, a set of rules for manipulating the statements to arrive at new statements. (Cohen, 1980, p. 171)
>
> Theory is a mental activity. . . . It is a process of developing ideas that can allow us to explain how and why events occur. Theory is constructed with several basic elements or building blocks: (1) concepts, (2) variables, (3) statements, and (4) formats. (Turner, 1986, pp. 4–5)
>
> Behavioral theories are composed of interrelated propositions, based on stated assumptions that tie selected constructs together and create a parsimonious system for explaining and predicting human behavior. (DiClemente, Crosby, & Kegler, 2002, p. 3)

When examined further, these definitions also refer to scientific theories' three main goals, purposes, or functions:

- *Description.* Theories should facilitate the description (and understanding) of the phenomena being studied. The scientist/social scientist must be able to "describe the phenomenon he [sic] is studying so that others can repeat his descriptions with a high degree of agreement" (Denzin, 1970, p. 31).
- *Explanation.* Scientific theories allow "the construction of a system of interrelated propositions that permits the scientist to 'make sense' out of the events observed" (Denzin, 1970, p. 31).
- *Prediction.* The utility of scientific theories extends beyond mere description and explanation, however. "If a [scientist/social scientist] claims to have explained why a given set of variables occurs together, he must be able to predict the future relationships" (Denzin, 1970, p. 31).

This, in simple terms, is how scientific theories are often defined and characterized. Scientific theories explain phenomena in a logical, ordered, interconnected manner. Like commonsense theories, scientific theories represent attempts to make sense of reality through descriptions, explanations, and predictions of events and circumstances.

The definition proposed by Turner (1986, p. 4) places theory in the world of words or ideas (a mental activity), highlighting the power of language to create and shape human reality. Cohen's (1980, p. 171) proposition also includes an important characteristic of scientific theories. To earn the status of being scientific, theoretical explanations need to go together, connect according to specific rules, and follow a unique grammar. Denzin (1970) called this set of rules, or this grammar, a deductive system. Explanations of cause and effect, by themselves, do not constitute a theory: They are merely explanations. What lends these explanations the status of theory is the manner in which the explanations are connected, derived from, or related to each other. Denzin (1970) explains it this way: "A theory must contain a set of propositions or hypotheses that combine descriptive and relational concepts. . . . Unfortunately, a set of propositions taken alone does not constitute a theory either. The set must be placed in a deductive scheme" (p. 34).

This particular feature of scientific theories (relationships among explanations or constructs) is similar to the craft of quilting. Quilting consists of sewing fabric together, usually combining large squares of material with different textures and colors to form an intricate pattern. This craft offers a very useful image for the process of theory building because it helps one see how, depending on the way the blocks of fabric are connected, entirely different images can emerge (see **Figure 4–1**).

The designs displayed in the last row of Figure 4–1 were all formed by combining the top square into blocks of four squares each (shown in the second row). The variation in shape is a result of how the original block is combined with other identical blocks. The same idea applies to scientific theories: String the data or facts together using a certain logic or set of beliefs as the starting point, and

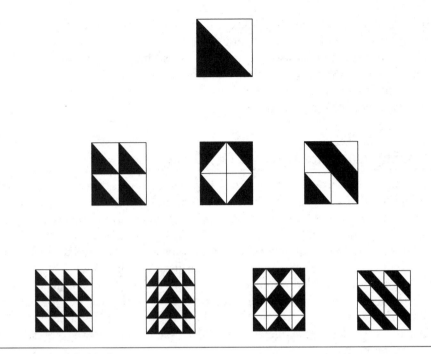

**FIGURE 4–1   Quilt blocks.**
*Source:* Goodson P. (2010). *Theory in Health Promotion Research and Practice.* Burlington, MA: Jones & Bartlett Learning.

one set of explanations emerges; combine them within another logic, structure, or paradigm, and the resulting explanations might look very different. The important point to remember from this illustration is that individual blocks of fabric do not make a quilt. Similarly, a scientific theory is not developed until various explanations are weaved within a logic pattern.

Surprisingly, in neither the hard sciences nor the social sciences do scholars share a single agreed-upon view of what a theory is, nor do they care to reach consensus over a single definition (Cohen, 1980; Turner, 1986). Although for some people the term *theory* may refer to a "set of tested empirical generalizations" or to a "unified, systematic causal explanation of a diverse range of social phenomena" (Schwandt, 2001, p. 252), others may view theory as broad "theoretical orientations or perspectives (e.g., functionalism, symbolic interactionism, behaviorism)" or, more specifically, as a single theory (e.g., critical theory) (Schwandt, 2001, p. 252).

At the same time, various types of ideas, speculations, hypotheses, models, criticisms, conceptual frameworks, and propositions, when interconnected with words (and even scholars' personal beliefs), are sometimes called theories in certain disciplinary fields (Cohen, 1980; Denzin, 1970). Therefore, despite the apparent rigor, order, logic, and systematic thinking needed in scientific theorizing, social scientists themselves use the term *theory* to mean many different things.

Far from indicating that these scientists are incorrect in their use of the term, this lack of consensus reinforces the notion that theory is a complex, multidimensional phenomenon that resists attempts to be simplified, unidimensionalized, and boxed into one specific container. The beauty of theory lies precisely in its intricate complexity, much like the beauty of a kaleidoscope, a fractal image, or the inner workings of the human body.

## Theorizing and Theoretical Thinking

The way that some authors attempt to simplify theoretical thinking, to reduce it to its bare bones, to skeletonize the phenomenon, and thus to distance the person from the forces involved in its creation, implementation, and refinement is perhaps merely an attempt to be didactic. In trying to help readers understand, authors have instead figuratively taken readers into an anatomy lab, made them look at a cadaver, and declared, "Here is what life looks like."

The problem is that definitions of scientific theories ignore a crucial element within the theory domain—the theorizing *process*. To think about theory is to think about explanations, descriptions, and predictions, but it is more than that. It means also considering the questions and the reasoning that lead to these explanations, descriptions, and predictions.

I define theorizing or theoretical thinking as the dynamic process of asking and answering specific types of questions. Theory may be defined also as the end result, the outcome, or the outgrowth from this operation. Theorizing implies movement, dynamics, and dialogue—a volleying between questions and replies. Theory is the answer part of the equation. This conception of theory and theoretical thinking is diagrammed in **Figure 4–2**.

Within this framework, scientific theories are characterized by questions focused on causes and with explanations or answers that attempt to tell the story of why phenomena occur as they do. Theoretical questions in scientific-type thinking about health promotion, for example, ask the questions, "What influences or determines healthy behaviors among older adults?" "Do attitudes lead to behavior change among adolescents?" "Why is education level associated with certain health outcomes?" Scientific theories—when they have already been proposed and tested—provide clean, decluttered answers to these questions. They have been carefully thought out, tentatively proposed (at first), and repeatedly tested to see whether the explanations will hold over time and across various contexts. Only after much tweaking, adjusting, and testing do these explanations gain the status of a scientific theory, and, in science, all of the tweaking, adjusting, and testing follow carefully outlined protocols. In other words, they are done in a systematic way, following principles and procedures of scientific practice (Pedhazur & Schmelkin, 1991).

Other types of theories (policy, ethics, nursing, and commonsense theories) ask different types of questions. They are not cause and effect theories, but rather they focus on questions such as the following: "What is the ultimate end of health

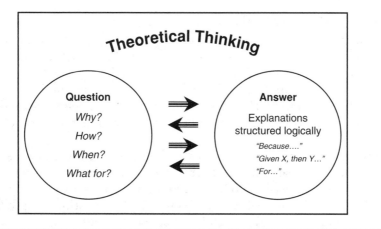

**FIGURE 4–2  The theorizing process.**
*Source:* Goodson P. (2010). *Theory in Health Promotion Research and Practice.* Burlington, MA: Jones & Bartlett Learning.

promotion?" "Why should healthier lifestyles be promoted?" "Are the means being used to promote health healthy themselves?" "Which nursing interventions result in patient well-being?" "Is health a human right to which all human beings are naturally entitled?" "How can a country's public health system protect its populations against potentially dangerous illnesses?" "What can be expected from globalization, in terms of its effects on health promotion, on a worldwide basis?"

# Theory as Practice

## What Does Theory Do?

Setting aside the differences between commonsense and scientific theories, it is evident that both categories have a pivotal common element: meaning attribution. This is precisely the job of theoretical thinking. It is exactly what theory—or more precisely, theorizing—does (Nealon & Giroux, 2003). Theory-type questions and their answers lend meaning, provide explanation, impose order, and organize logically the events that engulf healthcare professionals. Theorizing, in other words, leads practitioners to take the following steps:

- *Ask* certain types of questions
- *Question* the status quo
- *Seek* the most plausible and meaningful answers
- *Build* a narrative or logical structure for the questions and the answers

Theory should be viewed as a type of practice precisely because theorizing involves all of these actions. It is important to keep this point in mind: *Theory is practice.* If practice is action or doing, then theory does quite a lot more than might first be suspected. Thinking theoretically is, indeed, engaging in very practical tasks.

## What Does Theory Look Like?

If one views theoretical thinking as a process of asking specific types of questions and obtaining certain kinds of answers, then scientific theories and commonsense theories become merely different manifestations—different "looks"—of the theorizing process. They appear different, but the difference lies on the surface, in the types of questions raised. The bottom-line processes of sense making, meaning attribution, explanation, and description remain the same for both (for all) types of theories.

Many scholars defend the notion that humankind's most universal strategy for making sense of reality is that of creating and telling stories. "We are storied selves," according to Nash (2004, p. 8). Because theories are one way to explain and attribute meaning to reality, theories undeniably constitute a specific type of story (Hoffmann, 2003). Edberg (2007) described the notion well:

> It could be said that a key characteristic of modern humans from prehistoric times has been the creation of tales, myths, and stories that, for example, describe an entire cosmological system, explain the creation of society, explain how men and women came to be what they are, and so on. These are all theories in the broad sense, for they present a coherent account from which more specific judgments and conclusions can be drawn. (p. 26)

When theories are compared with stories, it does not mean that theories are the product of fantasizing about make-believe worlds. Rather, theories themselves are built following certain narrative structures, certain "story-building rules" and purposes. What these stories or theories "look like" depends on whether they are scientific theories, public policy theories, nursing theories, ethics theories, commonsense theories, or conspiracy theories. Packaged in different formats, they all represent ways to provide accounts of phenomena in orderly, logical, and meaningful ways (Lemert, 1993). In this sense, theories are stories. Notice how Frank (1995), author of *The Wounded Storyteller*, described the book in which he analyzed the human experience of disease by focusing on his and others' personal stories of illness:

> This book [*The Wounded Storyteller*] is a *work of theory*, but it is equally a collection of stories and a kind of memoir. For almost a decade I have been a wounded storyteller, and I have cultivated the stories of others who are wounded, each in different ways. The "theory" in this book elaborates my story and theirs.
>
> Charles Lemert introduces his social theory textbook calling theory "a basic survival skill" (Lemert, 1993). *The Wounded Storyteller* is a survival kit, put together out of my need to make sense of my own survival, as I watch others seeking to make sense of theirs. The wounded storyteller, like Lemert's theorist, is trying to survive and help others survive in a world that does not immediately make sense. (p. xiii)

If stories are crafted and told for sense-making purposes (for survival, Frank and Lemert might say), however, they have meaning only within a given context. The biblical story of the creation of the cosmos makes no sense within the context of physics and astronomy. Theories of health promotion that emphasize individual responsibility for wellness have little relevance in refugee camps, among victims of natural disasters, or among populations afflicted by wars. To understand what theory looks like or what kind of meaning it is creating, a theory must be understood within its particular context, against the backdrop of the particular stage on which it is enacted. Edberg (2007) stated:

> [Theories] are propositions that have meaning, validity, and truth (or falsity) within a specific context, such as a historical context, a social context, or a cultural context. Within their contexts, they are commonly held to be meaningful. Thus, to understand why a particular theory is meaningful or to evaluate its validity, you need to understand the contextual ground rules, so to speak. (p. 26)

It is important to note that theories will look different, depending on the context within which one searches for them. They will have unique appearances depending on the needs they were designed to meet at the time they were created. Furthermore, they will be considered true, valid, or even useful only after considering the historical, social, professional, and cultural circumstances within which they were developed.

If that context is the natural sciences in the 20th and 21st centuries, for example, theories will look very rigid or authoritative, and some will have gained the status of universal laws (e.g., the law of gravity). In this context, the need being met is that of discovering realities existing outside of human experience—of developing factual, predictable knowledge: hard-fast, lasting, and stable rules that are efficient at prediction and control.

In contrast, if the context is the behavioral sciences within modern Western societies, theories will be numerous, varied, much more malleable, and almost none will have achieved the status of universal explanations despite much testing. Some of these theories will even question the theorizing or sense-making processes themselves, asking whether the search for meaning is, indeed, a universal trait among humans. Within the context of behavioral sciences—lying at the intersection of biological and social sciences—the need being met by scientific theories is both to explain or gain clarity (Buchanan, 2004) regarding humans as individuals and social beings, and to predict and control human behavior.

If the context is public policy, theories will be less concerned with the aim to understand human behavior and more directed toward facilitating healthy community living and protecting individuals within specific population groups. If the context is Western ethics, theories will focus on normative aspects of human lives (what should be done, what is ethically right or wrong) and the development of guidelines for seeking out the common good. In a nursing context, theories are focused on knowing how to achieve positive patient outcomes.

Thus the outcome of the theorizing process, as well as the theorizing process itself, will assume many personas; theories wear the clothing provided by their historical and practical contexts. Much in the same way that tofu takes on the taste of the sauce in which you cook it, theories take on the form, shape, language, norms, and values of the many contexts in which they are built and applied.

## Theory Versus Practice

In the fall of 2006, at the start of my "Behavioral Foundations of Health Education" class (an introductory, graduate-level health behavior theories course), I asked the students to jot down brief answers to this question: "What comes to mind when you hear the word 'theory'?" I told them that I was looking for emotions, beliefs, descriptions, or definitions that immediately surfaced when they thought about the term.

Not surprisingly, of the 14 responses I collected, none listed a single positive emotion. Half contained what I considered neutral or descriptive elements (such as "relationship," "explanation," "ideas," "hypotheses," "logical process," "concepts," "road map"). The remaining half of the class brought up negative or critical elements. Here are a few examples:

- Not factual
- Old—dating back many years and may or may not be improved or changed
- Hard to prove and understand
- Something abstract, difficult to understand
- Not useful
- Lack of concrete parameters and confusing guidelines/boundaries

My favorite response was this one: "Theory is complex, something I don't like thinking about . . . It's a lot of thoughts with no specific answers."

A recounting of my students' beliefs is not needed, however, to illustrate the negativity that some people exhibit regarding theory. These same attitudes are sometimes apparent in textbooks. Here is an example of a preface to a well-known book on theory-driven evaluations (Chen, 1990):

> I would be more sympathetic to [the author's] use of "theory" if that term did not carry with it such a load of unwanted meanings. For example, in sociology, "theory" is often equated with the abstract essays written by sociologists who are long dead. In other fields, theory is equated with sets of integrated mathematical statements concerning highly abstract properties. (p. 9)

Could it be that the separation between theory and practice is so pronounced because scholars and practitioners have applied the wrong types of theories to their practice? In other words, is it possible that researchers or academics (the theorists) have been asking theoretical questions that are not productive for understanding why human beings do what they do? Could they perhaps be theorizing about human health behaviors by asking the wrong types of questions? Theorists and researchers have insisted on asking what causes human behavior (in the same way they would ask what causes a certain cell to replicate or what causes a planet to maintain its orbit). Should they instead be asking questions about the purpose and the meaning of human behavior (Buchanan, 2000)?

In considering whether this might be possible, I invoke the words of Aristotle. Theorizing or philosophizing about human knowledge, Aristotle classified human experience into three types—*theoria, poiesis,* and *praxis.* Each of these types generates a specific kind of knowledge—*episteme, techne,* and *phronesis* (practical wisdom), respectively (Buchanan, 2000, p. 54). To this day, Western thinking about what knowledge is has been influenced by Aristotle's typology; in a way, it is helpful to understand the multiple ways in which humans experience reality and learn from such experience.

For Aristotle, *episteme*-type knowledge—or the type of knowledge gained from observing "events that are constant, universal, and eternal" (Buchanan, 2000, p. 54), the type of knowledge being generated in the natural sciences— is "inadequate and inappropriate for analyzing social situations." As Buchanan (2000) explained:

> Aristotle observed that human relationships are historical, contextual, and contingent. Action in the social domain must be responsive to the novel features of each situation, to contexts in which a limitless variety of features fluctuate in salience, and to the ethical relevance of the particular persons in the specific situation at hand. . . . While the force of gravity is uniform throughout the known universe (except, possibly, in black holes), Aristotle noted that relationships in the sociohistorical domain do not display the same invariability. On the contrary, how people respond to events depends on when and where they occur, who is present, and what the individuals hope to accomplish. (p. 54)

Thus the negative feelings that theory often generates among students and health-care practitioners may indeed be the product of approaching human behavior as resulting from fixed, universal forces (*theoria–episteme*). Negative views of theory may arise because people insist on asking the wrong questions, because they fail to admit that health behaviors lie in the domain of *praxis*-type experience (transient, fluctuating, contingent, contextual) and, therefore, lead to practical reasoning; that is, health behaviors involve *phronesis*-type knowledge, not *episteme*-type knowledge. Some current theories of health behavior, for example, provide "one size fits all" answers to questions such as "What causes people to choose a healthy lifestyle?" or "What may lead people to better manage their diets and eating habits?" Most of the answers available tend to be universal and fixed, blatantly ignoring that health behaviors are contingent on their sociocultural and socioeconomic contexts.

If this truly is the case, then why would practitioners want to use these theories that do not answer the "right here, right now" questions that they have? For example, if a nurse wonders, "How can I help Ms. Smith manage her diabetes, given the small retirement income she manages and the large family she always says 'comes first'?" then the answers provided by health behavior theories, such as "increase Ms. Smith's self-efficacy" (Bandura, 1997) and "increase her perception of the severity of diabetes" (Champion & Skinner, 2008), are totally irrelevant. In fact, if the nurse is not careful, focusing on these scientific answers can do more harm than good or become iatrogenic. Because Ms. Smith's context (low income, large family, and her place within this family network) seems to shape her health problems, intervention attempts to increase self-efficacy or perceived severity of the disease may actually exacerbate Ms. Smith's anxiety and guilt (Becker, 1993). The practitioner's intervention—if he or she is concerned about applying "one size fits all" health behavior theories to develop her educational program—may transform Ms. Smith from a "person at risk" into an "anxious person at risk," thereby worsening what has been dubbed an "epidemic of apprehension" (Becker, 1993, p. 2).

From this perspective, one might even conclude that it may, in fact, be positive for theory and practice to maintain a healthy distance from each other. Yet, I would argue that the current status of theory and practice in health care is a significant symptom of an underlying illness that has been institutionalized among the healthcare professions. To separate theory and praxis (or theoretical thinking from action) is an artifact. There is nothing more valuable, more enlightening, and more empowering than the marriage of the right type of question with the appropriate answer—to build understanding, to shape professional practice, and to sharpen professional awareness. Theoretical thinking that is relevant is intricately tied to practice. Divorcing the two becomes nonsense (no sense). It is breaking something that is a unit, a one, a whole, into pieces and expecting the pieces to survive and perform on their own—like splitting a peanut butter and jelly sandwich by pulling apart the slices of bread. Try doing this, and nothing remains: not a peanut butter and jelly sandwich, not peanut butter and bread, not bread and jelly. If split, the final product is something else, but it is not a peanut butter and jelly sandwich.

Freire—the Brazilian critical theorist and philosopher of education whom health promoters have come to know well because of his contributions related to empowerment theories (Wallerstein, Sanchez-Merki, & Dow, 1997)—deftly articulated this unity between theory and practice. For him, the relationship is the same as the one between action and reflection. He called the relationship between theory and practice a dialogical one. For Freire, individual behavior and the way people live in society constitute a constant conversation or dialog between one's doing and thinking about what was done—the thinking about what was done, in turn, shaping what will be done next, and so forth in a continual iterative process.

Willinsky (1998), writing about theory in the context of teaching literature, argued this point quite eloquently:

> Try thinking of how we practice theory, that is, of how theory is a form of practice. After all, theory is practiced, whether by a young child facing a plate full of different foods or a teacher in front of a class on the first day. Theory takes practice. Theory shapes practice.
>
> Take this a step further and consider how this habit of naming one thing as "practice" and another as "theory" is in itself the work or practice of theory. It is a theoretical distinction. Such is the practice of theory. In this way, it seems fair to say that a theory of the world is what enables us to work with it. Or to put this another way, the world makes little sense without a theory about it. Our practices exist by virtue of our theories. (p. 244)

When relevant questions and appropriate answers are developed and applied, what is generated is theory and practice as action and reflection, or reflexive praxis: two sides of the same coin. If one wants to use metaphysical images, this unity can be thought of as being similar to a person. People consist of a physical dimension (body) and a nonphysical dimension (spirit, mind, or whatever is not solely physical). If these two dimensions of a person were separated, the result would be disastrous. Similarly, if one tried to artificially separate theory from practice and action from reflection, the result would be deficient. It is not surprising that healthcare professionals and students complain that theory is dry, irrelevant, and boring. A comparison is a person walking around, interacting with others, with no personality, emotions, hopes, dreams, or quirks. The beauty in humankind lies in the dynamic life force within people, the interaction among all of the dimensions that constitute who they are.

When theorizing is viewed as an interplay, a dance, or a constant dialog between a specific type of question and its respective answers, when the questions asked and the answers given match, and when both emerge from action, theory/theoretical thinking and practice are one. This constant, dynamic dance/dialog of action and reflection, theory and practice, makes the two inseparable. It also reinforces the notion that theory or theorizing is itself a type of practice. Because theory questions actions, questions the status quo (the manner in which things are done), seeks the most plausible and meaningful answers, and builds a narrative in which to frame the questions and the answers, it does indeed require practitioners to engage in quite a bit of practical work.

Viewed in this way, theory has a necessary practical dimension. Without practice (understood as everyday living), theory would not happen—it would not exist. Conversely, without theory, living would be undefined and meaningless, merely biological subsistence. Therefore, to divorce theory from practice becomes detrimental to sense making: Practice and those things that are extremely relevant to practice cannot be explained, nor can the way of doing things be improved, because they are not questioned.

## Summary

I would like to add one final observation to the claims that scientific theories provide practitioners with the ability to predict behaviors, and I will use an example from my own specialty of health promotion. Similar comparisons can be made with nursing and other healthcare professions. Despite widespread dissatisfaction in the field with health behavior theories' power to describe, foretell, and prevent risky behaviors, the mere notion that theories aspire to predict behavior with precision and efficiency is, to me, very scary.

Imagine this scenario: A certain theory proposes that an individual's theoretical self-esteem (TSE—defined as the regard one has for oneself in terms of the ability to think theoretically) is associated with his or her theorizing behavior. If I—the theorizing expert—knew the TSE scores of a certain group of students, I could easily predict to what extent those students would practice theorizing behaviors, or better yet, I could devise educational or marketing strategies to enhance that group's TSE and, therefore, to wheedle more frequent theorizing behavior out of them. Fortunately, there is no such thing as TSE (interestingly enough, though, there is such a thing as "web-esteem," so it may not be long until we see TSE as a bona fide theoretical construct; see Brock, 2006).

While the construct of TSE is merely a product of my imagination and predictions of ability to think theoretically are not life threatening, the ability to predict behavior is not science fiction. It is, in fact, one of the main goals of scientific theorizing. As has been learned from the natural sciences, prediction of behavior is possible. But should it be done? Buchanan, for instance, argues that if health behavior theories and health promotion methods were to become ultraefficient at predicting and changing health behaviors, human beings' autonomy would be lost:

> To me, the quest to find such power is deeply disturbing. Whoever controlled these new behavioral technologies would have the power to control your and my behavior. If effective scientific models [or theories] were ever developed, then the government, for example, would have the power to decide whether I would eat that dessert, exercise today, smoke pot, have sex outside marriage, or change any other behavior that it wanted to control. If effective scientific models were ever developed, then the very foundations of human autonomy, responsibility, dignity, and respect would be destroyed. We would have no autonomy, no moral responsibility, and no dignity because (1) scientists would have identified the causes of the behavior in question, and ipso facto, (2) they would have the power to change or eliminate that behavior. It would, in short, be a brave new world, beyond freedom and dignity. (Buchanan, 2004, p. 150)

Theorists and researchers are quick to point out that prediction is not very precise at the level of the individual; thus I really cannot do a good job of anticipating a person's behavior. Prediction works best at the level of aggregate data—when dealing with averages—and with populations or groups, not with individual persons. Even so, if one considers that public policy is usually predicated on such averages and on target groups or populations, it can still be a scary thought that people would try to predict (and, therefore, control and tweak) other people's behaviors.

To end this chapter on a positive note, consider the words of Lemert (1993):

> Theory is a basic survival skill. This may surprise those who believe it to be a special activity of experts of a certain kind. True, there are professional . . . theorists, usually academics. But this fact does not exclude my belief that . . . theory is something done necessarily, and often well, by people with no particular professional credential. When it is done well, by whomever, it can be a source of uncommon pleasure. (p. 1)

## Discussion Questions

1. Conduct an informal survey of your colleagues. Ask them this question: "When I say the word 'theory' [or the phrase 'health behavior theories'], what comes to mind?" Assess whether their answers carry positive, negative, or neutral connotations.

2. Engage in a discussion with your colleagues regarding (1) which types of ideas have earned the label of "theory" in nursing and (2) whether nursing is asking the appropriate theoretical questions.

3. Discuss the ethical implications of using theory to predict and control behavior.

## References

Bandura, A. (1997). *Self-efficacy: The exercise of control.* New York, NY: W. H. Freeman.

Becker, M. H. (1993). A medical sociologist looks at health promotion. *Journal of Health and Social Behavior, 34*(1), 1–6.

Brock, R. (2006, July 21). Women diminish their web-surfing skills, but the sexes are even study finds. *Chronicle of Higher Education.* Retrieved from http://business.highbeam.com/434953/article-1G1-148314000/women-diminish-their-websurfing-skills-but-sexes-even

Buchanan, D. R. (2000). *An ethic for health promotion: Rethinking the sources of human well-being.* New York, NY: Oxford University Press.

Buchanan, D. R. (2004). Two models for defining the relationship between theory and practice in nutrition education: Is the scientific method meeting our needs? *Journal of Nutrition Education and Behavior, 36,* 146–154.

Champion, V. L., & Skinner, C. S. (2008). The health belief model. In K. Glanz, B. K. Rimer, & K. Viswanath (Eds.), *Health behavior and health education: Theory, research, and practice* (4th ed., pp. 45–65). San Francisco, CA: Jossey-Bass.

Chen, H. T. (1990). *Theory-driven evaluations.* Newbury Park, CA: Sage.

Cohen, B. P. (1980). *Developing sociological knowledge: Theory and method.* Englewood Cliffs, NJ: Prentice Hall.

Denzin, N. K. (1970). *The research act: A theoretical introduction to sociological methods.* Chicago, IL: Aldine.

DiClemente, R. J., Crosby, R. A., & Kegler, M. C. (Eds.). (2002). *Emerging theories in health promotion practice and research: Strategies for improving public health.* San Francisco, CA: Jossey-Bass.

Edberg, M. (2007). *Social and behavioral theory in public health.* Sudbury, MA: Jones and Bartlett.

Frank, A. W. (1995). *The wounded storyteller: Body, illness, and ethics.* Chicago, IL: University of Chicago Press.

Glanz, K., Rimer, B. K., & Viswanath, K. (2008). *Health behavior and health education: Theory, research, and practice* (4th ed.). San Francisco, CA: Jossey-Bass.

Hoffmann, R. (2003). Why buy that theory? *American Scientist, 91,* 9–11.

Kurtz, M. L. (2006). *The JFK assassination debates: Lone gunman versus conspiracy.* Lawrence, KA: University Press of Kansas.

Lemert, C. (1993). *Social theory: The multicultural and classic readings.* Boulder, CO: Westview Press.

Nash, R. J. (2004). *Liberating scholarly writing: The power of personal narrative.* New York, NY: Teachers College Press.

Nealon, J., & Giroux, S. S. (2003). *The theory toolbox: Critical concepts for the humanities, arts, and social sciences.* New York, NY: Rowman & Littlefield.

Pedhazur, E. J., & Schmelkin, L. P. (1991). Theories, problems, and hypotheses. In E. Pedhazur & L. P. Schmelkin (Eds.), *Measurement, design and analysis: An integrated approach* (pp. 180–210). Hillsdale, NJ: Lawrence Erlbaum Associates.

Schwandt, T. A. (2001). *Dictionary of qualitative inquiry* (2nd ed.). Thousand Oaks, CA: Sage.

Turner, J. H. (1986). *The structure of sociological theory.* Chicago, IL: Dorsey Press.

Wallerstein, N., Sanchez-Merki, V., & Dow, L. (1997). Feirian praxis in health education and community organizing: A case study of an adolescent prevention program. In M. Minkler (Ed.), *Community organizing and community building for health* (pp. 195–211). New Brunswick, NJ: Rutgers University Press.

Willinsky, J. (1998). Teaching literature is teaching in theory. *Theory Into Practice, 37*(3), 244–250.

CHAPTER

5

# Components and Levels of Abstraction in Nursing Knowledge

*Janie B. Butts*

## Introduction

This chapter is a to-the-point summary for graduate students and advanced practice nurses. It is not a comprehensive review of nursing knowledge development, conceptual models, theory, or empirical indicators. Rather it is an overview of the components and levels of abstraction in nursing knowledge. The backdrop is the structural holarchy of contemporary nursing knowledge described by Jacqueline Fawcett. Her internationally recognized expertise on theory, her duration and experience in studying theory, and, especially, the significance and value of her work on theory and knowledge development continue to attract many advanced practice nurses and scholars to her work.

Graduate nursing students, who are at the stage of relearning components of nursing knowledge and theory in more detail, often become confused as they attempt to interpret different authors' terminology, especially when trying to distinguish uses for different aspects of nursing knowledge and the levels of abstractness involved in thinking. Graduate nursing students, who are earning degrees in a Doctor of Nursing Practice program or Master of Science in Nursing program, focus on theory, at varying levels of specificity and detail, and the translation of theory to practice; likewise, so do advanced practice nurses. The American Association of Colleges of Nursing (2006) specified in *Essential I, Scientific Underpinnings for Practice* in *Essentials of Doctoral Education for Advanced Nursing Practice* that scientific-based theories and concepts will be used for nursing practice and the evaluation of outcomes. *Essential I* is relevant to the content in the holarchy of contemporary nursing knowledge.

## Components of Nursing Knowledge

Nurses and others often pose the question "What do nurses *do?*" in an attempt to understand the nature of nursing and nursing practice. In reality, another question, "What do nurses *know?*", is more critical to the development of knowledge for the discipline of nursing (Rodgers, 2005, pp. 1–2). The development of nursing as a discipline and a profession in the past century has been extraordinary. It is beyond the scope of this chapter to explore the historical development of nursing knowledge, but Rodgers' discussion of the history of nursing knowledge development is an excellent source. Knowledge today is "the culmination of the integration of what is known and understood through learning and experience. Knowledge is dependent on theory and research to provide a cumulative, organized, and dynamic body of current information that can be used to answer questions, solve problems, explore phenomena, and generate new theory" (Johnson & Webber, 2005, pp. 11–12). Nursing knowledge development and practice must be in a constant state of evolution so that nurses will be equipped to fulfill the ever-changing societal needs.

Fawcett (2005a, 2005b) recognized nursing as a distinct discipline with a structural holarchy of contemporary nursing knowledge in which all components are functionally integrated into an order of wholeness or unity, where the largest whole makes up the scheme of nursing knowledge. Nursing knowledge is acquired by levels of abstraction, from the most abstract to the most concrete thinking, and vice versa. The holarchy described by Fawcett consists of five components that make up nursing knowledge, each of which is both a whole in itself and also one part of a larger whole (see **Figure 5–1**): (1) metaparadigm (most abstract); (2) philosophy; (3) conceptual model; (4) theory; and (5) empirical indicator (most concrete).

### The Knowledge Holarchy

In formulating his own beliefs about the predicament of the human condition, Arthur Koestler (1975/1967) coined the term *holarchy* as an intended substitution for the word *hierarchy*. A holarchy is a type of fractal that consists of conceptual arrangements such as the one presented in Figure 5–1. Numerous depictions of other holarchies can be found in the literature. Additionally, several creative representations of holarchies based on others' perceptions of how entities work in the world can be located on the Internet. Koestler (1975/1967) used the ancient term *holon* (originating from the pre-Socratic Greek word *holos*) in his book *The Ghost in the Machine* as a way to explain humans' predicament of having to live divided between emotion and reason and to point out how that predicament affects humans' personal and larger involvement in social and political processes and in war. As a side note, Ken Wilber (1996) later adapted Koestler's concept of holarchy and integrated his own view of it in his "chain of being" philosophy.

One can think of a holon as a node that functions independently but also interacts with other holons or nodes (wholes, or wholes within wholes) in an

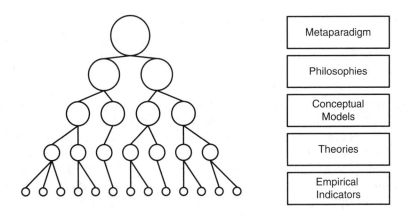

| | Metaparadigm |
| :--- |
| Philosophies |
| Conceptual Models |
| Theories |
| Empirical Indicators |

**FIGURE 5–1   Holarchy of nursing knowledge.**

holarchical structure. Through their own cognitive processes, holons coordinate and include holons of a subordinate level and transmit the information necessary "to conform the superordinate level, thereby producing an evolutionary dynamic process" (Mella, 2009, p. 27). In other words, a holarchy is not just a two-directional vertical interactive connection (top-down, bottom-up) made up of successive holons that transcend and include all holons to the point of succession from the direction of the interactions. Koestler (1975/1967) and Mesarovic, Macko, and Takahara (1970) suggested that some holons also interact with other holons in their environment (how the philosophy component interacts within the holarchy is discussed later in this chapter). If individuals were viewing these interactions, they would see how holons relate to one another as the point of focus moves up, down, or across the nodes (holons) of the holarchy; these interactions change with individual eye movement and interpretation.

Two other ways of mentally viewing the nursing knowledge holarchy provided in Figure 5–1 are possible. To create these mental images, think about theory development, for instance. There are two ways that knowledge development takes places in theory: testing theory (top-down) and generating theory (bottom-up). Both of these processes are accomplished by research.

The first mental image of the holarchy focuses on *testing theory*. Testing theory is accomplished by research through deductive reasoning and thinking, from a broad generalization to a specific entity. To think deductively about the holonic interaction, imagine being on top of the holarchy, above the metaparadigm component, and looking downward. Looking at the holarchy as a whole, you would see each of the components as one unit (wholes within the whole). Then you would see the metaparadigm as the inner "ring" or core, which is the most abstract component. As your eye moved outward, the rings would progress from the most abstract, general ring (metaparadigm) to the ring with the most concrete, specific entities (empirical indicators).

*Generating theory* is a second mental image of the holarchy. Generating theory is accomplished by research through inductive reasoning and thinking, from a concrete specific entity to an abstract broad generalization. To think inductively about the holonic interaction, imagine being on top of the holarchy and looking straight down. Inductively, you would first see the most concrete specific entities of the outer ring (empirical indicators) of the holarchy, and moving inward you would see the most abstract inner ring (metaparadigm).

Imagining these rings by levels of abstractness clarifies one's perspective on the knowledge components of the holarchy. Any of the ways of viewing the holarchy, whether seeing it in Figure 5–1 or imagining it deductively or inductively, provides some degree of reference to help facilitate understanding of the levels of abstractness in thinking about nursing knowledge development and the ways in which to acquire and process that knowledge.

In several publications (e.g., 2005a, 2005b), Fawcett framed the components of nursing knowledge (metaparadigm, philosophy, conceptual model, theory, and empirical indicator) around the notion of the holarchy. In some of her earlier work (e.g., 1999 and previously), she used the term *hierarchy*; in later publications, she adopted the term *holarchy* as part of her framework. In many of her publications (e.g., Fawcett, 1999, 2005a, 2005b; Fawcett & Garity, 2009), Fawcett discussed the components in the holarchy of nursing knowledge in relation to how the C-T-E (conceptual–theoretical–empirical) structures are linked by means of research analysis of data (discussed briefly in the section on functions of theory in this chapter).

## Metaparadigm

A *metaparadigm* is the world view of a discipline—the view that distinguishes the focus of a discipline. A metaparadigm, which is thought to be the most abstract viewpoint of a discipline, is made up of concepts that define the discipline. The most accepted nursing metaparadigm concepts are *human beings* (also known as persons), *environment, health,* and *nursing,* initially identified by Fawcett (1978a, 1978b, 2005b) as essential units of nursing. Several theorists have presented variations of the terms and concepts for the metaparadigm. Kim (1997), for example, defined the typology of the four domains as client, client–nurse, practice, and environment. King (1984) identified the primary concepts as man, health, role, and social systems. Other theorists, such as Morse (1996), recommended that nurses concentrate on formulating and using theories that they can directly link to practice instead of using an overarching metaparadigm that is possibly too abstract to be applied to practice.

To be a discipline obliges us to have a metaparadigm, and to have a metaparadigm obliges us to call nursing a discipline. The general consensus in nursing is that nursing is a discipline with a metaparadigm. Donaldson and Crowley (1978) defined a *discipline* as "a distinct way of viewing all phenomena, which ultimately defines the limits and nature of its inquiry" (p. 113). In terms of the overall function of a metaparadigm, Fawcett said, "Articulation of the metaparadigm brings a certain unity to a discipline" (2005b, p. 4). Being able to articulate the central focus of the nursing discipline means that nurses can communicate who they are and who they are not, what they do and what they do not do, and what they are about and what they are not about.

## Philosophies

Philosophers question and search for explanations and analyze common reason in an effort to enrich our lives and to increase our understanding about the very existence and experiences of human beings. Scholars in the discipline of philosophy ask many questions, such as "Who are we?," "Where do we come from?," "Why do we exist?," and "What is the nature of our existence?" The same or similar questions are asked by nursing scholars and philosophers as they seek understanding not just of human beings from a global perspective, but also of the substance revealing the nature of our existence as a discipline. For years, nursing scholars have searched for and documented the existence and nature of phenomena that identify nursing as a discipline.

Although slight language variations can be discerned in the definitions of philosophy, all in all philosophy is the searching for and communicating of a viewpoint. Fawcett (2005b) defined philosophy as "a statement encompassing ontological claims about the phenomena of central interest to a discipline, epistemic claims about how those phenomena come to be known, and ethical claims about what the members of a discipline value" and noted that the function of a philosophy is "to communicate what the members of a discipline believe to be true in relation to the phenomena of interest to that discipline" (pp. 11–12).

Answers to empirical questions cannot explain any discipline's ontological, epistemic, and ethical philosophical questions that serve as a discipline's foundation for science, mainly because philosophy is concerned with questions of a second-order nature. Second-order questions are asked by philosophers as part of their search for the meaning and nature of the first-order acquired knowledge (Edwards, 2001). Examples of inquiry by way of second-order knowledge include "What is meant by sexual abstinence?", "What is the nature of sickness?", "What is meant by health?", and other "What is meant by . . . ?" and "What is the nature of . . . ?" questions.

The four philosophical areas of inquiry are *ontological*, *epistemology*, *ethics*, and *logic*. The *ontological* area (study of reality or the metaphysical) is inquiry along the lines of "What is said to exist or be?" and "If it exists, what is there to it?" In nursing, ontology is what we believe to be "true" in terms of the central interest to the discipline; it answers the question, "What is it that we believe exists?" The *epistemology* area (study of knowledge) is inquiry into the creation, dissemination, and categorization of knowledge. In nursing, this area includes questions such as "What can we know?", "How do we know what we know about the phenomena of interest?", and "In which category does the knowledge belong?" The *ethics* area (moral philosophy) is normative inquiry about what is valued by a discipline in terms of actions and practices. In nursing, we ask normative moral questions such as "What *ought* I do as a nurse", "How *ought* I act to be ethical in practice?", and "What *ought* we do as a profession?" The *logic* area is a *method* of inquiry or logical reasoning through which arguments are presented and evaluated.

Nursing scholars communicate and disseminate their ontological, epistemological, and ethical assertions about the discipline of nursing by developing a philosophical view about the world and human beings. Fawcett (2005a, 2005b) identified three world views that have materialized from the work of nursing scholars: (1) reaction world view, (2) reciprocal interaction world view, and (3) simultaneous action world view. These world views are further explained in **Table 5–1.**

## The Philosophy Connection to the Holarchy

At first glance, the philosophy component appears to fall in line (in Figure 5–1) directly under the metaparadigm and directly before the conceptual model component. However, this is not the case. Remember that a holon, such as philosophy, can interact up and down or all around its own environment with other holons. Fawcett (2005b) made the following statement about the philosophy component:

> [T]he metaparadigm of a discipline identifies the phenomena about which ontological, epistemic, and ethical claims are made. The unique focus and content of each conceptual model then reflect certain philosophical claims. The philosophies therefore are the foundation for other formulations, including conceptual models, grand theories, and middle-range theories. (p. 22)

## Conceptual Models

The terms *conceptual framework*, *conceptual system*, *paradigm*, and *disciplinary matrix* often are used interchangeably with the term *conceptual model*. Fawcett (2005b) defined a conceptual model as follows:

> [A] set of relatively abstract and general concepts that address the phenomena of central interest to a discipline, the propositions that broadly describe those concepts, and the propositions that state relatively abstract and general relations between two or more of the concepts. (p. 16)

The overall function of a conceptual model is to characterize relationships of phenomena in a coherent format in order to shape a distinctive frame of reference. Specifically, conceptual models assist us in communicating concept links that we believe exist and then in communicating those concepts with some degree of assurance that we understand what we are conveying to one another (Shoemaker, Tankard, & Lasorsa, 2004).

Conceptual models have practical value because they guide research and practice. A "reciprocal relationship" exists between conceptual models and nursing practice in that conceptual models provide the characterization and structure for nursing practice. In turn, the outcomes of nursing practice supply evidence

**TABLE 5–1 Three World Views of Nursing**

| World View | Foundation | Perspectives |
| --- | --- | --- |
| Reaction world view | Mechanistic | Human beings are bio-psycho-social-spiritual beings. |
| | Persistence | Human beings react to external environmental stimuli in a linear, causal manner. |
| | Totality | Change occurs only for survival and as a consequence of predictable and controllable antecedent conditions. |
| | Particulate-deterministic | Only objective phenomena that can be isolated, observed, defined, and measured are studied. |
| Reciprocal interaction world view | Organismic | Human beings are holistic and parts are viewed only in the context of the whole. |
| | Simultaneity | Human beings are active, and interactions between human beings and their environments are reciprocal. |
| | Totality | Change is a function of multiple antecedent factors, is probabilistic, and may be continuous or may be only for survival. |
| | Change | Reality is multidimensional, content dependent, and relative. |
| | Persistence | |
| | Interactive-integrative | |
| Simultaneous action world view | Organismic | Unitary human beings are unified by pattern. |
| | Simultaneity | Human beings are in mutual rhythmical interchange with their environments. |
| | Change | Human beings change continuously, unpredictably, and in the direction of more complex self-organization. |
| | Unitary-transformative | The phenomena of interest are personal knowledge and pattern recognition. |

Adapted from Fawcett, J. (2005). *Contemporary nursing knowledge: Analysis and evaluation of nursing models and theories* (2nd ed., pp. 12–13). Philadelphia, PA: F. A. Davis. Used with permission.

**TABLE 5-2   Conceptual Models of Nursing**

| Conceptual Model | Publication Dates and Revisions |
| --- | --- |
| Johnson's behavioral system model | 1959, 1980, 1990 |
| King's conceptual system | 1968, 1971, 1981 |
| Levine's conservation model | 1969, 1991, 1996 |
| Neuman's systems model | 1982, 1995, 1996 |
| Orem's self-care framework | 1971, 1983, 1987, 2001 |
| Rogers' science of unitary human beings | 1980, 1990, 1994 |
| Roy's adaptation model | 1971, 1976, 1999 |

Adapted from Fawcett, J. (2005). *Contemporary nursing knowledge: Analysis and evaluation of nursing models and theories* (2nd ed., pp. 1–48). Philadelphia, PA: F. A. Davis. Used with permission.

for theorists to determine the degree to which a conceptual model has credence (Fawcett, 1992; Kahn & Fawcett, 1995).

A unique facet of each conceptual model is that it provides an individual with the ability to interpret and characterize reality from that particular model (Fawcett, 2005b). Each discipline does not have just one reality, but rather multiple realities. The seven conceptual models of nursing recognized by Fawcett enable nurses to view the world and its functions in different ways (see **Table 5–2**). Each conceptual model of nursing gives the discipline a unique perspective of the metaparadigm concepts and provides a path for concrete theories (specifically, middle-range theories) to be generated and tested for practice.

Fawcett (1995, 2005b) has always contended that individuals cannot view the world and make observations about the world apart from a conceptual model frame of reference. Philosophers such as Karl Popper (1959) have noted that we see, hear, and process information through some determinate frame of reference, or belief and value system, painting everything we perceive and influencing how we interpret it. Fawcett (2005b) emphasized that because nurses see the world and their observations about the world through some frame of reference, choosing a credible conceptual model is central to expert practice.

Fawcett (2003) was resolute in her statement on the essentialness of conceptual models to the discipline of nursing: "Conceptual models . . . are the foundation on which claims of disciplinary status for nursing rests" (p. 229). For several years, Fawcett has communicated her concern about whether the discipline of nursing will survive given that many nursing researchers no longer use, support, or value conceptual models as integral to the viability of the discipline (Fawcett, 2003, 2008; Fawcett & Alligood, 2005; Fawcett, Newman, & McAllister, 2004). Without specific nursing conceptual models for guiding research and nursing practice, Fawcett (2003) has expressed her worry that the discipline will become extinct and nurses will regress to no more than "skilled tradespeople" (p. 229).

Nursing must have its own identity with its own conceptual models, and not borrow from other disciplines. As a discipline, it has reached a bifurcation point where a decision must be made. Without using our own conceptual models of nursing, we stand to lose nursing's identity.

***Conceptual Models Versus Theories.***    More than 30 years ago Fawcett (1978b) distinguished conceptual models and theories by the level of abstraction. Since then she has built on this distinction as part of her work. Along the way, she devised a rule for making this distinction, based on a determination of the purpose of the work being examined (Fawcett, 2005b). This can be referred to as *if–then determinations* (**Box 5–1**). Such determinations are useful for advanced practice nurses and students as they attempt to decipher the level of abstractness required for each work being examined. To answer the questions related to Determinations 1 to 3 in Box 5–1, the advanced practice nurse would examine the purpose

---

### Box 5–1 *If–Then* Determinations: Is It a Conceptual Model or a Theory?

| Determination | If | Then |
|---|---|---|
| **Determination 1** | *If* the purpose of the work is to articulate a body of distinctive knowledge for the whole of the discipline of nursing | *Then* the work is probably a conceptual model |
| **Determination 2** | *If* the purpose of the work is to further develop one aspect of a conceptual model | *Then* the work is probably a grand theory |
| **Determination 3** | *If* the purpose of the work is to describe, explain, or predict concrete and specific phenomena | *Then* the work is probably a middle-range theory |
| **Determination 4** | *If* the work requires that one must work through four steps to directly link the concepts to empirically testable hypotheses | *Then* the work is probably a conceptual model |

*(Continues)*

## Box 5–1 *If–Then* Determinations: Is It a Conceptual Model or a Theory? *(Continued)*

| Determination | If | Then |
|---|---|---|
| **Process Steps to Linking** | *If* three steps are required | *Then* the work is probably a middle-range theory |

Step 1: Create the conceptual model.

Step 2: Derive the middle-range theory.

Step 3: Identify empirical indicators.

Step 4: Identify empirically testable hypotheses.

Adapted from Fawcett, J. (2005). *Contemporary nursing knowledge: Analysis and evaluation of nursing models and theories* (2nd ed., pp. 1–48). Philadelphia, PA: F. A. Davis. Used with permission.

of the work in terms of three different *if–then* conditions. Determination 4 has to do with the number of steps required for one to work and think through the process of formulating concepts and translating them into empirically testable hypotheses. These steps are embedded within the components of the holarchy.

Fawcett (2005b) specified the level of abstractness of conceptual models in more detail:

> The concepts are too abstract and general for direct observation of phenomena to occur. The concepts are not restricted by anyone—individuals, groups, situations, or events. The propositions are too abstract and general for direct empirical observation to occur. The related concepts are stated in an abstract and general manner.

Fawcett and Garity (2009) mentioned an additional condition for a conceptual model to be designated as such: A conceptual model must be complete in terms of the four concepts of the metaparadigm. The three theories they listed as "grand" contain only three of four metaparadigm concepts that designate a conceptual model (see **Table 5–3**).

### *Distinction Between Conceptual Models and Other Models for Middle-Range Theories.*
Fawcett and Garity (2009) found that nursing scholars from time to time incorrectly refer to a conceptual model as a grand theory or theoretical framework, and vice versa, or refer to a schematic diagram for middle-range theories as a conceptual model. An important point to consider is that Fawcett's description of a conceptual model is not the same as a model for middle-range

**TABLE 5–3    Grand Theories of Nursing**

| Grand Theory | Publication Dates and Revisions |
| --- | --- |
| Newman's theory of health as expanding consciousness | 1979, 1986, 1994, 1997 |
| Parse's theory of human becoming | 1981, 1987, 1992, 1994, 1996, 1997, 1998 |
| Leininger's theory of culture care, diversity, and universality | 2006 |

Adapted from Fawcett, J. (2005). *Contemporary nursing knowledge: Analysis and evaluation of nursing models and theories* (2nd ed., pp. 1–48). Philadelphia, PA: F. A. Davis and from Fawcett, J., & Garity, J. (2009). *Evaluating research for evidence-based nursing practice.* Philadelphia, PA: F. A. Davis, pp. 57–71. Used with permission.

theory often seen in some nursing articles and in other disciplines, such as in the social sciences and philosophy of science.

Fawcett (2005b) articulated the differences between a conceptual model and a model for a middle-range theory. Unlike Fawcett's description of a conceptual model, a *model for middle-range theory* is a schematic diagram of theories, a representation of testable theories, or a graphic representation that helps one to comprehend the theory. Shoemaker and colleagues (2004) called a model a "theoretical tool" that is used to represent a theory; a theory can talk to a model, and a model can talk to a theory. Models not only suggest relationships, but they also can imply relationships in middle-range theory; nevertheless, these are the models of middle-range theories and not conceptual models.

In contrast, each conceptual model has its own distinctive language of its concepts and propositions, and the definition of each term and phrase is directly connected to the essence and meaning of the conceptual model (Fawcett, 2005b). A conceptual model is extremely abstract and represents the physical, psychological, and logical processes of the world (Neuliep, 1996).

## Theories

Theorists and metatheorists define, classify, and stack theories in different ways. These differences are evident in nursing, for example. Some theorists do not try to place conceptual models and theories in echelons, whereas others do place them in echelons but in differing ways. Graduate nursing students who are at the stage of relearning theory in more detail could become confused as they try to interpret different authors' terminology, especially when trying to sort out the answers to questions such as "What is the difference between a conceptual model and a theory?", "Should theories be categorized?", "How are theories sorted?", "Which way is right?", and "Who is right?" Much of this chapter has followed Fawcett's way of distinguishing theory; refer to Box 5–1 for the *if–then* determinations that allow for differentiating a conceptual model from a theory.

Fawcett (2005b) defined a theory as "one or more relatively concrete and specific concepts that are derived from a conceptual model, the propositions that narrowly describe those concepts, and the propositions that state relatively concrete and specific relations between two or more concepts" (p. 34).

Meleis (2007, pp. 38–39) found six different ways that theory is defined, where each type is based on how it is defined:

1. Based on structure (McKay, 1969)
2. Based on practice goals (Dickoff & James, 1968)
3. Based on tentativeness (Barnum, 1998)
4. Based on research (Ellis, 1968)
5. Based on creativity in developing and connecting concepts and the use of theory in practice and research (Chinn & Kramer, 2004, 2008)
6. Based on progression from conceptual models to theory (Fawcett, 2005b)

***Functions of Theory: Theory to Practice.***    The function of theory is closely connected to "how good" the theory is. According to Jaccard and Jacoby (2010), a good theory is one that helps us better understand the world. Fawcett and Garity (2009) note that each theory is evaluated in terms of how good it is for guiding research and practice; thus, if we are to judge whether a theory is good, we must evaluate its *utility*. Shoemaker and colleagues (2004) stated the function of theory in a concise way: Its major purpose, they say, is to "condense and store knowledge . . . and put our discoveries of the nature of the world into statements" (p. 169). To accomplish this goal, the information within the theory must be good.

Fawcett (2005b) detailed the functions of theory development as twofold: (1) *research* inquiry based on theory-testing or theory-generating research and (2) research-supported theory translated into *practice*. In an article published in 1992, she emphasized that a reciprocal relationship exists between conceptual models and nursing practice (see the section on conceptual models in this chapter). The *conceptual–theoretical–empirical* (C-T-E) formalization for theory development has been presented by her in many publications. The C-T-E formalization is a way to analyze research by systematically testing or generating theory; it is sometimes called *theoretical substruction*, a term still used today by a few scholars and educators (Fawcett, 1999). Within the C-T-E formalization, there are two major C-T-E structures: (1) one C-T-E formalization for theory-testing research (top-down) and (2) one C-T-E formalization for theory-generating research (bottom-up). These functions of theory are noted throughout Fawcett's discussion of the C-T-E structures.

Conceptual models inform and transform practice by systematically providing evidence; in turn, the systematic use of the conceptual model provides information that is used for modifications of the conceptual model and documentation of outcomes (Fawcett, 1992, 2005b). Fawcett (1992) summed it up by saying, "Indeed, the reciprocal relationship between a conceptual model and nursing practice progresses from the abstract content of the conceptual model to the real world of clinical practice back to the conceptual model" (p. 226).

***Theory by Levels of Abstractions.***    Fawcett (2005a, 2005b) categorized theories based on their levels of abstraction and scope, with grand theory being more abstract with a broad scope, but less abstract than a conceptual model, and middle-range theory being more concrete and narrower in scope. It is important to note that Fawcett only mentioned grand theory and middle-range theory as the two categories in the theory component of the holarchy of nursing knowledge. Metatheory and practice theory were not named components of Fawcett's holarchy of nursing knowledge, but they are briefly defined in this section to familiarize advanced practice nurses with these terms and the way in which some theorists view them.

*Metatheory* is not a named level of abstraction of Fawcett's theory component in the holarchy of nursing knowledge, possibly because metatheory is philosophical study about theory and is not itself theory content. As described by Meleis (1997), metatheory is a theory of theories. Metatheory encompasses a philosophical stance, debate, or evaluation about theory and its methods and processes for generating knowledge (Chinn & Kramer, 2008). Metatheory involves scholars debating theory in an effort to move the discipline toward a coherent body of knowledge. A *metatheorist* "talks" theory, analyzes theory, and develops processes for theory development, whereas a *theorist* develops the actual theory and its content (Meleis, 1997). Some scholars refer to metatheory as being the highest level of abstraction of theory.

*Grand theory* is a named level of abstraction of Fawcett's theory component in the holarchy of nursing knowledge. This kind of abstract, broad theory consists of concepts and propositions that are less broad and abstract than a conceptual model but not as specific and concrete as middle-range theory (Fawcett, 2005b). Grand theory is sometimes referred to as macro theory, meaning that the theory is far too abstract to state relationships or hypotheses in empirical terms or to specify actions and processes for nursing practice (McKenna & Slevin, 2008). Fawcett recognized three theories in nursing as grand theories (see Table 5–3). Grand theories are derived from conceptual models and often become "the starting points for middle-range theory development" (Fawcett, 2005b, p. 19). A grand theory sometimes can be used as the "C" (conceptual) of the C-T-E structure, replacing the conceptual model in this structure (Fawcett & Garity, 2009). It should be noted here that middle-range theories also frequently originate directly from conceptual models (discussed in the next section).

*Middle-range theory* is a named level of abstraction of Fawcett's theory component in the holarchy of nursing knowledge. It is less abstract, narrower in scope, and has fewer concepts and propositions than grand theory. Numerous middle-range theories have been formulated in the past 15 years because they provide elements that especially align with practice in nursing (Peterson, 2009). Robert Merton (1957/1949), a sociologist who is known for his position on middle-range theory, stated that theories of this level guide research and have specificity for practice; according to Merton, theories of the middle range are strongly supported by empirical data (indicators).

Fawcett's long-term aims have been to express (1) the importance of middle-range theories to practice; (2) how middle-range theories fit in the holarchy, specifically with the conceptual model component; (3) how middle-range theories

**TABLE 5-4    Middle-Range Theories of Nursing**

| Middle-Range Theory | Publication Dates and Revisions | Type |
| --- | --- | --- |
| Theory of deliberative nursing process | Orlando 1961, 1972 | Predictive middle-range theory |
| Theory of interpersonal relations | Peplau 1952, 1987, 1989 | Descriptive middle-range theory |
| Theory of human caring | Watson 1979, 1985, 1996, 2001 | Explanatory middle-range theory |
| Theory of goal attainment | King 1981, 1995 | Derived from King's conceptual system (1981) |
| Theory of adaptation during childbirth | Tulman and Fawcett 2003 | Derived from Roy's adaptation model (1981, 1999) |

Adapted from Fawcett, J. (2005). *Contemporary nursing knowledge: Analysis and evaluation of nursing models and theories* (2nd ed., pp. 1–48). Philadelphia, PA: F. A. Davis and from Fawcett, J., & Garity, J. (2009). *Evaluating research for evidence-based nursing practice*. Philadelphia, PA: F. A. Davis, pp. 73–88. Used with permission.

can be tested, evaluated, and translated into practice; and (4) how they signal the onset of a maturing discipline. In her book of contemporary nursing knowledge, Fawcett (2005b) highlighted three middle-range theories that were derived from conceptual models but noted that many middle-range theories have been derived from conceptual models of nursing (see **Table 5-4**). Two other examples are King's theory of goal attainment (1981, 1995), which is derived from King's conceptual system (1981), and Tulman and Fawcett's (2003) theory of adaptation during childbirth, which is derived from Roy's adaptation model (Roy & Andrews, 1999; Roy & Roberts, 1981).

Conceptual models guide the direction of the propositions and empirically testable hypotheses used to create or refine middle-range theories. As stated previously in this chapter, every person views the world and how it works from a frame of reference (i.e., a conceptual model). Popper (1959) maintained that everything a person observes is screened and interpreted through that person's conceptual backdrop. The implicit understanding of this view is that nurses have assumptions about the world and the way the world functions based on their historical and cultural underpinnings. Those assumptions guide nurses toward their choice of a credible conceptual model of nursing for use in practice.

When theorists develop middle-range theories, they do so from a chosen conceptual model that aligns with their own assumptions about the world. Many middle-range theories come from the same conceptual model. As Fawcett (2005a) noted, "Many middle-range theories are needed to deal with all of the phenomena encompassed by any one conceptual model because each theory deals with only a limited aspect of the total reality encompassed by a conceptual model" (p. 36). Thus, when many middle-range theories have emerged from a conceptual model, there is more detail and specificity to that particular model. Because grand theories are also derived from conceptual models, many grand theories are also needed to detail and specify any one conceptual model (Fawcett, 2005b).

Middle-range theory is categorized in similar but slightly different ways. Fawcett (2005a) specified three types of middle-range theories: (1) descriptive, (2) explanatory, and (3) predictive. McKenna and Slevin (2008) defined four types of scientific theories: (1) descriptive, (2) explanatory, (3) predictive, and (4) prescriptive, and concisely designated them as "information presenting," "knowledge building," "knowledge confirming," and "knowledge utilization," respectively (p. 30). *Descriptive theory*, the most basic type of theory usually involving one concept, is "information presenting" in the sense that phenomena are classified and described. For descriptive theory, "an explanation is called for but not yet available" (McKenna & Slevin, 2008, p. 30). *Explanatory theory*, or "knowledge building," attempts to explain how two or more concepts relate to each other. *Predictive theory*, or "knowledge confirming," predicts cause and effect relationships between two or more concepts. *Prescriptive theory* is "knowledge utilization" that goes beyond the predictive cause and effect relationships. This type of theory builds on descriptive, explanatory, and predictive theory. McKenna and Slevin emphasized the strength of prescriptive theory:

> We must have considered the evidence for the cause–effect relationship. We must have considered the "expected utility" of one or some actions as opposed to others. And, we will have taken account of the context. (p. 31)

Some theorists label prescriptive theory as practice theory, which has a narrower scope than what is often labeled as middle-range theory (practice theory is discussed later in this section).

Other slight variations on types of theory exist as well. For example, Meleis (2007) defined theory by goal orientation and divided it into two major categories—descriptive and predictive. Within descriptive theory, she delineated two classifications: (1) "factor-isolating, category-formulating, or labeling theory" and (2) "explanatory" (p. 44). McEwen (2011) specified four types of theories: (1) descriptive theory as factor-isolating theory, (2) explanatory theory as factor-relating theory, (3) predictive theories or promoting or inhibiting theory as situation-relating theory, and (4) prescriptive theory as situation-producing theory.

A derivative of middle-range theory is *practice theory*, which is a very narrow theory resulting from empirical testing (Peterson, 2009). Practice theory is also known as prescriptive theory. Fawcett (2005b) does not compartmentalize practice theory or prescriptive theory apart from her middle-range theory category, but she does refer to descriptive, explanatory, and predictive theories as types of middle-range theories. Specifically, Fawcett and Garity (2009) refer to predictive theory as empirical, experimental theory for practice based on the effects of actions and processes on people and situations. This definition encompasses prescriptive theory.

As Peterson (2009) has explained, labeling any theory that is very concrete and narrow in scope can present challenges. Synonyms for practice theory include *situation-specific theory* and *micro theory* (Peterson, 2009). Dickoff and James (1968), who were noted for their stance that theory exists only for the sake of practice, categorized practice theory as goal-incorporating, prescriptive, and situation-producing theory.

The concepts of practice theory (or micro theory) are precisely defined for specific populations, desired situations, or fields of practice. Numerous practice theories exist, including these five theories:

1. The praxis theory of suffering (Morse, 2001, 2005)
2. The theory of postpartum depression (Beck, 1993)
3. The theory of breastfeeding (Nelson, 2006)
4. The theory of health promotion for preterm infants (Mefford, 2004)
5. The theory of dependent care in research with parents of toddlers (Arndt & Horodynski, 2004)

### Empirical Indicators

Fawcett (2005b) defined an *empirical indicator* as "a very concrete and specific real world proxy for a middle-range theory concept; an actual instrument, experimental condition, or procedure that is used to observe or measure a middle-range theory concept. The information obtained from empirical indicators is typically called data" (p. 21).

Empirical indicators provide a way for middle-range theories to be tested or generated, but there is no direct link between empirical indicators and conceptual models, philosophies, or the metaparadigm. The only way that empirical indicators are connected to theory is by way of an operational definition for each concept in the middle-range theory. Research instruments with data about concepts, nursing protocols, nursing practice quality indicators, and other outcome data used by nurses, among many other methods, can be used as empirical indicators. In turn, those empirical indicators can be used to test or generate middle-range theories.

## Using the Components in Practice

The C-T-E system is a whole system of nursing knowledge that is implemented for conceptual model-based or theory-based scientific practice. A conceptual model, a theory (or more than one), and empirical indicators are strongly linked to form a C-T-E system for application of a conceptual model or theory to nursing practice, research, and education. Fawcett (2005b) defined the C-T-E system as "service to the society guided by knowledge that is specific to the discipline of nursing, as articulated in conceptual models of nursing and nursing theories" (p. 32). Fawcett described two functions of the C-T-E system: (1) "to provide an intellectual lens" for human beings participating in nursing, their health, and their environment, and (2) "to provide a purposeful and systematic process for practice, that is, a practice methodology" (p. 33). The C-T-E system can be implemented by nursing departments within healthcare institutions, advanced practice nurses and other nurses working in private practice, and nursing educators to guide curriculum development or to teach students this system for practice. This section provides a brief synopsis of the substantive elements of the C-T-E system for practice.

Three substantive elements must be considered if the C-T-E system is adopted and used. Referring back to the discussion of the components of nursing knowledge will help clarify this section's meaning. **Figure 5–2** provides an overview of the holarchy translated into practice.

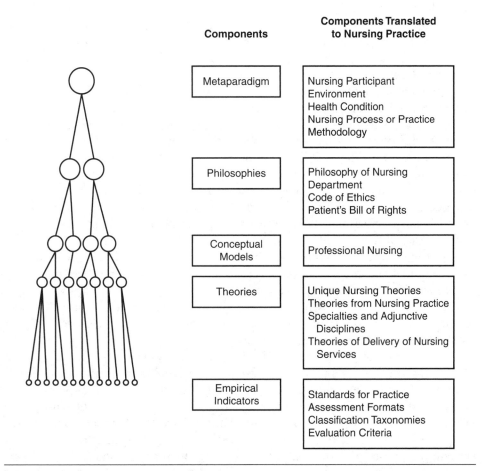

| Components | Components Translated to Nursing Practice |
|---|---|
| Metaparadigm | Nursing Participant<br>Environment<br>Health Condition<br>Nursing Process or Practice Methodology |
| Philosophies | Philosophy of Nursing Department<br>Code of Ethics<br>Patient's Bill of Rights |
| Conceptual Models | Professional Nursing |
| Theories | Unique Nursing Theories<br>Theories from Nursing Practice Specialties and Adjunctive Disciplines<br>Theories of Delivery of Nursing Services |
| Empirical Indicators | Standards for Practice<br>Assessment Formats<br>Classification Taxonomies<br>Evaluation Criteria |

**FIGURE 5–2    Holarchy of nursing knowledge.**
Adapted from Fawcett, J. (2005). *Contemporary nursing knowledge: Analysis and evaluation of nursing models and theories* (2nd ed., p. 34). Philadelphia, PA: F. A. Davis. Used with permission.

The first element is translation of the metaparadigm of nursing into practice. The metaparadigm includes the human beings requiring nursing care, meaning the participant, family, or community; the environment of the human beings requiring care and the nursing practice environment; the health status of the participant; and the nursing practice methodology. In healthcare institutions, the mission statement sets the tone of the institution, the scope of nursing practice and its methodology, and types of service.

The second element is translation of philosophies into nursing practice. As previously discussed, the philosophy is a world view about the beliefs and values of nursing as a discipline. The institution has a philosophy of its beliefs and values about human beings, the institution's environment, health, and nursing methodology. Some of the ways in which philosophy is communicated include the American Nurses Association's *Code of Ethics for Nurses* (2001) or other codes of conduct; the patient's bill of rights for the particular institution—for hospitals, for example, the American Hospital Association has written and adopted *The Patient Care Partnership* (2008) document, which has replaced its universal Patient's Bill of Rights; and the nursing department's philosophy statement that is uniquely formulated by each institution.

The third element is translation of the conceptual model, theories, and empirical indicators into a comprehensive "formal nursing knowledge system," the C-T-E system. This step "requires the linkage to a conceptual model, one or more theories, and one or more empirical indicators" (Fawcett, 2005b, p. 34). There are numerous ways that a C-T-E system becomes evident. The conceptual model can be the individual nurse's professional perspective on nursing and/or the institution's and nursing department's adopted conceptual model or theory. The practicing nurse works within the institution's or agency's conceptual model or professional practice model. Theories that are adopted include nursing theories and theories of delivery of nursing care and services. All theories used must be consistent with the adopted philosophy and the conceptual model. Once the conceptual model and the theories are congruent and in place, empirical indicators are adopted. Numerous empirical indicators could be used, along with documents that include their own empirical indicators. Sources for empirical indicators include standards for practice, assessment designs, taxonomies, protocols for intervention, and an evaluation program.

It is not within the scope of this chapter to present an in-depth discussion of the substantive elements of the C-T-E system. To read more about the C-T-E system and guidelines using the C-T-E system for practice, research, education, or administration, refer to Chapter 2 of the contemporary nursing knowledge book by Fawcett (2005b). In that same chapter, Fawcett offers a perspective on the process elements of the C-T-E system; successful implementation of a C-T-E system; the phases of evolution during the implementation, which is called perspective transformation; strategies to facilitate perspective transformation; and levels of integration of the C-T-E system.

# Summary

This chapter presents a review of the holarchy of nursing knowledge that was formulated by Fawcett. The components of nursing knowledge—that is, the metaparadigm, philosophy, conceptual model, theory, and empirical indicator—were discussed. According to Fawcett, middle-range theories must be strongly linked to nursing's conceptual models if nursing is to remain a viable and bona fide discipline. As Fawcett pointed out, nursing stands to lose its identity if nursing researchers and scholars continue to abandon nursing's own conceptual models in favor of models and theories of other disciplines. Linking conceptual models of nursing, theories, and empirical indicators to the C-T-E system is necessary for the application of a conceptual model of nursing and, therefore, for the translation of the components of nursing knowledge into real-world practice.

# Discussion Questions

1. Examine each of the components in the holarchy of nursing knowledge. Identify one conceptual model of nursing, one grand theory of nursing, and one middle-range theory of nursing. Either search this text for the content of each one, or search in the CINAHL or Medline databases. Using the *if–then* determinations in Box 5–1 of this chapter, explain the distinguishable levels of abstraction characteristics of each one (conceptual model, grand theory, and middle-range theory).

2. Which one of the three philosophical world views from Table 5–1 reflects your philosophical world view? Explore how your philosophical world view (reaction, reciprocal interaction, or simultaneous action) interweaves with the philosophical world view adopted by your workplace.

3. Determine which conceptual model of nursing you prefer. Then, choose a middle-range nursing theory that has been formulated or derived from your preferred conceptual model of nursing. Analyze the parts of your chosen middle-range theory that reveal the derivation characteristics from your chosen conceptual model of nursing. An example includes (but is not necessarily the model and theory that you will choose) King's theory of goal attainment (1995), which is a middle-range nursing theory derived in 1981 from King's conceptual system (1971).

4. Explore specific strategies that you or other advanced practice nurses can implement to advance the discipline of nursing. What is the critical nature of the relationship between conceptual models of nursing and middle-range nursing theories?

5. Analyze how the C-T-E structures translate into nursing practice (see Figure 5–2). Use actual examples. You may use the middle-range nursing theory and the conceptual model of nursing that you chose in Discussion Question 3. In addition, choose two or more empirical indicators that are consistent with your middle-range nursing theory and that can be translated into a testable hypothesis. Give an overview of this C-T-E structure process.

# References

American Association of Colleges of Nursing. (2006). *Essentials of doctoral education for advanced nursing practice.* Retrieved from http://www.aacn.nche.edu/publications/position/DNPEssentials.pdf

American Hospital Association. (2008, April 1). *The patient care partnership.* Washington, DC: Author. Retrieved from http://www.aha.org/aha/issues/Communicating-With-Patients/pt-care-partnership.html

American Nurses Association. (2001). *Code of ethics for nurses with interpretive statements.* Washington, DC: Author.

Arndt, M. J., & Horodynski, M. A. O. (2004). Theory of dependent-care in research with parents of toddlers: The NEAT project. *Nursing Science Quarterly, 17,* 345–350.

Barnum, B. J. S. (1998). *Nursing theory: Analysis, application, and evaluation* (5th ed.). Philadelphia, PA: Lippincott Williams & Wilkins.

Beck, C. T. (1993). Teetering on the edge: A substantive theory of postpartum depression. *Nursing Research, 42,* 42–48.

Chinn, P. L., & Kramer, M. K. (2004). *Integrated theory and knowledge development in nursing* (6th ed.). St. Louis, MO: Mosby.

Chinn, P. L., & Kramer, M. K. (2008). *Integrated theory and knowledge development in nursing* (7th ed.). St. Louis, MO: Mosby.

Dickoff, J., & James, P. (1968). A theory of theories: A position paper. *Nursing Research, 17*(3), 197–203.

Donaldson, S. K., & Crowley, D. M. (1978). The discipline of nursing. *Nursing Outlook, 26*(2), 113–120.

Edwards, S. D. (2001). The nature of philosophy of nursing. *Philosophy of nursing: An introduction.* New York, NY: Palgrave.

Ellis, R. (1968). Characteristics of significant theories. *Nursing Research, 17*(3), 217–222.

Fawcett, J. (1978a). The relationship between theory and research: The double helix. *Advances in Nursing Science, 1*(1), 49–62.

Fawcett, J. (1978b). The "what" of theory development. In J. Fawcett, L. T. Zderad, J. G. Paterson, J. M. Rinehart, & M. E. Hardy (Eds.), *Theory development, What, why, and how?* (pp. 17–33). New York, NY: National League for Nursing [Pub. No. 15–1708].

Fawcett, J. (1992). Conceptual models and nursing practice: The reciprocal relationship. *Journal of Advanced Nursing, 17,* 224–288.

Fawcett, J. (1995). *Analysis and evaluation of conceptual models of nursing* (3rd ed.). Philadelphia, PA: F. A. Davis.

Fawcett, J. (1999). *The relationship of theory and research* (3rd ed.). Philadelphia, PA: F. A. Davis.

Fawcett, J. (2003). Guest editorial: On bed baths and conceptual models of nursing. *Journal of Advanced Nursing, 44,* 229–230.

Fawcett, J. (2005a). Middle-range nursing theories are necessary for the advancement of the discipline. *Aquichan, 5*(001), 32–43.

Fawcett, J. (2005b). The structure of contemporary nursing knowledge. In *Contemporary nursing knowledge: Analysis and evaluation of nursing models and theories* (2nd ed., pp. 1–48). Philadelphia, PA: F. A. Davis.

Fawcett, J. (2008). Editor's choice: The added value of nursing conceptual model-based research. *Journal of Advanced Nursing, 61,* 583.

Fawcett, J., & Alligood, M. R. (2005). Influences on advancement of nursing knowledge. *Nursing Science Quarterly, 18,* 227–232.

Fawcett, J., & Garity, J. (2009). *Evaluating research for evidence-based nursing practice.* Philadelphia, PA: F. A. Davis.

Fawcett, J., Newman, D. M. L., & McAllister, M. (2004). Advanced practice nursing and conceptual models of nursing. *Nursing Science Quarterly, 17,* 135–138.

Jaccard, J., & Jacoby, J. (2010). Science as an approach to understanding. In *Theory construction and model-building skills: A practical guide for social scientists* (pp. 22–36). New York, NY: Guilford Press.

Johnson, B. M., & Webber, P. B. (2005). Language, meaning, and structure. *An introduction to theory and reasoning in nursing* (2nd ed., pp. 9–29). New York, NY: Lippincott Williams & Wilkins.

Kahn, S., & Fawcett, J. (1995). Continuing the dialogue: A response to Draper's critique of Fawcett's "Conceptual models and nursing practice: The reciprocal relationship." *Journal of Advanced Nursing, 22,* 188–192.

Kim, H. S. (1997). Terminology in structuring and development nursing knowledge. In I. M. King & J. Fawcett (Eds.), *The language of nursing theory and metatheory* (pp. 27–36). Indianapolis, IN: Sigma Theta Tau International Honor Society of Nursing.

King, I. M. (1981). *A theory for nursing: Systems, concepts, process.* New York, NY: Wiley.

King, I. M. (1984). Philosophy of nursing education: A national survey. *Western Journal of Nursing Research, 6,* 387–406.

King, I. M. (1995). The theory of goal attainment. In M. A. Frey & C. L. Sieloff (Eds.), *Advancing King's systems framework and theory of nursing* (pp. 23–32). Thousand Oaks, CA: Sage.

Koestler, A. (1975/1967). *The ghost in the machine.* New York, NY: Random House.

McEwen, M. (2011). Overview of theory in nursing. In M. McEwen & E. M. Wills (Eds.), *Theoretical basis for nursing* (3rd ed., pp. 21–45). Philadelphia, PA: Wolters Kluwer/ Lippincott Williams & Wilkins.

McKay, R. (1969). Theories, models and systems for nursing. *Nursing Research, 18*(5), 393–399.

McKenna, H. P., & Slevin, O. D. (2008). *Nursing models, theories and practice* (pp. 1–61). Oxford, UK: Blackwell.

Mefford, L. C. (2004). A theory of health promotion for preterm infants based on Levine's conservation model of nursing. *Nursing Science Quarterly, 17,* 260–266.

Meleis, A. I. (1997). Theoretical nursing: Definitions and interpretations. In I. M. King & J. Fawcett (Eds.), *The language of nursing theory and metatheory* (pp. 41–50). Indianapolis, IN: Sigma Theta Tau International Honor Society of Nursing.

Meleis, A. I. (2007). *Theoretical nursing: Development and progress* (4th ed.). Philadelphia, PA: Lippincott Williams & Wilkins.

Mella, P. (2009). *The holonic revolution: Holons, holarchies and holonic networks: The ghost in the production machine.* Pavia, Italy: Pavia University Press.

Merton, R. K. (1957/1949). *Social theory and social structure* (revised ed.). New York, NY: Free Press.

Mesarovic, M., Macko, D., & Takahara, Y. (1970). *Theory of hierarchical, multi-level systems.* New York, NY: Academic Press.

Morse, J. M. (1996). Nursing scholarship: Sense and sensibility. *Nursing Inquiry, 3,* 74–82.

Morse, J. M. (2001). Toward a praxis theory of suffering. *Advances in Nursing Science, 24*(1), 47–59.

Morse, J. M. (2005). Creating a qualitatively-derived theory of suffering. In U. Zeitler (Ed.), *Clinical practice and development in nursing* (pp. 83–91). Aarhus, Denmark: Center for Innovation in Nurse Training.

Nelson, A. M. (2006). Toward a situation-specific theory of breastfeeding. *Research and Theory for Nursing Practice, 20*(1), 9–27.

Neuliep, J. W. (1996). *Human communication theory: Applications and case studies.* Boston, MA: Pearson/Allyn & Bacon.

Peterson, S. J. (2009). Introduction to the nature of nursing knowledge. In S. J. Peterson & T. W. Bredow (Eds.), *Middle range theories: Application to nursing research* (2nd ed., pp. 3–45). New York, NY: Lippincott Williams & Wilkins.

Popper, K. (1959). *The logic of scientific discovery.* New York, NY: Basic Books.

Rodgers, B. L. (2005). *Developing nursing knowledge: Philosophical traditions and influences.* Philadelphia, PA: Lippincott Williams & Wilkins.

Roy, C., & Andrews, H. A. (1999). *The Roy adaptation model* (2nd ed.). Stamford, CT: Appleton & Lange.

Roy, C., & Roberts, S. L. (1981). *Theory construction in nursing: An adaptation model.* Englewood Cliffs, NJ: Prentice Hall.

Shoemaker, P. J., Tankard, J. W., & Lasorsa, D. L. (2004). *How to build social science theories.* Thousand Oaks, CA: Sage.

Tulman, L., & Fawcett, J. (2003). *Women's health during and after pregnancy: A theory-based study of adaptation to change.* New York, NY: Springer.

Wilber, K. (1996). *A brief history of everything.* Boston, MA: Shambhala Books/Random House.

# PART 3

# Interdisciplinary Philosophies and Theories

# Complexity Science and Complex Adaptive Systems

*Joan C. Engebretson*
*Joanne V. Hickey*

## Introduction

*Complexity science* is an emerging paradigm being integrated into the healthcare literature as a new approach from which to view clinical care and healthcare organizations (HCOs). Grounded in physics and mathematics, it offers a fresh approach for studying regularities that differ from traditional science. Unlike traditional science that incorporates laws of science, complexity science is based on the thought that complexity emerges from simple rules (Phelan, 2001).

The theoretical concepts of complexity have been broadened into a paradigm of science concerned with the interconnection between individual units or agents (Kauffman, 1995; Waldrop, 1992). Complexity science has expanded recently with the ability to analyze huge amounts of data through computers. Thus, it has expanded the view of scientific research beyond purely linear reductionism. It has been applied to fields such as weather forecasting, economics, and neuroscience, as well as social and organizational behavior. The term *complex adaptive system* (CAS) refers to a special application of complexity that bears some similarity to systems theory. As such, this framework will likely have an inherent resonance with nurses. The idea of nested systems from the individual patient, family, and community—as well as the healthcare unit, organization, and healthcare system— is familiar to most nurses.

CASs have recently been applied to health care in relation to physiology and medicine. Additionally, complexity frameworks have been applied to local healthcare systems (Anderson, Issel, & McDaniel, 2003; Crabtree, Miller, & Strange, 2001) and organizations.

Biomedical scientific frameworks of mechanism and reductionism, which have produced excellent medical advances, have not always been a good fit for nursing. This lack of fit has led to a long-standing problem for nursing professionals when they try to ground practice, research, and scholarship in reductive scientific approaches. In reality, many nursing activities could be better understood through a complex, dynamic systems framework. Therefore, it is important for nurses to understand this movement and become familiar with its basic concepts and principles (see **Table 6–1** for definitions). A word of caution is offered: Often, the vocabulary that supports complexity science is confusing, and the concepts sometimes seem to be inconsistent.

The purpose of this chapter is threefold: (1) to introduce the reader to the roots, common terminology, and basic concepts of complexity science and math, which serve as a foundation for understanding its application to nursing, health care, and HCOs (2) to explore the CAS, a special form of complexity particularly relevant for nurses; and (3) to discuss the implications of complexity science for practice and health care.

# Introduction to Complexity Science

Complexity science is not a single theory but rather an emerging field that is engaging scholars and scientists in a new paradigm of interdisciplinary study. Complexity, complexity science, and the CAS are being described in a number

---

**TABLE 6–1  Complexity Science: Terminology**

**Complexity science:** The science based in physics and mathematics that uses basic principles such as simple rules or functions to explain the relationship between variables, and that allows for variations and emergent behaviors that are not fully predictable. Computer modeling using these rules/functions has accommodated large amounts of data that allow for the study of phenomena on intermediate levels in dynamic systems.

**Nonlinear dynamics:** The mathematics used to understand complex deterministic systems with complex behavior.

**Complexity theories or concepts:** The basic principles or concepts from complexity science and complex adaptive systems that are *applied*, often metaphorically, to other biological and social systems.

**Complex adaptive systems (CASs):** The application of complexity theories and systems perspectives to living, dynamic systems in biology and other systems.

**Complex responsive processes (CRPs):** The application of complexity to organizations in which a CAS is not completely applicable based on organizational structure and the ways in which people learn and form mental models in structured organizations. Currently, new mathematical models are being applied to science at all levels and the language has begun to penetrate other areas.

of fields, including physics, mathematics, biology, economics, and the biological and social sciences. Complexity science is an emerging field of interest that is attracting a diverse group of scholars and scientists across disciplines to view phenomena of interest through a new lens. Many scholars have identified it as a new paradigm in science. A prominent physicist has stated recently that complexity is a technical scientific revolution that will change the focus of research in all scientific disciplines, including human biology and medicine (Baranger, 2009).

For the past century, science has been focused largely on an analytical/reductionist paradigm of breaking things down into smaller units and isolating the parts from their contexts in an effort to understand how things operate in nature. The reductionist approach has been very successful in many ways and has engendered tremendous progress in health-related fields. Nevertheless, this approach is not sufficient to understand nature, especially living things that are dynamic and adaptive. This limitation has been a concern in the nursing profession, which is oriented to a more holistic approach.

Several scientists from the physical and biological sciences have postulated that complexity science will be the preeminent science of the 21st century (Baranger, 2009). Robert Laughlin, Nobel laureate and physicist, has been quoted as stating that science has shifted from the *age of reductionism* to the *age of emergentism* (as cited in Kelso & Engstrom, 2006). This trend represents a fundamental shift away from breaking things down into the smallest parts and toward supplementing this approach with understanding of the behavior of the whole.

This paradigm shift is echoed by Sturmberg and Martin's (2009) speculation that the unilateral focus on reductionist thinking has resulted in some of the problems that we now face in health care. These authors call for the application of complexity systems thinking to address the social dimensions of health care. Their call is not to abandon the reductionist view, but rather to embrace both the holistic and reductionist perspectives to gain a new and more complete understanding of the world. This shift toward examining the whole, as well as appreciating the component parts and their relationship, combines the two views as a "both/and" perspective rather than an "either/or" approach in complexity science.

While complexity science is not a unified theory, its constructs have been applied to health care recently, and many of the general principles and concepts have an inherent resonance with nursing. The perspective of seeing the whole, which is perceived as more than the sum of its parts, is fundamental to nursing theory; therefore, this is an important opportunity for nurses to understand this movement and become familiar with its key concepts and principles. As emphasized previously, however, the vocabulary that supports complexity science is often confusing, and the concepts are defined inconsistently.

Complexity science has been applied to a number of fields, such as computing, economics, and earth sciences. Aspects such as agent-based modeling and computer simulations have recently been applied to health care in relation to physiology and medicine. Complexity frameworks have also been applied to local healthcare systems, social behavior, and organizations. These later applications have significant relevance to nursing, because many nursing theorists have a systems theory orientation. While notable debate has ensued about the relationship between complexity and systems theory, and especially in relation to some of the more recent advancements proposed by Richardson (2005), many authors point out that complexity science has many of the same elements of systems theory, which is a theory highly familiar to nursing. The systems orientation situates patients, families, and organizations within hierarchies of systems. With these systems orientations and theoretical frameworks, the biomedical scientific framework of mechanism and reductionism has resulted in not as good a fit for nursing as previously thought. The lack of fit has produced a long-standing problem for nursing researchers who are trying to ground practice, research, and scholarship in reductive scientific mechanisms. As is now being discovered, many nursing activities could be understood better through complex dynamic systems frameworks.

# Background

It may be helpful to differentiate between complexity science as the application of mathematical and physics science to large data sets and the use of computer modeling. CASs are special cases of complexity in which some of the basic constructs are used and generally thought of more as complexity theory or a conceptual framework. Complexity science is grounded in theoretical mathematics and physics and is concerned with the interconnection between agents (Kauffman, 1995; Waldrop, 1992). Agents are units or components of the system; they may consist of individual people, birds in a flock, bees in a hive, or a component of a human system such as genes or neurons. An example is the heart and circulatory system, both of which act as agents within a body.

Many of the complexity concepts come from chaos theory, quantum mechanics, and nonlinear mathematics. It is the interconnection between or among these agents that is the focus of complexity science. *Chaos theory* signifies a different concept from the common usage of the term chaos. In a chaotic system that conforms to chaos theory, behaviors may appear to be chaotic, random, or incoherent when analyzed in a linear fashion; in contrast, when analyzed using nonlinear approaches, the system exhibits dynamic *patterned* variation. For this reason, chaos theory is described as patterned complexity rather than being equivalent to the common usage of the terms chaos and random incoherence.

Complexity science provides language, metaphors, conceptual frameworks, models, and theories that can be applied to health care. A *metaphor* is a figure of speech in which a word or phrase literally denotes one kind of object or idea in place of another to suggest a likeness or analogy between them. Metaphors are useful in describing complicated concepts because they provide a good conceptual analogy, allowing us to communicate and think about abstract concepts.

For example, the metaphor of a machine is used to convey the idea of parts that can be identified and understood. This metaphor has been successfully applied to understanding the mechanisms of how things behave or operate.

The use of metaphors in complexity science also can help communicate abstract information. These metaphors shape our thinking and perspective by connecting an idea to a known concrete entity. In one sense, then, all scientific thinking is metaphorical because the metaphors influence which questions we ask and how we understand phenomena. The machine metaphor has been the predominant metaphor shaping our thinking about physiology and guiding medical research. Indeed, a large amount of medical research is devoted to understanding the mechanisms, whether they are at the genetic, biochemical, structural, or physiological levels. For example, clinical practice and research trials are predicated on understanding the mechanism of a disease or disorder, developing an intervention to repair function, or interrupting a disease process. The expected outcome is better function or a reduction in signs or symptoms of the disease. This linear process approach is a dominating factor in terms of the way we think about clinical research and patient care, with the outcomes being based on efficacy and efficiency.

The machine metaphor has not only been used to make sense of physiological functions of the body, but it has also been applied to social organizations. Although useful, this metaphor has limitations for understanding individual behavior and organizations. Complexity science, by comparison, provides a different metaphor that looks at living systems as complex, adaptive, self-organizing systems. Complexity science is concerned with the relationship among the units, components, or agents rather than just the components themselves. This perspective sheds light on how individuals and organizations behave and how change happens (Zimmerman, Lindberg, & Plsek, 1998). Physicists have identified laws of quantum mechanics on the micro (atomic and subatomic) and cosmic levels, which have been metaphorically applied at the intermediate levels (i.e., the behavior between the atomic and cosmic levels). Currently, new mathematical models are being applied to science at all levels, and the language has begun to penetrate other areas, including health care. Adding this perspective of understanding is most relevant to health care and to the profession of nursing.

Many healthcare disciplines are beginning to acknowledge the limitations of using only reductive approaches and the machine metaphor (Plsek & Greenhalgh, 2001; Sturmberg & Martin, 2009). Consider an example from the field of genetics. Researchers who identified human genes inspired new questions about how these genes are activated. Genetic researchers have become aware of the importance of understanding the gene and its molecular aspects (micro level) as well as the context, the environment, and the ecosystem of behavior (macro level) influencing gene behaviors. Elucidation of both levels is necessary for understanding how genes behave in a human organism related to expressions of health and disease. As noted previously, scholars are not suggesting that complexity science wholly replace analytical reductive science; rather, complexity science embraces both the reductive and complexity perspectives (Lindberg, Nash, & Lindberg, 2008). Using this approach in nursing allows us to begin to address the complex challenges of patient behaviors, work environments, and care environments.

# The Scientific Roots of Complexity Science

A brief introduction to the mathematical and scientific roots of complexity science is important to ground the understanding of the concepts, which then may be applied to other systems such as individual people, groups, and organizations. The following descriptions of nonlinearity are adapted from Liebovitz's (1998) explanations of fractals and chaos, with the concepts being simplified here for the life sciences. Another scientific application of complexity science lies in coordination dynamics, where mathematics is applied to reconcile the polarized world of contradictory pairs for the purpose of understanding the poles and the world between them.

## Nonlinear Mathematics

Nonlinear mathematics provides a language to explain complex dynamic changes over time and three-dimensional space (four dimensions); it focuses on the interactions among variables, rather than the variables themselves. Some of the major concepts are presented in this section, although a full discussion of the math and science concepts is beyond the scope of this chapter. Nonlinear approaches can be applied when the data do not follow a normal distribution pattern or when additional data do not fall close to the norm. Given that these concepts apply to the mathematical functions and patterns, one must be careful when applying them directly to other observed phenomena. Table 6–2 lists some nonlinear dynamics concepts.

### Focus on Simple Rules

These mathematical functions refer to the rule that describes the relationship. For example, in the common equation $1 + 1 = 2$, a linear approach would deductively examine the dependent variable as 2 and then focus on the two independent variables of 1. In contrast, the nonlinear approach focuses on the + symbol, which is the rule or mathematical function that explains the relationship between the variables.

---

**TABLE 6–2   Nonlinear Dynamics Concepts**

- Nonlinearity
- Focus on simple rules
- Coupling
- Deterministic
- Sensitivity to initial conditions
- Fractals and self-similarity
- Scaling
- Emergence

---

## Coupling

*Coupling* looks at the strength of the relationship between functional units. Additionally, the whole may be greater than the sum of the parts.

## Deterministic Systems

In a *deterministic system,* system behavior is not random but rather has coherence or a pattern. A small number of equations and the understanding of their variables from the past can be used to compute values in the short term. Computer modeling may be used to make these explanatory predictions. The simple rules/functions specify how these variables change over time and space, at least in the short run.

## Sensitivity to Initial Conditions and Perturbations

An initial condition is the starting point of a dynamic system, and a small difference in starting values can result in significantly different trajectories. To understand this concept, picture a plot on a graph where a minuscule difference in the starting point could alter the angle of the trajectory so that it would point in a different direction if you tracked it over time. These perturbations can disrupt a system or create new emergent behaviors.

## Fractals and Self-Similarity

A *fractal* is a geometrical pattern or structure that is self-similar and repeating. Similar patterns are repeated on different scales or resolutions. The similarity may be apparent, but when used strictly in math and science it is also mathematically similar so that the scales are proportional (i.e., self-similar). A common classic example from the discovery of fractal geometry is provided by Mandelbrot (1967, 1982). He described the coastline of England as a fractal because as it is observed from closer points of view (i.e., by changing the scale of magnification), the patterns appear to be repeated in a self-similar way. If you were to use binoculars and take repeatedly closer looks (different scales of resolution) at the entire coastline, you would likely see similar patterns, albeit on an even smaller scale. In complexity science, one finds self-similar mathematical patterns.

## Scaling

The different resolutions of measurement are referred to as *scaling.* Perhaps a more familiar example of fractals is the blood vessels networks or the branches of a tree, in which the patterns are repeated on different scales; in other words, patterns are repeated at increasingly finer and finer resolution. In complexity science, new information is apparent at finer resolutions. As the object is viewed under continually closer resolutions, it appears more complex rather than exactly the same. Liebovitz (1998) distinguished nonfractal objects from fractal objects when he stated, "As a non-fractal object is magnified, no new features are revealed. As a fractal object is magnified, ever finer features are revealed. The shapes of the smaller features are kind of like the shapes of the larger features" (p. 4).

### Emergence

The unpredictability of a complex system that allows for new and unexpected behavior that is generated by the system itself is called *emergence*.

## Coordination Dynamics

Another scientific application of complexity lies in *coordination dynamics*—the study of patterns of coordinated behavior in living things.

### Pattern Dynamics

Kelso and Engstrom (2006) stated in regard to coordination dynamics, "It is a set of context dependent laws or rules that describe, explain, and predict how patterns of coordination form, adapt, persist and change in natural systems" (p. 90). These dynamics exist between two points or between complementary pairs. In their book *The Complementary Nature*, Kelso and Engstrom explored many of the contraries or oppositional pairs that are ubiquitous in the way humans make sense of the world. Coordination dynamics are a way to begin to understand these dichotomies, dualities, and polar opposites.

### Complementary Pairs

Although by definition complementary pairs are opposed, they actually are coexistent, linked, and often mutually dependent. Kelso and Engstrom (2006) recommended that these dichotomized pairs be written with the symbol ∼ (tilde)—for example, mind∼body, random∼determined, objective∼subjective, local∼global, stability∼instability, and qualitative∼quantitative. In approaching complementary pairs, it is important to understand not only both poles of the pairs, but also the dynamics that occur between them. An important scientific example is the wave∼particle theory of light. The dynamics of waves and particles, as well as the interaction between them, are needed to describe light in a complete way.

Coordination dynamics offers a way to address the whole∼part phenomena. Using coordination dynamics harkens back to the appeal to think in terms of "both/and" rather than "either/or" or "black/white." Likewise, the study of living things can be studied by reductive/analytical∼emergent approaches. One key feature of coordination dynamics is control parameters, which can be either endogenous or exogenous, that can cause the system to adapt and change. Conversely, control parameters could be stabilizing to the system. Thus the control parameters may be described as stabilizing∼destabilizing-transformative. (Life is replete with ambiguities and paradoxes.)

## Complex Adaptive Systems

The term *complex adaptive system* refers to special cases of complex systems. CASs have been studied for more than 40 years, beginning at the Santa Fe Institute, where interdisciplinary researchers investigated the application of complexity science in physical, biological, computational, and social sciences. Other groups across the world also have engaged in the application of complexity science and CAS to real-world problems. The control within a CAS is decentralized and dispersed. Coherent behavior in the system arises from competition and cooperation among the agents (Waldrop, 1992). A CAS is a collection of individual agents with freedom to act in ways that are not always totally predictable and whose actions are interconnected so that the action of one part changes the context for other agents (Wilson, Holt, & Greenhalgh, 2001).

A CAS is a network consisting of many agents that follow simple rules, are in constant dynamic interaction with one another, and can generate complex structures. The CAS has the capacity to adapt and become a good fit within a changing environment. This ability to adapt allows the organism or organization to continually modify itself relative to a changing environment by changing the rules of interaction among component agents. The process of adaptation occurs through learning new rules or behaviors and accumulating new experiences. In this process, the organism/organization evolves through a process of self-organization, which in turn allows for creativity and lacks complete predictability. A cardinal aspect of a CAS is that small actions or inputs may have large effects; conversely, large inputs may have small effects.

A CAS has a high degree of adaptive capacity and is characterized by self-similarity, complexity, emergence, and self-organization. The concept of CAS has been used to describe a flock of birds, a school of fish, a hive of bees, a human body, a family, and a community in which each level is considered a system that is different from, and more than, the sum of its parts of components. Each of these CASs is embedded in larger contexts. Moreover, CAS concepts have been applied to human physiology, such as cellular networks, neural networks, and the cardiovascular system. It is clear that the application of a CAS perspective is broad and wide—and relevant to health care and nursing.

## Components of Complex Adaptive Systems

A CAS is composed of agents that interact within the system. These agents also may be considered a CAS embedded in a larger CAS. For example, an individual in a family is a CAS as well as an agent in the family. These agents act within the system according to patterned behavior. That behavior may self-organize at the CAS level, leading to new emergent behavior. The components of these networks are agents and patterns.

### Agents

*Agents* are units or components of the system, which as mentioned can be individual people, birds in a flock, bees in a hive, or a component of a human system such as genes or neurons. These agents interact in a particular way, and their interaction and the patterns of interaction are the focus of complexity science, rather than understanding the agent in isolation. The interaction enables the system to function in a way that could not be understood from the examination of only the components.

Each agent also may be a CAS and, in turn, is also part of a larger CAS. For example, a nurse in a clinic is a CAS as well as an agent in the CAS of the clinic. The nurse coevolves with the unit as the system emerges from the patterns of interactions. In this way, the nurse also contributes to and is affected by the organization of the unit.

Control of a CAS is highly dispersed and decentralized, and the overall behavior of the system is the result of multiple decisions by individual agents (Waldrop, 1992). The agents, as well as the system, are adaptive. Agents have fuzzy boundaries and simultaneously may be members of several systems. Examples include the immune system, a financial market, and a hospital unit.

### Patterns

*Patterns* are formed by agents acting from a set of internalized rules. In a biochemical system, these patterns can be a series of chemical reactions; in an organization, they comprise the behavior of individuals or groups. Patterns and behaviors are the focus of understanding the CAS. Again, the emphasis is the relationships among the agents, rather than the agents themselves. Agents within a CAS have patterns of behavior that evolve. They absorb their past history and experiences, as well as respond to endogenous and exogenous changes. The CAS can develop rules that shape the interaction of the agents. Such systems are capable of emergent patterns that may be incorporated into the CAS's future behavior.

## Characteristics of Complex Adaptive Systems

The following characteristics are part of the CAS. Many of these constructs are similar to some of the features of the math and science disciplines (see **Table 6–3** for a summary of CAS characteristics). Here, however, they are applied in a more conceptual or theoretical framework, which allows them to be applied to clinical situations, thereby demonstrating both a patient and an organizational focus.

## Connectivity

Agents or components of a system are connected to other components both within the system and within larger systems.

### Complex Adaptive Systems Are Dynamic and Adaptive

A key characteristic of a CAS is that it is *dynamic*—that is, the system can adapt to changes in both its internal and external environments. The organism or organization demonstrates transformations of behavior through multiple modes of behavior. According to general systems theory, a system that loses its ability to maintain its equilibrium may cease to exist. Lindberg and colleagues (2008) note that nurses, physicians, and other healthcare professionals often have an orientation toward homeostasis and strive to maintain the status quo both in

---

**TABLE 6–3   Complex Adaptive Systems Concepts**

Components
- Agents
- Patterns

Characteristics
- Connectivity
- CASs are dynamic and adaptive
- Simple rules allow CASs to function
- Emergence is a property of a CAS
- CASs are self-organizing
- Control is distributed rather than centralized
- Diversity maximizes self-organization
- CASs are deterministic
- CASs are exemplified by embeddedness (i.e., a CAS may be nested within a larger CAS)
- Coordination dynamics occur within a CAS
- CASs are sensitive to initial conditions
- Coevolution occurs with a CAS
- CASs are robust and adaptable

---

physiology and in organizations. A healthy system often features processes that keep the system in a balanced or dynamic state of equilibrium so that the system can adapt to both internal and external stimuli. Complexity exists in the dynamic balance between stability and instability.

Goldberger (1996) provided a physiological illustration of this balance through a discussion of heart rate, rhythm, and cardiac output. At one extreme is a patient who is stable but whose electrocardiographic tracing strip reflects heart failure with minimum variability. This lack of variability indicates a system that is unable to respond or adapt to changes or demands on the system. This is a most unhealthy, nonadaptive state. Conversely, fibrillation, in which the heart demonstrates chaotic, highly irregular, and unpatterned rhythms, is both dysfunctional and life threatening. These examples stand in contrast to a healthy cardiac system, which operates within the range of complexity so that there are continual alterations in the heart rate in response to small and large stimuli. Thus the heart is capable of adapting to its changing environment by adjusting output.

## Simple Rules Support Complex Adaptive Systems

It is posited in complexity science that a CAS operates by an adherence to a few *simple rules* that allow the system to function. These rules are not overly specific, written, or overt; rather, they are part of the function of the components of the system. A frequently cited example is used to illustrate some of the rules that allow a flock of birds to fly in a group. The following rules have been suggested by computer modeling: (1) maintain a minimum specific distance from other birds;

(2) match velocity with other birds in the flock; and (3) move toward the center of the mass of birds in the neighborhood. Imagine what it would take to give specific instructions to each bird, depending on the bird's location within the flock.

A different set of rules operate in a bee hive, where residents of the hive have different specific roles and each bee (the agent) adapts to certain environmental external and internal stimuli based on simple rules. When agents follow these rules, a form of collective behavior—a structure or a process that is more complex than the rules that produced it—emerges (Paley, 2007). These simple rules guide the CAS and allow it to act as a system. For example, an application of simple rules allows social insects such as bees to form a collective unit that enables them to behave like a single organism or system (Kauffman, 1995; Waldrop, 1992). Scientists and mathematicians have now begun to discover some of these rules and are seeking to construct mathematical models to understand the behavior of the CAS—namely, its ability to behave as a single organism with multiple agents.

## Emergence Is a Property of Complex Adaptive Systems

Emergence has been compared to novelty, flexibility, and the creative advancement of a system (Capra, 2002). Novel or new structures, patterns, properties, or processes can emerge during the process of self-organization in a CAS. Examples of emergence include the ways in which termites and ants build large complex structures that appear to have had an architect, designer, or structural engineer guiding the process. The human brain may operate in a similar fashion, as individual neurons (i.e., agents) operate locally and in networks through some simple patterns of reciprocal activation. In both cases, the collective structure or activity cannot be deduced from individual behaviors. These emergent behaviors can be innovative and creative. It is also a possibility that some emergent patterns will not be sustainable or adaptive over the long run.

## Complex Adaptive Systems Are Self-Organizing

A cardinal property of a CAS is that it is *self-organizing*. Most such systems operate on a stability~instability dynamic. Self-organization requires appropriate conditions, often described as far from equilibrium or on the edge of chaos. This terminology indicates a zone that is closer to the instability pole where change can occur. Given its ability to exhibit emergent collective behavior, the CAS can self-organize into novel or new patterns. In this way, it moves away from a simple equilibrium or stable state and activates the nonlinearity inherent in the system. This evolution may lead to a new pattern and change the dynamics of the system. The important idea here is that these activities, behaviors, or patterns come from the CAS without the imposition of a central grand plan or control, or an externally imposed plan.

## Control Is Distributed Rather Than Centralized

A characteristic of self-organization in a CAS is *distributed control*. This term implies that the agents or components do not act through a central agent or blueprint within or outside of the system. There is no central control that is responsible for the behavior or structures that emerge; rather, the CAS is a network of disparate agents exhibiting coherence and the ability to change without central direction or a single intelligent executive function. The commonality in the examples of emergence is that the activity or structure is produced by local interactions, without any central command center. This principle is often referred to as distributed control (Lindberg et al., 2008).

Unexpected complex results from the decentralized local interaction of agents often appear to mimic more centralized organized and planned activities that are evident in a growing number of disciplines (Paley, 2007). For example, the brain has approximately 100 billion individual neurons—agents interacting with one another through hormonal and other mediators, which are themselves often localized (Holt, 2004). The individual neurons have no cognitive capacity, but nonlinear interactions between them may generate higher-level cognitive functions. Distributed control is an important characteristic of self-organization. Nevertheless, the self-organization is not always independent of the environment, because often it is the environment to which the CAS adapts.

## Complex Adaptive Systems Have Diversity

*Diversity* has been identified as a characteristic that maximizes self-organization. The greater the diversity of the components or patterns, the more robust and adaptable the system can be. Having diversity allows for the use of multiple resources to respond to external stimuli and internal adaptations (Lindberg et al., 2008). Diversity in a system provides for novelty and is a source of the capability for adaption. It is a key to innovation and long-term viability in both individuals and organizations. In addition, diversity has been demonstrated to be an essential ingredient in healthy ecosystems (Wilson, 1992). When the ecosystem is unhealthy and the environment is ruined, civilizations can collapse.

## Complex Adaptive Systems Are Deterministic

CASs tend to have patterns that follow or are *determined by* earlier ones. This stands in contrast to stochastic or random systems, in which there is no predictability or coherent pattern from previous states. The CAS operates by simple rules, and often these patterns continue and are predictable in the short run. The tendency toward determinism can be cause for confusion, however, because this characteristic coexists with emergence and self-organization. Even in complex emergence, there is generally a pattern that is not totally chaotic, but rather demonstrates a self-similar pattern.

## Complex Adaptive Systems Are Exemplified by Embeddedness

Similar to the hierarchy of systems in systems theory, CASs exist in an ecological nest of *embeddedness*. Similar to systems theory, one can locate the level of the system as the focal system, with those systems within it being considered subsystems.

This system is embedded then in larger systems, which form its context. It is important to locate the level that one is addressing to discuss it. Complexity scientists often refer to the concept of embeddedness as levels that represent (1) an external level as the context, (2) the middle level as the focus of the interactions among the agents, and (3) the inner level as the agents and behaviors within the focal system. All actions and dynamics influence and are influenced by all three levels, with each level influencing all of the others. The degree of cohesion between the three levels depends on each nested system's behaviors. When one of the nested systems experiences a change or perturbation, the entire system is affected. An example of how changes in a system can alter the network of embedded systems can be seen with fluctuations in the stock markets. In 2008, when the U.S. stock market experienced a crisis, stock markets around the world experienced the effects.

### Coordination Dynamics Occur Within Complex Adaptive Systems

Coordination dynamics are context dependent and operate according to a three-part process of interaction between parts: (1) within a focal (or part of a) system, such as the firing of neurons within the brain; (2) between different parts of the same system, such as between the heart and the lungs; and (3) between other systems, the person, and the environment (Kelso & Engstrom, 2006). A significant amount of this interaction is related to self-organization. These coordinating elements interact with one another, as well as their surroundings, and they organize themselves into dynamic patterns.

### Complex Adaptive Systems Are Sensitive to Initial Conditions

Given these dynamics, one can see how initial conditions could have a great impact on outcomes. Even a small perturbation in the system has the capacity to greatly alter the future structures, patterns, and processes. Lorenz (1993), a leading figure in chaos theory, noted that a small change in the initial condition of a system might trigger a chain of events that could lead to large-scale alterations of outcomes. The metaphor of the *butterfly effect* has become very popular. As small an input as a butterfly flapping its wings in Brazil can, at a critical point, alter the weather system so that a tornado occurs in Kansas. This highly sensitive nature of the CAS underscores the difficulty of making long-term predictions. Indeed, a condition in a certain time or space may affect significantly the dynamics of the system under certain conditions, but not others. Thus small inputs may have large effects, and large effects may have simple causes. For example, a person may be exposed to multiple viruses many times yet never become sick; in contrast, at a different time and place, just a minimum exposure may result in sickness.

### Coevolution Occurs with Complex Adaptive Systems

When the environment includes other CASs, a process of reciprocal adaptive dynamics often occurs. In this case, two systems are simultaneously changing and self-organizing, a process termed *coevolution*. Many scientists cite coevolution and the adaptive changes that organisms and the universe have made as an explanation for evolution (Kauffman, 1995). An example might be the way in which a parasite and its host coevolve to form a single system, with each party benefiting from and adapting to the other, but evolving to a different system than either one independently (Lindberg et al., 2008).

## Robustness and Adaptability

Robust systems are able to continue to function and adapt to changes within the system as well as changes in the environment. A robust system can respond to external and internal changes while still maintaining the integrity and function of the system. Some of this adaptability is related to the coordination of stability with disruption/transformation.

# Complex Adaptive Systems, Complex Responsive Processes, and Organizations

Several authors have applied CAS concepts to organizations (Plsek, 1997), while others have made a distinction between CAS and complex responsive processes (CRPs; Stacey, 2001) in applying complexity to systems. CAS is the term more widely used in the United States when dealing with HCOs. The following sections provide brief discussions of organizations from both perspectives.

## Organizations as Complex Adaptive Systems

Plsek (as cited by the Institute of Medicine [IOM], 2001), in reference to organizational systems, defined a CAS as a system of individual agents who are interconnected yet have freedom to act in novel and unpredictable ways. One agent's action changes the context for other agents, which illustrates how control is dispersed throughout the interaction among agents.

Applying complexity to organizational structure was advocated by Plsek (2001). He illustrated his advocacy for complexity first with an example of the mechanistic approach and then contrasted it with an example of complex, self-organizing behaviors. A good surgical team operates via a mechanistic approach, such that their actions are predictable and ordered. This is seen as the only viable approach, because an "either/or" perspective fears any approach that is not ordered. Thus the choice in the operating room is strict control—an ordered mechanistic approach that has both benefits and limitations. Plsek contrasts that example with a unit that is more complex and self-organizes and emerges with creativity. In this area, new and novel behaviors occur. It is important to note that this emergent behavior can manifest as either innovation or error. Plsek advocated for an application of CAS concepts to describe a middle zone of complexity in which a CAS can act from a range of adaptability from highly ordered to an area of emergence, with the ability to adapt to different conditions.

Plsek (2001) criticized traditional management theory because of its emphasis on ways to establish order and control through the actions of a few people at the top of the organization hierarchy. Jordan and colleagues (2009) described order and structure, as well as innovation, spontaneously coming about through self-organization. Emergent properties can be produced from self-organization of agents at lower levels, which then leads to patterns and order at higher levels, which in turn can reinforce existing patterns or create systems change. Plsek (1997) described the perspective of viewing the organization through the lens of a CAS, which would avoid the limitations associated with over-controlled hierarchical organizations. By expressing general direction and a few basic principles, CAS leaders would allow enough flexibility for the adaptability and creativity of the organization to emerge.

It was contended that the organization would be able to achieve a balance by integrating a planned ordered approach with a more flexible approach. Plsek used the metaphors of clockware (planned, rational, repeatable, standardized, and measured) and swarmware (exploring new possibilities, trials, freedom, autonomy, and intuition) to describe this process. By working at the edge of knowledge and experience or near the edge of chaos, maximum flexibility and innovation can be realized. Operating from this edge of chaos allows creativity to emerge but at the same time creates a need to balance the tension fostered by simultaneously maintaining the status quo and allowing creative change. In advocating for this blending of approaches, Plsek emphasized a need for interaction among agents to work through the tensions of perspectives as well as allowing new ideas to emerge.

Plsek (2001) described how a few simple rules could be demonstrated in organizations that allow for both functional order and creativity, citing the Internet as a prime example. He highlighted the many successful high-tech firms that have fewer rules, structures, and policies than their less successful competitors. Plsek identified three types of simple rules that can apply to organizations: (1) rules that point to a general direction, such that management provides the general direction or goals for the organization; (2) prohibitions or regulatory and boundary-setting rules, which restrain and maintain standards and order; and (3) recourses, incentives, and permission-providing rules, which allow for innovation and rewards.

Lanham and colleagues (2009) also used the concept of CAS in an analysis of four studies dealing with primary care. These researchers found that CAS was a useful and comprehensive theory to explore emergence of systems-level properties arising over time from local interactions among agents. They determined that practice-level quality is viewed best in holistic ways as systems issues rather than individual components. Thus making an effort to improve the relationships among the members, rather than focusing on the individual components, allows for more effective strategies for improvement.

## Organizations and Complex Responsive Processes

Organizational theorist Ralph Stacey (2001) applied complexity thinking to organizations and coined a new term in doing so, the previously mentioned *complex responsive process*. Stacey objected to the systems approach, which he contended placed the organization and individuals at different explanatory levels. Instead, he focused on learning and knowledge creation. His premise is that organizational knowledge can be found in the relationships and conversations between people in an organization. The individual mind and the social world are the same process; thus knowledge is in perpetual construction. The potential for both continuity and change exist within these everyday conversations. Therefore, change comes from the interaction between or among individual people. The complexity concepts of self-organization, emergence, and nonlinear patterns of behavior are applied in this model as well.

## Complex Responsive Processes and Relationship-Centered Care

CRP approaches have been promoted by Suchman (2006) as part of *relationship-centered care* (RCC) and through *complex responsive processes of relating* (CRPRs). RCC is based on a Pew–Fetzer task force effort to advance humanism in medicine in order to combat the objectivist and reductive approach of science-based practice. RCC went a step further, by advocating the notion of patient-centered care and the biopsychosocial model. RCC is founded on four principles:

1. Relationships in health care include the personhood of the participant.
2. Affect and emotions are important components of these relationships.
3. Healthcare relationships occur in the context of reciprocal influence.
4. Genuine relationships in health care are morally valuable, and the patient–clinician relationship is central, but relationships of clinicians with one another, with the community, and within themselves are important as well (Beach, Inui, & The Relationship-Centered Care Research Network, 2006, p. 53).

Drawing on Stacey's work on CPR, Suchman (2006) used a process of CRPR to examine pieces of meaning and relating in each relationship encounter. These patterns reflect role structures, dominance hierarchies, and behavioral norms, as well as vocabulary, concepts, and knowledge (particular and specific). The self-organization of patterns in social process is ubiquitous. Self-organization at this level requires the simultaneous action of order~disorder and constraint~freedom. CRPR allows one to determine how these patterns are created and maintained. Suchman has applied this approach to patient–provider encounters, as well as to interprofessional relationships. These applications, which are often of a reciprocal nature, could have significant relevance to the relationships between nurses and patients.

# Implications for Practice

## Practice as Complex Adaptive Systems

The IOM (2001) noted that complexity in the practice setting is a leading variable in the "significant unpredictability and variation in clinical outcomes." One can think of practice from the perspective of various sizes of systems. Microsystems, mesosystems, and macrosystems are all CASs that are related and connected through relationships (Roussel, 2014). It is through the connections within these systems that providers and patients and providers and providers interact as CASs. The clinical microsystem, for example, is the frontline unit of care that interacts with the patient and that affects outcomes. High-performance clinical microsystems foster a positive culture of open and respectful interaction that is focused on the mutual patient and provider goal of optimal patient outcomes (Batelden, Nelson, Edwards, Godfrey, & Mohr, 2003). Clinical microsystems are dynamic and vulnerable to small changes, such as the attitude of one of its members, which can have a major influence on group dynamics and patient outcomes.

Any number of CAS microsystem interactions can be cited as examples, but one of great current interest is that of transitions in care. What happens when several clinical microsystems interact—as they do with transitions of care—in increasingly rapid cycles? Care transition is defined as hospital discharge, or movement from one healthcare setting to another (Geary & Schumacher, 2012). Many of these transitions occur in the context of increasingly fragmented care. One of the strengths of using a CAS approach to clinical situations is that CAS concepts can be integrated with other models and theories to elucidate understanding. One useful model is Meleis's (2010) middle-range transition theory. As Geary and Schumacher (2012) point out, combining CAS concepts from complexity science with transition theory provides a powerful new lens through which to view care transitions and ultimately to improve transition outcomes within the current context of limited continuity and consistency in care.

## Viewing Healthcare Organizations Through the Lens of Complexity

It is generally accepted that HCOs are examples of a high order of complexity systems because these organizations typically contain systems embedded within other systems. From a macrosystems perspective, each HCO is part of a larger entity. An individual healthcare facility could be part of a larger healthcare system that includes a number of other facilities. The individual facility or system is, in turn, part of the local and national healthcare system that provides for the comprehensive healthcare needs of the nation across care settings and services. From a microsystems perspective, the HCO is composed of a number of traditional administrative and service lines, all of which are divided into smaller units that provide a variety of focused services to specific populations.

In examining an organization such as an acute care hospital, the number of different units within larger units is striking. For example, major units on the organizational chart include nursing administration, nursing/patient care units, food services, pharmacy, rehabilitation services, diagnostics (laboratory and radiology), business management, and environmental services, to mention only a few. Each of these major units, in turn, has subunits. For example, patient care units may be organized around body systems, such as cardiovascular surgery, orthopedics, or neurology. Nurses who work on these units become highly specialized in the care of the target population. These nurses tend to develop expert knowledge related to the care of this population and create a culture that addresses and supports the special problems and needs of the population of interest. Such a unit is also part of the system of nursing services, with the unit and nursing service interacting. Additionally, each unit interacts with other nursing units and departments such as rehabilitation, radiology, and food services.

The overall purpose of HCOs is to deliver high-quality, comprehensive care that is coordinated, integrated, and cost-effective. In *Crossing the Quality Chasm: A New Health System for the 21st Century* (IOM, 2001), six recommendations to improve the current healthcare system are outlined: Health care should be (1) safe, (2) effective, (3) patient centered, (4) timely, (5) efficient, and (6) equitable. In preparing its report, the IOM committee was guided by the belief that care must be delivered by systems that have been designed carefully and consciously. The committee noted the following:

> Such systems must be designed to serve the needs of patients, and to ensure that they are fully informed, retain control and participate in care delivery whenever possible, and receive care that is respectful of their values and preferences. Such systems must facilitate the application of scientific knowledge to practice, and provide clinicians with the tools and supports necessary to deliver evidence-based care consistently and safely. (IOM, 2001, pp. 7–8)

When describing systems in the report, reference is made to all systems that affect healthcare delivery, such as regulatory, insurance, and HCOs; here, the focus is limited to HCOs, though we fully recognize that other systems interact with and influence HCOs and healthcare delivery. All systems must have at least two core values: to serve the needs of patients and to allow patients to retain control over and fully participate in their own health care. Viewing HCOs through the lens of complexity science provides a dynamic framework for examining HCOs as CASs.

## Healthcare Organizations as Complex Adaptive Systems

CASs are special cases of complex systems. No format or guideline exists to help one determine precisely what qualifies as a simple system or a complex system, although individual and collective wisdom are thought to make the distinction. In complex systems, unpredictability and paradox are ever present, and some things will inevitably remain unknowable (Plsek & Greenhalgh, 2001).

This section addresses some key issues related to the framing and understanding of HCOs in terms of contemporary and highly complex organizations. They include new models of HCOs, leadership, and research.

### New Models of Healthcare Organizations

Models of organizational development and change based on linearity, vertical organization, hierarchal decision making, and controlled change strategies are outmoded and do not work for contemporary HCOs. New models are needed to understand the dynamic fast-paced volatility of healthcare delivery changes that influence HCOs.

New mental models must replace outdated ones, and complexity science offers a new paradigm. Complexity science is as much a vehicle for change as it is for creating a lens to understand organizations and change (Norman, 2009). As defined by cognitive scientists, a *mental model* is a concept that refers to deeply held or ingrained assumptions or generalizations about external reality, which can take the form of patterns or images that, in turn, frame and focus how we understand the world (Werhane, 1999). Individuals construct mental models based on knowledge and experience gained in the past. These mental models are used then to understand the present, allowing the individual to make decisions and to act (Rouse & Morris, 1986). Two important points about mental models should be recognized. First, they are socially learned and, therefore, incomplete. Second, but more significantly, because they are socially learned, they are open to change (Chen, Mills, & Werhane, 2008). New mental models shape the way we see the world.

The past is populated with mental models that primarily represent only linear thinking. In fact, the complexity of modern-day HCOs and healthcare delivery make simple linear thinking obsolete. To manage the escalating complexity in HCOs and healthcare delivery, healthcare professionals must abandon the unitary approach of linear models, accept unpredictability, respect and make use of autonomy and creativity, and respond flexibly to emerging patterns and opportunities (Plsek & Greenhalgh, 2001). This transformation requires incorporating a complexity perspective to understand better the dynamics of these organizations. As previously emphasized, a "both/and" perspective rather than an "either/or" assumption is appropriate.

## New Models of Leadership

Leadership styles change in a culture of complexity. An understanding of the organization as a CAS allows its leaders to accommodate their leadership style by engaging the natural dynamics of groups to self-organize to new situations and changes in both the ecosystem and the internal system. One such model applied in a CAS milieu is sometimes referred to as an *emergent model of leadership*. In CAS networks, leaders are open, responsive catalysts; they are collaborative co-participants who are connected and adaptable and who acknowledge paradoxes. These leaders value people and are engaged, continuously emerging, and able to shift as processes unfold. They decrease the burden imposed by rules, help others, and are good listeners.

By contrast, in many traditional hierarchical linear-oriented systems, leaders value position and structure; they are controlling, in charge, autonomous, self-preserving, and disengaged; and they hold and value formal positions, set rules, make decisions, and repeat the past. This system bears little resemblance to a CAS, in which there are a few simple rules and the self-organizing dynamics are understood, thereby allowing for emergent adaptive behavior.

Leaders who embrace complexity and the CAS perspective view their roles differently. With a vision that allows the system to evolve, they support and encourage emergence and self-organization, rather than being controlling and dictatorial. Creativity is stimulated and encouraged. Key stakeholders are supported as they work to find solutions to problems affecting them. The vertical authority gradient of the top-down hierarchy is flattened, and new collegial partnerships based on respect, trust, and values replace autocratic leadership.

To facilitate the creation of such leaders in this new age of complexity science, major changes must occur in how leadership is perceived and prepared through formal educational processes and mentorships. This effort will also require a receptive organizational environment with a new vision of an organizational culture.

## *New Models for Research*

Viewing HCOs from a reductionistic perspective and using the machine as a metaphor to understand dynamic and adaptive systems have clear limitations. The randomized controlled trial (RCT), often described as the gold standard of research design, comes from the tradition of reductionism and, therefore, is not sufficient for the nonlinear and dynamic nature of the CAS. This is not to say that RCTs and other research designs based on a reductionist foundation are not useful; rather, the key point is that envisioning these designs as the only approach to understanding is knowledge limiting. It is important for researchers to apply the appropriate model to the area of interest and be open to expanding paradigms and methods.

Researchers McDaniel, Lanham, and Anderson (2009) emphasize that because HCOs are CASs, the phenomena of interest tend to be dynamic and unfold in unpredictable ways, and these unfolding events are often unique. Most current research designs and methodologies fail to capture either the dynamic nature of the area of interest or the unpredictable unique occurrences. McDaniel and colleagues (2009) note that the traditional classification of research as either qualitative or quantitative is distracting and often not helpful in this setting, because both approaches begin with a question, build or test models, and aim to understand or explain phenomena of interest. Neither category alone is a perfect match for CAS, although the use of mixed-methods models in conjunction with new methodologies will more likely capture the richness of CAS and lead to better understandings. Using qualitative~quantitative research embraces a "both/and" approach rather than an "either/or" philosophy.

One recently emerging approach comprises *action research,* in which researchers incorporate action perspectives to change organizational patterns by actively engaging stakeholders in the change process (Koch & Kralik, 2006). Researchers are also using other techniques, such as *positive deviance*, to discover, for example, a unit within an organization that has significantly better outcomes or better approaches with similar resources and constraints and in which others hold the view that the unit or area is exceptional. A positive deviance approach can be used as a model for change in other areas of the organization. Another approach, *appreciative inquiry*, is used by researchers to discover and then amplify what works "well" within an organization and to discover the direction that the organizational team wants to take based on what has transpired in the past. When this strategy is employed, a culture of positive innovation can flourish.

The state of the science of CAS research is developing as well. Bar-Yam (2000) developed techniques to study nonlinear dynamics in complex systems. McDaniel and Driebe (2001) applied CAS theory to the analysis of HCOs. Agar (2004) combined ethnographic approaches with agent-based modeling to understand social systems. Nonreductionist strategies also have been frequently applied to understand large-scale systems such as hurricanes (Sornette, 2006).

Maguire, McKelvey, Mirabeau, and Oztas (2006) conducted a survey of complexity science and organizational studies. The 2009 issues of the *Journal of Evaluation in Clinical Practice* include a collection of articles on complexity science, and an ongoing section will appear in forthcoming issues. The interest in HCOs and CASs is growing, and new research methodologies are emerging to support this interest.

Recently, complexity has been applied to clinical research. Understanding the human as a complex system has led to new approaches to clinical research. Systems biology, which examines the network structures and dynamics with regard to regulatory circuits, is exploring the system's robustness in regard to adaptation to external forces, internal stability, and graceful degradation, which allows for a gradual aging process (Kitano, 2002). Complexity has been applied to multiple organ dysfunction syndrome (Seely & Christou, 2000) and sepsis (Mann, Engebretson, & Batchinsky, 2013). Research techniques that track multiple points of physiological data using computers to analyze very large data sets are now available. One example of computational analysis of these large data is analyses of fractal dynamics and presence of loss of complexity. Research in complexity is generally conducted with multidisciplinary teams, representing clinical, biological, mathematical, and computational expertise.

# Application to Health Care and Nursing

## Application to Clinical Care

With the advent of computers and the corresponding ability to manage large amounts of data quickly, interdisciplinary teams have begun to apply complexity concepts to physiology and the management of patient care. West (2008), a physicist, advocated a medical application of a complexity approach, using it to program life-support equipment to a more appropriate variability in healthy people. For example, he suggested that the patterns of respirations be studied and that the finer variability be programmed into respirators, rather than relying on a mechanically regular pulsation. Use of the complexity concept in this way addresses the adaptive pattern that can be predicted in the short run. This kind of agent-based modeling simulates the operations of complex physiological behavior in an attempt to re-create and predict the appearance of complex phenomena.

A key notion is that simple behavioral rules generate complex behavior. This principle facilitates developing supportive interventions to mimic that pattern. The pattern can be drawn from theory or from actual empirical data of an individual patient. In another application, a team of researchers in the Veterans Administration used detailed monitoring of heart rate variability in trauma victims to identify early changes in the autonomic nervous system, thereby allowing for earlier intervention than was possible with the existing technology (Salinas, 2010). This is also applied in some intensive care units, where panels of biomarkers are fed into computers that can generate patterns that might indicate a loss of complexity, allowing earlier detection of the patient's condition. Other researchers have advocated the use of complex systems modeling as a means to obtain a better understanding of the obesity epidemic (Hammond, 2009).

## Application to Nursing

Complexity science and its application to nursing, health care, and HCOs is emerging as a new paradigm capturing the interest of scholars across a number of diverse disciplines (see **Box 6–1**). The use of computers has assisted researchers in refining the research of complexity science, which in turn has inspired a new paradigm in scientific thinking. This shift in the paradigm has influenced the way that people interpret the world.

---

### Box 6–1 Complexity Science Application to Health Care

In this chapter, advanced practice nurses (APNs) are introduced to an important paradigm through which to view clinical practice and care environments in new ways. Clinically, nurses need to be aware of a new spectrum of thought that can capture the details and complexities of human physiology. Adoption of this paradigm will enable the APN to provide more individualized care to augment the adaptive capacity of the human body. Because new research findings based on complexity science are becoming available daily, it is important for APNs to understand the terminology and conceptual framework so that they can apply this new knowledge to patient care. In addition, this paradigm shift will spawn numerous applications of emergent technologies in patient care.

The complexity paradigm has major implications for health care through its application to organizations and work environments. As organizations struggle to be more responsive to internal and external issues, the ability to be flexible, adaptive, and innovative becomes essential for survival. Many organizations are beginning to apply complexity science at all levels. Nurses at all levels must understand this important framework of CAS if they are to maximize their ability to function both individually and as part of groups to sustain a dynamic and relevant organization posed for innovation and change in response to the ever more complex healthcare environment.

---

**TABLE 6–4    Sources for Further Reading**

General References of Interest

Kauffman, S. (1995). *At home in the universe: The search for laws of self-organization.* New York, NY: Oxford University Press.

Kelso, J. A. S., & Engstrom, D. A. (2006). *The complementary nature.* Cambridge, MA: MIT Press.

Stacey, R. (2001). *Complex responsive processes in organizations.* New York, NY: Routledge.

Waldrop, M. M. (1992). *Complexity: The emerging science at the edge of order and chaos.* New York, NY: Simon & Schuster.

Zimmerman, B., Lindberg, C., & Plsek, P. (1998). *Edgeware: Lessons from complexity science for health care leaders.* Bordentown, NJ: Plexus Press.

Specific to Nursing

Lindberg, C., Nash, S., & Lindberg, C. (2008). *On the edge: Nursing in the age of complexity.* Bordentown, NJ: Plexus Press.

Website

Plexus Institute: http://www.plexusinstitute.org

## Summary

The concepts of complexity are pervading many areas of study and have multiple applications to health care. A paradigm based on complexity science is congruent with the holistic paradigm that is so familiar to nursing. The ability to apply the science as well as the associated change in thinking about physiology, human beings, groups, and organizations has significant implications for the discipline of nursing. In keeping with the holistic approach, it is important to remember that the complexity perspective is complementary to the reductionistic model. Together, they offer a more complete and holistic view of the world. For further reading on complexity science and CAS, see **Table 6–4.**

## Discussion Questions

1. How does more diversity in the nursing profession relate to CASs?
2. How could some of the agent-based modeling concepts be applied to individual patient-centered care?
3. How could local units in a hospital or clinic setting apply concepts of self-organization to become more adaptive to situational demands?
4. How could the APN apply the concepts of a CAS to individual patient care?
5. Reflect on a professional or personal experience when a seemingly small incident had a much larger impact than expected. What did you learn from this experience?

# References

Agar, M. H. (2004). We have met the other and we're not all nonlinear: Ethnography as a nonlinear dynamic system. *Complexity, 10*(2), 16–24.

Anderson, R. A., Issel, L. M., & McDaniel, R. R. (2003). Nursing homes as complex adaptive systems: Relationship between management practice and resident outcomes. *Nursing Research, 52*(1), 12–21.

Baranger, M. (2009). *Chaos, complexity and entropy: A physics talk for non-physicists.* Unpublished manuscript, Massachusetts Institute of Technology.

Bar-Yam, Y. (Ed.). (2000). *Unifying themes in complex systems: Proceedings of the International Conference on Complex Systems.* Cambridge, MA: Perseus Books.

Batelden, P. B., Nelson, E. C., Edwards, W. H., Godfrey, M., & Mohr, J. J. (2003). Microsystems in health care: Part 9. Developing small clinical units to attain peak performance. *Joint Commission Journal on Quality and Patient Safety, 11*, 575–585.

Beach, M. C., Inui, T., & The Relationship-Centered Care Research Network. (2006). Relationship-centered care: A constructive reframing. *Journal of General Internal Medicine, 21*, S3–S8.

Capra, F. (2002). *The hidden connections.* New York, NY: Doubleday.

Chen, D. T., Mills, A. E., & Werhane, P. H. (2008). Tools for tomorrow's health care system: A systems-informed mental model, moral imagination, and physicians' professionalism. *Academic Medicine, 83*(8), 723–732.

Crabtree, B. F., Miller, W. L., & Strange, K. C. (2001). Understanding practice from the ground up. *Journal of Family Practice, 50*(10), 881–887.

Geary, C. R., & Schumacher, K. L. (2012). Care transitions: Integrating transition theory and complexity science concepts. *Advances in Nursing Science, 35*(3), 236–248.

Goldberger, A. (1996). Non-linear dynamics for clinicians: Chaos theory, fractals and complexity at the bedside. *Lancet, 347*, 1312–1314.

Hammond, R. A. (2009). Complex systems modeling for obesity research. *Preventing Chronic Disease: Public Health Research, Practice and Policy, 6*(3), 1–10.

Holt, T. (2004). *Complexity for clinicians.* Oxford, UK: Radcliffe Medical Press.

Institute of Medicine. (2001). *Crossing the quality chasm: A new health system for the 21st century.* Washington, DC: National Academy Press.

Jordan, M. E., Lanham, H. J., Crabtree, B. F., Nutting, P. A., Miller W. L., Strange, K. C., & McDaniel, R. R. (2009). The role of conversation in health care interventions: Enabling sensemaking and learning. *Implementation Science, 4*(15). Open access BioMed Central. Retrieved from http://www.implementationscience.com/content/4/1/15

Kauffman, S. (1995). *At home in the universe: The search for laws of self-organization.* New York, NY: Oxford University Press.

Kelso, J. A. S., & Engstrom, D. A. (2006). *The complementary nature.* Cambridge, MA: MIT Press.

Kitano, H. (2002). Systems biology: A brief overview. *Science, 295*(560), 1162–1664.

Koch, T., & Kralik, D. (2006). *Participatory action research in health care.* Malden, MA: Blackwell.

Lanham, H. J., McDaniel, R. R., Crabtree, B. R., Miller, W. L., Strange, K. C., Tallia, A. F., & Nutting, P. A. (2009). How improving practice relationships among clinicians and nonclinicians can improve quality in primary care. *The Joint Commission Journal on Quality and Patient Safety, 35*(9), 457–466.

Liebovitz, L. S. (1998). *Fractals and chaos simplified for the life sciences.* New York, NY: Oxford University Press.

Lindberg, C., Nash, S., & Lindberg, C. (2008). *On the edge: Nursing in the age of complexity.* Bordentown, NJ: Plexus Press.

Lorenz, E. N. (1993). *The essence of chaos.* Seattle, WA: University of Washington Press.

Maguire, S., McKelvey, B., Mirabeau, L., & Oztas, N. (2006). Complexity science and organization studies. In S. R. Clegg, C. Hardy, T. B. Lawrence, & W. R. Nord (Eds.), *The Sage handbook of organization studies* (2nd ed., pp. 165–214). London, UK: Sage.

Mandelbrot, B. B. (1967). How long is the coast of Britain? *Science, 156,* 636–638.

Mandelbrot, B. B. (1982). *The fractal geometry of nature.* San Francisco, CA: W.H. Freeman.

Mann, E., Engebretson, J., & Batchinsky, A. (2013). A complex systems view of sepsis: Implications for nursing. *Dimensions of Critical Care Nursing, 32*(1), 12–17.

McDaniel, R. R., & Driebe, D. J. (2001). Complexity science and health care management. In J. D. Blair, M. D. Fottler, & G. T. Savage (Eds.), *Advances in health care management* (Vol. 2, pp. 11–36). Stamford, CT: JAI Press.

McDaniel, R. R., Lanham, H. J., & Anderson, R. A. (2009). Implications of complex adaptive systems theory for the design of research on health care organizations. *Health Care Management Review, 14*(2), 191–199.

Meleis, A. (2010). *Transitions theory: Middle range and situation specific theories in nursing research and practice.* New York, NY: Springer.

Norman, C. D. (2009). Health promotion as a systems science and practice. *Journal of Evaluation in Clinical Practice, 15*(5), 868–872.

Paley, J. (2007). Complex adaptive systems and nursing. *Nursing Inquiry, 14*(30), 233–242.

Phelan, S. E. (2001). What is complexity science, really? *Emergence, 3*(1), 120–136.

Plsek, P. E. (1997). *Creativity, innovation, and quality.* New York, NY: McGraw-Hill.

Plsek, P. E. (2001). Redesigning health care with insights from the science of complex adaptive systems. In Institute of Medicine, Committee on Quality of Health Care in America, *Crossing the quality chasm: A new health system for the 21st century* (pp. 322–335). Washington, DC: National Academy of Sciences.

Plsek, P. E., & Greenhalgh, T. (2001). The challenge of complexity in health care. *British Medical Journal, 323,* 625–628.

Richardson, K. A. (2005). Systems theory and complexity: Part 3. *Emergence: Complexity & Organization, 7*(2), 104–114.

Roussel (2014) should follow Rouse & Morris (1986) per alpha order.

Rouse, W. B., & Morris, N. M. (1986). On looking into the black box: Prospects and limits in the search for mental models. *Psychological Bulletin, 100,* 349–363.

Roussel, L. A. (2014). The nature of the evidence: Microsystems, macrosystems, and mesosystems. In H. R. Hall & L. A. Roussel, *Evidence-based practice: An integrative approach to research, administration, and practice* (pp. 171–184). Burlington, MA: Jones & Bartlett Learning.

Salinas, J. (2010). *Analysis, classification, and complexity of physiologic signals to support medical decision support: Why is my computer smarter than me????* Presentation at University of Texas–Houston School of Nursing, February 2, 2010.

Seely, A. J. E., & Christou, N. V. (2000). Multiple organ dysfunction syndrome: Exploring the paradigm of complex nonlinear systems. *Critical Care Medicine, 28*(7), 2193–2200.

Sornette, D. (2006). *Critical phenomena in natural sciences: Chaos, fractals, self-organization and disorder: Concepts and tools* (2nd ed.). Berlin, Germany: Springer-Verlag.

Stacey, R. (2001). *Complex responsive processes in organizations.* New York, NY: Routledge.

Sturmberg, J. P., & Martin, C. M. (2009). Complexity and health: Yesterday's traditions, tomorrow's future. *Journal of Evaluation in Clinical Practice, 15*(5), 543–548.

Suchman, A. (2006). A new theoretical foundation for relationship-centered care: Complex responsive process of relating. *Journal of General Internal Medicine, 21*, 40–44.

Waldrop, M. M. (1992). *Complexity: The emerging science at the edge of order and chaos.* New York, NY: Simon & Schuster.

Werhane, P. H. (1999). *Moral imagination and management decision making* (pp. 11–12). New York, NY: Oxford University Press.

West, B. (2008). A physicist looks at physiology. In C. Lindberg, S. Nash, & C. Lindberg, *On the edge: Nursing in the age of complexity* (pp. 97–123). Bordentown, NJ: Plexus Press.

Wilson, E. O. (1992). *The diversity of life.* Cambridge, MA: Belknap Press.

Wilson, T., Holt, T., & Greenhalgh, T. (2001). Complexity science: Complexity and clinical care. *British Medical Journal, 323*, 685–688.

Zimmerman, B., Lindberg, C., & Plsek, P. (1998). *Edgeware: Lessons from complexity science for health care leaders.* Bordentown, NJ: Plexus Press.

# Critical Theory and Emancipatory Knowing

*Peggy L. Chinn*

## Introduction

This chapter provides an overview of emancipatory knowing and the critical philosophy and theory upon which emancipatory knowing is founded. Emphasis is placed on the importance of critical perspectives for best practices in nursing. The chapter provides specific guidelines for developing and evaluating nursing practice based on critical approaches.

*Emancipatory knowing* in nursing is a term that refers to a pattern of knowing that has conceptual roots in critical social theory and practice. Critical social theory is a general perspective that uncovers social, historical, and ideological forces and structures that limit human potential and that produce injustice and inequity in society. Emancipatory knowing in nursing is defined by Chinn and Kramer (2010) as "the human capacity to be aware of and critically reflect on the social, cultural, and political status quo, and to figure out how and why it came to be that way." In short, emancipatory knowing is a central, critical, and necessary pattern of knowing that underpins the development of all nursing knowledge and that shapes all nursing practices that flow from nursing's disciplinary knowledge.

The critical philosophical perspective of emancipatory knowing frames social problems as circumstances that are unjustly created by humans. Furthermore, it posits that humans can change these circumstances. All too often, however, the social order is taken for granted and assumed to just be "the way things are." In fact, social structures have developed over generations and are well entrenched. Thus, they typically have been thought not to be open to challenge, even when the structure sustains serious injustices and harm.

Politics is the process of exercising one's values and desires in a social situation. Critical perspectives view all human activities as political, in the sense that what humans do and say inevitably affects others. When human actions harm or disadvantage others, or limit human potential in any way, those actions are inherently wrong and need to be changed so that no member of the society is harmed or disadvantaged.

Despite the persistent assumption that nurses shy away from political matters, the fact remains that nursing practice, by definition, is inherently and deeply political. Put simply, a fundamental goal of nursing is to bring about maximum health and well-being for every individual, family, and community. This goal is intentionally aimed at establishing an explicit value in a social community. To accomplish this goal, nurses must remain constantly vigilant in identifying circumstances that impede its achievement. The more deeply nurses probe to identify and address the underlying causes or circumstances that create barriers to maximum health and well-being, the closer they come to identifying social, cultural, and political barriers that limit the potential for maximum health (Kagan, Smith, Cowling, & Chinn, 2009).

Consider, for example, a relatively simple low-tech nursing activity—setting up and conducting a clinic to provide health screening, monitoring, and supervision for elders served by a community senior center. Such a clinic is assumed to contribute to the health and well-being of the people to be served, and to promote their achievement of optimal health. Typically, establishing such a clinic represents an effort to change something about the kinds of services the people can access and to provide a social network of support that was not available in the community previously. To get the clinic set up and functioning, myriad community-based arrangements are required, including the very political activities involved in working with various agencies and individuals to gain their cooperation in making the clinic a reality. Once the clinic is functioning, each individual who comes to the clinic brings with him or her huge packages of personal and social circumstances that nurses must take into account if their practice is to actually achieve the goal of improving the health of the individual and the community.

The package of individual circumstance that individuals bring with them to the clinic is, in turn, wrapped in a complex network of social factors that influence the effectiveness of nursing care. For example, if patients have trouble understanding their condition and the things they need to do to take care of themselves, the nurse is drawn to consider various things that might be contributing to this challenge—for example, media messages, family and cultural belief systems, overriding economic concerns, and unspoken fears based on misperceptions. Each possible barrier is not simply an individual's problem; it has roots in social relations and circumstances, and effective nursing approaches must address those underlying roots.

This chapter begins with an overview of the fundamental patterns of knowing in nursing. It then provides a brief explanation of the underlying philosophy and theory on which emancipatory knowing is based, with a particular emphasis on how the philosophy and theory are made visible in advanced nursing practice.

Next, the chapter outlines criteria for assessing and developing advanced nursing practice from an emancipatory perspective. The final sections of the chapter offer an explanation of the necessity of emancipatory knowing approaches to achieve the essential competencies required for advanced nursing practice.

## Nursing's Patterns of Knowing

Barbara Carper (1978) conducted a philosophical analysis of early nursing literature and identified four fundamental patterns of knowing in nursing: (1) empirics, the science of nursing; (2) ethics, the component of moral knowledge in nursing; (3) the component of personal knowing in nursing; and (4) aesthetics, the art of nursing. Carper's analysis opened the way for a broad, comprehensive, and holistic view of nursing knowledge and nursing practice beyond the constricted confines of empirics or science alone.

However, as nurse scholars and practitioners began to delve further into the broader fundamental understandings that form a foundation for nursing, it became increasingly clear that there is yet another pattern of knowing that has long been a foundation for nursing practice. This realm of knowing, first identified in the literature by Jill White (1995), was identified as sociopolitical knowing. Later, Chinn and Kramer (2007) developed a conceptualization of emancipatory knowing that embraced White's conceptualization but expanded it to emphasize the nature of this pattern of knowing as expressed in nursing. In addition, Chinn and Kramer used the term *emancipatory* to emphasize the driving force underpinning this pattern of knowing—the universal human longing for liberation from those circumstances that limit human potential.

All patterns of knowing in nursing have both a *knowing* dimension and a *being/doing* dimension. The knowing (epistemological) dimension addresses how we come to know or understand things and what is required to admit something as knowledge. In all disciplines, methods and standards for conducting those methods exist so that the members of the discipline can agree on what is valid knowledge and what is not (meaning those things that are considered myths, falsehoods, or misconceptions). In nursing, practitioners rely on fundamental knowledge that has been verified as valid and reliable in related disciplines, as well as knowledge that has been verified within nurses' own discipline related to phenomena identified as central to processes of achieving maximum health. For example, in nursing, Mishel (1990, 1997) developed knowledge of uncertainty from her practice observations and research focusing on people's experiences of illness.

The being/doing (ontological) dimension addresses how what nurses know is manifested in who they are and what they do. This is the very practical dimension of nursing that brings knowledge and practice together as one. Nurses have a long history of sensing that knowledge (theory) and practice need to be fully integrated. Unfortunately, theory and practice have often seemed to dodge integration because nursing theory development and academic research have tended to be a dominant focus in discussions of nursing knowledge. Recognizing the crucial doing (ontological) dimension of knowing and knowledge development is a major step toward a more complete integration of theory and practice.

For example, consider what it means to know and understand Mishel's theory of uncertainty. One can read all that has been written about this theory, including the reports of the research studies that were conducted to develop aspects of the theory. Nurses would probably think about what all this might mean for their practice. Understanding the theory might shift their perceptions of who they are and how they respond when working with someone who is struggling to cope with a difficult illness experience. As nurses experience this shift in practice, they become more aware of things about the experience that are as yet poorly understood; in response, they may seek new evidence, or knowledge, concerning this experience. This scenario is a circle of knowing and doing—a close connection between practice and theory that is not often acknowledged but that often enters into daily nursing. This kind of connection is increasingly being recognized and promoted by recent movements toward evidence-based practice, practice-based evidence, and translational research.

## Philosophical and Theoretical Foundations of Emancipatory Knowing in Nursing

Emancipatory knowing and the methods that flow from this pattern of knowing are grounded in several fundamental assumptions:

- *There is no ahistorical, value-neutral knowledge.* All knowledge is constructed by humans and is saturated with value-laden and culturally situated perceptions. That which is taken as "true" or "real" is shaped by humans and can shift over time and over different contexts.
- *Research is a political activity.* Even the act of forming a research question is grounded in human values, intentions, and vested interests. The choice of research focus and the results that flow from this activity shape human actions and interactions.
- *Power relations inform knowledge development.* Those who conduct knowledge development activities have the privileges of a certain kind of academic experience and the economic privilege that is required for this experience. Their social position in society carries with it a privileged lens that shapes all knowledge development activities.
- *Language is constructed to carry power meanings.* Modern English discourse is saturated with militaristic, adversarial, and confrontational metaphors and expressions. Most of this language is not even recognized as carrying power meanings, but these meanings do, in fact, shape our perceptions and attitudes.
- *Social oppressions are not natural or fixed.* Social structures are constructed by humans and can be changed. In fact, social structures evolve and change over time, shaped by emerging contexts and circumstances.

People can let change happen, but it is in their best interest to help shape the course of change in a direction of creating justice for all.

These fundamental assumptions are shared by a number of philosophers and theorists who are generally recognized as advocating a critical social perspective (Kagan et al., 2009). The ideas of two significant philosophers who have formed the foundation for nursing's emancipatory critical perspective—Jürgen Habermas and Paulo Freire—are summarized in the following sections.

## Habermas's Critical Social Philosophy

Habermas's (1973, 1979, 1981) critical social philosophy is concerned with everyday life and the practices that sustain people on a daily basis. A very pragmatic philosophy, it is one of the first philosophical approaches to recognize that understanding of the world requires a number of different approaches. These traits make this line of thought particularly appealing from a nursing perspective. After all, nursing deals with the most ordinary, and yet deeply significant, realities of life—illness, death, activities of daily living, and human relationships. In addition, nursing is grounded in the recognition that daily human experience is complex and requires many different approaches in order to be understood in ways that support effective nursing practice.

Habermas's works are massive and complex and cover immense philosophical, political, and theoretical territory. The brief discussion presented here touches on central ideas that form the foundation for the concept of emancipatory knowing. This philosopher's ideas are centrally concerned with the public sphere and the communicative action that sustains public life. Communicative competence is a unique human capacity that has evolved over time to create social and political structures that are necessary for social coexistence. However, forces that create dominance and advantage for some, and disadvantage and injustice for others, have suppressed capacity for communicative competence. Habermas's philosophy and theory are intended to provide a framework for emancipation from such social forces of injustice.

Habermas described three human interests that are fundamental to everyday life: technical, practical, and emancipatory. Each interest demands its own method and involves a particular kind of knowledge that makes human survival possible.

*Technical interest* involves the human interest and capacity to work with and create tools and systems that make it possible to carry out daily activities of living. It is rooted in the human interest in predicting and controlling the environment. Technical interest requires empirical methods that measure things, predict outcomes based on statistical significance, and calculate probabilities of natural phenomena. A significant portion of nursing and health care involves our technical interest—for example, drugs and interventions to treat illness, knowledge and use of nutrition for maintaining health, and knowledge and use of physical activity as it relates to health and well-being.

*Practical interest* is concerned with what Habermas termed *communicative* functions of life—the ways that people seek to get along with one another and to understand themselves within the context in which they live. Practical interest is vital to survival, to getting along with others, and to forming meaningful connections with acquaintances, friends, and family. Practical interest requires interpretive/philosophical methods that provide interpretive insight into the illusive yet vital human experiences of interacting with one another. The significant aspects of nursing that involve our caring relationships with individuals, families, and communities—the art of nursing—all involve professionals' practical interest.

*Emancipatory interest* is the human capacity to recognize that something in the social milieu is wrong, unjust, or failing, and subsequently the human impulse to make things right. Emancipatory interest also involves the capacity to recognize self-deception and the ideologies that shape human perception of the world. This feat requires the use of critical methods to probe for underlying patterns that arise from ideologies, often shaping circumstances of inequality and injustice. Critical methods seek understanding of social structures and interactions that create and sustain unjust circumstances within the status quo. Nursing concerns for promoting health and well-being for individuals and communities require our emancipatory interest.

## Freire's Theory of Human Liberation

Paulo Freire's theory of human liberation was developed from his experience of instituting an unorthodox form of literacy education among sugar cane workers in Brazil during a time when literacy was required to vote. His approach to education is described in his classic book *Pedagogy of the Oppressed* (Freire, 1970), which remains the foundational work for all critical approaches in education, as well as in other disciplines.

Freire explained the conditions that sustain privilege for some and disadvantage for others and outlined specific propositions that point these parties in the direction toward liberation and freedom. Along the way, Freire identified certain traits that tend to dominate the life space of those who are privileged, who are called *the oppressor* in his early works:

- The dominant group is powerful and unified.
- Those who are privileged fail to recognize others as human, meaning that .those who are not part of the dominant group are assumed to be "others" and are subject to manipulation and control.
- Those who are privileged have a consciousness and ethic of self-interest, and they use their power and privilege to sustain their own interests.
- The dominant group prescribes and defines reality for all, often in subtle ways, so that the status quo ends up being viewed by all as "the way things are" (hegemony).
- The dominant group exploits and manipulates others without apology.

By contrast, those who are disadvantaged (termed *the oppressed* in Freire's early works) exhibit traits that complement the traits of the dominant group and that serve to help sustain the circumstances of their disadvantage:

- The oppressed are powerless and divided. Their lack of unity contributes to their powerlessness, which in turn sustains the privilege enjoyed by the dominant group.
- Because they are not granted the rights and responsibilities of full humanity, the oppressed are prevented from being authentic; they are barred from realizing their full human potential.
- Those who are disadvantaged think and behave according to the prescribed norms of the dominant group and assume that those norms are natural or fixed.
- Those who are disadvantaged deny the self; instead, they internalize the consciousness of the oppressor.
- Those who are disadvantaged are exploited and manipulated and because they deny the self, they do not typically recognize their own exploitation.

These complementary characteristics of the dominant and disadvantaged groups exist not by individual will or intention, but rather because of systematic conditions inherent in the social structure that sustain injustice. Even those who are privileged often do not recognize their own self-interest and the actions that sustain exploitation of others.

Within an unjust social system, those with power and privilege can seem generous when they demonstrate even small, insignificant acts of generosity, which, in fact, do little or nothing to change the injustice of the system. Educational opportunities are distributed unequally, with those who are relatively oppressed being denied access to adequate education. Specifically, oppressed groups are not taught their own history; as a consequence, they are not able to see their circumstance in its historical context, and they do not understand the roots of the divisiveness that exists in their own group. People who are disadvantaged tend to avoid forming associations with members of their own group—they do not join organizations with others of their own group, but instead they invest time and energy into becoming involved in the activities of those who are privileged.

Individuals in the oppressed group are vulnerable to being used as tokens, because they believe the illusion that pleasing or serving the oppressor will eventually garner more power and privilege for those who are relatively disadvantaged. When members of the oppressed group do achieve some relative status (usually by token acts of generosity), they tend to become the oppressors of those who are now subordinate to them.

Furthermore, systematically embedded conditions make action toward liberation very difficult in these circumstances. The relative power of those who are privileged conveys the illusion that they are right, that their perspective is good and to be desired. Related to the internalization of this notion that those who are privileged are right, disadvantaged groups tend to see themselves as incapable of taking risks and sometimes even as deserving of their present situation. It is also a frightening prospect to challenge the status quo and to seek freedom, because examples exist of the dangers that come to those who act. For example, when individuals do begin to act in a manner seeking liberation from disadvantage, they are often subjected to danger, ridicule, firing from a job, or other feared outcomes. The message to the oppressed is clear: It is safer to not "rock the boat."

What is required for liberation, for moving toward freedom from the constraints of disadvantage, is actually quite simple yet very difficult to do. First, disadvantaged groups must become aware of their situation, of the limits of the context in which they exist. This process, which has been termed *consciousness raising* in feminist and other activist groups, involves coming to realize one's own consciousness and becoming aware of the actual circumstances of one's own situation. Beyond the basic consciousness of the limits of the situation, liberation requires *consciousness of actions* that are feasible but have not yet been tried or tested—the untested feasibilities.

To take action requires unity with others who are also disadvantaged—it is not possible to take action alone (see **Box 7–1**). Together, groups of people begin to test the feasibility of possible actions. Most important, it is essential for the steps toward liberation to be fully and consciously grounded in love for self *and* for those who are privileged—the oppressor. It is this grounding in love, for both self and the oppressor, that makes it possible for people to move toward liberation without becoming, in turn, the oppressors of those subordinate to them (Freire, 1970).

## Implications of the Philosophy and Theory for Practice

If you are a reader who has typically thought of philosophy and theory as unrelated to practice, ideally the discussion so far has conveyed a sense of how vitally important one's own philosophy and theoretical perspective are in shaping the nature of one's practice. Because an emancipatory approach is so dramatically different from the traditional approaches to both theory and practice, it requires a more complete explanation than other individual-focused perspectives on which practice and theory are based. Once an emancipatory perspective is brought to bear on an individual's practice, several shifts become possible. The shifts include, but are not limited to, viewing the problems that people bring to health care as intrinsically linked to social and political processes, recognizing the need for action to change social circumstances, and recognizing the potential for every person to become an agent for change. The following sections detail the various ways in which an emancipatory perspective shapes the reality of nursing practice.

### Emancipatory Nursing Practice

Joyce Fontana (2004) conducted an analysis of the foundations of critical/emancipatory scholarship and the various published works in nursing that were conducted using critical approaches. She identified seven traits that characterize critical

## Box 7–1 Application of Freire's Theory of Liberation

Jane and her best friend Sue have worked together on a surgical unit for more than 10 years. To celebrate their long and close working relationship, they plan an overnight getaway at a spa, where they can be pampered with great meals (cooked by someone else!), saunas, massages, pedicures, and manicures. When they arrive at the spa late in the afternoon on Friday, they begin with massages and some relaxing time in the sauna. They then enjoy an exquisitely prepared dinner. Over dinner, Jane shares with Sue that she has enrolled in a Doctor of Nursing Practice (DNP) program to become an advanced practice nurse. Sue is shocked; usually Jane tells her about something like this long before it actually happens. The news that Jane has already decided, and has enrolled, throws her off balance. Sue gathers her composure and offers a toast to Jane's new adventure, and they continue to enjoy their good time together.

When Sue arrives home, she becomes aware of her growing resentment that Jane has made this decision. She decides to talk to Jane about it when they take their break on Monday. When Sue brings up the subject, she explains that she wishes Jane had told her about what she was doing. Sue says, "Jane, you know I can't afford to go into the DNP program, and I wish you well, but I wish you had told me you were thinking about this. But, most of all, I hope that this change in your life won't interfere with our friendship." Jane brushes off the comment and assures her that they will remain close friends.

Sue and Jane do remain close for a while, but gradually Jane begins to be critical of everything that Sue and other staff nurses are doing, and they begin to see Jane as having a chip on her shoulder and acting in a "holier than thou" manner. Eventually Jane moves on to a private practice, but occasionally she comes back to the unit to see her patients. She is cordial, but she makes demands on the staff nurses as if she had never been part of their life. The staff nurses, in turn, resist following Jane's orders and try to avoid her as much as possible. When one of them does cooperate with Jane, the others tend to view their staff nurse colleague as "sucking up" to Jane, and resentment builds among the staff nurses.

Based on Freire's theory of liberation, consider the following questions related to this situation:

1. What, theoretically, is going on here?
2. What needs to happen for this situation to change?
3. What is the most important factor for real change to occur?
4. How would you feel if you were one of the staff nurses hearing this theoretical explanation?
5. If you were Jane, how would you feel if someone explained this situation to you in terms of Freire's theory?

work in nursing: (1) critique, (2) context, (3) politics, (4) emancipatory intent, (5) democratic structure, (6) dialectic analysis, and (7) reflexivity. These seven traits are explained in the following subsections in relation to nursing practice. Fontana focused on critical research, but critical methods do not draw a firm line of distinction between research and practice. Because critical emancipatory approaches require participation by those who are disadvantaged and aim to achieve change in their lives, a research project is also *practice*.

Drawing on Fontana's conceptualization, the sections that follow describe the features of emancipatory practice in relation to nursing. Examples are drawn from the Nurse Manifest projects, which were designed to explore the circumstances of practice that limit nurses' ability to practice nursing as they themselves wish to practice (Jacobs, Fontana, Kehoe, Matarese, & Chinn, 2005; Jarrin, 2006; *Nurse Manifest Research Study Report*, 2002). Examples are also drawn from a project in which a nurse engaged adolescent girls in examining the experience of menarche, which illustrates an emancipatory approach in practice (Hagedorn, 1995).

## Critique

Assuming that people have a desire to be free of constraints that limit them, critique is central to critical methods in emancipatory nursing practice. From a critical perspective, this activity involves much more than simply taking stock of a situation to figure out what is wrong (as in problem solving). Rather, critique requires an analysis that exposes the political and social structures that sustain patterns of injustice and imbalance (Fontana, 2004). In practice, it typically requires a group of people who first examine their experiences of a situation on an individual basis and then, working as a group, begin to identify the common dynamics of each of their unique experiences. Given the assumption that all humans have an emancipatory interest, as soon as people recognize the conditions of their experience that constrain their human potential, they shift to figuring out how to eliminate these barriers and change the situation.

For example, in the project reported by Hagedorn (1995), adolescent girls shared stories of their own menarche. When they did so, they began to realize that—contrary to their preconceived assumption—they were not alone in their experience. Their critique of their experiences led them to examine the social and political forces that shaped their experience, including the roles of culture, the influence of the for-profit corporate entities that sell menstrual care products, and the lack of appropriate education for girls related to menarche.

## Context

Emancipatory methods are fully situated in the circumstances of daily life. As a consequence, the people who are directly affected by the conditions of disadvantage and injustice play central roles as active participants (not subjects), whether it is a research project or a clinical project (Fontana, 2004). Allies who are relatively advantaged, or at least not seriously disadvantaged in the situation, can join with those who are directly experiencing injustice or limitations, but allies are always present only to facilitate, encourage, and support those who are the central actors in the situation (Chinn & Kramer, 2010).

The process of taking the project to the people and their context was demonstrated in powerful ways in Freire's (1970) early work, which, as mentioned, focused on teaching Brazilian sugar cane workers to read. Freire and his fellow teachers went into the villages and spent time simply experiencing the conditions of the lives of the workers. Through this effort, they developed a stance of complete love and respect for the people and a fuller understanding of their lives. Rather than announcing at the outset that they were there to teach the people to read, the teachers began by inviting small groups of workers to examine photos and drawings of ordinary life experiences in the village and simply asked the question, "What is going on in this picture?" Freire called the pictures "codifications"—things that illustrated the ordinariness of daily life.

As people began to discuss what was going on, they recognized dynamics of their situation that were not right and needed to change. Their recognitions did not necessarily differ from what the teachers might have identified, but their personal, inner recognition brought with it a realization of their own authentic consciousness—not a consciousness based on what someone else told them to think or see.

## Politics

Critical approaches, in contrast to most mainstream approaches to research and practice, acknowledge up front the value basis of the work. Philosophically, critical science is based on the assumption that all research and all human actions are political in the sense that they enact values in the world and, by doing so, affect the world and others who inhabit that world. However, most scientists, scholars, and practitioners do not overtly acknowledge their value stance or their political intentions, and they may not be consciously aware of this aspect of their work. In contrast, those who work from a critical perspective make explicit their fundamental intent to expose injustice and discrimination and their plan to initiate steps to correct these conditions.

For example, in the various Nurse Manifest projects, the facilitators of each project conveyed to potential nurse participants their concern for the contexts in which nurses are practicing—the strained economy, the shortage of nurses, the demands placed on nurses to work long hours, and so forth—and their hope that the project would lead to new ideas about how to change those situations. The groups began their discussion based on a simple question concerning their experience of practicing nursing: "What is it like to practice nursing today?" (Jarrin, 2006).

## Emancipatory Intent

Closely related to politics is the emancipatory intent that is explicit in any critical approach. This intent shapes an emancipatory approach from the outset, requiring that the people who are most directly affected by a situation of injustice be central. Their perceptions and voices must dominate any discourse and must be fully respected. This intent is fully disclosed at the outset, but with the clear understanding that the facilitators or caregivers do not come with preconceived ideas about what is required to make the situation better for those who are involved. Rather, people are assured that any ideas or solutions or actions that might come from their discussion will be their ideas, and that the role of any ally or facilitator will be to support their exploration of what is feasible as they test the various options for action that might be considered.

The actions that arose from the Nurse Manifest projects were typically not large or earth-shattering, but they were significant in a very practical sense. The outcomes included (but were not limited to) significant shifts in awareness among the participating nurses concerning the historical and political contexts of their work, awareness of the importance of working together and supporting one another, increased respect for nurses and nursing, renewed determination to gain control over their own priorities, and working toward finding nursing's own voice in the healthcare system (Jarrin, 2006).

Likewise, in the project in which adolescent females explored their experience of menarche, the immediate outcome was an educational video that the young women made themselves, which both reported the findings of their discussions and fact-finding projects and sought to educate younger women about the experience of menarche. Their primary conclusion was that menarche education should not be provided by the corporations that sell menstrual care products, but rather should be designed and conducted by "peers"—adolescent girls who best understand the challenges of the experience and can best convey to younger girls what to expect and how to manage their menstruation once it starts (Hagedorn, 1995).

## Democratic Structure

All who participate in an emancipatory project are equal agents; the processes used are collegial, with every participant learning from others and also teaching others. There is no one voice of authority. Instead, all aspects of the project are negotiated among equals, and leadership shifts based on the needs of the group and the particular capabilities of each participant. Given that this approach is not the way in which most people are accustomed to working together, accomplishing a democratic structure that places everyone on equal footing requires conscious effort and willingness by each participant to own responsibility for the process itself and to turn the critical lens inward to better shape the democratic ideal.

In the Nurse Manifest projects, groups used variations of the processes described in *Peace and Power* (Chinn, 2013). When groups convene for discussion using this process, each person has equal opportunity to speak. A discussion begins with everyone checking in to share their intentions for the discussion; it ends with each person speaking to share critical reflections on the discussion and ideas for what that individuals hopes will happen next. During the discussion, a process of "rotating chair" is used, in which the person who is speaking recognizes the next person to speak (instead of a single "chair" calling on people to speak). Jacobs and her colleagues (2005) described the role of the researcher or leader in a group using this process, illustrating how a leader can shape a genuinely democratic process without imposing the leader's own will on the group:

> The role of the researchers was to engage the participants in the initial identification of codifications, to respectfully hear the views of all participants, pose questions, and suggest possibilities to assist in discovering background awareness of the dialectical relations between two or more dimensions of reality. (p. 10)

The experience of participating in a group that functions in this manner is itself an experience of empowerment and change, and adapting this approach to group interactions was the major recommendation of the Jacobs report (Jacobs et al., 2005).

## Dialectic Analysis

Emancipatory approaches focus on understanding the many contradictory elements of any social structure, but particularly the contradictions between the ideal and the real. A critical approach assumes that the totality of the world involves contradiction, or seemingly opposing sides that in actuality constitute the whole—day and night, front and back, general and specific, abstract and concrete, thought and action, subjective and objective, global and local. Each component of a contradiction must be understood if one is to understand the whole.

In the Nurse Manifest projects, nurses realized that they already knew the ideal but that they had lost sight of what might be possible because of their immersion in the realities of daily nursing. Exploring the ideal brought into better focus the situation of their real-world practice and engendered new realizations of ways in which the ideal could be feasible. The simple yet challenging personal project of gaining a sense of respect for other nurses and finding ways to support one another gradually became viewed as actually possible. Through this process, participants come to see themselves as active agents, rather than passive objects subject to others' dominance (Jacobs et al., 2005).

## Reflexivity

Reflexivity means examining not only what the nurse and the group are doing, but examining how you are doing what you are doing. The central question that focuses this kind of reflective commitment is "Do I know what I do, and do I do what I know?" Given the democratic nature of this approach, each individual engages in this kind of personal reflection, and the group also discusses and shares individual insights with one another concerning the activities of the group.

In groups that use the processes outlined in *Peace and Power* (Chinn, 2013), critical reflections shared at the end of each gathering serve to bring this ideal into reality. This exercise becomes one of the most valuable aspects of working together to create change. Everyone in the group respects each member's reflections on how the group is functioning and how well their shared intentions and values are expressed in their actions. Each shared perspective reveals insights for everyone about the struggle of overcoming the tendencies associated with the dominant power structure and the challenges of creating social and political change.

## Emancipatory Knowing and the Essentials of Advanced Nursing Practice

Emancipatory knowing, and the approaches that flow from this pattern of knowing, are essential for anyone who is a nurse, whether one is practicing as a staff nurse, nurse manager, administrator, educator, researcher, or advanced practice nurse in a specialty area. Most of the nursing literature that describes emancipatory approaches focuses on research methods (see, for example, Fontana, 2004; Jarrin, 2006; Kagan et al., 2009) or nursing education (see, for example, Anthony & Landeen, 2009; Falk-Rafael, Anderson, Chinn, & Rubotzky, 2004; Falk-Rafael, Chinn, Anderson, Laschinger, & Rubotzky, 2003).

Emancipatory knowing lies at the heart of nursing practice, even though it is not typically acknowledged explicitly. Bringing forth awareness of this vital component of knowing and action provides a bridge to actualize the ideals of nursing practice, particularly the ideals of advanced nursing practice. To illustrate, consider the *Essentials of Doctoral Education for Advanced Nursing Practice* (2006), which the American Association of Colleges of Nursing formulated as a guide for the development of advanced nursing practice roles. The first seven of the *Essentials* address competencies for advanced nursing practice in all specialties:

1. Scientific underpinnings for practice
2. Organizational and systems leadership for quality improvement and systems thinking
3. Clinical scholarship and analytical methods for evidence-based practice
4. Information systems/technology and patient care technology for the improvement and transformation of health care
5. Healthcare policy for advocacy in health care
6. Interprofessional collaboration for improving patient and population health outcomes
7. Clinical prevention and population health for improving the nation's health

The following subsections outline ways in which an emancipatory approach can vitally strengthen each of these essential competencies.

### Essential I: Scientific Underpinnings for Practice

An emancipatory lens is essential in determining adequate scientific underpinnings for practice. This determination requires questioning the value and worth of what is taken to be a scientific underpinning. An *emancipatory critique* goes deeper than simply determining the methodological strengths and weaknesses of research reports and begins to ask questions like these:

- What ideology does this report reflect?
- Which biases and implied assumptions shaped the design and outcomes of this study?
- Who benefits if these findings are used as a basis for practice?
- Does this report adequately account for the social and political context of the people for whom I provide care?

These questions are not only posed by individual nurses, but they are also used as a basis for discussion among members of the team evaluating scientific worth.

## Essential II: Organizational and Systems Leadership for Quality Improvement and Systems Thinking

Emancipatory knowing and the approaches that flow from this pattern of knowing are, by definition, *systems thinking*. This pattern of knowing demands not simply a local systems approach, but a global, social, and political systems approach. The emancipatory processes described in *Peace and Power* (Chinn, 2013) provide a kind of leadership that moves organizations and systems to seek quality improvement constantly on a level that goes beyond something that can be easily measured. When teams of individuals who are providing care come together in small, meaningful discussions to examine not only what they are doing but also how they are doing it, each person becomes invested in the processes required to improve the care that is provided, as well as the conditions of their own experience in the workplace.

This kind of emancipatory leadership is facilitative rather than prescriptive and supportive rather than demanding. During work with nurses involved in daily nursing care roles, it becomes clear that nurses deeply yearn to create conditions in which they can provide the highest quality of care. Leadership that facilitates the impulse to bring this ideal into reality is, indeed, transformative.

## Essential III: Clinical Scholarship and Analytical Methods for Evidence-Based Practice

Clinical scholarship that is founded in an emancipatory approach brings together scholarship and practice in ways that are not possible with research approaches that lack this perspective. Emancipatory approaches do not prescribe a method; rather, any research method can be employed as a component of an emancipatory project.

For example, the adolescent women who explored their experience of menarche used their group discussion as a basis for undertaking a qualitative analysis of the common elements of their unique experience. From this discussion, however, they grew curious about the larger social, historical, and cultural forces that had shaped their experience. Once they realized that the corporations that sell menstrual care products also produced all of the educational materials they had been given about menarche, they gathered evidence of the corporate motives (profit) that shaped the approaches and content that were presented in these materials. The young women's findings led them to engage in a more critical appraisal of the educational materials that are produced by these companies. For example, the adolescents sought evidence of the nature of the menarche experience in cultures other than their own and discovered that this event in a young woman's life was treated as a sacred event in Native American cultures, leading to their realization of the mutability of their own Eurocentric experiences. They interviewed their mothers and grandmothers to gain a sense of the generational roots of their own experiences. They conducted a survey of all schools in their district to determine if there was variability between and among schools in how menarche education was conducted. They accomplished all of this research and produced the video documenting their experience, in the course of one semester (Hagedorn, 1995).

In addition to the diversity of methods that can be employed, the example of the adolescent women's project illustrates the kinds of questions that arise from an emancipatory perspective, which tend to broaden and deepen the exploration of what might be considered evidence for practice. Emancipatory scholarship demands asking questions such as "Who will benefit if we base our practice on this evidence?," Who will be disadvantaged?," and "Which ideology (or stereotype) does this evidence sustain?"

### Essential IV: Information Systems/Technology and Patient Care Technology for the Improvement and Transformation of Health Care

Several critical questions that an emancipatory lens focuses on technology are vital in determining the worth and desirability of technological tools:

- Is this technology appropriate for the people we serve and in the context in which we work?
- What are the underlying motivations in adopting and using this technology?
- Who actually benefits from this technology?
- Does this technology actually improve and transform care, or does it serve other interests, such as profit or aggrandizement for some at the expense of others?

### Essential V: Healthcare Policy for Advocacy in Health Care

The policy initiatives that emerge from a grassroots level, which by definition is inherent in emancipatory approaches, are those that best serve the interests of the people. Allies and advocates are essential in the policy-making process, of course. Rather than imposing policy on groups of people, emancipatory approaches take the discussion to the people, and allies and advocates follow the will of the people. When examining policy initiatives, the questions posed from an emancipatory perspective can guide both grassroots activists and allies/advocates in selecting and refining the ideals they seek through policy:

- Who benefits?
- Who is disadvantaged?

- Which social values does this policy reflect?
- From which motives does this policy arise?
- Is this policy good for the health of all members of our community?

## Essential VI: Interprofessional Collaboration for Improving Patient and Population Health Outcomes

Emancipatory approaches demand the involvement of all who are party to a situation. Therefore, all members of a healthcare team or provider unit, as well as people served in the community, must collaborate in any project that arises from an emancipatory perspective. The initial commitment, and then the subsequent effort required to make this happen, are immense—but the benefits are immeasurable. When every voice is heard, when people have a meaningful role to play in a situation, and when people are given the opportunity to understand a situation from the outset, the chances of achieving good cooperation and collaboration in providing high quality care are significantly increased.

## Essential VII: Clinical Prevention and Population Health for Improving the Nation's Health

Because emancipatory thinking is an upstream approach, by definition it leads to prevention and population health. A parable-like story is often used to illustrate upstream thinking: A small group of people were walking along a river, and they saw a child being swept downstream, desperately struggling to get out of the current and reach the shore. One of the walkers dove into the river and pulled the child to shore. Before long, another child came along being swept by the current, then another, and another. Finally, one of the walkers said, "I am going to walk upstream and find out who is throwing these children into the water, and stop what they are doing." Emancipatory approaches ask the fundamental question: What is happening upstream to create the patterns of injustice, discrimination, and disadvantage?

This approach seeks to understand patterns within a social and political structure that are much less obvious than children being swept down a river. An emancipatory lens also brings the patterns into focus as a social construction that can be changed. Understanding the social structures that create and sustain such patterns is essential to change what is happening and, in turn, is key to successful prevention efforts aimed at improving population health.

## Summary

Clearly, the challenges inherent in modern-day nursing and health care are immense. Emancipatory perspectives provide a lens that may seem to make the challenge more complex and more difficult, in that this approach shifts to a more global, deeper probing of the issues and problems than is required from other perspectives. Even so, given the assumption that the challenges are created and sustained within a social and political structure, the most effective approaches for addressing the challenges must lie within the realm of the social and political. Emancipatory knowledge, and the approaches that flow from it, provides a means to move in this direction and, in turn, to better meet the needs of those who receive nursing care.

## Discussion Questions

1. Think about a recent situation in nursing that you recognized as needing to change in some way and share your reflections with others in your group.

2. Did you take action to change the situation in Question 1? If not, why not? If so, consider the following:

   a. Who did you connect with in some way to create change?
   b. What were the barriers that you faced in making the change?
   c. What facilitated getting something done?
   d. Looking back, what would you do differently next time around?

3. Identify an object, painting, or picture that represents to you the current practice of nursing. Identify another object, painting, or picture that represents to you what the practice of nursing should or could be at its best. Share what each of these representations means with others in your group and identify common ground that you all have related to nursing as it is and nursing as it could be.

4. Identify a situation in nursing that you encounter frequently, preferably one that you experience as frustrating or unsatisfying. Write a brief account of a recent experience you had with this type of situation. After you have written this account, think about what tends to go through your mind as the situation unfolds and what you think needs to happen differently the next time. Imagine the situation occurring but with the changes you imagine; if possible, try to enact the situation as you imagine it might be. Share your experience with others in your group and invite them to help you imagine a different kind of experience in this situation.

5. Think about the relationships you experience (or have experienced in the past) with your coworkers. Write a brief synopsis of these relationships and then do the following:

   a. Identify the groups (or individuals) who are the most advantaged or privileged in the work environment.
   b. Identify the groups (or individuals) who are the most disadvantaged. You might identify more than two layers of relative advantage.
   c. Describe the traits of those who are advantaged and disadvantaged in light of Freire's theory of liberation.

d. Write a brief action plan, based on Freire's theory, describing what could happen to change the work situation.

e. Discuss your insights with your group, and invite their suggestions about how to change this kind of situation.

# References

American Association of Colleges of Nursing. (2006). Essentials of doctoral education for advanced nursing practice. Retrieved from http://www.aacn.nche.edu/DNP/pdf/Essentials.pdf

Anthony, S. E., & Landeen, J. (2009). Evolution of Canadian nursing curricula: A critical retrospective analysis of power and caring. *International Journal of Nursing Education Scholarship, 6*(1), 1–14. Retrieved from http://www.degruyter.com/view/j/ijnes.2009.6.1/ijnes.2009.6.1.1766/ijnes.2009.6.1.1766.xml?format=INT

Carper, B. A. (1978). Fundamental patterns of knowing in nursing. *Advances in Nursing Science, 1*(1), 13–23.

Chinn, P. L. (2013). *Peace and power: New directions for building community* (8th ed.). Burlington, MA: Jones & Bartlett Learning.

Chinn, P. L., & Kramer, M. (2007). *Integrated theory and knowledge development in nursing* (7th ed.). St. Louis, MO: Mosby.

Chinn, P. L., & Kramer, M. (2010). *Integrated knowledge development in nursing* (8th ed.). St. Louis, MO: Mosby.

Falk-Rafael, A. R., Anderson, M. A., Chinn, P. L., & Rubotzky, A. M. (2004). Peace and power as a critical feminist framework for nursing education. In M. H. Oermann & K. T. Heinrich (Eds.), *Annual review of nursing education* (Vol. 2, pp. 217–235). New York, NY: Springer.

Falk-Rafael, A. R., Chinn, P. L., Anderson, M. A., Laschinger, H., & Rubotzky, A. M. (2003). The effectiveness of feminist pedagogy in empowering a community of learners. *Journal of Nursing Education, 42*(12), 1–9.

Fontana, J. S. (2004). A methodology for critical science in nursing. *Advances in Nursing Science, 27*(2), 93–101.

Freire, P. (1970). *Pedagogy of the oppressed* (M. B. Ramos, Trans.). New York, NY: Seabury Press.

Habermas, J. (1973). *Theory and practice* (J. Viertel, Trans.). Boston, MA: Beacon Press.

Habermas, J. (1979). *Communication and the evolution of society* (T. McCarthy, Trans.). Boston, MA: Beacon Press.

Habermas, J. (1981). *Theory of communicative action* (T. McCarthy, Trans.). Boston, MA: Beacon Press.

Hagedorn, S. (1995). The politics of caring: The role of activism in primary care. *Advances in Nursing Science, 17*(4), 1–11.

Jacobs, B. B., Fontana, J. S., Kehoe, M. H., Matarese, C., & Chinn, P. L. (2005). An emancipatory study of contemporary nursing practice. *Nursing Outlook, 53,* 6–14.

Jarrin, O. F. (2006). Results from the Nurse Manifest 2003 study: Nurses' perspectives on nursing. *Advances in Nursing Science, 29*(2), E74–E85.

Kagan, P. N., Smith, M. C., Cowling, W. R., & Chinn, P. L. (2009). A nursing manifesto: An emancipatory call for knowledge development, conscience, and praxis. *Nursing Philosophy, 11,* 67–84.

Mishel, M. H. (1990). Reconceptualization of the uncertainty in illness theory. *Image: The Journal of Nursing Scholarship, 22, 256.*

Mishel, M. H. (1997). Uncertainty in acute illness. In J. J. Fitzpatrick & J. S. Norbeck (Eds.), *Annual review of nursing research, 15,* 57–80. New York, NY: Springer.

Nurse Manifest 2002 research study report. (2002). Retrieved from http://www.nursemanifest. com/research_reports/2002_study/2002_study.htm

White, J. (1995). Patterns of knowing: Review, critique, and update. *Advances in Nursing Science, 17*(4), 73–86.

CHAPTER

8

# Feminist Ethics: Some Applicable Thoughts for Advanced Practice Nurses

*Rosemarie Tong*

## Introduction

Feminist approaches to ethics provide professionals in the field of nursing with nontraditional ways to examine moral issues critically, apply moral principles judiciously, and call forth human emotions appropriately. Myriad in number, these moral perspectives fall into two basic groups: *care-focused approaches* and *power-focused approaches* (Code, Mullett, & Overall, 1988; Gilligan, 1982; Jaggar, 1992; Noddings, 1984; Ruddick, 1989; Sherwin, 1992). Care-focused feminists are particularly attentive to the moral dramas that play out in the private realm. As they see it, a feminine style of moral reasoning that works to weave and maintain good human relationships is just as valid as a masculine style of moral reasoning that aims to establish just and fair universal laws. Care-focused feminists claim that individuals should try to meet others' genuine needs simply because everyone is subject to the same vicissitudes of human carnality and the inevitability of human mortality. In contrast to care-focused feminists, power-focused feminists are more intent on understanding the moral implications of power relationships, asking questions about why women usually have less social standing, economic wealth, and political clout than men. The latter feminists are generally very active politically, seeking ways to develop strategies and policies to eliminate or at least ameliorate discrimination against women and other groups of people who experience unfair and systematic subordination.

Importantly, both care-focused and power-focused feminists agree with feminist thinker Alison Jaggar (1992), who suggested that any approach to ethics that calls itself feminist must meet the following criteria: (1) view men and women as having fundamentally dissimilar life situations; (2) provide ways to undermine the "systematic subordination of women"; (3) offer methods for dealing with issues that arise in the private sphere, but particularly in domestic life; and (4) "take the moral experience of all women seriously, though not, of course, uncritically" (p. 364). Interestingly, neither care-focused nor power-focused feminists maintain that gender oppression is necessarily the worst form of human oppression. On the contrary, they assert that oppression rooted in race, class, age, nationality, health status, and so forth can be equally pernicious. Even so, gender oppression has a universality that other forms of oppression may lack. Women everywhere, to some extent or another, have less power, authority, and autonomy than men do. Because this state of affairs stubbornly persists, feminists ally with one another in an attempt to transform familial relationships, political structures, economic policies, social norms, and cultural attitudes. They insist that women—no less than men—are full human persons and, as such, deserve the same respect and standing that men have. This chapter examines several feminist perspectives in the hope that nurses may find them of use in their lives and work.

## Care-Focused Feminist Approaches to Ethics

Care-focused feminists spend considerable time explaining the differences between an *ethics of justice* (rights) and an *ethics of care* (responsibilities and relationships). They also devote energy to developing paradigms for appropriately caring relationships. Importantly, most care-focused feminists believe that women's caregiving skills are far more developed than men's. For example, in the United States, 91.7% of registered nurses are women (U.S. Department of Labor & U.S. Bureau of Labor Statistics, 2008). The fact that most men avoid fields of work such as nursing is a worrisome state of affairs that care-focused feminists seek to address. For men generally to dismiss care work as "women's work" is, in some ways, for men to devalue this essential human labor as beneath them. Indeed, one study revealed that some men would prefer not to work at all rather than to do "women's work" (Williams, 2000, p. 309).

Probably the most well-known thinker who has promulgated a care-focused feminist approach to ethics is moral psychologist Carol Gilligan (1982). She argued that because women have traditionally focused on meeting the needs of children, elderly family members, and people with illnesses or disabilities, they have developed a language of care that helps create and maintain a thick web of loving (or at least friendly) human relationships. In contrast, because men have traditionally thrust themselves into the marketplace and the civic arena, they have developed a language of justice that shapes and maintains contractual agreements between supposedly rational and free adults eager to specify and protect their respective rights. Gilligan also maintained that scales that measure moral development privilege the ethical language of justice over the ethical language of care. For example, Lawrence Kohlberg's widely used six-stage moral development scale relegates care considerations to the lower stages of moral development and justice considerations to the higher stages of moral development (as cited in Tong, 1993, p. 82).

Thinking about Kohlberg's ladder of moral development, Gilligan asked why women rarely get past stage 3, whereas men usually get to stage 4 or even 5. Hypothesizing that Kohlberg's scale is constructed in ways that favor men, Gilligan watched Kohlbergian researchers at work. She noted that they usually asked their research subjects to resolve hypothetical moral dilemmas. The case of Heinz, a husband whose wife's life depends on him stealing an expensive drug for her, was typical of these dilemmas. Heinz's wife desperately needs a drug, but he cannot afford to purchase it. The moral question is: "Should Heinz steal the drug under these circumstances?"

When Jake and Amy, two 11-year-old children, were asked this question by Kohlbergian researchers, they gave very different answers. Jake approached the question as a math problem. He said Heinz should steal the drug because the right to life trumps the right to property. In contrast to Jake, Amy did not view Heinz's dilemma as a conflict between competing rights. Instead, she viewed it as a relationship issue: how Heinz's theft of the drug might affect him and his wife in the long run. Commented Amy:

> If he stole the drug, he might save the wife then, but if he did, he might have to go to jail, and then his wife might get sicker again, and he couldn't get more of the drug, and it might not be good. So, they should really just talk it out and find some other way to make the money. (Cited in Tong, 1993, p. 83)

Importantly, the Kohlbergian researchers gave a higher test score to Jake than to Amy. If one thinks about it, though, Amy's answer was probably the better one, all things considered. Certainly, it opened up the possibility of discussing what might really be morally wrong with Heinz's situation—namely, a pharmaceutical industry that overprices drugs, the lack of affordable healthcare insurance, or the absence of a welfare safety net for people like Heinz and his wife.

Gilligan contrasted Jake's and Amy's differing responses not to negate Jake's style of moral reasoning, but rather to affirm Amy's style of moral reasoning and to set the stage for more deeply understanding it. As the result of several empirical studies, including interviews with 29 relatively diverse women who were deciding whether to have an abortion, Gilligan concluded that women's *ontologies* and *epistemologies*, as well as *ethics*, typically diverge from men's. Focusing on the different roles of intimacy and self-individuation in men's and women's lives, Gilligan observed that the importance of individuality and autonomy for men often leads them to center discussions of morality on issues of justice, fairness, rules, and rights. In contrast, the importance of family and friends for women prompts them to center discussions of morality on people's wants, needs, interests, and aspirations. Gilligan also claimed that for women—much more than for men—moral development means learning how to integrate other-directed demands with self-centered concerns. During the process of their moral development, women supposedly move between three levels of moral reasoning: an overemphasis on self (Level 1), an overemphasis on others (Level 2), and a proper emphasis on self in relation to others (Level 3). Although a woman's moral development is always in process, as a woman morally matures, an increasing number of her decisions will exhibit Level 3 characteristics (as cited in Tong, 1993, p. 85).

Comparing Gilligan's and Kohlberg's diverging accounts of moral development, it is easy to understand why Gilligan thought Kohlberg's account reflected men's moral development rather than everyone's moral development. She claimed that a "formal logic of fairness" informs Kohlberg's mode of reasoning and style of discourse; his scale interprets moral phenomena in terms of a set of rights and rules. In contrast, a "psychological logic of relationships" informs Gilligan's mode of reasoning and style of discourse; her scale interprets moral phenomena in terms of a set of responsibilities and connections. To be sure, Gilligan's scale is no more a scale of human moral development than is Kohlberg's. Rather than denying this fact, however, Gilligan asked nurses to reflect on the different ways in which men and women describe their distinctive moral journeys, viewing them as alternative ways to achieve the ultimate goal of a morality that requires both rights (justice) and responsibilities (care) (as cited in Tong, 1993, p. 87).

Like Gilligan, Nel Noddings, a philosopher of education (as cited in Tong, 1998, pp. 132–135), suggested that ethics is about creating and maintaining caring relationships. She claimed that traditional Western ethics is so fixated on "principles and propositions" and values such as "justification, fairness, and justice" that it fails to recognize the importance of "human caring and the memory of caring and being cared for" (as cited in Tong, 1993, p. 108). Convinced that traditional ethics had gone wrong by emphasizing justice and deemphasizing care, Noddings proposed to set it right by injecting "eros, the feminine spirit" into "logos, the masculine spirit." Although women are just as capable of rational moral reasoning as men are, in Noddings' estimation, most women still prefer to consult their "feelings, needs, impressions, and . . . sense of personal ideal" when they make moral decisions (p. 109).

According to Noddings, sentiments of sympathy and empathy are innate in all human beings, but they need to be cultivated if they are to guide everyday moral decisions. Noddings identified two sorts of human caring: *natural caring* and *ethical caring*. As she saw it, caring comes easily to us when we are young. We want to help others because they matter to us and we want their love and approval at all costs. Later, said Noddings, it becomes more difficult for us to help others because our own self-interest begins to dominate. We want our own way, even if getting it separates us from others. To the extent that this happens, said Noddings, we need to remember how others have cared for us. Noddings claimed that it is through this process of "remembrance" that ethical caring—the kind of caring that expresses itself as "I *must* care"—comes into existence. This form of caring is more deliberate and less spontaneous than what Noddings termed natural caring (as cited in Tong, 1993, p. 112). It comes into being when our feelings are dormant, distant, or otherwise temporarily diminished.

Importantly, Noddings did not think that ethical caring should replace caring. Rather, she suggested that our "oughts" should build on our "wants." Commented Noddings, "An ethics built on caring strives to maintain the caring attitude and is thus dependent upon, and not superior to, natural caring" (p. 112). When we engage in ethical caring, we are not denying, negating, or renouncing ourselves in an effort to affirm, posit, or accept others. Rather, we are acting to fulfill our "fundamental and natural desire to be and to remain related" (p. 112).

In an attempt to further elucidate why care is fundamentally about connection, Noddings wrote a book about evil (1989). In it, she argued that for women, an evil event is a bad event—something that harms someone. By comparison, for men, an evil event is a rule-breaking event—a violation of God's commandments or the state's laws. Noddings wanted to replace the father's idea of evil as sin, guilt, impurity, and fault with the mothers' experience of evil as "that which harms or threatens harm" (as cited in Tong, 1993, p. 113). Noddings insisted that evil is not about disobeying authority figures. Rather, it is about experiencing, in a wide variety of ways, the kind of pain, separation, and helplessness we all experience shortly after being born. In Noddings' estimation, this new conception of evil, and its concomitant stress on relationships, may make it easier for us to resist evil throughout our lives, but especially as we grow older (p. 113).

Noddings used Doris Lessing's novel *The Diary of a Good Neighbor* to better articulate women's understanding of evil. In the novel, Jane, a middle-aged, well-heeled novelist and magazine editor, tries to alleviate the suffering of Maudie, a skinny, unkempt, lower-class, 90-year-old woman. A cadre of nurses and nurse's aides (all women) assist Jane in her work. In contrast to a male physician who views Maudie as a "case," the women view Maudie as a unique individual who needs their help as she suffers through the infirmities of old age. They do not find abstract meaning in Maudie's suffering, because her pain serves no healing purpose. Nor do they speak of God's will, as if Maudie's suffering were the price she must pay for her past transgressions. On the contrary, they simply work "to relieve her pain, alleviate her loneliness, and preserve—as nearly as they can—her autonomy" (as cited in Tong, 1993, p. 114).

Using the story of Maudie as a specific example of evil, Noddings proceeded to construct a phenomenology of evil. As she sees it, evil is not an abstract phenomenon, but rather a concrete reality that takes at least one of the three following forms:

1. Inflicting pain (unless it can be *demonstrated* that doing so will or is at least likely to spare the victim greater pain in the future)
2. a. Inducing the pain of separation
   b. Neglecting relation so that the pain of separation follows or those separated are thereby dehumanized
3. a. Deliberately or carelessly causing helplessness
   b. Creating elaborate systems of mystification that contribute to the fear of helplessness or to its actual maintenance (Cited in Tong, 1993, p. 122)

These actions, said Noddings, are evil, as many people in the nursing profession know all too well. No higher or better good can ever justify causing another person unnecessary pain or rendering another person separate or helpless (p. 122). Ethics is about overcoming pain, separation, and helplessness—a task that requires human beings to relate to one another as people whose goodness requires a sense of community.

To read *Women and Evil* together with *Caring* is to realize that Noddings espoused a relational ethics that is built on a relational ontology. According to Noddings, most individual dilemmas are, in fact, *relational* dramas that require dialog, not monologue. Seeking to make her point more concretely, Noddings claimed that patients, for example, should not make healthcare decisions ordinarily—and particularly end-of-life decisions—unilaterally. Rather, they should make these decisions in consultation with their families and friends. Noddings suggested that the process of someone dying can be an opportunity for family members to draw closer to one another, although she also realized that some families ruin this opportunity as they play out old rivalries and engage in power struggles. Under such strained and stressful conditions, patients who are competent must determine whether their own needs outweigh those of their families and friends. There are some things one person is not entitled to ask another person to do. Dying is one; not dying is another. Relationships are important, but so is the individual. In other words, any viable relational ethics must resist the tendency to make the relationship something individuals must serve no matter what. A self that is disconnected from others may be a solipsistic atom, but a self that is totally welded to others is no longer a self.

Although nurses may find an ethics of care valuable in their workplace, it is not a flawless ethics. A nurse can care or be expected to care too much. The phenomenon of nurse burnout attests to this fact. Sometimes caring is taken to its limits in the nursing profession. Commented Allethaire Cullen (1995):

> The *nursing system* itself contributes to burnout by presenting as "normal" the kinds of situations most people would find uncomfortable and frightening. How many people, for example, would feel comfortable holding babies born addicted to drugs or children who have died? Nurses do these things routinely as part of their role and care to patients. Few people in other professions are directly responsible for another person's life, yet nurses shoulder this responsibility daily. (p. 25)

In expressing concern about the dangers of caring too much, Gilligan's critics echoed Elizabeth Cady Stanton's 19th-century warning that, given society's tendency to take advantage of women, it is vital that women make self-development, rather than other-directed self-sacrifice, their first priority. Even so, it is important not to overemphasize the problems associated with caring too much. Whatever weaknesses an ethics of care may have, the world would be a worse place were women—and especially women in the caring professions—suddenly to stop meeting the physical and psychological needs of those who depend on them. Care is worth rescuing from the power structures that misshape it. If it is to be rescued, however, we need to recognize the differences between what feminist Sheila Mullett (1988) termed *distortions of caring* on the one hand and *undistorted caring* on the other hand.

According to Mullett, a person cannot truly care for someone if she is economically, socially, or psychologically coerced to do so. In other words, genuine or fully authentic caring cannot occur under conditions characterized by unfairness, domination, and subordination. Only under conditions of equality and freedom can women in the caring professions, for example, tend to patients' needs without being diminished, disempowered, or disregarded. Absent such ideal conditions, women in the caring professions must care cautiously, asking themselves whether the kind of caring in which they are engaged is:

- Care that fulfills the one caring
- Care that calls upon the unique and particular individuality of the one caring
- Care that is not produced by a person in a role because of gender, with one gender engaging in nurturing behavior and the other engaging in instrumental behavior
- Care that is reciprocated with caring, and not merely with the satisfaction of seeing the ones cared for flourishing and pursuing other projects
- Care that takes place within the framework of consciousness-raising practice and conversation (Cited in Tong, 1993, p. 103)

Care can be freely given only when the person caring is not taken for granted (p. 104).

Reasoning much like Gilligan and Noddings, so-called maternal thinkers have used the mother–child relationship as a springboard for discussing the necessary and sufficient conditions for truly moral human relationships. Specifically, feminist Sara Ruddick argued that from the work mothers do for their children emerges a distinct mode of moral reasoning best termed *maternal thinking* (as cited in Tong, 1993, pp. 136–137). To meet the three fundamental goals of maternal practice—namely, the preservation, growth, and social acceptability of children—mothers or persons who engage in motherly behavior must cultivate a multitude of very specific virtues, the most important of which is the metavirtue of attentive love. This metavirtue, which is at once cognitive and affective, enables mothers to really know their children. Realizing what is bad as well as good about their children, "good" mothers try to help their children eliminate their vices and weaknesses, slowly replacing them with virtues and strengths.

Concerned that men of goodwill might feel that, by virtue of their XY chromosome, they cannot think maternally, Ruddick noted that all human beings are capable of thinking in terms of preserving one another, helping one another grow, and making one another socially acceptable. To survive as a human species and to thrive as individual human beings, we all need to think maternally. Ruddick hypothesized that because women were largely excluded from the public realm until relatively recently, maternal thinking has not made its way into the public realm's power-wielding central offices. Instead, a very nonmaternal kind of thinking has dominated the public realm—the kind of thinking that leads to ecological disorder, social injustice, and even war.

People who do not think like mothers, said Ruddick, do not see like mothers. They do not make a connection, for example, between war as an idea and war as a reality. For them, war is about winning, defending one's way of life, and establishing one's position of power. For a maternal thinker, war is about conceivably destroying the child one has spent years preserving, nurturing, and training: a unique human person who cannot be replaced. In summary, for a maternal thinker, war is about killing—about canceling out the "product(s)" of maternal practice, and such a realization catapults maternal thinkers in the direction of peace activities (as cited in Tong, 1993, pp. 382–383).

Building on Ruddick's work, feminist philosopher Virginia Held (1993) noted that just because a maternal ethics exceeds the "moral minimum" of taking everyone's rights seriously, that does not mean it is free to dispense with this "moral minimum." Mothering persons must be fair, as well as compassionate, rational, and emotional, and able to make generalizations about human relationships as well as to articulate their specific features. A maternal thinker who says that no two human relationships are ever alike invites moral chaos. Like principles, relationships can be qualified as good, better, or best (bad, worse, or worst), and that which is subject to *qualification* is also subject to *evaluation*. In the same way that we can ask what makes a principle good or bad, so we can ask what makes a relationship good or bad.

Held (1993) stressed that both men and women can be mothering persons. Inviting girls but not boys to do caregiving work, she noted, produces boys with personalities "in which the inclination toward combat is overdeveloped and the capacity to feel for others is stunted" (p. 146). Because bellicose, unfeeling boys usually mature into bellicose, unfeeling men in positions of power, Held claimed that human survival may depend on society's ability to get men as well as women to care for children and, by parity of reasoning, for other vulnerable people (p. 146).

Despite the fact that Held believed that both men and women can mother, she nonetheless suggested that there could be a *qualitative* difference between female mothering and male mothering. The fact that women bear children as well as rear children could signal that "women are responsible for the existence of new persons in ways far more fundamental than are men" (p. 146). Women need men to begin a pregnancy, but they do not need men to end a pregnancy. Through abortion or suicide, women can say a definite "no" to life.

Even if rearing a child to adulthood is overall more taxing and demanding than the process of pregnancy and giving birth, Held asserted that the birthing act should not be discounted as if it had no special effect on subsequent parent–child relationships. In suggesting that biological experiences may influence "the attitudes of the mother and father toward the 'worth' or 'value' of a particular child"

(p. 147), Held sought to explore the relationship between the kind of feelings women and men have for their children on the one hand and the kind of obligations they have to them on the other hand. If ethicists assume that natural male tendencies play a role in determining men's moral rights and responsibilities, then they should likewise make the same assumption about natural female tendencies:

> Traditional moral theories often suppose it is legitimate for individuals to maximize self-interest, or satisfy their preferences, within certain constraints based on the equal rights of others. If it can be shown that the tendency to want to pursue individual self-interest is a stronger tendency among men than among women, this would certainly be relevant to an evaluation of such a theory. And if it could be shown that a tendency to value children and a desire to foster the developing capabilities of the particular others for whom we care is a stronger tendency among women than among men, this too would be relevant in evaluating moral theories. (Cited in Tong, 1993, p. 147)

Held joined Gilligan and Noddings in their condemnation of the biblical character Abraham, who was willing to kill his son, Isaac, to honor God's command. Women who birth children—who preserve, nurture, and train them—are not likely to believe that obeying a command, including one from God, is more sacred than preserving the very lives of their children. To be sure, from the standpoint of traditional ethics, a mother's refusal to subordinate the concrete life of her child to the abstract commands of duty or higher law may indicate her underdevelopment as a moral agent. Yet, in an age where a blindness to interconnection has led to the destruction of the environment and a perilous buildup of the war arsenal, it can be argued reasonably that a focus on connections rather than rights may constitute a higher and better morality than traditional ethics (Tong, 1993, pp. 145–148).

As a result of her awareness of how socioeconomic as well as physical and psychological conditions affect women's (and men's) ability to care, Eva Kittay (1998), another proponent of care ethics, focused on dependency workers—people who take care of people (most often for pay) but who view their job as more than a mere job—as the paradigm for caregivers. Nurses and other paid careworkers fall into this class of workers in a marked way. Kittay used Sasha, the woman who cared for her severely developmentally disabled daughter for more than 25 years, as her prime example of a dependency worker. In describing how Sasha's "labor of love" enabled her to succeed as a scholar and teacher, Kittay made the general point that we need to understand how people are interrelated. Without careworkers, domestic laborers, public health workers, and the like, human beings could not survive. Yet we often take our support systems for granted, paying meager salaries to the people (mostly women) who tend to our wounds, clean our bodies, and remove our dirt. Worse, we often view our caregivers as somehow less equal—less deserving of respect—than those who rule over us on Wall Street or in the White House.

It was this thought that pushed Kittay to use the mother–child paradigm to articulate the bottom-line rationale of her ethics of care. She thought of her mother, who used to sit down to dinner after serving her and her father, pointedly asserting: "After all, *I'm* also a mother's child" (Kittay, 1998, p. 25). In this statement—"I, too, deserve to eat"—is contained the fundamental source of human equality, according to Kittay. We are all equal because we are all the product of some mother's labor. We are the same not in our independence, but rather in our dependence.

# Power-Focused Feminist Approaches to Ethics

Although power-focused feminist approaches to ethics appreciate the value of care, they are interested primarily in analyzing practices, policies, systems, structures, ideologies, and attitudes that contribute to the oppression of women and other groups that suffer equal or even worse forms of damaging subordination (Card, 1999). The ultimate goal of power-focused feminist ethicists is to transform a world burdened by covert and overt forms of sexism, racism, classism, ableism, heterosexism, ethnocentrism, and colonialism into a world in which all people are treated equally. In a transformed world, caregiving tasks would be equally distributed, and caregivers would receive as much care as they give.

Power-focused feminist approaches to bioethics can generally be divided into two groups: (1) those that emphasize the ways in which political, economic, and social forces systematically cause gender oppression and other forms of human oppression; and (2) those that stress the ways in which ideology, identity issues, and cultural forces account for women's (and other marginalized groups') second-class status. Liberal feminists belong to the first group, whereas radical, multicultural, global, and third-wave feminists are members of the second group.

## Liberal Power-Focused Feminists

*Liberal feminists* have their historical roots in Mary Wollstonecraft's (1988) *A Vindication of the Rights of Woman*, John Stuart Mill's (1970) "The Subjection of Women," and the women's suffrage movement of the 19th century. Among the organizations with which contemporary liberal feminists are most aligned is the National Organization for Women (NOW). Liberal feminists maintain that the primary cause of women's remaining subordination to men is a set of lingering social norms and formal laws that have made it hard for women to succeed in the public world. When a woman chooses to be a nurse today, for example, this decision is not made because she cannot be a physician. Rather, it is because she wants to be a nurse, not a physician. One hundred years ago, a woman would not have had such a choice. The doors of medical schools would have been closed to her.

Although many people think that liberal feminism is passé and that the ethical issues that preoccupied them have been resolved, the fact of the matter is that as of 2010, the Bill of (Women's) Rights, which was first articulated by NOW in 1967, had yet to be fully implemented. Furthermore, U.S. women's reproductive rights are still not secure (the right to have an abortion remains under siege), and the Equal Rights Amendment has yet to pass. If the goal of liberal feminism is to push women full force into the public world and catapult them into its higher orbits, then its work is far from done.

## Radical Power-Focused Feminists

Pointing to what they perceive as the central weakness of liberal feminism—the view that "I can be a man, too"—*radical feminists* claim that women's fundamental strength rests in their differences from men. Radical feminists do not think it is in women's best interest to become part of a system that devalues, among other things, caregiving practices and occupations. On the contrary, they think women should reject this system because its values—power, dominance, hierarchy, and competition—breed injustice. Not only must patriarchy's legal, political, educational, and economic structures be overturned, in radical feminists' estimation, so too must its sexual and reproductive practices and institutions be challenged.

Although all radical feminists focus on issues related to gender, sex, and reproduction, they do so in different ways depending on whether they are *radical-libertarian feminists* (the chapter author's terminology) on the one hand or *radical-cultural feminists* (also the chapter author's terminology) on the other hand. With respect to gender-related inequities, radical-libertarian feminists think that both men and women suffer when women are required to exhibit feminine characteristics only (e.g., "interdependence, community, connection, sharing, emotion, body, trust, absence of hierarchy, nature, immanence, process, joy, peace and life," as cited in Tong, 1993, p. 163) and men are required to exhibit masculine characteristics only (e.g., "independence, autonomy, intellect, will, wariness, hierarchy, domination, culture, transcendence, product, asceticism, war and death," p. 163). As radical-libertarian feminists see it, this enforced divide between the feminine and the masculine deforms both women and men, rendering both sexes deficient. Thus it is vital for society to permit both men and women to be androgynous—to exhibit a full range of masculine and feminine qualities. Men should be permitted to explore their feminine dimensions and women their masculine ones. No person should be forbidden the sense of wholeness that comes from combining his or her masculine and feminine dimensions. Such a view would enable more men to feel at home in the caring professions, and the terms *male nurse* and *female physician* would cease to exist.

Disagreeing with radical-libertarian feminists that a turn to androgyny would be a liberating strategy for women, radical-cultural feminists argue against this move. Some anti-androgynists maintain that the problem is not femininity in and of itself, but rather the low value that patriarchy assigns to feminine qualities and the high value that it assigns to masculine qualities. They claim that if society learned to value the feminine side of human existence as much as the masculine side of human existence, women's oppression would end. Other anti-androgynists disagree. They claim that femininity, as it is commonly understood, is a problem because it was constructed by men to achieve patriarchal purposes. To be liberated, they say, women must give new gynocentric meanings to femininity. According to this view, femininity should no longer be understood as those traits that deviate from masculinity and those traits that equip women to serve men's needs and desires. Rather, femininity should be reinterpreted as an authentically female way of being designed to support, delight, and satisfy women.

Radical feminist thought is as diverse on issues related to reproduction as it is on matters related to gender. Radical-libertarian feminists claim biological motherhood drains women both physically and psychologically. Women should be free, they say, to use both the old reproduction-controlling technologies of contraception, sterilization, and abortion and the new reproduction-assisting technologies of in vitro fertilization, egg donation, and surrogate motherhood on their own terms—to prevent or terminate unwanted pregnancies or, alternatively, to initiate pregnancies that require third-party intervention. Women should be able to have children when they want to, how they want to (in their own womb or that of another woman), and with whom they want to (a man, a woman, or alone through reproductive cloning). Some radical-libertarian feminists take this position even further, however. They look forward to the day when *ectogenesis* (extracorporeal gestation in an artificial placenta) entirely replaces the natural process of pregnancy and women no longer have to experience the physical discomforts that accompany gestation and/or the birthing process.

Objecting to radical-libertarian feminists' celebration of assisted reproduction, radical-cultural feminists caution that technology is not necessarily women's friend. According to these theorists, technology is breaking the links between conceiving, gestating, birthing, and rearing a child. Women had best keep an eye on technology lest it push them into the kind of dystopia Margaret Atwood imagines in *The Handmaid's Tale*. In Atwood's novel, some women serve men as sexual toys; other women clean their homes. Still other women called handmaidens breed their children, and another group of women rear their children. Following a birth, the central character, Offred—a handmaiden whose name literally means "to be of Fred"—recalls better times and speaks in her mind to her mother, who had been a feminist leader: "Can you hear me? You wanted a woman's culture. Well, now there is one. It isn't what you meant, but it exists. Be thankful for small mercies" (as cited in Tong, 2009, p. 81).

## Multicultural, Global, and Third-Wave Power-Focused Feminist Ethics

*Multicultural* and *global feminists* add new thoughts to those of liberal and radical feminism. They believe that women need to focus on the ways in which race, ethnicity, nationality, sexual identity, gender identity, age, religion, educational level, profession or occupation, marital status, health, and so forth contribute to some women being more powerful, free, and well-off than other women. Being a nurse in the United States, for example, is far different from being a nurse's aide in the United States or being a nurse in the Philippines or Kenya.

Audre Lorde (1992), Bell Hooks (1990), and Patricia Hill Collins (2008) were among the first multicultural feminists who stressed the ways in which some women are multiply jeopardized. The way for a marginalized woman to liberate herself from thoughts that she is deviant or inferior, said Lorde, is for her to "integrate all the parts of who [she is], openly, allowing power from particular sources of [her] living to flow back and forth freely through all [her] different selves, without the restrictions of externally imposed definition" (as cited in Tong, 2009, p. 539). Women must fight the enemy without—the political, economic, legal, and social systems and structures that keep women oppressed—but they also must fight the enemy within.

Global feminists are particularly attuned to the ways in which women in the so-called "First World" countries (i.e., heavily industrialized and market-based countries located primarily in the Northern Hemisphere) often unknowingly take advantage of women living and working in "Third World" countries (i.e., economically developing countries located primarily in the Southern Hemisphere). According to these feminists, relatively wealthy women in the upscale urban homes should think twice before buying inexpensive goods produced by poor women in global sweatshops. To be sure, purchasing such goods may be morally justifiable in the short run so that the women who make them now can survive; yet in the long run, this short-term remedy may actually prevent Third World women from organizing the kind of protests necessary to effect major social change.

Truth be told, reliance on immigrant women to do low-paid care work seems to be the order of the day. First World countries increasingly view Third World countries as a source of female caregivers willing to work for next to nothing. For example, in the United Kingdom, 35% of the nurses who work in the eldercare environment are immigrants. In London, more than 60% of the people who do eldercare work are immigrants (Cangiano, Shutes, Spencer, & Leeson, 2009, p. 182). These immigrant workers are nearly exclusively women, and they come mostly from Zimbabwe, Poland, Nigeria, the Philippines, and India. Their employers like their work ethic and their "warmth, respect, empathy, trust and patience in the care relationship" (p. 184). They also like the fact that they are willing to work for wages that native-born eldercare workers find outrageously low.

As in the United Kingdom, there is an exceptionally high demand for immigrant careworkers in Taiwan. Since the early 1980s, significant numbers of immigrant women without legal papers have worked in Taiwanese households (Lan, 2002, p. 188), thereby enabling Taiwanese women to remain in the paid workforce. Comments Pei-Chan Lan, "The filial duty of serving aging parents is transferred first from the son to the daughter-in-law (a gender transfer); later, it is outsourced to migrant careworkers (a market transfer)" (p. 188). As a result of citizens' increasing demand for inexpensive eldercare workers for their aged relatives, the Taiwanese government decided to legalize large numbers of immigrant careworkers. Specifically, in 1992, Taiwan started to grant work permits to domestic caretakers who agreed to care for severely ill or disabled people, children younger than the age of 12, or elders older than the age of 70 (p. 171). Moreover, the country's leaders began to describe the importation of eldercare workers from the Philippines and Indonesia in particular "as a solution to the growing demand for paid care work among both nuclear households and the aging population" (p. 172).

Interestingly, Taiwanese female employers sometimes bond with their Filipina employees. They ally with them against husbands who are often viewed as tyrannical or extensively demanding. For the most part, however, no such bond is created and the Filipina employee may suffer accordingly. She may be abused verbally or discriminated against on account of her race, for example. Not having any real way to defend herself against mistreatment, the Filipina employee, like other immigrant eldercare workers, may do what she is told to do and leave it at that. The fact that she has legal documents does not mean she can quit and secure another job that pays well enough to support herself and her family back home.

If it is easy to take advantage of immigrant eldercare workers with proper legal documents, it is far easier to intimidate, harass, or bully immigrant eldercare workers without legal documents. Fearing deportation, undocumented eldercare workers are a particularly vulnerable group of careworkers. One rich New York businesswoman described her ideal careworker as a person who "basically [did] not have a life" of her own and who had nowhere to turn for help (Chang, 2006, pp. 43–45). The words of this wealthy woman are, of course, disconcerting. They clearly reduce the ideal careworker to a mere means—that is, a thing or instrument to serve one's own interests with no concern for the interests of the person one is using.

Although multicultural and global feminism are still alive and very well (Howard & Allen, 2000), these perspectives have been joined by yet another form of feminism: *third-wave feminism*. Contradiction, including self-contradiction, is expected and even willingly welcomed by third-wave feminists. So, too, is conflict. Two leading third-wave feminists, Leslie Heywood and Jennifer Drake (1997), commented:

> Even as different strains of feminism and activism sometimes directly contradict each other, they are all part of our third-wave lives, our thinking, and our praxes: we are products of all the contradictory definitions of and differences within feminism, beasts of such a hybrid kind that perhaps we need a different name altogether. (p. 3)

Heywood and Drake's suggestion that feminism may be passé is perhaps troubling, but it is understandable.

Being a feminist in a society where a growing number of people can literally choose their gender or racial/ethnic classification is different from being a feminist in a society where one's identity is more of a given and is difficult, if not impossible, to escape. Moreover, engaging in feminist action is extraordinarily challenging in a global context. According to third-wave feminist Chilla Bulbeck (1997), women in the First World have a lot of learning to do about women in the Third World. She stressed that the term *Third World* is "double valenced" (p. 35); that is, the Third World can be understood either negatively as a backward, poor, and bad place to live, or positively as "a subversive, immense repressed voice about to burst into centre stage of the globe" (p. 35).

Yet, however great the positive potential of the Third World is in Bulbeck's estimation, it still works against the women who live in it. Most Third World women are disadvantaged, as are women in the Fourth World (1997, p. 34), the world in which indigenous people in settler societies live—for example, the world of Native American women in the United States. Also disadvantaged are women in the Fifth World (O'Keefe & Chinouya, 2004), the world of migrants and immigrants who have left their native lands either because they wanted to or because they had to—for example, immigrant African women in the United Kingdom. Thus third-wave feminists realize just how elusive the concept of some sort of universal sisterhood is.

In addition to being open to women's different social, economic, political, and cultural differences, third-wave feminists are open to women's sexual differences. In the 1970s, feminists debated whether sex between heterosexuals and lesbians always needed to be egalitarian, feeling, and gentle, or whether it could sometimes be mechanical, rough, and violent. Even more specifically, they wondered about the appropriateness of women working in the sex industry as porn models, call-girls, lap dancers, exotic dancers, and prostitutes. Were these women the victims of sexual objectification and dire economic conditions, or were they instead cagey entrepreneurs who realized they could make far more money selling their sexual services than working as waitresses at local diners? Although some second-wave feminists were willing to applaud women who used their sexuality in ways that served their self-reported interests, the general consensus of most second-wave feminists was that the dangers of sex were greater than its pleasures and that women had best steer clear of violent sex and commercialization of their bodies.

In contrast to most second-wave feminists, third-wave feminists are less prescriptive about what counts as good sex for women. They are also more comfortable with women who enhance their bodies to meet cultural expectations about what counts as beautiful. If a woman wants to wear make-up, have cosmetic surgery, and wear sexually provocative clothes, then, as far as many third-wave feminists are concerned, she should feel free to do so provided that she feels empowered by her actions and not somehow demeaned, diminished, or otherwise objectified by them. Unlike most second-wave feminists, third-wave feminists think that a woman can be both a feminist and a star in porn flicks. The apparent contradiction in the term *feminist porn queen* does not seem to bother third-wave feminists. Likewise, these feminists are very comfortable living in a transgendered world, in which people can change their sex or present themselves in a way that resists gender categorization.

Third-wave feminists are shaping a new kind of feminism that is not as interested in getting women to want what women should want as it is in responding to what women say they want and not judging whether their wants are authentic or inauthentic. Indeed, third-wave feminists describe the context in which they do feminism as one of "lived messiness" (Heywood & Drake, 1997, p. 8). Theorist

Rebecca Walker has speculated that because many third-wave feminists grew up "transgender, bisexual, interracial, and knowing and loving people who are racist, sexist, and otherwise afflicted" (Walker, 1995, p. xxxiii), they are not as judgmental as second-wave feminists were. She stressed that because "the lines between Us and Them are often blurred," third-wave feminists seek to create identities that "accommodate ambiguity" and "multiple positionalities" (p. xxxiv).

Clearly, the openness of third-wave feminists is generally appealing and, in many instances, particularly liberating. When Walker (1995) said her third-wave feminist goal is to "debunk the stereotypes that there is one lifestyle or manifestation of feminist empowerment" (p. xxxiii) and instead offered "self-possession, self-determination, and an endless array of non-dichotomous possibilities" (p. xxxiv) to women, most young nurses would likely second her views. Yet just because third-wave feminists are able to deal with difference in admirable ways, it does not mean that third-wave feminism is flawless.

Whereas the challenge for second-wave feminists was to see and use women's differences productively to overcome the idea that all women are necessarily the same or some sort of victims, the challenge for third-wave feminists is to recognize that to have feminism, one has to believe that women constitute a distinct social group (Ferguson, 1989, p. 352) and that just because some women feel empowered does not mean all women feel this way. Thus it is troubling when second-wave feminism is dismissed as unalloyed victim feminism and third-wave feminism is celebrated as unalloyed power feminism.

In the hands of third-wave feminists such as Heywood and Drake, as well as Walker, power feminism seems inviting enough. Conversely, in the hands of other thinkers, sometimes described as third-wave *postfeminists*, power feminism gets very mean-spirited. Specifically, third-wave postfeminists such as Katie Roiphe (1993), Camille Paglia (1992), and Rene Denfield (1995) insisted that nowadays women are free to be whomever they want to be and to do whatever they want to do. Women's only possible enemy is themselves, they implied. Forgetting how much their power is connected to their advantaged position, Roiphe, Paglia, and Denfield have failed to recognize the vulnerability and victimization of disadvantaged women in the United States and elsewhere. For every nurse who loves her job, there is another one who hates it; and for every nurse who heads a team, there is another one who knows better than to disagree with a physician, an administrator, or even a demanding patient. This is not the time for women to reject the label feminist—far from it, it is the time for women, especially women in the caring professions, to embrace it more enthusiastically lest women's progress not reach a dead end as it has in the past. Think about all the women who are leaving their careers because they cannot handle both career and family responsibilities; more specifically, think of all the nurses who are leaving nursing because their workplaces are anything but female-friendly, paradoxical as that claim may seem.

All women, but especially women in the caring professions, should rally around the feminist flag to call attention to their caregiving powers. This statement is not intended to dismiss the important roles played by men in the nursing professions and men who proudly call themselves feminist. Rather, the intention is to agree with feminist theorist Christine di Stephano, who claimed, "Gender is basic in ways that we have to fully understand, . . . it functions as 'a difference that makes a difference,'" even as it can no longer claim the legitimating mantle of the difference (di Stephano, 1990, p. 70). If any group of people—including men—can figure out what this difference is, it is nurses; nursing is almost an intractably gendered field, and we would all do well to understand why this is so.

# References

Atwood, M. (1985). *The handmaid's tale*. Toronto, Canada: McClelland & Stewart.

Bulbeck, C. (1997). *Re-orienting Western feminisms: Women's diversity in a postcolonial world*. New York, NY: Cambridge University Press.

Cangiano, A., Shutes, I., Spencer, S., & Leeson, G. (2009). *Migrant care workers in ageing societies: Research findings in the United Kingdom*. Oxford, UK: COMPAS: ESRC Centre on Migration, Policy, and Society, University of Oxford.

Card, C. (1999). *On feminist ethics and politics*. Lawrence, KS: University Press of Kansas.

Chang, G. (2006). Disposable domestics: Immigrant women workers in the global economy. In M. K. Zimmerman, J. S. Litt, & C. E. Bose (Eds.), *Global dimensions of gender and care-work* (pp. 39–47). Stanford, CA: Stanford Social Sciences.

Code, L., Mullett, S., & Overall, C. (Eds.). (1988). *Feminist perspectives: Philosophical essays on method and morals*. Toronto, Canada: University of Toronto Press.

Cullen, A. (1995). Burnout: Why do we blame the nurse? *American Journal of Nursing, 95*(11), 22–28.

Denfield, R. (1995). *The new Victorians: A young woman's challenges to the old feminist order*. New York, NY: Routledge.

di Stephano, C. (1990). Dilemmas of difference. In L. J. Nicholson (Ed.), *Feminism/postmodernism* (pp. 63–82). New York, NY: Routledge.

Ferguson, A. (1989). Sex and work: Women as a new revolutionary class. In R. S. Gottlieb (Ed.), *An anthology of Western Marxism: From Lukacs and Gramsci to socialist-feminism* (pp. 348–372). Oxford, UK: Oxford University Press.

Gilligan, C. (1982). *In a different voice*. Cambridge, MA: University Harvard Press.

Held, V. (1993). *Feminist morality: Transforming culture, society, and politics*. Chicago, IL: University of Chicago Press.

Heywood, L., & Drake, J. (Eds.). (1997). *Third wave agenda: Being feminist, doing feminism*. Minneapolis, MN: University of Minnesota Press.

Hill Collins, P. (2008). *Black feminist thought: Knowledge, consciousness, and the politics of empowerment*. New York, NY: Routledge Classics.

Hooks, B. (1990). *Yearning: race, gender, and cultural politics*. Boston, MA: South End Press.

Howard, J. A., & Allen, C. (2000). *Feminisms at a millennium*. Chicago, IL: University of Chicago Press.

Jaggar, A. M. (1992). Feminist ethics. In L. Becker & C. Becker (Eds.), *Encyclopedia of ethics* (pp. 363–364). New York, NY: Garland.

Kittay, E. F. (1998). *Love's labor: Essays on women, equality, and dependency*. New York, NY: Routledge.

Lan, P. C. (2002). Among women: Migrant domestics and their Taiwanese employers across generations. In B. Ehrenreich & A. R. Hochschild (Eds.), *Global woman: Nannies, maids, and sex workers in the new economy* (pp. 169–189). New York, NY: Metropolitan Books.

Lessing, D. (as J. Somers, pseudonym). (1983). *The diary of a good neighbor.* New York: Alfred A. Knopf.

Lorde, A. (1992). Age, race, class, and sex and women redefining difference. In M. L. Anderson & P. H. Collins (Eds.), *Race, class, and gender* (2nd ed., pp. 503–509). Belmont, CA: Wadsworth.

Mill, J. S. (1970). The subjection of women [1869 orig pub by Mills]. In A. S. Rossi (Ed.), *Essays on sex equality* (pp. 123–243). Chicago, IL: University of Chicago Press.

Mullet, S. (1988). Shifting perspectives: A new approach to ethics. In L. Code, S. Mullett, & C. Overall (Eds.), *Feminist perspectives: Philosophy essays on methods and morals* (pp. 109–126). Toronto, Canada: University of Toronto Press.

Noddings, N. (1984). *Caring: A feminine approach to ethics and moral education.* Berkeley, CA: University of California Press.

Noddings, N. (1989). *Women and evil.* Berkeley, CA: University of California Press.

O'Keefe, E., & Chinouya, M. (2004). Global migrants, gendered tradition, and human rights: Africans and HIV in the United Kingdom. In R. Tong, S. Dodd, & A. Donchin (Eds.), *Linking visions: Feminist bioethics, human rights, and the developing world* (pp. 217–234). Lanham, MD: Rowman & Littlefield.

Paglia, C. (1992). *Sex, art, and American culture: Essays.* New York, NY: Random House.

Roiphe, K. (1993). *The morning after: Sex, fear, and feminism on campus.* New York, NY: Little, Brown.

Ruddick, S. (1989). *Maternal thinking: Towards a politics of peace.* Boston, MA: Beacon Press.

Sherwin, S. (1992). *No longer patient: Feminist ethics and health care.* Philadelphia, PA: Temple University Press.

Tong, R. (1993). *Feminine and feminist ethics.* Belmont, CA: Wadsworth.

Tong, R. (1998). The ethics of care: A feminist virtue of care for healthcare practitioners. *Journal of Medicine and Philosophy, 23*(2), 131–152.

Tong, R. (2009). *Feminist thought: A more comprehensive introduction* (3rd ed.). Boulder, CO: Westview Press.

U.S. Department of Labor & U.S. Bureau of Labor Statistics. (2008). Women in the labor force: A databook. *Report, 1011,* 31.

Walker, R. (1995). *To be real: Telling the truth and changing the face of feminism.* New York, NY: Anchor Books.

Williams, C. L. (2000). The glass escalator: Hidden advantages for men in the "female" professions. In M. S. Kimmel & A. Aronson (Eds.), *The gendered society reader* (pp. 294–310). New York, NY: Oxford University Press.

Wollstonecraft, M. A. (1988) [C. H. Polston, Ed.]. *Vindication of the rights of woman.* New York, NY: W. W. Norton.

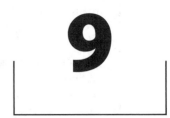

# Theories and Methods in Ethics

*Karen L. Rich*

## Introduction

The first purpose of this chapter is to analyze the theoretical nature of ethics—that is, to provide a framework to answer the question, "Do ethical theories really exist?" The reader should be an active participant in answering this question. To conduct this analysis, the nature of philosophy, ethics, science, and theory are each explored. The second purpose of the chapter is to discuss several important approaches to ethics. In the literature, these approaches often are referred to as *theories of ethics*. Before reading further, visit **Box 9–1** to begin an analysis of theory in the field of ethics.

## Philosophical Inquiry

*Philosophy,* translated literally, means the love of wisdom. One of the oldest scholarly disciplines, it retains at its roots an effort to understand the abstract questions about the nature of *knowledge* and *being* and a search for *truth*. The discipline remains esoteric, but it has evolved over the years to include formal systems and principles such as those used in the practice of logic.

   *Philosophical inquiry* can be grouped into content areas, which may differ slightly among philosophers. Three main content areas or types of inquiry in philosophy are (1) *epistemology*, the study of knowledge; (2) *ontology* (metaphysics), the study of the nature of being; and (3) *axiology*, the study of values. Ethics is concerned with axiological inquiry. Philosophy provides a method of studying

## Box 9–1  Ethics-Focused Inquiry

In *Essentials of Doctoral Education for Advanced Nursing Practice* (American Association of Colleges of Nursing [AACN], 2006), it is stated that Doctor of Nursing Practice programs prepare graduates to "integrate nursing science with knowledge from" other sciences and disciplines "as the basis for the highest level of nursing practice" (p. 9). Advanced practice nurses (APNs) need to be able to think critically about, question, and analyze epistemological, ontological, and empirical matters. Probing the following questions and considering possible answers is an exercise in preparing to integrate knowledge into practice. *Ethics* can be defined simply as the study of ideal ways of being and behavior. With this in mind and before reading this chapter, reflect on and use your current knowledge to answer the following questions:

1. Is ethics a science? What does one have to know to answer this question?
2. As a field of study, is ethics suitable for theory development and use? Why or why not?
3. Which methods of inquiry or research do you believe are appropriate for ethics?

and, consequently, knowing something about the nature of knowledge, reality, and existence, and what is highly desirable, good, or useful.

Billington (2003) divided philosophy into areas that focus on questions of "Why?"—that is, epistemology, metaphysics, and logic—and questions of "How?" or "What?"—which focus on decisions about behavior, priorities, and relationships. According to Billington, ethics belongs in the second category of focus.

Durant (1933) included five fields of study and discourse within the discipline of philosophy: (1) logic, (2) esthetics, (3) ethics, (4) politics, and (5) metaphysics. The first four of these fields constitute a study of the *ideal,* which is described as the study of ideal "method in thought and research," "form or beauty," "conduct," and "social organization," respectively (p. 3). According to Durant, metaphysics does not fit the same pattern as other forms of philosophy. Specifically, it does not focus on trying to accommodate the real with the ideal. Instead, metaphysics is a study of ultimate reality. Included in metaphysics is a study of the nature of mind (philosophical psychology), matter (ontology), and knowledge (epistemology).

No matter how ethics is classified, whether as a primary field of philosophy or as a field subsumed within another field, ethics is always considered to be a subdivision of philosophy. Because it is a branch of philosophy, ethics resides in the tier of the most abstract approaches to studying and understanding the nature of human beings and reality. Ethics means different things to different people. When the term is narrowly defined according to its historical use, ethics is the study of ideal human behavior and ideal ways of being. The approaches to ethics and the meanings of related concepts have varied over time among philosophers and ethicists. For example, Aristotle believed that ideal behaviors are those practices that lead to the end goal of *eudemonia*, which is synonymous with a special or high level of happiness or human well-being, whereas the 18th-century philosopher and ethicist Immanuel Kant (1785/2012) believed that ideal behavior entails acting in accordance with one's duty. Human well-being, according to Kant, is having the freedom to exercise self-determination (autonomy), being respected, and having the capability to think rationally.

As a field of study, ethics is a systematic approach to understanding, analyzing, and distinguishing matters of right and wrong, good and bad, and admirable and deplorable and how these matters relate to the well-being of and the relationship among sentient beings. Ethics is an active process rather than a static condition. Therefore, some ethicists prefer to use the phrase *doing ethics* to describe work in this field. When people are doing ethics, they need to support their beliefs and assertions with sound reasoning. In other words, even if people believe that ethics can be done subjectively, they must be able to justify this position through logical, rational arguments.

As contrasted with ethics, *morals* are specific beliefs, behaviors, and ways of being derived from doing ethics. As a practical matter, these terms are often used interchangeably.

## Science: The Daughter of Philosophy

Philosophy has been practiced since ancient times, when Plato declared that philosophers would be kings in ideal republics. Lovers of wisdom provided much of the means of humans' intellectual progress for hundreds of years. Eventually, it was philosophy that inevitably gave birth to science (Magee, 2001) as people sought more certainty to explain their external environment and human nature. As people moved out of the Middle (Dark) Ages and into the Age of Enlightenment, those in the Western world began to feel confident that human nature and the material world could be explained, predicted, and controlled.

> After Newton, science reigned as the authoritative definer of the universe, and philosophy defined itself in relation to science—predominantly supportive, occasionally critical and provocative, sometimes independent and concerned with different areas, but ultimately not in a position to gainsay the cosmological discoveries and conclusions of empirical science, which now increasingly ruled the Western world view. (Tarnas, 1991, p. 280)

Russell (1945) called philosophy an intermediate discipline between theology and science. Philosophy has commonalities with both: Like theology, philosophy is speculative and provides no definitive answers; like science, philosophy is based on reason rather than on dogma and tradition. In what he called the "no man's land" of philosophy, Russell contended that the most interesting questions of speculative minds reside there. Science cannot answer these questions, and theologians no longer hold the authority that they did in past centuries.

Philosophy can enrich the lives of people because it is focused on this no man's land of questions that have confounded humans for ages. "Philosophizing is thinking hard about life's most fundamental questions" (Lund, 2003, p. 2). Thinking hard, using reason, and evaluating arguments about the fundamental questions of life liberates one from dogma and small-minded customs. Although many philosophers have religious beliefs, good philosophizing does not resort to the use of religion to support philosophical positions (Magee, 2001). Instead, good philosophy is an attempt to "see how far reason will take us" (p. 7). In **Box 9–2** the reader is asked to consider some of the questions related to the ideas proposed in this paragraph.

Although both philosophers and scientists search for truth using rational thought processes, the answers to the questions of philosophical inquiry are neither well defined nor unequivocal. Scientists, however, use experiments in an

---

### Box 9–2  How Do We Know What We Know?

In *Essentials of Doctoral Education for Advanced Nursing Practice* (AACN, 2006), it is stated that "the [APN] scholar applies knowledge to solve a problem via the scholarship of application (referred to as the scholarship of practice in nursing)" (p. 11). But how do nurse scholars know what they know? Reflect on the following questions posed by Magee (2001, p. 7). How would you answer them?

1. Can we ever really know, in the sense of being sure of, anything? If so, what?
2. Even if we do know, how will we be able to be sure that we know? In other words, can we ever know that we know?

Now compare and contrast your answers to these questions as they relate to moral knowledge and scientific knowledge. Consider the following quote in your process of answering these philosophical questions:

> It is a conclusion which—like all other philosophical conclusions—we shall require good reasons for believing. We shall not be willing just to accept it on spec, or on faith, or because we have an intuition to that effect: we shall want to know why we should believe it to be true. (Magee, 2001, p. 8)

attempt to elucidate them. Of course, there is no experiment that can answer some of society's most fundamental ethical questions, such as "What is the meaning of good?" and "How beneficent are people or nurses required to be?"

Philosophy is used to address problems that are prescientific or nonscientific, problems such as the determination of good and evil (Durant, 1933). Science begins with a hypothesis that is tested with the scientific method; if the scientist is successful, doing science ends with a practical achievement. Philosophy, by comparison, "is a hypothetical interpretation of the unknown (as in metaphysics), or of the inexactly known (as in ethics or political philosophy)" (p. 2). Durant used a military metaphor to compare philosophy and science. In a siege of truth, philosophy occupies the most forward trench, whereas science represents the captured land. However, philosophy "leaves the fruits of victory to her daughters the sciences" (p. 2).

Science should be conducted impartially and objectively; it is focused on fact finding. Philosophy, although conducted with rational thinking, is value laden and is used to interpret and synthesize ideal possibilities, meanings, and the significance of experience. Science breaks the whole into parts, and then philosophy puts the parts back together again in a form that is better than the original whole. According to Durant:

> Science tells us how to heal and how to kill; it reduces the death rate in retail and then kills us wholesale in war; but only wisdom—desire coordinated in the light of all experience—can tell us when to heal and when to kill. (p. 2)

## Methods and Outcomes of Inquiry

Scientists generally use the scientific method to conduct *scientific inquiry*. Some of the characteristics of scientific inquiry are objectivity, generalizability, reproducibility, and being able to achieve outcomes of practical importance. In his classic book *A Primer in Theory Construction*, Reynolds (1971) listed five characteristics that a scientific body of knowledge should provide: (1) typology, (2) predictions, (3) explanations, (4) understanding about causes (i.e., independent variables' effects on dependent variables), and (5) control.

Often the outcomes of philosophy as compared to science provide knowledge and satisfaction for its own sake rather than for its practical benefits (Lund, 2003). In referring to medical ethics, Sulmasy and Sugarman (2001) stated that it is not always clear whether work done in the field of ethics by disciplines such as nursing, medicine, sociology, economics, law, and others is scholarly work. Three accepted scholarly methods of ethical inquiry or thinking that relate to ethics exist: *normative ethics*, *meta-ethics*, and *descriptive ethics* (Frankena, 1973). Sulmasy and Sugarman contended that "normative ethics [inquiry] is at the core of scholarship in ethics" (p. 4).

## Normative Ethics

Normative ethics is an attempt to decide or prescribe values, behaviors, and ways of being that are right or wrong, good or bad, and admirable or deplorable. When using the method of normative ethics, inquiries are made about how humans should behave, what ought to be done in certain situations, or which type of character one should have or how one should be. Outcomes of normative ethics are the prescriptions derived from asking normative questions. These prescriptions include accepted moral norms, standards, and codes.

One such accepted moral standard is the *common morality* (Beauchamp & Childress, 2009). The common morality consists of normative beliefs and behaviors about which the members of society generally agree and that are familiar to most human beings. For example, the belief that robbing a bank is wrong is part of the common morality in the United States. In contrast, because of the many and varying positions about the rightness or wrongness of abortion, accepting abortion as a moral act is not a part of our common morality. A normative belief in the nursing profession is that nurses ought to be compassionate—that is, nurses should work to relieve suffering. This claim is supported by the *Code of Ethics for Nurses with Interpretive Statements* (American Nurses Association, 2001) and *The ICN Code of Ethics for Nurses* (International Council of Nurses, 2006).

## Meta-Ethics

The focus of meta-ethics, which means "about ethics," is not an inquiry about what ought to be done or what behaviors should be prescribed. Rather, meta-ethics is concerned with understanding the language of morality through an analysis of the meaning of ethically related concepts and theories, such as the meaning of good, happiness, and virtuous character. For example, a nurse who is engaging actively in a meta-ethical analysis might try to determine the meaning of a good (i.e., moral) nurse–patient relationship.

## Descriptive Ethics

Of the three methods of inquiry, descriptive ethics comes closest to a scientific method of inquiry as opposed to philosophical ethical inquiry. This approach is used when researchers or ethicists want to describe what people think about morality or how people actually behave (i.e., their morals). Professional moral values and behaviors can be described empirically through nursing research using traditional descriptive research methodology. An example of descriptive ethics is the outcome of research that identifies nurses' attitudes regarding telling patients the truth about their terminal illnesses.

## The Fact/Value Distinction

In conducting ethical inquiry, one should be aware of the "fact/value" distinction to avoid the pitfall in moral reasoning called the "is/ought" gap. During the 18th century, the philosopher David Hume (1711–1776) made an important point about good moral reasoning, when he argued that there is a distinction between facts (for example, scientific or descriptive findings) and values (normative beliefs) when moral reasoning is considered. Not being sensitive to the "fact/value" distinction can leave one with an "is/ought" gap. A skeptic, Hume suggested that people should not acknowledge a fact of what is and then believe that they can legitimately prove the rightness or wrongness of a value judgment based on that fact. In other words, one logically cannot take a fact of what is and then extrapolate an ethical judgment of what ought to be.

If Hume's argument is accepted as valid, people should refrain from making the following assumption: (1) I see Sara practicing hard paternalism with her terminally ill cancer patient; (2) many bioethicists caution that a hard form of paternalism is unethical; therefore, (3) Sara ought not practice paternalism because it is unethical (a value statement). According to people who believe in the truth of the "fact/value" distinction, it is a fact that Sara is acting paternalistically toward her cancer patient, and it is a fact that many bioethicists believe that paternalism is unethical. However, the two facts in this example do not prove the moral nature of Sara's act of paternalism. The conclusion that Sara's act of paternalism is unethical is only a feeling that places a certain value on a particular act. Although Hume's "fact/value" distinction requirement for doing ethics precludes being able to prove the rightness or wrongness of value statements, it does not minimize the need for people to support their moral positions (value judgments) with valid arguments. Nevertheless, accepting Hume's argument does mean that identifying the truth in value statements is an interminable endeavor.

## Perspectives on Theory

The meaning and purposes of theory have been described and analyzed differently among myriad people both within and outside of nursing. Different perspectives about theory are discussed briefly in this section. Rather than providing a definitive conclusion about whether theories of ethics exist, and if they exist, the type of theory into which moral theory can be classified, readers are encouraged to draw their own conclusions about these points. It is important to note that most ethicists and other writers do refer to theories of ethics or moral theory when discussing ethics; however, most ethicists do not typically analyze the theoretical nature per se of ethical approaches.

Reynolds (1971) referred to "scientific theory" (p. 10) in his primer. He proposed that three primary forms of theories exist: (1) set-of-laws, (2) axiomatic, and (3) causal process. The first form is composed of theories that can be classified as scientific laws; the second includes sets of definitions, existence statements, and relational statements; and the third form is composed of sets of definitions, existence statements, and causal statements. Axiomatic theories are rare in social and human phenomena. Plane geometry is a good example of an axiomatic theory. Reynolds acknowledged that the following are sometimes considered to be other forms of theory: "1) vague conceptualizations or descriptions of events or things, 2) prescriptions about what are desirable social behaviors or arrangements, or 3) any untested hypothesis or idea" (p. 11). Nevertheless, he avoided a discussion of these latter forms of theory in his classic theory primer.

Some nurse authors and theorists distinguish nursing philosophies from nursing theories (McEwen, 2007; Tomey & Alligood, 2006). The structural holarchy of contemporary nursing (Fawcett, 2005) is depicted visually with a figure that lists the following elements in top to bottom order, although no assumption should be made that these elements exist linearly: metaparadigm, philosophies, conceptual models, theories, and empirical indicators. Fawcett defined theory as "one or more relatively concrete and specific concepts that are derived from a conceptual model, the propositions that narrowly describe those concepts, and the propositions that state relatively concrete and specific relations between two or more of the concepts" (p. 18).

Meleis (2005) defined theory as "an organized, coherent, and systematic articulation of a set of statements related to significant questions in a discipline that are communicated in a meaningful whole" (p. 12). These statements are used to describe, explain, predict, or prescribe "events, situations, conditions, or relationships" (p. 12). According to Meleis, a theory should contain concepts related to a discipline's phenomena of interest.

The philosophers Dickoff and James (1968) argued that theory for the practice discipline of nursing should be of the highest level—a type of theory that these authors called situation producing. They outlined the following characteristics of *situation-producing theory*: (1) it is invented for a purpose; (2) it includes specific goal content aimed at the outcome of some activity; (3) it is prescriptive in nature; and (4) it contains a survey list of aspects of related activity. Beckstrand (1978, 1980) specifically criticized Dickoff and James' conception of situation-producing theory as being too personal in nature, as well as being unnecessary for nursing. Although the term *evidence-based practice* was not in vogue when she wrote her articles, Beckstrand contended that when nurses use situation-producing theory, they essentially decide on their own goals for patient care without subjecting the goals to consensus or examining evidence for and against the goals. Beckstrand's other criticism is discussed later in this section.

Wiedenbach (1970), who wrote and worked with Dickoff and James, also developed a philosophy-based practice theory for nurses that she classified as prescriptive. Wiedenbach defined theory as follows:

> [A]n abstract phenomenon. It develops within the mind but derives from reality and influences action. It is the outgrowth of an intellectual process set in motion by observations. From them, ideas are generated. Then, by means of the intellect, the ideas—we'll call them concepts—may be consciously brought into meaningful relationship with one another for such purposes as to identify or isolate factors, to characterize or classify them, to predict effect from cause, or to prescribe a course of action by which to obtain desired results. (p. 1057)

Wiedenbach (1970) asserted that nurses use theory to guide practice, which can be interpreted as a personal use, and to improve nursing practice, which can be interpreted as a use for the common good of the profession. According to Wiedenbach, each nurse must identify (theorize about) what underlies his or her practice. To meet this challenge, the nurse must answer three questions: (1) "What needs to be accomplished?", (2) "How will it be accomplished?", and (3) "In which context will it be done?" When these questions are answered, the nurse has the information needed to identify a prescriptive theory for practice. The three essential characteristics of the prescriptive theory are (1) the nurse's professional commitment (purpose), (2) the prescription for achieving the nurse's purpose, and (3) the realities that affect the process and, ultimately, the outcomes of the nurse's actions. In regard to the first characteristic, nurses need to specify their beliefs. Wiedenbach's prescriptive form of practice theory is subject to the same criticism that Beckstrand (1980) used in evaluating Dickoff and James' situation-producing theory—namely, it might be viewed as too subjective.

In 1978, Beckstrand asserted that while much buzz focused on developing a practice theory for nursing, such as the situation-producing theory suggested by Dickoff and James (1968), the profession does not really need a practice theory at all. She argued that nurses have access to scientific and ethical theories and that all other knowledge needed by nurses is reducible to these two fields. Science is needed "to describe, to explain, and to predict natural and social phenomena" and "the purpose of ethical or normative theory is to describe and to predict what actions and characteristics will lead to the realization of morality and goodness" (Beckstrand, 1978, p. 606). Nursing practice is focused on changing entities so that more good can be achieved. Beckstrand distinguished ethical theory useful to nursing as being of the normative type. She discussed important ethical knowledge in terms of moral obligations and moral values. Also essential to justify the goals of nursing practice is knowledge about theories of nonmoral value, which can be evaluated in terms of utility or being intrinsic, extrinsic, contributory, or instrumental. Ultimately, Beckstrand concluded that scientific theory and ethical theory (including nonmoral value theory) are sufficient to guide nursing practice without the development of additional practice theories.

According to Vaughn (2010), "moral theories are meant to explain what makes an action right or a person good" (p. 43). Thus Vaughn's position indicates that moral theory is of the explanatory type, but he added that moral theory also "must be filled out with details about how to apply them in real life and the kinds of cases to which they are relevant" (p. 31). This means that moral theory is prescriptive as well as explanatory. He divided moral theories into those that focus on right action and those that focus on good or bad character. To identify the best theory for determining what is right and good, three criteria were proposed: "consistency with our considered moral judgments, consistency with the facts of the moral life, and resourcefulness in moral problem solving" (p. 44).

Vaughn (2010) called morality a "normative, or evaluative, enterprise" (p. 5) that can be distinguished from nonmoral norms, which also are applied in everyday life. Moral norms are different because they possess the following characteristics: (1) *normative dominance*—accepting the practice of allowing moral norms to dominate or override nonmoral norms; (2) *universality*—recognizing that certain moral norms should be applicable across all comparable situations; (3) *impartiality*—the notion that all individuals' interests should be considered equally (note: this characteristic has been debated among ethicists depending on preferred theories, such as in feminist ethics and communitarianism); and (4) *reasonableness*—norms having sound support in good moral reasoning.

The ethicists Beauchamp and Childress have been highly influential in the development of the field of bioethics. Beauchamp and Childress (2009) proposed that the following characteristics may be used to describe ethical or moral theory: "1) abstract moral reflection and argument, 2) systematic presentation of the basic components of ethics, 3) an integrated body of moral principles, and 4) a systematic justification of moral principles" (p. 333). Major moral theories include a hypothesis that offers a moral framework. These authors distinguish two conceptions of ethical theory, which are separated temporally. The task of ethical theory in the older conception (late 18th to early 20th century) "is to locate and justify general norms as a system" (p. 334). In the more recent conception, which is less well formed, ethical theory is tasked with reflecting "critically on actual and proposed moral norms and practices" (p. 334).

Beauchamp and Childress (2009) have outlined eight conditions against which ethical theories can be evaluated: (1) clarity (clearness), (2) coherence (no conceptual inconsistencies or contradictory statements), (3) comprehensiveness (accounts for a sizable number of justified moral norms or judgments), (4) simplicity (narrows morality to only a few basic norms), (5) explanatory power (helps people understand morality), (6) justificatory power (provides new grounds for beliefs or a justified criticism of defective beliefs), (7) output power (produces new moral judgments), and (8) practicability (requirements of the theory are not too demanding to make it unfeasible to use). It is not expected that all ethical theories will be able to fulfill all eight of these conditions.

The next section of this chapter covers specific approaches to ethics that most ethicists call theories. Before reading this section, review **Box 9–3** and begin to formulate your positions about theory as it relates to ethics.

## Theoretical Approaches to Ethics

Assuming that ethical or moral theories exist, they generally are considered to be normative in nature. Normative ethical theories function as moral guides to answer the questions, "What should I do or not do?" and "How should I be?" A moral theory can provide individuals with guidance in moral thinking and reasoning, as well as offering justification for moral actions.

> ## Box 9–3  Evaluation of Theory for Ethics
>
> Formulate answers to these questions before reading the final section of the chapter. After reading the final section, revisit these questions and continue to refine your judgments. Supplementary information may be needed to accomplish this activity, especially additional readings about specific moral theories or approaches.
>
> 1. Do ethical or moral theories exist? Support your answer.
>
> 2. Which type of classification best fits the purpose of ethical theories or approaches (for example, prescription, explanation, prediction, or control)? Support your answer.
>
> 3. How do ethical theories or approaches differ from nursing theories? Compare and contrast.

The descriptions of the theories in this section are not all inclusive, nor do they necessarily include all variations of the theories that are discussed. Theories of ethics overlap and often are quite abstract and difficult to study. Therefore, the theories discussed in this chapter, because of their brief presentation, provide a somewhat oversimplified view. The goal was to include enough discussion to illustrate the major concepts important to the content of each theory. Readers are encouraged to seek more information about each theory, consider related concepts, and construct propositional statements that are reasonable given what is included in discussions of the theories in ethics literature.

## Rule-Based Theories
### Natural Law Theory
Most modern versions of natural law theory have their basis in the philosophy of St. Thomas Aquinas (ca 1225–1274). People who adhere to natural law theory believe that the rightness of actions is self-evident because morality is determined by inherent human nature, not by customs and preferences. According to this theory, the law of reason is incorporated within the order of nature (usually thought to be implanted by God), and this law provides the rules or commands for human actions. Consequently, natural law theory is often associated with rule-based Judeo-Christian ethics. Natural law theory is the basis of religious prohibitions against acts that some people consider to be unnatural, such as homosexuality, the use of birth control, and fertility procedures.

### Rights Theory
Since the time of Thomas Hobbes (1588–1679), the concepts of individualism and liberalism have been associated with a rights-based theory of ethics (Beauchamp &

Childress, 2009). "Rights are *justified claims* that individuals and groups can make on other individuals or on society" (p. 350). Decisions about allowing or disallowing rights come from a society's normative framework. In the United States, legal rights stem from the Constitution and federal, state, and local legal systems. Moral rights are less well defined. For example, in the United States, groups continue to argue about whether health care is a right or a privilege. Libertarians believe in market justice—that is, they believe that people should earn and pay for the benefits that they receive; in contrast, communitarians believe that health care for all citizens contributes to the common good of the community.

Disagreements also exist about whether moral rights are always absolute or whether they sometimes are *prima facie* claims that must give way to other rights. To exercise one's rights ethically, it is generally accepted that a person should not violate the rights of other people. An example of an absolute right is the right to choose one's religion, whereas a *prima facie* right is the right to autonomy. Sometimes one's autonomy must be overruled when, for instance, it might cause an infringement on another person's right to health.

## *Deontology*

Deontology, literally the study of duty, is an approach to ethics that focuses on duties and rules. The most influential philosopher associated with the deontological way of thinking was Immanuel Kant (1724–1804). Kant (1785/2012) defined a person as a rational, self-legislating (autonomous) being with the ability to know universal, objective moral laws and the freedom to decide to act morally, which means to act according to one's duty. Kantian deontology prescribes that each rational being is ethically bound or obligated to act first and foremost from a sense of duty. When deciding how to act, the consequences of one's actions are considered to be irrelevant.

According to Kant, only dutiful actions have moral worth. Even when individuals do not want to act from a motivation of duty, Kant believed that they are required ethically to do so. In fact, having one's actions motivated by duty is superior to acting from a motivation of love. Because rational choice is within one's control, whereas one has only tenuous control over personal emotions, only reason—and not emotion—is sufficient to lead a person to moral actions. In Kantian deontology, the only intrinsically good thing is a good will that motivates dutiful actions.

Kant believed that people are ends in themselves and should be treated accordingly. Each autonomous, self-directed person has dignity and is due respect. An individual should never act in ways that involve using other people as a means to his or her personal ends. In fact, when people use others as a means to ends, even if they believe that they are using persons to reach ethical goals, Kant believed that a person's dignity is harmed. An example would be a failure to obtain full, informed consent from a research participant even though the researcher steadfastly believes that the research will be beneficial to the participant.

Kant identified rules to guide people in thinking about their obligations. In doing so, he drew a distinction between two types of duties or obligations: the *hypothetical imperative* and the *categorical imperative*. Hypothetical imperatives are optional duties or rules that people ought to observe or follow if certain ends are to be achieved. Such statements are sometimes called *if–then* imperatives, which means that they involve conditional or optional actions—for instance, "If I want to eat tonight, then I should go to the grocery store today."

However, where moral actions are concerned, Kant believed that duties and laws are absolute and unconditional. He proposed that people ought to follow a universal, unconditional framework of maxims, or rules, as a guide to know the rightness of actions and one's moral duties. According to Kant, these absolute and unconditional duties constitute categorical imperatives. When deciding about matters of ethics and acting according to a categorical imperative, one needs to ask the question, "If I perform this action, could I will that it should become a universal law for everyone to act in the same way?" No action can ever be judged as right, according to Kant, if it is not reasonable that the action could become a binding, ethical law for all people. For example, Kant's ethics imposes the categorical imperative that one should never tell a lie, because a person cannot rationally wish that all people should be able to pick and choose when they have permission not to be truthful. Another example of a categorical imperative is that suicide is never acceptable. A person, when committing suicide, cannot rationally wish that all people should feel free to commit suicide or the world would become chaotic.

Kantianism is valued highly in Western medicine because of the focus on individual rights, autonomy, and informed consent. In the U.S. healthcare system and in Western bioethics, the choices of rational individuals generally are respected. In public health, however, practitioners often must balance the rights of individuals against the rights of populations and communities. Sometimes navigating this delicate balance can be controversial or generate dilemmas, such as considering appropriate actions that may breach confidentiality when a person with a stigmatizing communicable disease may jeopardize the health of other people. This situation results in a need to balance the need to respect the autonomy and protect the confidentiality of one person against the need to protect the safety of other persons.

## Consequentialism

Consequentialists, as distinguished from deontologists, do consider consequences to be an important indication of the moral value of one's actions. *Utilitarianism* is the most well-known consequentialist theory of ethics. Under utilitarianism, actions are judged by their utility—that is, they are evaluated according to the usefulness of their consequences. When people use the theory of utilitarianism as the basis for ethical behavior, they attempt to promote the greatest good (happiness or pleasure) and to inflict the least amount of harm (suffering or pain) that is possible in a situation. In other words, utilitarians believe that it is useful to society to achieve the greatest good for the greatest number of people who may be affected by a rule or action. People who use a utilitarian approach to ethics place great emphasis on what is best for collective groups, not individual people, although each individual's happiness is worthy of equal consideration as compared to every other individual in a group.

The British philosopher Jeremy Bentham (1748–1832) was an early promoter of the principle of utilitarianism. During Bentham's life, British society functioned according to aristocratic privilege. Poor people were mistreated by people in the upper classes and were given no choice other than to work long hours in deplorable conditions. Bentham tried to develop a theory that could be used to achieve a fair distribution of pleasure among all British citizens. He went so far as to develop a systematic decision-making method that relied on mathematical calculations. Bentham's method was designed to determine ways to allocate pleasure and to diminish pain by using the measures of intensity and duration. His approach to utilitarianism has been criticized, however, because Bentham equated all types of pleasure as being equal.

Another Englishman, John Stuart Mill (1806–1873), challenged Bentham's views when he pointed out that particular experiences of pleasure and happiness clearly do have different qualities and that different situations do not necessarily produce equal consequences. For example, Mill stated that the higher intellectual pleasures may be differentiated from lower physical pleasures. The higher pleasures, such as enjoying a work of art or a scholarly book, are considered to be better because only human beings, not other animals, possess the mental faculties to enjoy this higher level of happiness.

According to Mill, happiness is measured by quality and not quantity (duration or intensity). In making these distinctions between higher and lower levels of happiness, Mill's philosophy focuses more on ethics than does Bentham's philosophy, which was devised as a means to change social or political policy. Mill believed that communities usually agree about what is good and about those things that best promote the happiness of the most people. An example of an application of Mill's utilitarianism is mandatory vaccination laws, under which individual liberties are limited so that the larger society is protected from diseases. The consequence is that people generally are happier because they are free of diseases. Because of the emphasis on population-focused care, utilitarianism is one of the most widely used ethical approaches in public health practice.

People using Mill's form of utilitarian theory often can defer to widely supported traditions to guide them in deciding which rules and behaviors will probably produce the best consequences for the most people, such as the maxim, "Stealing is wrong." Through experience, humans generally have identified many behaviors that will produce the most happiness or unhappiness for society as a whole.

## Communitarianism

"All communities have some organizing vision about the meaning of life and how one ought to conduct a good life" (Wildes, 2000, p. 129). Communitarian ethics is based on the position that "everything fundamental in ethics derives from communal values, the common good, social goals, traditional practices, and cooperative virtues" (Beauchamp & Childress, 2001, p. 362). Communitarian ethics is relevant to moral relationships in any community.

The notion that communitarian ethics is based on the model of friendships and relationships that existed in the ancient Greek city-states described by Aristotle was popularized in modern times by the philosopher and ethicist Alasdair MacIntyre (1984) in his book *After Virtue*. In general societal ethics and in bioethics, the valuing and consideration of community relationships have come to mean different things to different people, however (Beauchamp & Childress, 2001). Communitarian ethics is distinguished as an ethical approach in that the epicenter of communitarian ethics is the community, rather than any one individual (Wildes, 2000). The value of discussing and articulating an approach to communitarian ethics lies in the benefit that can be gained from illuminating and appreciating the relationships and interconnections between people that are often overlooked in everyday life.

According to this philosophy, although personal moral goals, such as the pursuit of personal well-being, are significant, the importance of forming strong communities and identifying the moral goals of communities must not be neglected if both individuals and communities are to flourish. An important distinction that legitimately can be drawn between communitarian and other popular ethical approaches, such as rule-based ethics, lies in communitarian ethicists' proposal that it is natural for humans to favor the people with whom they live and have frequent interactions. Kantian deontologists base their ethics on an impartial stance toward the persons who experience the effects of their morally related actions. However, using a communitarian ethic and valuing partiality as a way of relating to other people do not necessarily exclude caring about people who are personally unknown to moral agents. Although it is often easier for people to care about and have compassion for people who are relationally closest to them, it is not unrealistic to believe that people can develop empathy or compassion toward people who are personally unknown to them. Such behavior and expectations are an integral part of Christian and Buddhist philosophies, for example. Accepting the notion that humans usually are more partial to those people with whom they are most closely related, while at the same time believing that it is possible to expand the scope of their empathy and compassion to unknown others, broadens the sphere of morality in communitarian ethics.

The education of communities often occurs through role modeling (Wildes, 2000). Members of communities learn about what is and is not accepted as moral through personal and group interactions and dialog within their communities. Nurses share narratives about the lives of exemplars, such as Florence Nightingale and Lillian Wald, to illustrate moral living. By her efforts to improve social justice and health protection through environmental measures and her efforts to elevate the character of nurses, Nightingale exhibited moral concern for her local

**TABLE 9–1**

| Theory | Concepts |
|---|---|
| Natural Law | Self-evident; nature; natural; inherent |
| Rights | Justified claim; individualism; liberalism; absolute right; *prima facie* right |
| Deontology | Categorical imperative; duty; ends and means; good will |
| Utilitarianism | Happiness; consequence; greatest good; utility |
| Communitarianism | Common good; flourishing; traditional practices; cooperative virtues |

society, the nursing profession, and people remote from her local associations, such as the population of soldiers affected by the Crimean War. Likewise, Lillian Wald was an excellent role model for members of communities because of her efforts to improve social justice through her work at the Henry Street Settlement. When learning from the examples of Nightingale and Wald, communitarian-minded nurses are in an excellent position to educate the public and other nurses and healthcare professionals about why they, in many ways, should assume the role of being their brothers' and sisters' keepers. (For a summary of the theories discussed in this section, see **Table 9–1**.)

# Summary

Rather than providing in-depth information about a variety of theories of ethics, this chapter seeks to raise awareness about the philosophy of ethics and the ways in which related theories are constructed and classified. Doing ethics is a significant part of advanced nursing practice, as is using appropriate theory in practice. Being moral and acting in moral ways is not accidental. Aristotle believed that morality (for him, virtue) can be taught and must be ingrained through habit. With Aristotle's position in mind, readers are reminded to learn more about ethics and consciously develop moral habits grounded in reasonable moral theories.

# Discussion Questions

1. Choose one ethical theory discussed in this chapter. Define the related concepts outlined in Table 9–1. Examine literature about the theory and identify and define other concepts used in the theory.

2. Use the concepts that you defined for Question 1 and develop proposition statements specific to the ethical theory.

3. Compare your chosen theory to Beauchamp and Childress's and Vaughn's criteria discussed in this chapter. What are your conclusions?

4. Analyze your chosen theory using Fawcett's criteria.

5. Do you agree with Beckstrand's argument that all knowledge in nursing is reducible to theories in the fields of science and ethics? Support your position.

# References

American Association of Colleges of Nursing. (2006). *Essentials of doctoral education for advanced nursing practice*. Washington, DC: Author.

American Nurses Association. (2001). *Code of ethics for nurses with interpretive statements*. Silver Springs, MD: Author.

Beauchamp, T. L., & Childress, J. F. (2001). *Principles of biomedical ethics* (5th ed.). New York, NY: Oxford University Press.

Beauchamp, T. L., & Childress, J. F. (2009). *Principles of biomedical ethics* (6th ed.). New York, NY: Oxford University Press.

Beckstrand, J. (1978). The notion of a practice theory and the relationship of scientific and ethical knowledge to practice. *Research in Nursing and Health, 1,* 131–136. Reproduced in L. H. Nicoll (1997), *Perspectives on nursing theory* (3rd ed., pp. 605–613). Philadelphia, PA: Lippincott.

Beckstrand, J. (1980). A critique of several conceptions of practice theory in nursing. *Research in Nursing and Health, 3,* 69–70. Reproduced in L. H. Nicoll (1997), *Perspectives on nursing theory* (3rd ed., pp. 620–631). Philadelphia, PA: Lippincott.

Billington, R. (2003). *Living philosophy: An introduction to moral thought* (3rd ed.). New York, NY: Routledge, Taylor & Francis.

Dickoff, J., & James, P. (1968). A theory of theories: A position paper. *American Journal of Nursing, 17*(3), 197–203.

Durant, W. (1933). *The story of philosophy*. New York, NY: Simon & Schuster.

Fawcett, J. (2005). *Contemporary nursing knowledge* (2nd ed.). Philadelphia, PA: F. A. Davis.

Frankena, W. K. (1973). *Ethics* (2nd ed.). Retrieved from http://www.ditext.com/frankena/e1.html

International Council of Nurses. (2006). *The ICN code of ethics for nurses*. Geneva, Switzerland: Author.

Kant, Immanuel. (Trans. M. Gregor). (1785/2012). *The groundwork of the metaphysics of morals*. Cambridge, MD: Cambridge University Press.

Lund, D. H. (2003). *Making sense of it all*. Upper Saddle River, NJ: Prentice Hall.

MacIntyre, A. (1984). *After virtue: A study of moral theory* (2nd ed.). Notre Dame, IN: University of Notre Dame Press.

Magee, B. (2001). *The story of philosophy*. New York, NY: Dorling Kindersley.

McEwen, M. (2007). Theory development: Structuring conceptual relationships in nursing. In M. McEwen & E. M. Wills (Eds.), *Theoretical basis for nursing* (2nd ed., pp. 73–94). Philadelphia, PA: Lippincott Williams & Wilkins.

Meleis, A. I. (2005). *Theoretical development and progress* (3rd ed. rev. reprint). Philadelphia, PA: Lippincott Williams & Wilkins.

Reynolds, P. D. (1971). *A primer in theory construction*. Indianapolis, IN: Bobbs-Merrill Educational.

Russell, B. (1945). *The history of Western philosophy*. New York, NY: Simon & Schuster.

Sulmasy, D. P., & Sugarman, J. (2001). The many methods of medical ethics (or, thirteen ways of looking at a blackbird). In J. Sugarman & D. P. Sulmasy (Eds.), *Methods in medical ethics* (pp. 3–18). Washington, DC: Georgetown University Press.

Tarnas, R. (1991). *The passion of the Western mind.* New York, NY: Ballantine.

Tomey, A. M., & Alligood, M. R. (Eds.). (2006). *Nursing theorists and their work* (6th ed.). St. Louis, MO: Mosby Elsevier.

Vaughn, L. (2010). *Bioethics: Principles, issues and cases.* New York, NY: Oxford University Press.

Wiedenbach, E. (1970). Nurses' wisdom in nursing theory. *American Journal of Nursing, 70*(3), 1057–1062.

Wildes, K. M. (2000). *Moral acquaintances: Methodology in bioethics.* Notre Dame, IN: University of Notre Dame Press.

# CHAPTER 10

# Educational and Learning Theories

*Margaret M. Braungart*
*Richard G. Braungart*

## Introduction

To learn is to gain knowledge, understanding, or skills through experience. Learning is fundamental to human development. It may be formal or informal, direct or indirect, or consciously or unconsciously acquired. From a psychological perspective, learning involves a relatively permanent change in an individual's thinking, emotions, attitudes, or behavior. A lifelong process, the key to learning is experience. Much of an individual's identity is based on what he or she has learned through family, schools, and culture, while growing up during a particular era in history. Not only are people challenged to learn new information and skills throughout their lives, but they may also need to unlearn or relearn behaviors, emotions, and attitudes—challenges that are especially evident in the healthcare field.

Nurses spend a significant amount of their time and energy involved with learning and teaching, whether acquiring new information as part of their professional and continuing education or instructing others in health care. Advanced practice nurses, in particular, are concerned with teaching and learning in numerous ways. In part, this focus reflects their leadership roles in healthcare education, administration, and planning. For example, how can a nursing instructor motivate a classroom of diverse students to learn when many are juggling the demands of education with the burdens of work and family? How can nurses in management and policy-making positions address the need to change staff behavior regarding ethical breaches, medical mistakes, infection control, and workplace conflicts? And how might nurses construct and implement an effective hospital or community education campaign to improve health behaviors?

These examples from nursing and health care suggest three fundamental questions about learning:

1. What are effective ways to learn new information or change attitudes and behaviors in health care?
2. How can people be motivated to learn, and which kinds of experiences facilitate learning?
3. What are effective ways to teach so that information and skills will be remembered rather than forgotten and will transfer correctly outside the immediate learning situation?

This chapter examines learning from an educational, psychological, and research-based perspective by reviewing the basic principles of learning theories and suggesting how they can be applied to advanced nursing practice. Learning theory is defined and discussed in relation to nursing, and the most widely used learning theories are described and illustrated with examples from health care. Neuropsychology research on the underlying physiological dynamics of learning is mentioned briefly as well. The perspectives on learning are then pulled together into a general model of learning, followed by a discussion of how nurses can decide which theories and principles to use and how the three fundamental questions about learning pertain to nursing practice.

## Learning Theory

Learning theory in education is rooted in the field of psychology. Psychology is the scientific study of mental processes and behavior and represents a research-based approach to understanding human behavior. Educational psychology is a specialty area devoted to the study of learning, teaching, and assessment (Ormrod, 2007; Woolfolk, 2001). Reflecting different schools of psychology, the principal learning theories were formulated during the first half of the 20th century to describe, explain, and predict how learning occurs. Learning theories are useful for understanding how people gain knowledge and skills, as well as how emotions, attitudes, and behaviors are acquired and can be changed. These theories are highly applicable and provide the foundation for educational practices, counseling, advertising, workplace management, and rehabilitation.

To help nurses understand the various dimensions and dynamics of learning, the chapter summarizes four learning theories that are widely recognized in psychology and education: (1) behaviorist theory, (2) cognitive theory, (3) psychodynamic theory, and (4) humanistic theory. Behaviorist and cognitive theories were prominent in education during the first half of the early 20th century; by the 21st century, however, cognitive theory had begun to dominate academic research and practice in psychology and education. Nonetheless, principles of behaviorist theory continue to be useful in education, the workplace, counseling, health care, and other areas in society. While not always considered learning theories per se, psychodynamic and humanistic theories are included in the discussion presented in this chapter because they highlight emotional learning and emphasize the importance of the teacher–learner relationship (Hilgard & Bower, 1966). Illness and health care are often highly charged experiences. Consequently, nurses conducting health education and endeavoring to achieve behavior change should not ignore the role of emotions in the learning process.

Each of the four theories discussed here reflects a different perspective on learning and comprises a distinct set of constructs and principles. The theories include information regarding the kinds of experiences that motivate learning and how to maximize the likelihood that learning will be remembered and can be transferred to a variety of settings. The theories differ in terms of whether the learner is viewed as more passive or active; whether the focus of the theory is on external environmental influences or on internal processes within the learner; and whether the principal route to learning is through behavior, thinking processes, or emotions and feelings. These days, learning theory cannot be fully discussed without including information from neuropsychology research, which helps educators sort out conflicting claims of learning theories. Principles of learning can be applied to nursing, patient, staff, and community education, as well as to changing attitudes and behavior in a variety of circumstances. Healthcare research data reveal that using learning theories to design professional education and intervention programs enhances their success (Clark, Mitchell, & Rand, 2009; Ferguson & Day, 2005; Leinster, 2009; Sargeant, 2009).

This chapter is organized as follows. An overview of each learning theory is presented, including its origins, basic constructs, and principles. Focus is given to each theory's perspective on motivation, practice, retention, and transfer, as well as to which kinds of teaching approaches and experiences aid or hinder learning. Criticisms of the theories are also offered. The theories and principles selected for discussion are considered useful to advanced practice nurses. Behaviorist and cognitive theories are emphasized, and psychodynamic and humanistic theories are viewed as supplementing and strengthening nursing education and professionalism. For organizational clarity, each theory is presented as a unit. In practice, the theories are often used in combination. To help nurses make decisions about how to use learning theories, a general model of learning is offered, and the three fundamental questions raised earlier about learning and teaching are addressed in relation to nursing practice. Learning theories provide a toolbox of approaches from which nurses can select the appropriate option to address problems related to nursing and health education or to modify attitudes and behavior in a variety of settings.

## Behaviorist Learning Theory

According to behaviorist theory (also referred to as behaviorism), given that there is no way to know accurately what is going on within a person's mind, the focus should be on only what is directly observable. What is observable in any learning situation are the stimulus conditions (S) in the environment and the behavior (movements, acts, actions) that is exhibited in response (R) to stimulus conditions (O'Donohue & Kitchener, 1999). In this model, learning is relatively simple; it is based on the associations people make between *stimuli* and *responses* (termed the *S–R model of learning*), and the belief that life is largely a matter of habit that requires little thinking. For example, people learn their health habits, such as their responses to foods, their physical exercise patterns, and their reactions to stress. For better or worse, much behavior is learned in the family through socialization and is passed from generation to generation.

According to behaviorists, what is learned can be unlearned by modifying stimulus conditions in the environment or changing the response to stimuli. The route to learning, then, goes through behavior and action—the learning is in the doing—rather than through inner processes such as thinking and feeling. Changes in thinking and feeling, in fact, may come about by first changing behavior; thoughts and emotions then follow. For instance, if nurses who lack self-confidence are given responsibilities where they can perform well, their self-confidence may improve over time. Thus the route to personal change proceeds through behavior and practice.

Behaviorist principles are useful for breaking bad habits, designing practice sessions for sports and rehabilitation, and working with people who are more comfortable engaging in actions than reflecting on thoughts and emotions. Behaviorism provides the foundation for behavior modification programs, behavioral medicine, commercial advertising, and some therapies. The principles of the behaviorist model of learning can be applied to animals as well as people.

To promote learning, behaviorists change the stimulus–response (S–R) associations the learner makes in the environment and may follow a learner's response with some kind of reinforcement. To learn, of course, people must be motivated to make a response. Motivation is based on drive reduction—that is, having a drive that needs to be alleviated or satisfied. Primary drives are unlearned, such as the drive for food, warmth, sleep, sex, and avoidance of pain. In contrast, secondary drives are learned, such as the drive for financial security, popularity, or achievement. Culture plays an important role in learning secondary drives. It is difficult to encourage people to learn if there is no drive to be reduced, such as when people are satisfied, complacent, and satiated, or when another drive overpowers the drive to learn.

According to behaviorist learning theory, the process of learning proceeds as follows. Once a primary connection is made between the stimulus and the response, learning can be said to have occurred, which is somewhat of an "all or nothing" experience (e.g., not being able to ride a bike, then suddenly being able to steer and ride the bike; not being able to insert an intravenous [IV] line after many tries, then suddenly inserting it correctly). Most initial learning needs to be strengthened with practice. According to behaviorists, memory and retention are helped by repeating S–R connections, although there is a point at which practice becomes redundant and a waste of time. In its early stage, learning tends to be generalized to similar objects, situations, and stimuli. With additional and varied experiences, however, learners begin to make more sophisticated distinctions, called *discrimination learning*. In a sense, advanced practice nursing education is an exercise in discrimination learning.

The goal of most learning is to be able to transfer what is learned to other settings, such as teaching self-care to patients in the hospital—learning that is intended to be transferred to the home and workplace once patients have been discharged from the hospital. Transfer of learning is enhanced when the stimulus conditions and responses in the practice session and in the transfer situation are similar. Thus, working with patients in a hospital or rehabilitation center is necessary, but it may not be sufficient for the transfer of patients' learning outside the institution.

In the behaviorist model, the learner is relatively passive. The teacher or instructor plays a significant role in influencing learning through astute observation of S–R conditions and learners' reactions. Teachers are also responsible for the selection of motivating and well-chosen experiences to maximize learning, retention, and transfer. Likewise, the effectiveness of teaching depends on identifying appropriate stimulus conditions, reinforcement, practice, and feedback to ensure learning.

Two behaviorist perspectives on how learning occurs have had a significant impact on education and promoting behavior change: (1) classical conditioning and (2) operant conditioning. Conditioning is a powerful tool of learning, largely because little, if any, thinking is required in the learning process.

## Classical Conditioning

*Classical conditioning*, sometimes referred to as respondent conditioning or Pavlovian conditioning, is a simple model of learning identified by Russian physiologist Ivan Pavlov in the late 19th century. Pavlov's classical experiment demonstrated how organisms become conditioned or learn their responses to stimuli. Simple conditioning works as follows. Take a naturally occurring S–R connection that did not have to be learned (an unconditioned stimulus–unconditioned response connection). In Pavlov's experiment, hungry dogs salivate when presented with food; in this case, food is the unconditioned stimulus (UCS) and salivation is the unconditioned response (UCR).

Pavlov then decided to introduce a neutral stimulus (NS) into the experiment; a NS is an arbitrary stimulus that has no natural connection to the UCS–UCR association. In one experiment, he used a bell as the NS. Initially, when Pavlov rang the bell, it did not signal anything in particular to the dog. To demonstrate how simple learning occurs, he decided to condition the dog to salivate at the sound of the bell. As Pavlov presented food (UCS) to the dog, he rang the bell (NS), and the dog salivated (UCR); the salivation occurred in response to the presentation of the food at this time. Pavlov then repeated the UCS–NS–UCR sequence. After several repeated trials, he rang the bell but did not present food, and the dog salivated. The dog's reaction demonstrated that learning had occurred—the bell had become the conditioned stimulus (CS) and salivation the conditioned response (CR). In other words, the once NS that had no meaning to the dog had been learned as a signal for food that the dog responded to by salivating (CS–CR). Pavlov later conditioned the dog to respond to a light as a signal, demonstrating how diverse neutral stimuli can become associated with responses.

A pervasive example of classical conditioning in health care in the United States occurs with prescription drug advertising. (Only the United States and New Zealand currently permit direct-to-consumer prescription drug advertising.) Each pharmaceutical company attempts to condition potential customers to prefer its drug over competitors' drugs to treat the same medical condition. In the ads, a company's drug is the NS, which is then paired with a naturally occurring association, such as images of patients' happiness about relief from pain, their comfort and attractiveness in being able to perform normal functions, or their ability to remain active and independent. The drug's brand name is repeated a number of times so that it becomes associated with images of relief, attractiveness, or independence, and consumers are urged to ask their doctor about the brand-name drug. To see how this association changes depending on the target audience, compare ads for a particular prescription drug in commercial trade magazines with ads for the same drug in medical journals. In medical journals, prescription drugs are often associated with images of physician power, authority, or even magical healing abilities.

Classical conditioning has been used to demonstrate how emotions such as fear can be learned. In fear conditioning, an NS is paired with an aversive stimulus (e.g., pain, loud noise, shock, traumatic experience) until the NS alone comes to elicit the fear response (freezing, stress reaction, agitation, and anxiety). Behaviorists have shown that fear can be taught (conditioned) in animals and in people, which represents one explanation for how anxiety, phobias, and delayed-stress syndrome may be learned. As an illustration, people may learn to genuinely fear hospitals if they have several unfortunate or painful (physical or emotional) experiences with hospitals as a patient or a visitor.

What has been learned can be unlearned, according to the behaviorists. Indeed, over the years behaviorists have shown how principles of conditioning can be used to extinguish negative emotions (fears, anxieties, rage) and break bad habits (unhealthy behaviors) simply by changing S–R connections and practicing the new response. Note that in classical conditioning, rewards are not needed.

A first step in this type of effort is to carefully assess the stimulus conditions or cues in the environment that automatically trigger the undesirable response. Some of the following procedures may be used to extinguish problematic emotions or unhealthy habits:

- Introduce the fear- or anxiety-producing stimulus (e.g., fear of heights, dark spaces, or a certain animal; anxiety about public speaking or social situations) at a low level so the client does not respond negatively. Gradually increase the strength of the fearful or anxious stimulus presented until the client can be in its presence without being afraid or agitated. For instance, someone with a fear of dogs might be shown pictures of dogs first, be given a cute toy dog, then view a live dog at a distance, slowly moving the dog closer until the client pets the dog. This conditioning technique, which is termed *systematic desensitization*, may take several sessions and is useful for extinguishing many fears, phobias, and anxieties. Clients are sometimes taught relaxation techniques so they can remain relatively calm (not anxious) in the presence of a fearful or threatening stimulus.

- Rechain events (S–R connections) by identifying the stimuli or cues that trigger unwanted behavior and then constructing a new chain of responses that does not include the unwanted behavior in response to the cues. This approach is useful for dieters, procrastinators, and persons with anger management issues, among others. To illustrate, procrastinating students often engage in a host of distracting tasks once they arrive home. Studying is postponed until late at night when they are tired. As part of their retraining, students realize the S–R chain starts when they enter the door at home, and their first task in rechaining events is to study for at least an hour before performing other tasks. Practicing this sequence of events for several weeks can help students' procrastination decrease and their studying behavior improve at home.

- Interfere with an S–R association, which can be accomplished in two ways. First, one can create new stimulus conditions. People who abuse alcohol, for example, may need to change friends and avoid stimulus environments (e.g., bars, cocktail parties, restaurants serving alcohol) that increase the likelihood of substance abuse. Second, one can substitute a healthy response for the unhealthy response to existing cues. If individuals with an alcohol problem need to be in situations where people are drinking alcohol, they could change their response to the stimulus situation by drinking sparkling water or juice in a cocktail glass. Building a new S–R association takes time; practice is required to form new habits. This technique may be useful for dieters, smokers, and persons struggling with substance abuse, anger management, or worry and anxiety.

- "Fatiguing the response" involves performing the unwanted behavior repeatedly until the client has a negative reaction and manifests a different response. For instance, chain smokers may be told to stand in a corner and smoke cigarette after cigarette. As the smoke blows back in their face, they become disgusted or feel ill and demand to stop. When this behavior is practiced over several days, the once pleasurable cigarettes become associated with an unpleasant physical reaction. There are risks with this technique, however, and it does not apply well to many problem behaviors.

It takes much longer and is more difficult to unlearn or extinguish a response than it is to learn the response. Moreover, although a response may appear to be extinguished, it can return at any time (termed *spontaneous recovery*), especially under similar stimulus conditions when the response was often performed in the past. If the response resurfaces, it may recover at full strength. For example, people who have smoked cigarettes and quit can easily experience spontaneous recovery. They may not have had a cigarette for months or years, yet at a party accept and smoke one. Their smoking habit then may return at full strength. The problem of spontaneous recovery needs to be given serious attention in any health program to change behavior, such as substance abuse, weight loss, or nutrition.

## Operant Conditioning

*Operant conditioning* is another widely recognized behaviorist approach. Popularized by B. F. Skinner (1974), operant conditioning gives less attention to stimulus conditions and more attention to a response and what happens to an individual after he or she responds. According to operant conditioning principles, behavior is most effectively influenced or changed by following an individual's response with some kind of reinforcement. A *reinforcement* is defined as a stimulus that increases the probability that a response will occur again under similar stimulus conditions.

According to operant conditioning principles, learning can be enhanced and behaviors increased or decreased simply by applying reinforcement on a proper schedule. Often working with animals such as rats and pigeons, Skinner formulated a well-organized way to understand how desirable and undesirable responses are learned, and how to change behaviors using scheduled reinforcement. Operant conditioning principles lie at the heart of behavioral modification programs in institutions, as well as instructional technologies where learners teach themselves by using teaching machines or computer programs.

Four types of reinforcement can be applied after a response is made to either increase or decrease the likelihood of the response being performed in the future: (1) positive reinforcement—applying a pleasant stimulus; (2) negative reinforcement—removal of an unpleasant stimulus; (3) nonreinforcement—not applying any kind of pleasant or unpleasant stimulus; and (4) punishment—applying an unpleasant stimulus. Of these four types of reinforcement, positive reinforcement is the most powerful way to promote learning.

### Increasing a Response

To increase a response, apply (1) positive reinforcement or (2) negative reinforcement.

*Positive reinforcement* entails providing a pleasant stimulus or reward after a response is made, which increases the likelihood that the response will be performed in future similar situations. Keep in mind that both desirable and undesirable behaviors may be strengthened with positive reinforcement. For instance, acknowledging a staff member's cooperative behavior increases the likelihood that he or she will continue to act in cooperative ways. Operant conditioning also helps us understand why people engage in unhealthy, annoying, or damaging behaviors. For example, smokers, attention-getters, and angry people are receiving some kind of positive reinforcement for their behavior, which explains why they keep making the same unwanted responses. To change behavior, identify what is positively reinforcing to the person, make sure not to reinforce the undesirable behavior, and then positively reinforce the person's desirable responses. As an example, if a principal goal of patient care is to help patients be independent, then individuals should not be rewarded when they complain or act in a dependent manner; instead, every attempt should be made to recognize and reward them when they strive for independence. For some patients, the more active they become, the less they are concerned with pain, and the experience of pain appears to lessen. This approach may not work with all patients, however.

*Negative reinforcement* involves removing an unpleasant stimulus, which acts to increase a response in similar situations. Two types of negative reinforcement are distinguished: escape conditioning and avoidance conditioning. The difference between the two relates to their timing.

*Escape conditioning* occurs when an unpleasant stimulus is applied (e.g., a clinical instructor chastises a student) and the person (student) makes a response (cracks a joke) that stops the unpleasant stimulus from being applied (the instructor ceases chastising and laughs at the joke). In this case, the student has escaped the unpleasant stimulus (being chastised). Consequently, humor is the response that is likely to be increased the next time the student is in a difficult situation.

*Avoidance conditioning* occurs when aversive stimuli are anticipated but not yet applied. In particular, when people want to avoid an unpleasant situation (e.g., a test or a job interview), they may say they are sick. If they continue to claim they are sick to avoid difficult situations, they may actually become ill when they feel threatened or anxious. Sick behavior is the response that has been increased through avoidance conditioning.

## Decreasing a Response

To decrease a response, apply (1) nonreinforcement or (2) punishment.

*Nonreinforcement* involves ignoring behavior (not applying any kind of reinforcement), which acts to lessen the frequency of a response. Attention-getting behaviors, temper tantrums, and attempts to upset people emotionally may be reduced when no reinforcement is given. Ignoring desirable behavior may also result in its decline. In a healthcare setting, if nurse managers preoccupy themselves with problem behaviors and fail to reward those nurses who are performing well, the frequency of this desirable behavior may decrease.

*Punishment* involves applying an unpleasant or aversive stimulus, which serves to reduce the likelihood of a behavior. Punishment is used only as a last resort if nonreinforcement and other techniques do not work. Physical punishment should not be employed for obvious reasons. Verbal confrontation, removing disruptive individuals from situations where they can get attention, and imposing penalties (e.g., fines, being grounded, "three strikes and you're out") are some examples of unpleasant stimuli that might be used. If punishment is utilized, keep the focus on the behavior that needs to be changed and avoid personal disparagement (i.e., punish the behavior, not the person).

Punishment is risky, with behaviorists finding that punishment may not weaken responses or decrease behavior in the long run (Hilgard & Bower, 1966; O'Donahue & Kitchener, 1999). This tactic also arouses emotions that may work against learning what needs to be learned and may well create a negative attitude toward the punisher. Even so, there are situations when it becomes necessary to apply an unpleasant stimulus to decrease a response. An illustration is the punishment administered by hospital committees and state boards that deal with unethical, irresponsible, and harmful behavior by health professionals. The behavior may be punished by putting professionals on probation or even suspending their license to practice. Dealing with frequent medication errors and blatant disregard for infection control are other behaviors where nonreinforcement hardly seems a viable option.

How, when, and which kind of positive reinforcement to use are important considerations in operant conditioning. First, in initial learning, it is necessary to reinforce the learner after each response (continuous reinforcement); once the response is established, one must then move to intermittent reinforcement (sufficient to keep the response functioning). Second, the reinforcement has to be of value to the particular learner, and unhealthy rewards (e.g., sweet or fattening foods, large amounts of money, risky pleasures) should not be used. Third, administrators need to know that rewarding the group is not as effective in maintaining positive behavior as rewarding the individual. Saying "Good job—I am very proud of all of you" has less impact than acknowledging each staff member, because rewards are more effective if they are personal and directed individually.

There are many criticisms of behaviorist learning theory. Foremost is the ethical concern about who is to decide what the desirable behavior should be. Should it be docile patients who give the staff little trouble, or passive students who do not take issue with or criticize others? Second, the emphasis on rewards and gains may foster materialism and manipulation. Should students be given tangible rewards for studying, or should they study to develop a genuine love of learning? Third, research indicates behaviors learned through classical and operant conditioning techniques may fade away quickly once the individual moves to a different setting—perhaps the same kind of environment and irrational reinforcement system that got the person in trouble in the first place. Finally, when working with people in the classroom or in the healthcare setting, it seems unrealistic to ignore learners' inner processing, such as their thoughts, emotions, motivations, and interpretations.

## Cognitive Learning Theory

Cognitive learning theory focuses on the perceptions, thinking, reasoning, memory, developmental changes, and processing of information that transpire within the learner (Matlin, 2005; Sawyer, 2006). Taking issue with the behaviorists, researchers advocating this perspective undertook a series of cognitive experiments that demonstrated a number of factors related to learning, such as reward is not necessary to learn, and thinking and reasoning develop in stages over the course of childhood and adolescence. Researchers also documented that learning is an active process in which learners perceive, interpret, and respond to the environment in their own ways, with social factors having a strong influence on each learner's construction of reality.

The introduction of several important subtheories has contributed to the advancement of cognitive theory over more than a century, with cognitive theory currently influencing much of educational practice. Cognitive theory is useful for appreciating the different ways that individuals approach and respond to any learning situation, recognizing the complexity of learning, and prompting instructors to take their cues from learners to be effective.

According to the basic principles of cognitive theory, the way individuals approach any learning situation reflects their level of cognitive development, their past experiences, the way they perceive and process information, and the way they think about themselves and respond to instruction. Attention is the key to learning, with each learner incorporating, organizing, and interpreting new information in relation to what he or she already knows. Learners have an awareness of how they acquire knowledge and think—a capacity termed *metacognition*. The ability to alter his or her thoughts, beliefs, and behavior rests on the learner discovering some kind of insight that causes him or her to reorganize these perceptions and thoughts. Thus a change in one's perception and thinking may lead to behavior change.

In cognitive theory, motivation is based on the learner's goals and expectations, which create disequilibrium and a tension to act. People without goals or with low expectations for themselves are not motivated to act. Conversely, people whose goals and expectations are too high may be at risk for disappointment and becoming discouraged about education and learning. Research suggests that having realistic goals (goals that stretch accomplishment but are achievable for the person) and taking responsibility for one's actions (internal locus of control) result in better academic performance, compared to having unrealistic goals (too high or too low) and blaming outside forces for one's success or failure (external locus of control).

In using cognitive theory, the educator's job is to assess readiness to learn; provide a variety of meaningful, developmentally appropriate experiences; and allow individuals to discover what they learn for themselves. Teachers and other students may provide feedback to correct faulty conceptions. Thus, according to this view, education is a social experience that benefits from human interactions. Sharing different perceptions and ways of thinking enhances learning and fosters an appreciation for the rich diversity in human thought.

When operating from a cognitive perspective, instructors need to be organized, with clear goals and expectations and a well-structured approach to presenting information. It may be helpful to provide a framework for understanding (advance organizers) to prepare learners for maneuvering through information on their road to discovery and insight. Creativity and original thought contribute to the excitement of learning and are encouraged—creativity is engendered by a novel and insightful reorganization of information and experience. Practice for the sake of practice is not helpful, such as boring repetition, rote memory, and demanding that thinking conform to instructor expectations and remain "inside the box." Instead, offering diverse experiences linked to learning is a more beneficial kind of practice.

Memory and retention are facilitated by the organization and meaningfulness of the educational material, along with proper pacing and time to reflect on the information. Recognition must be given to the various ways that individuals approach and respond to what is to be learned. Because learning is subject to social and personal influences within a cognitive framework, it is important to determine how information has been perceived, interpreted, and stored. It may be helpful to offer techniques that aid memory and transfer (Matlin, 2005).

When a cognitive theoretical approach is used, it is essential to give feedback to learners so they can make adjustments in how they process information. The transfer of learning to future situations is not likely to be total, however, given that every experience and situation where learning is to be performed will have its own set of differences and anomalies. Thus, the emphasis is on fortifying learners' abilities to solve problems by providing a variety of experiences, encouraging flexibility in thinking and creativity, and promoting feelings of competence or self-efficacy. Such training prepares learners to adjust to new cognitive patterns and changing situations—and it explains why clinical experiences need to be carefully selected and structured for nursing students. Having students rotate through different kinds of healthcare facilities broadens their clinical education.

The remainder of this section profiles some useful concepts and principles from the leading subtheories within cognitive theory.

## Gestalt Theory

Gestalt theory was formulated in the early 20th century around the same time as the behaviorists were gaining influence in psychology. This theory stresses the importance of sensory perception, attention, and the unique ways in which people may organize information and experiences. Gestalt means *configuration*; thus gestalt experiments demonstrate how people can encounter the same event yet perceive, interpret, and respond to it differently (Murray, 1995). According to gestalt theorists, people feel a tension to try to make sense out of confusing reality and to structure events in personal and sometimes idiosyncratic ways.

Some useful principles from gestalt theory are highlighted here, with examples from health care being used to illustrate each principle:

- Given the wealth of stimuli at any one time, people pay attention (orient) to some information while screening out (habituate to) other information. For example, patients may not attend to the health information a nurse presents because they are focused on their personal worries, other people in the room, or various social distractions.

- Perception strives for simplicity, equilibrium, and regularity. When patient education is conducted, patients and their families endeavor to make the information easy to understand, to remain balanced or be comfortable with the information, and to relate the information to something familiar. Imagine what it is like for someone from a non-Western culture to be sick or injured in a U.S. hospital and how stressful it is to strive for simplicity, equilibrium, and regularity in such an unfamiliar environment! Young children or older patients hospitalized for the first time may have reactions similar to a foreigner.

- Perception is selective in terms of what is screened out and what is attended to; thus, perceptions and interpretations may be distorted or at odds with those of other individuals in the same situation. Patients and their doctors may selectively pay attention and interpret information in their own ways, which can be a source of misunderstanding. As an illustration, well-meaning doctors may tell patients they have a 95% probability of surviving their disease or operation, yet some patients may then stay awake all night worrying that they have a 5% chance of dying.

- Perception is influenced by structure and directed toward organization and closure—"the whole is greater than the sum of the parts." For example, when a diagnosis is unclear, patients may go to great lengths to find information (e.g., from books, the Internet, journals, friends) that can suggest a diagnosis for their condition. The diagnosis may not be accurate, but patients may organize their symptoms into an identifiable pattern and find comfort in having some kind of answer to bring closure to their tension. Clearly, certain people have a much greater need for perceptual structure and meaning than others.

- The patterns that people select and perceive in events are strongly influenced by their background, past experiences, needs, aspirations, and emotional attachments. Patients with the same disease may view their illness and react quite differently because of differences in their culture, age, religion, and gender. Anne Fadiman's book *The Spirit Catches You and You Fall Down* (1997), which illustrates the perplexing dilemmas of a Hmong family caught up in the California healthcare system, exemplifies these differences in perspective.

With regard to teaching, while gestalt theorists believe that discovery learning encourages retention, creativity, and problem solving, they stress that the way the material is presented and framed/structured can make all the difference in learning. The goal of learning is understanding, not rote memory and drill.

Presenting material in various ways—appealing to multiple senses, employing different methods and techniques—acknowledges the diverse ways that information and experiences are subjectively perceived and organized by each learner.

Looking at the same problem in different ways encourages flexibility in thinking and creativity in problem solving. Presenting an issue in incomplete form invites learners' involvement as they strive for insight, originality, and meaning. Relearning or retraining involves motivating a structural reorganization into a new configuration.

Although not much is written about gestalt theory in education these days, it remains the backbone of cognitive theory and has spawned many ideas in education about how to teach and learn. The importance of structuring perception using well-known gestalt principles is reflected also in medical and drug advertising.

## Cognitive Development Theory

Cognitive development theory focuses on changes and advancements in perception and thought that occur from infancy through old age. Demonstrating that children's reasoning progresses sequentially through a series of stages from early childhood through adolescence, Jean Piaget's work represented a significant breakthrough in how to understand and work with children (Piaget & Inhelder, 1969). By observing, asking questions, and listening to children try to solve problems, Piaget identified four stages of cognitive development:

1. In the *sensorimotor* stage, infants learn to coordinate sensory information with motor activity.
2. Once they begin to be able to represent mentally what is not present, children move to the second or *preoperational* stage, where the use of symbols and language advances rapidly. At this stage, the child remains egocentric (only able to perceive the world from their own perspective and deal with one dimension at a time).
3. The third stage, called *concrete operations,* occurs around school age as children become able to grasp more than one dimension and deal with relationships among objects, such as "greater than" and "less than," and manipulate concepts and numbers.
4. As children become adolescents, they are able to begin to think abstractly, termed the *formal operations* stage.

While Piaget initially attached approximate ages to the four stages, he subsequently decided that it was the sequence of development that was important. Indeed, research has shown that some adults may never reach formal operations and can reason in only concrete terms; a few adults may function at a preoperational stage.

Piaget described two central processes involved in learning. The first is *assimilation,* in which information is incorporated and made to fit the existing cognitive framework or schema. The second process is *accommodation,* where the information taken in actually changes the schema. Given the limitations of young children's perception and reasoning, much of what they do is to assimilate information and interpret it in their own way. Accordingly, young children may think the moon or a mountain follows them around, and school-age children do not deal well with abstractions such as literary criticism, philosophy, and ideas about universal morality. Adults, too, engage in assimilation and accommodation, sometimes evident when confronting prejudice, bias, and religious or political beliefs.

Cognitive development theory seriously challenged the behaviorists' view of learning and had significant implications for understanding and teaching children. Comparing children to little scientists, Piaget advocated active discovery learning, claiming that perception rather than language was the key to learning. Another cognitive development theorist, Lev Vygotsky (1986), agreed that teaching must be in keeping with the child's level of understanding but suggested that language was most critical to learning and that social interaction facilitates learning. Vygotsky advocated that teachers exercise a stronger role in guiding children's learning than Piaget recommended. According to Vygotsky, adults give meaning and provide understanding to children's actions. Of course, some children may respond better to discovery learning, whereas other children may benefit from social interaction and guidance. Both Piaget and Vygotsky's views of learning continue to have a significant impact on education.

Piaget's theory goes no further than adolescence in describing cognitive development—so what about cognitive development in adults? Research in psychology, gerontology, and education needs to be considered for those in health care working with young, middle-aged, and older adults. First, research indicates it may not be until late adolescence and early adulthood—if ever—that abstract thinking functions well. Teenagers have been characterized as engaging in black and white thinking, and they may behave in risky experimental ways without giving forethought to the possible consequences of their actions (Adelson, 1986). Second, adult cognitive processing may advance beyond the characteristics of formal operations to become more adept at synthesizing experiences, integrating information, and dealing with contradictions (Kramer, 1983). For this reason, adult learners require special consideration in education. They need to be treated with respect; they learn more effectively if allowed to discuss learning with others (cooperative and collaborative learning) and bring their own experiences to bear in a learning situation. Adults like independence and taking an active role in determining what and how they learn (Tennant, 2006).

Cognitive change in older adulthood is the subject of considerable research in gerontology and aging. Relative to health care, some older adults are burdened with cognitive deficits that may come with disease, medications, depression, or lack of interest in dealing with life's challenges. Other older adults may progress to an advanced stage of cognitive development where they demonstrate excellent judgment, a sophisticated perspective based on their years of experience, and a desire to give to others (Hooyman & Kiyak, 2007). In general, reaction time slows down and sensory declines occur with age. Thus, nurses attempting to educate older patients need to slow the pace of instruction and gear it to the patient's best sensory functioning. Relating new information to what is familiar to older persons may be helpful. As Sparks and Nussbaum (2008) urged, healthcare providers need to communicate at appropriate levels and meaningfully with older adults caught up in a healthcare system that demands high levels of literacy. Motivation can be a problem for older adults for a host of reasons, so it may be necessary to work to get their attention and involvement to solve problems.

## Information-Processing Theory

Information-processing theory provides another cognitive perspective on learning and teaching. Explicit attention is given to how information is encountered, taken in, stored, and remembered. Information-processing theory is especially useful in trying to understand what is going on within each learner, discovering how to structure a learning situation to facilitate retention, and learning why distortions and errors occur in faulty learning or behavior (Sternberg, 2006). The stages in processing information and learning are described next and illustrated with examples from health care:

- *Attention stage:* This is the initial crucial stage when learners decide whether to pay attention to the relevant information to be learned. If individuals are habituating to the information being presented and orienting to something else, then the intended learning will not occur. For example, it is generally a waste of everyone's time to try to educate patients when distractions (e.g., noisy setting, hallways and rooms bustling with human activity, people talking, television turned on, or patients feeling tired, nauseated, or worried) are present.
- *Sensory memory stage:* The information is taken in and quickly processed by the senses. For example, patients and students generally have preferred sensory modes for encountering and remembering information—for some persons, it may be visual; for others, the preferred mode is auditory; for still others, the need to touch and manipulate is paramount to learning best. When dealing with a group of learners, it is helpful to present pertinent health information in several different modes. Of course, sensory deficits must be factored in when deciding how to present and structure information.
- *Short-term* or *working memory stage:* Information is transferred from sensory memory to short-term memory, where it is encoded. Encoding is the form in which sensory information is transferred, such as the various ways people may briefly remember a telephone number—visualizing the numbers, remembering the numbers as a rhythm, or repeating the numbers vocally. Information lasts only seconds or less in short-term memory and then is either discarded and forgotten or transferred to long-term memory. As an example, teaching at too rapid a pace and presenting too many ideas in quick succession work against memory and retention. Unfortunately, physicians, instructors, health educators, and those charged with obtaining informed consent ("consenting the patient") may be more concerned with getting through all the information in a restricted time

period than with making sure that information is fully processed, understood, and remembered.

- *Long-term memory stage:* Information is organized by the learner for
  storage. Efficient learners may already have effective ways to structure
  and retain information. If they do not, instructors and health educators
  may provide learning strategies to aid effective storage, such as mnemonic
  devices, heuristics, rehearsal techniques, and memorable metaphors,
  among others (see Matlin, 2005).

- *Information retrieval stage:* The final stage involves retrieving information
  that is to be used—a feat that, as any student knows, can be problematic.
  It is not uncommon for nursing students to know the necessary information yet be unable to reproduce it when called on to do so on a test or in
  class. Older people, who generally have stored considerable information,
  may face issues of recognition versus recall. They may recognize something and know "they know it," but cannot recall it. For instance, they
  may know they take a medication for arthritis and can describe exactly
  what the pills look like, but they cannot recall the name of the drug when
  asked. The converse situation is where someone really does not know the
  information but is able to provide a correct answer or guesses correctly.
  The issue of competence versus performance is at the crux of any learning
  situation.

Information-processing theory encourages both students and teachers to organize
information and make it meaningful so that the information can be remembered.
Instructors need to be aware that what happens right before or right after information has been given may interfere with accurate storage and retrieval. Also, it
is not sufficient merely to teach information; time must be provided for learners
to demonstrate mastery of the information. Both students and patients may want
to appear intelligent and agreeable, so they may say they understand information
when, in fact, they do not. Instructors must check whether the information is accurately retained and can be performed. Feedback may need to be given to correct
faulty learning, and the learner must demonstrate at a later time that the information was retained and can be performed correctly.

Information-processing theory is especially useful when teaching patients
self-care, cautions about their medications, and behaviors to avoid so that they
can heal properly. It is also useful when teaching students skills such as cardiopulmonary resuscitation, inserting IVs, providing information for informed consent,
and a host of other professional skills.

## Social Learning Theory

Social learning theory was developed largely by psychologist Albert Bandura
(1977, 2001) over several decades and remains widely used today. Bandura (1977)
observed that people do not need to have direct experience to learn; much of learning is based on observing others and what happens to them after they behave in

particular ways. Initially, his theory reflected a behaviorist perspective on learning, in that Bandura demonstrated the power of role models on learning and behavior. Role models are persons in positions where their behaviors are likely to be both observed and copied, such as parents, teachers, and those in authority.

Observers are attuned also to whether the role model is rewarded for behavior, which Bandura termed *vicarious reinforcement*. Role model behavior that is positively reinforced is likely to be copied. Yet, in a disturbing finding, role models engaged in undesirable behavior but perceived to be rewarded were more likely to be copied than role models behaving properly and rewarded. No wonder organizational behavior can deteriorate quickly when executives and administrators behave in devious or destructive ways yet are perceived as rewarded for their actions. The predictions are that such results will prove damaging, with the unethical behavior being copied by others throughout the organization.

Principles of social learning theory have been widely adopted in health care. For example, they are evident in mentoring programs where inexperienced health professionals work closely with experienced members of their profession as a way to teach clinical skills and performance in the workplace.

In the next stage of theory development, Bandura (1977) became more interested in the role of the learner and shifted toward a cognitive perspective. As Bandura noted, the learner exercises a strong degree of control (self-regulation) over what is learned and how it is perceived, interpreted, and stored. Just because a role model is viewed as being rewarded does not mean the behavior will be copied. Much depends on the learner's internal processes. Accordingly, Bandura identified four processes or phases within the learner:

1. In the *attentional* phase, the learner decides whether to pay attention to a role model—high-status, attractive, compelling role models and role models who have similar characteristics as the learner are more likely to be copied.
2. In the *retention* phase, the learner engages in storage and retrieval of what was observed.
3. In the *reproduction* phase, the learner copies the role model's behavior. Rehearsal and feedback are important at this stage.
4. In the *motivational* phase, the learner may or may not be motivated to perform the role model's behavior. In deciding whether to copy a behavior, the motivational phase is very important. It is strongly affected by the likelihood of positive reinforcement or punishment, the learning situation, and the learner's evaluation of subsequent situations where the behavior might be performed.

In his more recent work on social learning theory, termed *social cognitive theory*, Bandura (2001) includes sociocultural factors in his model and conceptualizes the individual as an agent exerting considerable control over the learning process. Reflecting the interaction among the environment, the person, and behavior, the emphasis is on the learner's role in mediating and filtering social and cultural influences through the self-system to produce behavior. Personal selection, intentionality, self-regulation, self-efficacy, and self-evaluation come into play and affect both learning and performance. Bandura found self-efficacy to be especially salient in this respect. Self-efficacy has a strong cultural component, such as what stereotypes communicate about competence (e.g., men versus women, youth versus adult, employed versus unemployed). Thus one goal of behavior change and wellness in health care is to promote feelings of self-efficacy in clients trying to break bad habits or cope with their illness and a shifting sense of self. More explicit attention is given to the impact of social factors on learning in several additional cognitive theories, summarized next.

## Social Constructionism, Social Constructivism, and Social Cognition Theories

Social constructionism, social constructivism, and social cognition theories are a series of theories from the fields of sociology, psychology, and education that highlight the importance of social influences on learning and behavior. All three theories reflect the idea that knowledge is socially constructed. *Social constructionism* emphasizes the impact of the social context on molding a shared reality. *Social constructivism* stresses the individual's structuring of learning based on culture and social interaction. *Social cognition theory* focuses on how individuals try to make sense out of the social world (Fiske & Taylor, 1991; Matlin, 2005). While there are some differences between these three social theories, the emphasis in this chapter is on the general contribution of socially oriented theories to understanding learning and utilizing the information when charged with teaching others.

Individuals give organization and meaning to what they learn, with this process being strongly affected by social influences. In keeping with their cultural background and group affiliations, learners may misperceive, misrepresent, and distort information as they attend to it, incorporate it, store it, or retrieve it. More specifically, social factors such as gender, class, ethnicity, religion, and group memberships can affect what information is attended to and what is ignored, or what is and is not learned. Feelings of self-worth, competence, and efficacy can be critical in remembering and in performance. Given the diverse social backgrounds of people encountered by health professionals, social constructionism, social constructivism, and social cognition theories can help explain some of the widely varying—even irrational—attitudes and behavior exhibited in healthcare settings.

While cognitive theory is widely heralded in psychology and education, it is challenging for instructors to try to determine what is going on in the minds of learners. Also, many of the terms and concepts associated with this theory are not easily operationalized and measured for research purposes.

Another criticism of cognitive theory is that not much attention has been given to the role of emotions in learning until recently. First, a clue about the importance of emotions in learning has been provided by neuropsychological studies based on brain imaging of subjects as they engage in various activities.

Researchers found that along with thinking and reasoning, emotional areas of the brain become activated as subjects perform various tasks, including making moral judgments (Benjamin, de Belle, Etnyre, & Polk, 2008; Greene, Sommerville, Nystrom, Darley, & Cohen, 2001). Second, cognitive psychologists have recognized the importance of self-regulation not only in learning and studying, but also in being able to control emotions from early childhood throughout life (Baumeister & Vohs, 2007).

A third area incorporating emotions into cognitive functioning is *emotional intelligence*, which some have argued is more important in successful lives than cognitive intelligence. Emotional intelligence includes attributes such as self-motivation, managing personal feelings, and making wise judgments, as well as being able to read other people's feelings and working effectively in interpersonal relationships (Goleman, 1995; Mayer, Roberts, & Barsade, 2008).

Izard (2009) incorporated emotions into cognitive theory because of their impact on motivation, perception, and cognitive processes in affecting behavior outcomes. For example, emotional schemas can lead to psychopathology when learning has fostered connections among emotional feelings and maladaptive cognitions and actions. Although emotions are accorded some consideration by cognitive theorists, a more explicit focus is given to the effects of emotions on learning and behavior in psychodynamic and humanistic theories, which are discussed next.

# Psychodynamic Learning Theory

Psychodynamic theory evolved from Sigmund Freud's (1995/1938) theory of personality development, which is primarily directed toward understanding and treating dysfunctional behavior in light of childhood and past experiences, emotional conflicts, and motivational forces. Psychoanalysis is a method of treatment in which the patient freely describes his or her history, relationships, and anxieties, which the therapist then helps the patient interpret. The goal is for the patient to gain insights about the self and work through problematic emotional issues.

Mainly applied to personality pathology and abnormal behavior, psychodynamic theory had a profound impact on psychiatry and psychology in the early to mid-20th century. Subsequently, the psychodynamic perspective lost favor, both as a personality theory and as an approach to therapy. From a practical standpoint, however, some of the concepts from psychodynamic theory contribute to a fuller understanding of learning and teaching (Hilgard & Bower, 1966) and are especially useful to those working in health care and professions such as social work (Bower, 2005). This theory may be helpful for identifying barriers to learning and healthy behavior, promoting more positive attitudes, and recognizing some of the destructive dynamics in teacher–student and other power relationships. In health care, psychodynamic theory is especially useful for appreciating the role of emotions and motivation in patients, staff, and self and for becoming attuned to interpersonal and intrapersonal conflicts that may hinder productivity and functioning in any setting.

Largely a theory of motivation, psychodynamic theory highlights not only conscious aspects of behavior, but also unconscious motivations. It gives less emphasis to thoughts and thinking than to emotions, tensions, and conflict as driving forces in people's behavior. According to this theory, individuals are motivated to seek pleasure and to avoid pain, an idea termed the *pleasure principle*—a simple generalization that explains a lot of behavior in health care. Personality is conceptualized as having three basic components that motivate actions: the *id* (primitive drives that seek immediate gratification); the *superego* (internalized social values, norms, and standards); and the *ego* (the mediator between the id and the superego, which is grounded in reality). Some of Freud's followers emphasized the importance of healthy ego development, which helps individuals function realistically in an environment full of conflicts, contradictions, and challenges to the self.

As Freud conceived it, personality develops from infancy through adolescence in stages, with each stage involving a psychosexual conflict. Difficulties in adulthood are attributed to problems rooted in one or more childhood stages. Erik Erikson (1968), another psychodynamic personality theorist, later modified and expanded Freud's developmental model. According to Erikson, personality develops in eight stages throughout life, with each stage revolving around a specific psychosocial crisis to be resolved: (1) trust versus mistrust, (2) autonomy versus shame and doubt, (3) initiative versus guilt, (4) industry versus inferiority, (5) identity versus identity diffusion, (6) intimacy versus isolation, (7) generativity versus stagnation, and (8) integrity versus despair.

Research generally has supported Erikson's personality theory (Steinberg & Morris, 2001). The implication is that both teaching and caring relationships should be geared to enhancing personal and social development at every stage of life. Problems in learning or behavior are traced to difficulties in resolving issues during previous stages of development. For instance, growing up in an irresponsible family may result in offspring having problems with the very first crisis of trust versus mistrust. As adults, they may need to work through the issue of trust that is getting in the way of their optimal functioning.

Although not a learning theory per se, psychodynamic theory has some useful applications that can bring an interesting perspective to the dynamics of learning. It can be particularly helpful in understanding why someone may be having difficulty acquiring information or acting in healthy ways. According to psychodynamic theory, learners are motivated to do what is pleasurable and to avoid what is painful, which has several ramifications for healthcare educators. While learning need not be made a miserable experience, students must nevertheless be able to delay gratification and perhaps struggle to learn difficult material on their own.

Students with healthy ego development are more likely to work independently to truly understand what they are supposed to learn, whereas students motivated largely by id impulses may procrastinate, fail to show up for class or turn in assignments on time, and engage in a host of behaviors that ultimately set them up for failure. They may or may not be aware of their own dynamics. If they are not aware, they need to be encouraged to become cognizant of the consequences of their actions and to work for healthier ego development so they can function more effectively.

Equally important, some students with an overdeveloped superego may approach learning by demonstrating heightened anxiety, obsessing over grades, being unhappy over the challenges they need to meet, and becoming angry when they do not receive the grade they think they deserve. Clearly, they are not enjoying learning—and this negative attitude may endure throughout life. From an analytical perspective, the root of people's difficulties with learning can be traced to previous failures and past experiences with parents and other authorities. This suggests that problems with learning may have more to do with emotional conflicts than with cognitive abilities.

Memory and retention are, of course, central goals of learning, but according to the psychodynamic view, memory can be faulty or even inaccessible. In addition, memory lapses and mistakes can be significant and may represent unconscious conflicts and motivations (motivated forgetting). Why, for instance, is it difficult to remember a certain patient's name, or why does a particular nurse continue to make medication errors?

Anxiety can be another reason for difficulties in either learning or recalling information. To many students and for numerous reasons, education can be an anxiety-producing process. Even so, anxiety is not necessarily detrimental, because it may spur people to do a conscientious job or perform better, and life will always supply stressful and anxiety-producing situations that must be overcome. It is the ego's job to manage anxiety. As a consequence, it is crucial that the ego be able to differentiate objective anxiety that is realistic from anxiety that is unrealistic (not probable, overblown, or perhaps highly probable but ignored). When events are stressful, the ego may protect itself by employing defense mechanisms. In the short run, these defense mechanisms may help the self come to grips with a difficult situation. If they are overused or continued too long, however, the same coping strategies may become dysfunctional.

Because both education and health care can be stressful, it is worth reviewing some of the commonly employed ways of defending the self against threat. Examples from health care illustrate each mechanism in the following list:

- *Denial:* ignoring or refusing to acknowledge a threat (patients who refuse to believe their diagnosis and ignore treatment)
- *Rationalization:* excusing or explaining away a threat (staff members who make medical mistakes, which they excuse as caused by circumstances rather than their error)
- *Regression:* returning to a less mature stage as a way of coping with threat (administrators whose ideas are voted down and who then sulk and act like angry children)

- *Repression:* burying unacceptable impulses and thoughts from conscious awareness (nurses who claim they never met a patient they did not like)
- *Displacement:* rather than directing anger at the source of a threat, taking out aggressions on others as a way to release tension and anxiety (receptionists who snap at patients and give them a hard time for no good reason)
- *Projection:* perceiving one's own unacknowledged unacceptable characteristics or desires in others (staff members who gossip about lots of people having sexual affairs or whom they claim are gay)
- *Intellectualization:* minimizing anxiety by responding to threat in a detached, abstract, cold manner (physicians who act like technicians or absorbed scientists, failing to establish any rapport with patients)
- *Compensation:* making up for weaknesses by excelling in other areas (staff members who are refused admittance to medical school and subsequently become successful health professionals)

Two of these defense mechanisms, in particular, are endemic in health care and will be briefly discussed here: denial and intellectualization.

*Denial* is prevalent in professional education and health care and is a way of dealing with bad news that may seem overwhelming. Students may be in a state of denial about how poorly they are doing in a course, for example. Denial is the first stage in Elisabeth Kübler-Ross's (1969) stages of death and dying. This defense mechanism is understandable as a way to cope with a serious threat initially, but if continued it may keep students from addressing the need to study and find help, or it may hinder patients from seeking treatment for themselves or their children.

*Intellectualization* can be an occupational hazard in medicine, where health-care professionals protect themselves by being emotionally detached rather than genuinely engaging with patients needing support. Films such as *The Doctor* (also a book) and *Wit* (also a play) have dramatized the issue of intellectualization in medicine and its impact on patients.

Psychodynamic theory offers an insightful perspective on power relationships (teacher–student, doctor–nurse, nurse–patient). *Transference* is a term from psychodynamic theory describing the situation in which students, patients, or those in a dependent position project their feelings, conflicts, and reactions onto authority figures—often reacting to the authority figure as they would their parents. The reaction may result in hostility and rebellion or in heightened reliance and over-identification with the authority. There is a significant responsibility for those in authority not to exploit or manipulate a transference relationship. At the same time, a student or patient may remind a health professional of a person from their past, creating a *countertransference* reaction, in which the person in authority reacts to certain students or patients as if they were someone other than who they really are. This reaction could be either highly favorable or highly unfavorable. The problem is that the relationship becomes distorted and plagued with bias, which makes communication, learning, and treatment problematic.

Knowledge of psychodynamic theory in education and health care reminds teachers and those in authority to pay close attention to their own and others' emotions, anxieties, and conscious and unconscious motivations so that they can function in a safe, realistic manner. The goal is to promote the emotional development of patients, staff, colleagues, and self by recognizing the irrational aspects of human behavior. The psychodynamic approach has been found to be helpful in attempting to understand human trauma, patient and family noncompliance, palliative care, student anxieties, and some of the emotional undercurrents involved in caregiving and long-term care. As an example, Ferns' (2006) nursing study indicated that psychodynamic theory was useful in trying to comprehend and control bullying and abusive behavior by nurse managers, as well as the failure of nurses to report mistakes, highly unethical behavior, and incidents of violence.

Psychodynamic theory has been criticized vehemently for decades. Much of the theory rests on murky constructs and symbolism that is subject to interpretation, and some of Freud's concepts have been proven wrong or are outdated. In addition, this theory is criticized for being speculative and difficult to operationalize and measure. The data are based on descriptive anecdotal case studies of patients with emotional and behavioral problems. As a result, the findings may not be generalizable and are considered less meaningful than the conclusions reached in more rigorous, quantitative, large-sample studies (Bower, 2005). As a therapy modality, psychoanalysis may require years of expensive counseling and has not been demonstrated to be as effective as other therapies. Nevertheless, some aspects of psychodynamic theory add an important dimension to understanding the complexity and emotional nature of learning and the challenges in attempting to change behavior.

## Humanistic Learning Theory

Humanistic learning theory in psychology was developed during the mid-20th century, partially in reaction to the dominance of behaviorism and cognitive theory. The humanists argued that these two theories ignored or dismissed the role of emotions in learning and were more concerned with methodology, experimentation, and survey research findings than with people as unique individuals and human beings. Moreover, they criticized the psychodynamic approach for its negative focus on psychological pathology and dysfunction and its ready adoption of an emotionally detached medical model of treatment (Schneider, Bugental, & Pierson, 2001; Snowman & Biehler, 2006).

To the humanists, the purpose of psychology in general, and of education and therapy in particular, is to foster the growth, self-development, and creativity of each individual. Unfortunately, achieving positive self-development is made difficult in a highly technological, materialistic, bureaucratic society that devalues humanity and the human experience. Under the humanist framework, education is criticized for promoting conformity rather than creativity and for sapping enthusiasm for learning with boring curricula, formal lectures, and rote exercises. Moreover, individuals who are viewed as different are seen as being stigmatized by society, such as people with mental health problems, disabilities, or a host of characteristics that relegate entire groups of people to lesser status in the human community. Criticism is also directed at medicine for its hierarchical professional "know it all" approach, often referred to as *medicalization*, which treats people who seek help for their suffering in routine, mechanistic ways that do little to heal the person or the spirit.

Humanistic theory, in contrast, emphasizes a person-centered approach and stresses the importance of feelings over thoughts. The subjective human experience of each individual is seen as being of value, and human relationships depend on being spontaneous, authentic, and empathetic. The goal is to help individuals express their inner creativity, reach their human potential, and strive for personal growth. Motivation is derived from a person's needs, feelings about the self, and desire for positive self-development. Learning is facilitated by allowing people freedom and choices, by supporting their expressiveness and efforts at creative problem solving, and by making learning enjoyable. To achieve these goals, teachers, therapists, and health professionals need to engage in a collaborative relationship with students and patients based on authentic behavior, honest dialog, and genuine therapeutic listening. When learners are encouraged to make wise choices and are free to pursue creative interests, the retention and transfer of information are more likely than in an authoritarian approach to education. Education, therapy, and healing all need to take place within a nurturing context.

Humanistic theory was given considerable impetus by the work of Abraham Maslow (1954, 1987), whose hierarchy of needs concept of motivation engendered widespread attention and had significant implications for education and health care. According to Maslow, individuals are motivated to act on the basis of their needs, where the lowest-level needs must be met before higher-order needs are pursued. A student who is financially distressed, hungry, and tired is not likely to be oriented toward pursuing competitive academic achievement at school. A fearful, anxiety-ridden patient who is worried about money, his or her job, and family may not be concerned with learning about his or her disease and self-care. Maslow's hierarchy is conceptualized as moving from lowest- to highest-level needs:

- *Physiological needs:* meeting basic survival needs of food, warmth, sleep, and thirst
- *Safety needs:* meeting the need for security, protection, and freedom from fear
- *Belonging and love needs:* meeting the need to give and receive affection
- *Esteem needs:* meeting the need to be perceived as competent; to have confidence and independence; and to have status, appreciation, and recognition
- *Self-actualization needs:* meeting the need to fulfill one's potential as a creative human being

Although Maslow's model has intuitive appeal, Pfeffer (1985) concluded that this theory is not well supported by research. For one thing, the ranking of Maslow's hierarchy of needs does not appear to hold up under scrutiny. For example, creative people may not meet lower-level needs such as warmth and safety, yet they nonetheless manage to self-actualize.

Another important construct in humanistic theory is self-concept. Educator and therapist Carl Rogers (1961, 1994) argued that what people want most is "unconditional positive self-regard"—that is, to be loved for who they are as persons rather than for what they have or can do. Individuals who are threatening, judgmental, or coercive undermine people's self-concept and desire to learn. Rogers maintained that instructors and counselors should act as facilitators by using a person-centered approach with their patients and students. With this strategy, they spend more time listening than talking and convey the idea that they genuinely value and respect each learner as a person. Teachers also need to attend to learners' interests and recognize the importance of communicating and interacting in an honest and authentic manner. A teacher–student relationship based on mutual trust and enjoyment of learning lies at the heart of meaningful education according to humanistic theory.

The humanistic approach to learning fits well with an emphasis on holistic health, wellness, complementary medicine, and health promotion. Creative openness—a hallmark of humanistic theory—furthers healing through activities such as visualization, art, music, therapeutic listening, and communication. Humanists are not afraid to borrow from Buddhism, Chinese medicine, or alternative medical practices to soothe a sick or suffering person's mind, body, and spirit. Being in touch with one's sense of self and emotions, valuing empathetic understanding, and enjoying patients and families are especially critical for anyone in the healing professions. To the humanists, knowing is different from feeling, and feelings may well be more crucial than cold, hard facts. Humanistic principles are fundamental to self-help groups, wellness programs, hospice, and palliative care. In the spirit of humanism, health professionals need to be accepting and encouraging to those who are diagnosed with mental illness, are homeless, or have HIV/AIDS or other dreaded diseases.

While humanistic psychology does not enjoy as prominent a place in the theoretical armamentarium as it once did, its principles have had a clear impact on education and counseling, particularly in regard to its view of the student and patient as central to the mission of learning and therapeutic change. However, the constructs and principles in humanistic psychology are not easily measured and quantified, and the research conducted in this area is considered weak methodologically. Humanistic psychology has been criticized also for fostering narcissism and self-centeredness in learners, with critics charging that it does not prepare students to appreciate the benefits of constructive criticism. In addition, humanists have tended to dismiss the value of expert guidance, memorization, facts, practice, and drill in education, despite research indicating that these activities have their place in learning and can further knowledge, skill acquisition, and performance (Gage & Berliner, 1992).

More popular today than humanistic psychology is positive psychology (Snyder & Lopez, 2002), which is less oriented to learning than to topics such as health and well-being, happiness and life satisfaction, positive emotions, and optimism. Positive psychology also has been targeted by a growing number of critics, however (Ehrenreich, 2009; Hedges, 2009).

## Neuropsychology and Learning

Neuropsychology is a branch of psychology concerned with the scientific study of the brain in relation to mental processes and behavior. A relatively new and flourishing area of investigation, it has attracted scientists from a variety of fields, such as physiology, neurology, psychology, cognitive science, and medicine, among other disciplines (Benjamin et al., 2008; Sawyer, 2006). Although not a learning theory per se, the findings of neuropsychology are providing an accumulating body of knowledge about underlying brain structures and activity that come into play in attention, perception, information processing, making decisions, and taking action.

Basic research is fundamental to neuropsychology, derived from a variety of sources, including animal studies, work with neurologically impaired patients and people with physical and mental disabilities, and laboratory experiments with healthy subjects engaged in specific tasks. The rapid development of the field of neuropsychology has been greatly aided by advancements in brain imaging technology. Methodological tools include electrical recording (electroencephalography and event related potential technique), standardized neuropsychological tests, surgery, paper and pencil tests, and computer software. Neuropsychology research results pertain to a variety of topics and are found scattered among a number of disciplines and scientific journals.

An important contribution of neuropsychology research has been its documentation of the significant role of emotions in learning, information processing, memory, and recall. Emotions range from positive to negative (*valence*) and vary in intensity (*arousal*). In general, emotion has been found to modulate attention, learning, memory, and the brain's executive function (Warren, Miller, & Heller, 2008). As an illustration, in classical conditioning studies of fear, a number of brain structures pertaining to emotions have been identified, including the amygdala, hippocampus, and medial prefrontal cortex. Moreover, fear conditioning does not occur without an intact amygdala (Atkins & Reuter-Lorenz, 2008). As another illustration, arousing events—whether negative or positive—are remembered better than neutral events, with the amygdala exercising a prominent role in memory storage.

Today, the study of memory is one of the largest areas of research in neuropsychology. For example, emotional areas of the brain are clearly involved in memory storage and retrieval. Moreover, by mapping the circuitry activated in doing memory tasks, researchers have identified several independent memory systems. For example, Polk (2008) reported that working memory relies on different neural structures than long-term memory and sensory memory. Atkins and Reuter-Lorenz (2008) described two types of memory: (1) *implicit memory* (procedural memory or how to do tasks), which is mostly not accessible to conscious awareness; and (2) *explicit memory* (long-term memory and semantic memory), which is accessible to conscious awareness and verbal report. Studies also indicate that the depth of processing (i.e., how well the material is processed) is more important in learning and memory than the amount of repetition, rehearsal, or practice (Simon, 2008). These findings suggest that memory is more complex than often conceptualized. In the healthcare realm, when nurses expect students, patients, or family members to remember, they may need to employ different strategies for procedural memory than for long-term memory tasks. No one should be rushed through memory processing if the goal is to have information accurately remembered.

Another area of interest in memory research is aging and changes in memory and central nervous system functioning, which affect both communications with older people and their performance. The sensory declines and expected slowdowns in processing that come with age decrease reaction time along with all facets of information processing, retrieval, and performance. Lustig and Flegal (2008) noted that older adults have more difficulty with executive processes and screening out distractions and irrelevant information, although many develop effective strategies to compensate for this difficulty. Anyone working with older adults needs to be attuned to the many physiological changes that accompany aging that may affect attention, learning, memory, and performance.

Motor learning and skill acquisition is another research interest in neuropsychology. This is an important area in medicine and health care, where patients may need to learn self-care skills, providers may need to learn caregiving skills, patients may need to relearn motor skills because of injury or disease, and health professionals must acquire the skills necessary to manipulate medical instruments and equipment. Although skill learning has been studied for decades, identifying the underlying neural basis of skill learning is a relatively new endeavor—and one made possible thanks largely to the introduction of new technologies and methodologies (Bo, Langan, & Seidler, 2008). Information gained from mapping connections between brain and motor skill acquisition is expected to lead to better treatments and teaching strategies. For example, motor learning is not an entirely mechanical process; cognition and emotions are involved, especially in the early stages of learning or relearning. Eventually, however, the skills become more automatic. While practice is essential in learning motor skills, a number of issues and considerations surrounding the amount, type, frequency, variation, and spacing of practice sessions must be resolved to ensure effective learning.

Neuropsychological research has provided concrete evidence supporting a number of constructs and principles proposed as part of the various learning theories. In general, research has confirmed the validity of Piaget's concepts of constructivism, assimilation, and accommodation. The information-processing model of learning appears accurate, and Freud's notions of conscious and unconscious forces motivating learning and behavior have been supported by neuropsychology research as well. The humanists' emphasis on the importance of emotions in learning has been verified with evidence, as have many cognitive theory principles. Moreover, not only do brain structures affect learning, but learning, experience, and practice also change brain structures—a concept termed *plasticity* (Reber, 2008). The brain turns out to be much more flexible than once conceptualized, which has important implications for relearning.

The contributions of neuropsychology research suggest some of the following generalizations about learning. Learning is an active process that entails attention and perception, transforming information into preferred modes for encoding, short-term memory, and storage. The dynamics of assimilation and accommodation account for how new information is incorporated into existing structures. Emotions color all aspects of learning, and learning can occur without awareness or thought. Because brain processing is different for each learner, gaining the learner's attention, controlling the pace of learning, and identifying the specific mechanisms that enhance or inhibit learning are important challenges for any instructor. What is clear is that the learner exerts considerable control over whether learning occurs, what is learned, whether it is accurately learned, and whether learning acquired in one setting transfers to other settings.

Neuropsychology research is diverse, fragmented, scattered, and relatively new, and thus it is subject to some criticism relative to learning. First, the subjects used in neuropsychological studies typically are animals, people with disabilities and injuries, and convenience samples of volunteers willing to participate in research. The question then becomes, do the research results generalize to most people? Second, neuropsychology experiments and laboratory studies often involve contrived and relatively simple tasks, which raises concerns about validity and suggests caution when translating findings into the real world of classrooms, health education, or any place where teaching and learning occur on a regular basis. Third, the emphasis on biological mechanisms of learning is considered reductionistic—it oversimplifies learning and ignores the complexity of learning in diverse social environments. Moreover, the humanists caution that the individuality and humanity of learners is buried by science, while infatuation with the latest expensive technology can be a distraction from the actual worth and applicability of the project and its findings.

## Using Learning Theories in Advanced Nursing Practice

The learning theories discussed in this chapter have implications that extend beyond classroom instruction. Indeed, they may be particularly useful to advanced practice nurses in their leadership roles in education, management, or organizational and lifestyle change.

Taken together, the theories share common features that suggest some general advice about learning. Most theories indicate that learning is an active process, in which individuals have the ultimate control over what is learned and how well it is learned. Self-concept, feelings of self-efficacy, and the ability to self-regulate may need to be buttressed to improve knowledge acquisition or the confidence to change feelings, thoughts, and behaviors. Neuropsychology research documents that emotions are intertwined with learning, memory, decision making, and behavior and, therefore, must be considered in any learning situation. Social science research demonstrates that a significant amount of learning is affected by environmental influences and filtered through each learner's personal lens, which can distort perceptions, information processing, and interpretations. In addition, learning is a social experience, with many adults and some children acquiring information more effectively through social interaction.

In pulling together the learning theories, the following general model for learning is proposed (also see **Box 10–1**):

Learning experiences → learner processing → learning outcomes

A multidimensional approach to learning more accurately represents the complexity involved in learning, where the following three dimensions exist:

1. *External learning experiences:* environment or situation, stimuli, structure and configuration of teaching materials and approach, role models, and social influences
2. *Internal processing within the learner:* perceptions and cognitions; emotions and feelings; conscious and unconscious motivations; past experiences and cognitive and emotional developmental stage and schema; notions of self-efficacy, self-regulation, and self-concept; personality development and ego strength
3. *External outcomes and observable results of learning:* responses, behavior, actions, performance, transfer, feedback, and problem solving

---

## Box 10–1 General Learning Model

| External Learning Experiences | Internal Learner Processing | External Learning Outcomes |
|---|---|---|
| Environment | Attention | Responses |
| Situations | Perceptions | Behavior |
| Stimuli | Thoughts | Actions |
| Teaching materials | Memory (retention) | Performance |
| Teaching approach | Emotions | Choices |
| Role models | Motivation | Transfer |
| Social influences | Cognitive development | Feedback |
| Culture | Schema | Problem solving |
| Social interaction | Personality development | |
| | Ego development | |
| | Self-efficacy | |
| | Self-regulation | |
| | Self-concept | |
| | Transference | |

What becomes evident is that the learning theories work together, with each theory proving helpful in dealing with specific considerations and problems encountered when attempting to instruct others; break bad habits; or improve studying, behavior, and performance. In addressing the three fundamental questions raised in the beginning of the chapter, the following subsections cover some of the principal issues about learning in relation to nursing practice.

## 1. What Are Effective Ways to Learn New Information or Change Attitudes and Behavior in Health Care?

Research for nearly a century in education and psychology suggests that there is no "one size fits all" approach to learning. The question then becomes, how are advanced practice nurses supposed to decide which theories to utilize in their practice? Part of the decision-making process involves considering the situation, assessing the learner(s), and using the theories in combination to influence learning outcomes. Decisions about how to change behavior (unlearning–relearning) must also be addressed. Multiple applications of the learning theories to situations and people are described in the following section (also see **Box 10–2**).

- *Consider the situation.* One theoretical approach may be preferable to others in certain situations. For example, behaviorist theory is useful when dealing with simple behaviors, such as increasing study time, changing unhealthy habits, and promoting better organization and responsiveness in the workplace. Yet when knowledge acquisition is at stake (e.g., nursing education, patient education, or staff education), cognitive theory is essential in recognizing the control that the learner has over what is learned. Instruction must be given appropriately and in keeping with learners' developmental level, and teachers must remain attuned to the many considerations related to processing and retention within learners (e.g., pacing, organization, allowing time for reflection). Psychodynamic theory is helpful when learning and behavioral problems become evident and in promoting healthy ego development to cope more realistically with life's challenges. Humanistic theory reminds instructors of their role as facilitators in being respectful, encouraging, and supportive of learners.
- *Consider the learner(s).* People may learn more effectively with certain approaches than with others. Some patients, students, and staff members prefer to discover for themselves, whereas others do better with guidance and find that social interaction aids their learning. Individuals who are not cognitively oriented and need structure may learn better using behaviorist principles, whereas people who are self-motivated and verbal might learn more effectively using cognitive principles. Those who lack confidence can gain from a humanistic approach, as long as they do not need much structure and are self-directed. Students and staff members who encounter barriers to learning and do not function effectively might benefit from a psychodynamic approach where they can talk about their

## Box 10–2 Applications of Learning Theories to Situations and People

| Learning Theory | Applications to Situations and People |
| --- | --- |
| Behaviorist learning theory | Simple behaviors, skill learning, and nonverbal tasks<br>Breaking unhealthy habits<br>Organizational behavior and workplace performance<br>Medical advertising and public health campaigns<br>People who are not cognitively oriented<br>People who like to learn by doing and action<br>People who need clear structure, guidance, and rewards |
| Cognitive learning theory | Acquiring knowledge, complex learning, and understanding<br>Memory processing, problem solving, and creativity<br>Understanding distortions, misperceptions, and bias<br>People who are verbal and cognitively oriented<br>People who like challenges, problem solving, and creativity<br>Some people learn best by discovery, others by guidance<br>Some children and many adults learn well through social interaction<br>Consider the individual's stage in life and cognitive processing |
| Psychodynamic learning theory | Conflict situations: interpersonal and intrapersonal conflicts<br>Understanding conscious and unconscious motivation<br>Dealing with ego development and personality development<br>People exhibiting problems with learning or relationships<br>People overly motivated by the id or the superego<br>People who need to be in better touch with reality<br>Power relationships: transference and countertransference |
| Humanistic learning theory | Correcting situations that dehumanize and depersonalize<br>Palliative care, wellness, and emotional healing<br>People who are creative, self-directed, or seeking fulfillment<br>People with negative self-concepts or unhealthy needs<br>People stigmatized by society |

problems and, in the process, become more aware of their motivations, defensive behaviors, and consequences of their actions.

- *Consider how to use learning theories in combination to enhance learning outcomes.* Whether the goal is knowledge acquisition or behavior change, utilizing multiple learning theories can be more effective in influencing learning outcomes than relying on a single learning theory. For example, cognitive-behavioral therapy has been formalized as an approach to changing behavior. Reflecting a combination of behaviorist and cognitive principles, the emphasis with this approach is on assessing the effects of thoughts and feelings on behavior, changing responses through conditioning and reinforcement techniques, and practicing responses until an effective one has been discovered (Dobson & Dobson, 2009). However, nurses may achieve better outcomes by carefully assessing a learning situation themselves and developing a plan by thoughtfully selecting learning principles to apply to a specific situation and person(s). Try the plan, evaluate it, and, if it does not work, formulate another plan and evaluate it. Being comfortable and flexible in employing learning theories requires understanding, application, practice, and assessment—a perspective that is in keeping with an evidence-based approach to nursing, medicine, and health care. Assessment of students, patients, or staff is critical at the learning outcomes stage, where nurses might employ before–after measures of performance, qualitative and quantitative methods, and/or indicators of learner and instructor accountability.

Advanced practice nurses spend a significant amount of their professional time concerned with changing behavior—for example, with patients and community residents who may have learned little or incorrect health information, with those needing to alter their lifestyles, or in the scenario of unhealthy organizational behavior. Thus, it may be helpful to review how learning theories can be used to replace old habits with new ways of thinking and behaving.

The simplest way to modify behavior is to have individuals alter their responses to stimulus situations; over time and with practice, attitudes and behaviors may change. As the behaviorists suggest, there are several ways to effect such a change: (1) change the environment or situation in ways that will elicit desirable responses; (2) if the environment cannot be changed, substitute a healthier response to the environmental conditions; and (3) change responses to the situation by not reinforcing undesirable behaviors while positively reinforcing desirable behaviors. It can be helpful also for role models to demonstrate what is expected, such as through mentoring programs, visits to well-run healthcare facilities and offices, or meeting with people who successfully accomplished behavioral or organizational changes.

Another option is to work to change perceptions, thoughts, emotions, and attitudes within learners in the hope that behavior change will follow. Reflecting cognitive, psychodynamic, and humanistic theories, this aim may be accomplished by helping learners become more aware of unrealistic motivations, expectations, and goals, as well as negative thoughts, misperceptions, and damaging feelings (perhaps by journaling, keeping a diary or log, or videotaping). The next step is to encourage learners to formulate more realistic goals and motivations and then develop a plan (means) to change their perceptions and achieve their goals. Learners may need to work on what they tell themselves internally about what is contributing to dysfunctional attitudes and behavior. Both the psychodynamic and humanistic perspectives emphasize the need to achieve a balance between personal drive and desire relative to social pressures. The focus then becomes identifying and making mature choices, and practicing healthy responses to develop a better sense of self to cope with difficulties more effectively. Feedback and evaluation are critical along the way. Opportunities to discuss such changes with others may be helpful to some learners (e.g., self-help groups, group study sessions).

In keeping with the general model of learning, working on both external and internal dynamics of learning may be the wisest approach.

### 2. How Can People Be Motivated to Learn, and Which Kinds of Experiences Facilitate Learning?

Motivation can be the chief obstacle to acquiring knowledge or changing behavior. People may not be motivated for a host of reasons: They do not have a drive to learn, their equilibrium has not been disturbed and they are complacent, they lack self-discipline and cannot defer gratification for the long-term gain, or they lack self-confidence (self-efficacy) in their abilities. Students, patients, and staff may go through the motions of seeming to appear that they are learning when they have actually not learned, so it is important to evaluate what they have learned and to provide appropriate feedback.

This feedback can consist of a simple check with patients to ask them to repeat instructions or have them perform self-care several times until they feel comfortable. It may also help to assess learners' goals and expectations, although behaviorists and psychoanalysts might warn that what people identify as their goals may be less reliable than what their actions and nonverbal behavior indicate. Other factors to assess are feelings of self-efficacy and self-concept. Carl Rogers (1961) noted that it may be easier for people with low self-esteem to confirm a negative self-concept than to think of themselves in positive ways. Teaching is much like coaching, in that encouragement can help some people pull through low periods and buttress their motivation. To be successful, however, such encouragement must be genuine rather than merely saying the right things without demonstrable emotional warmth, rapport, or care.

Given the need to promote active learning, an instructor's main job is to provide experiences that excite learners' motivation. However, the experiences must be at an appropriate level and sufficiently diverse to encompass the numerous ways that learners have of perceiving, interpreting, and responding to information. Given that emotions are involved in all phases of learning, it is sensible to make learning pleasurable (psychodynamic), enjoyable (humanistic), rewarding (behaviorism), and meaningful (cognitive). Both cognitive theory and neuropsychology research indicate that processing information intensively (through reflection, relating to what is familiar, discussion, and criticism) is likely to lead to better retention and transfer. Learners need time to mull over experiences and opportunities to act on their newly learned information. Providing experiences where learners can discover by doing or engaging in hands-on action is recommended as an aspect of several theories. A Chinese proverb says, "I hear and I forget; I see and I remember; I do and I understand."

As an illustration, students may gain a fuller understanding (cognitively and emotionally) of poverty and the impact of low income on patient health by trying to fill out an application for Medicaid or going to a grocery store to see if they could buy healthy food for a family of four with the amount of money allotted for food stamps than by simply reviewing statistics. Other recommendations are to employ gestalt and cognitive principles in structuring experiences to excite learner motivation and to invite learners' involvement by disturbing their equilibrium. Some suggestions are to create dissonance with contradictory information, set up an experience where learners will want to bring closure, or give learners a problem to solve on their own before presenting information. What is learned initially must be assessed at a later time to make sure it has been learned accurately and can be transferred to situations where it needs to be performed. Therefore, one-shot learning experiences are not likely to be effective; feedback and follow-ups are essential.

## 3. What Are Effective Ways to Teach So That Information and Skills Will Be Remembered Rather Than Forgotten and Will Transfer Correctly Outside the Immediate Learning Situation?

In applying the learning theories' lessons regarding retention and transfer, a planned approach to teaching is suggested. Readers may want to formulate their own list of advice points about teaching for retention and transfer utilizing learning theories, but the following is a start:

- *Prepare to teach*. Observe learners to determine their level of cognitive development, identify what they respond to and what is familiar to them, and perhaps get to know learners at a personal level by listening while they describe themselves and their goals for learning. Also, determine readiness to learn by assessing learner motivations, attention (including distractions in the environment), and possible barriers to learning such as fatigue, anxiety, preoccupation with other thoughts, or being in pain, nauseated, or ill—all of which affect attention and concentration.

- *Present information*. Help individuals prepare their schema and framework for learning by providing advance organizers to inform them about the goals of the educational session and topics to be covered. Seek reactions from learners to find out what is familiar to them; this information can then be used to relate the substantive material to be presented. Pose a question, contradiction, or problem for learners to solve to heighten their interest and involvement, and prod learners' motivation. Ideally, the material needs to be presented in ways that activate different sensory modes and in keeping with learners' metacognition and ways of processing information. It can be helpful to break complex material into units or understandable chunks to make it easier to process and store—perhaps offering some memory techniques to aid retention. Pacing and time for reflection encourage deep processing and retention.

- *Construct a way for learners to act on the information.* Some suggestions are for learners to ask questions, participate in small discussion groups, and perform an exercise to apply the information. Learners may need time for chance discovery, reflection, and creative application, and they may also need to practice the information over time. The information may need to be repeated in different ways to increase the likelihood that it will be remembered and transferred. It is helpful if the material presented in a learning session can be practiced in settings similar to those in which it is likely to be transferred.

- *Evaluate the effectiveness of learning.* Learning can be assessed through tests, short quizzes, oral discussion, projects, and problem-solving opportunities. Learners must feel free to ask for clarification and help, and instructors need to be attuned to barriers to learning and information transfer, such as weak motivation, problems with self-efficacy and self-regulation, or faulty processing and possible rewards for not learning.

- *Provide remediation as soon as possible for weak or inaccurate learning.* Teachers may want to utilize computer technology for self-teaching and correction or have students or patients teach one another as practice (the best way to learn is to teach). In addition, some socially oriented students might benefit by working with others to remediate their learning. Perhaps some learners may not understand initially the value of acquiring certain information and, therefore, need a clearer rationale for learning, or perhaps they may benefit from having a direct experience that demonstrates the value of learning. Some students may need positive reinforcement. When difficulties in learning arise, it is essential to uncover what is inhibiting learners' processing and performance. Psychodynamic and humanistic learning theories can be helpful when remediation is an issue. Serious problems may require referral to formal counseling and therapy (see Box 10–2).

## Summary

As this review of educational and learning theories demonstrates, learning is a multidimensional process that involves external learning experiences, the internal processing within each learner, and the resulting learning outcomes as evidenced by behavior, actions, and performance. Learning theories provide a toolbox of approaches that advanced practice nurses can apply to educational activities, organizational management, medically related lifestyle and behavior change, and health communications. Research studies confirm that utilizing learning theories to formulate educational experiences in health care enhances advanced nursing practice.

Learning theories and theories in social psychology provide the rationale for successful continuing education programs to foster interprofessional collaboration and communication in preventing medical errors and ensuring patient safety (Sargeant, 2009). Graduate-level nursing programs increase in effectiveness when students are able to transfer theories and methods from classroom information about quality of care and patient safety to the wider healthcare setting (Jones, Mayer, & Mandelkehr, 2009). Equally important, when these precepts are applied to clinical education programs, students benefit by being actively engaged with patient care and receiving timely feedback (Leinster, 2009). By implementing educational and learning theories in their work, advanced practice nurses can be at the forefront of improved health care for patients, students, staff, and the human community.

## Discussion Questions

1. Which learning theories and principles do you think are the most useful to advanced practice nurses, and why?

2. Based on the learning theories discussed in this chapter, make a list of suggestions to help nurses do an effective job with patient education. You do not need to identify which theories you are using, but your suggestions should clearly reflect important learning principles.

3. Applying the learning theories discussed in this chapter, develop a step-by-step program to decrease the frequency of medical mistakes in hospitals, and cite the learning theories or principles that back up each step of your program. (Alternatively, choose a different application, such as decreasing workplace conflict, improving communication between physicians and nurses, reducing medication errors, or some other organizational problem confronting health care.)

4. Devise a step-by-step program for altering the lifestyles of patients who have serious health problems because of an unhealthy habit or habits (e.g., smoking, obesity, substance abuse, high stress levels, or some other unhealthy habit). Decide which specific habit or habits you want to address in your program, and then describe your program. Anchor the rationale for each step in learning theories and principles, and indicate which learning principles apply to each step.

5. As an alternative to Question 4, develop a step-by-step program to change a specific health behavior of your choice (e.g., smoking, obesity, healthier nutrition for people with diabetes, lack of exercise for cardiac patients, or

some other health problem). In your program, address the elements of the three fundamental questions discussed at the beginning of this chapter—effective ways to change health behaviors, ways to motivate program participants, experiences that might encourage learning, and teaching so that information and skills will be remembered and transferred outside of the classroom.

6. Using your own experience and knowledge, explain how a multidimensional approach employing learning theories is superior to a unidimensional approach in resolving health problems.

7. How has neuropsychology research improved our understanding of the general model of learning described near the end of the chapter?

8. As mentioned at the beginning of the chapter, knowledge of the role of emotions in learning and behavior is crucial in the highly charged field of health care. How can information from each of the four learning theories and neuropsychology research help advanced practice nurses include considerations related to emotions in patient education, nursing education, and organizational behavior?

# References

Adelson, J. (1986). *Inventing adolescence: The political psychology of everyday schooling*. New Brunswick, NJ: Transaction Books.

Atkins, A. S., & Reuter-Lorenz, P. A. (2008). Learning and memory for emotional events. In A. S. Benjamin, J. S. de Belle, B. Etnyre, & T. A. Polk (Eds.), *Human learning: Biology, brain, and neuroscience* (pp. 125–135). Boston, MA: Elsevier.

Bandura, A. (1977). *Social learning theory*. Englewood Cliffs, NJ: Prentice Hall.

Bandura, A. (2001). Social cognitive theory: An agentic perspective. *Annual Review of Psychology, 52*, 1–26.

Baumeister, R. F., & Vohs, K. D. (Eds.). (2007). *Handbook of self-regulation: Research, theory, and application*. New York, NY: Guilford Press.

Benjamin, A. S., de Belle, J. S., Etnyre, B., & Polk, T. A. (Eds.). (2008). *Human learning: Biology, brain, and neuroscience*. Boston, MA: Elsevier.

Bo, J., Langan, J., & Seidler, R. D. (2008). Cognitive neuroscience of skill acquisition. In A. S. Benjamin, J. S. de Belle, B. Etnyre, & T. A. Polk (Eds.), *Human learning: Biology, brain, and neuroscience* (pp. 101–123). Boston, MA: Elsevier.

Bower, M. (Ed.). (2005). *Psychoanalytic theory for social work practice: Thinking under fire*. New York, NY: Routledge.

Clark, N. M., Mitchell, H. E., & Rand, C. S. (2009). Effectiveness of educational and behavioral asthma interventions. *Pediatrics, 123*, S185–S192.

Dobson, D., & Dobson, K. S. (2009). *Evidence-based practice of cognitive-behavioral therapy*. New York, NY: Guilford Press.

Ehrenreich, B. (2009). *Bright-sided: How relentless promotion of positive thinking has undermined America*. New York, NY: Metropolitan Books.

Erikson, E. (1968). *Identity: Youth and crisis*. New York, NY: W. W. Norton.

Fadiman, A. (1997). *The spirit catches you and you fall down: A Hmong child, her American doctors, and the collision of two cultures*. New York, NY: Farrar, Straus and Giroux.

Ferguson, L., & Day, R. A. (2005). Evidence-based nursing education: Myth or reality? *Journal of Nursing Education, 44*, 107–115.

Ferns, T. (2006). Under-reporting of violent incidents against nursing staff. *Nursing Standard, 20*, 41–45.

Fiske, S. T., & Taylor, S. E. (1991). *Social cognition*. New York, NY: McGraw-Hill.

Freud, S. (1995/1938). *The basic writings of Sigmund Freud* (Modern Library Series, A. A. Brill, Trans.). New York, NY: Random House.

Gage, N. L., & Berliner, D. C. (1992). *Educational psychology* (5th ed.). Boston, MA: Houghton Mifflin.

Goleman, D. (1995). *Emotional intelligence*. New York, NY: Bantam Books.

Greene, J. D., Sommerville, R. B., Nystrom, L. E., Darley, J. M., & Cohen, J. D. (2001). An fMRI investigation of emotional engagement in moral judgment. *Science, 293*, 2105–2108.

Hedges, C. (2009). *Empire of illusion: The end of literacy and the triumph of spectacle*. New York, NY: Nation Books.

Hilgard, E. R., & Bower, G. H. (1966). *Theories of learning* (3rd ed.). New York, NY: Appleton-Century-Crofts.

Hooyman, N., & Kiyak, H. A. (2007). *Social gerontology: A multidisciplinary perspective* (8th ed.). Boston, MA: Allyn & Bacon.

Izard, C. E. (2009). Emotion theory and research: Highlights, unanswered questions, and emerging issues. *Annual Review of Psychology, 60*, 1–25.

Jones, C. B., Mayer, C., & Mandelkehr, L. K. (2009). Innovations at the intersection of academia and practice: Facilitating graduate nursing students' learning about quality improvement and patient safety. *Quality Management in Health Care, 18*(3), 158–164.

Kramer, D. A. (1983). Post-formal operations? A need for further conceptualization. *Human Development, 26*, 91–105.

Kübler-Ross, E. (1969). *On death and dying*. New York, NY: Scribner.

Leinster, S. (2009). Learning in the clinical environment. *Medical Teacher, 31*(2), 79–81.

Lustig, C., & Flegal, K. (2008). Age differences in memory: Demands on cognitive control and association processes. In A. S. Benjamin, J. S. de Belle, B. Etnyre, & T. A. Polk (Eds.), *Human learning: Biology, brain, and neuroscience* (pp. 137–149). Boston, MA: Elsevier.

Maslow, A. (1954). *Motivation and personality*. New York, NY: Harper & Row.

Maslow, A. (1987). *Motivation and personality* (3rd ed.). New York, NY: Harper & Row.

Matlin, M. W. (2005). *Cognition* (6th ed.). Hoboken, NJ: Wiley.

Mayer, J. D., Roberts, R. D., & Barsade, S. G. (2008). Human abilities: Emotional intelligence. *Annual Review of Psychology, 59*, 507–536.

Murray, D. J. (1995). *Gestalt psychology and the cognitive revolution*. New York, NY: Harvester Wheatsheaf.

O'Donahue, W., & Kitchener, R. (Eds.). (1999). *Handbook of behaviorism*. San Diego, CA: Academic Press.

Ormrod, J. E. (2007). *Human learning* (5th ed.). Upper Saddle River, NJ: Prentice Hall.

Pfeffer, J. (1985). Organizations and organizational theory. In G. Lindzey & E. Aronson (Eds.), *Handbook of social psychology: Vol. 1. Theory and method* (3rd ed., pp. 379–440). New York, NY: Random House.

Piaget, J., & Inhelder, B. (1969). *The psychology of the child* (H. Weaver, Trans.). New York, NY: Basic Books.

Polk, T. (2008). Introduction: Cognitive neuroscience of learning and memory. In A. S. Benjamin, J. S. de Belle, B. Etnyre, & T. A. Polk (Eds.), *Human learning: Biology, brain, and neuroscience* (pp. 75–76). Boston, MA: Elsevier.

Reber, P. J. (2008). Cognitive neuroscience of declarative and nondeclarative memory. In A. S. Benjamin, J. S. de Belle, B. Etnyre, & T. A. Polk (Eds.), *Human learning: Biology, brain, and neuroscience* (pp. 113–123). Boston, MA: Elsevier.

Rogers, C. (1961). *On becoming a person.* Boston, MA: Houghton Mifflin.

Rogers, C. (1994). *Freedom to learn* (3rd ed.). New York, NY: Merrill Press.

Sargeant, J. (2009). Theories to aid understanding and implementation of interprofessional education. *Journal of Continuing Education in Health Professions, 29*(3), 178–184.

Sawyer, R. K. (Ed.). (2006). *The Cambridge handbook of the learning sciences.* New York, NY: Cambridge University Press.

Schneider, K. J., Bugental, J. F. T., & Pierson, J. F. (Eds.). (2001). *The handbook of humanistic psychology: Leading edges in theory, research, and practice.* Thousand Oaks, CA: Sage.

Simon, D. A. (2008). Scheduling and learning. In A. S. Benjamin, J. S. de Belle, B. Etnyre, & T. A. Polk (Eds.), *Human learning: Biology, brain, and neuroscience* (pp. 61–72). Boston, MA: Elsevier.

Skinner, B. F. (1974). *About behaviorism.* New York, NY: Vintage Books.

Snowman, J., & Biehler, R. (2006). *Psychology applied to teaching* (11th ed.). Boston, MA: Houghton Mifflin.

Snyder, C. R., & Lopez, S. J. (Eds.). (2002). *Handbook of positive psychology.* New York, NY: Oxford University Press.

Sparks, L., & Nussbaum, J. F. (2008). Health literacy and cancer communication with older adults. *Patient Education and Counseling, 71*(3), 345–350.

Steinberg, L., & Morris, A. S. (2001). Adolescent development. *Annual Review of Psychology, 52,* 83–110.

Sternberg, R. J. (2006). *Cognitive psychology* (4th ed.). Belmont, CA: Thomson/Wadsworth.

Tennant, M. (2006). *Psychology and adult learning* (3rd ed.). New York, NY: Routledge.

Vygotsky, L. S. (1986). *Thought and language.* Cambridge, MA: MIT Press.

Warren, S. L., Miller, G. A., & Heller, W. (2008). Emotional facilitation and disruption of memory. In A. S. Benjamin, J. S. de Belle, B. Etnyre, & T. A. Polk (Eds.), *Human learning: Biology, brain, and neuroscience* (pp. 45–59). Boston, MA: Elsevier.

Woolfolk, A. E. (2001). *Educational psychology.* Boston, MA: Allyn & Bacon.

# Health Behavior Theories

*Karen Glanz*
*Lora E. Burke*
*Barbara K. Rimer*

## Introduction

This chapter focuses on contemporary theoretical bases for health behavior change for disease prevention and management and their applications to advanced nursing practice. It first introduces key concepts related to the application of theory in understanding and improving health behavior. It then describes several current theoretical models that can be helpful in planning and conducting patient and family education and behavioral interventions. Finally, it highlights important issues and constructs that cut across theories.

Health behavior is central to disease prevention and management. Nurses' roles in health behavior change, including patient education and health promotion, are pivotal because of nurses' centrality in health care and their credibility as patient educators. Contemporary evidence-based recommendations advise including intensive behavioral counseling for adult patients with known behavioral risk factors for chronic disease, noting that such counseling can be provided by physicians or other clinicians such as nurses. Also, some behaviors can be improved through brief, low-intensity counseling delivered by nurses and other health professionals. Further, nonclinical community sites such as work sites, churches, and community centers are becoming increasingly important as settings for health behavior interventions, especially with the growing and widespread prevalence of obesity and diabetes. Nurses may play leadership roles in these settings as well.

# The Evolution of Health Behavior Theory

The earliest known applications of health behavior theory occurred while social psychologists working in the U.S. Public Health Service were trying to understand how to increase participation in programs designed to prevent and detect disease (Hochbaum, 1958). Theories of health behavior reflect an amalgamation of approaches, methods, and strategies from social and health sciences. They draw on the theoretical perspectives, research, and practice tools of such diverse disciplines as psychology, sociology, anthropology, communications, nursing, economics, and marketing (Glanz, Rimer, & Viswanath, 2008). Health behavior and its close relative, health education/promotion, are also dependent on epidemiology, statistics, and medicine.

Many kinds of professionals contribute to and conduct health behavior and health education research and programs. Collaborations among professionals drawn from different disciplines, each of whom is concerned with the behavioral and social intervention process and its application to health issues, ensure the best blend of perspectives. For example, nurses bring to health behavior and health education their unique expertise in working with individual patients and patients' families to facilitate learning, adjustment, and behavior change, and to improve quality of life. Psychology brings to health education a rich legacy of more than 100 years of research and practice on individual differences, motivation, learning, persuasion, and attitude and behavior change (Matarazzo, Weiss, Herd, Miller, & Weiss, 1984), as well as the perspectives of organizational and community psychology. Other health, education, and human services professionals contribute their special expertise to health behavior and health education as well.

# Trends in the Use of Theories and Models

Theories that gain recognition in a discipline shape the field, help define the scope of practice, and influence the education and socialization of its professionals. No single theory or conceptual framework dominates research or practice in contemporary health behavior and health education, although a relatively small number of theories and models are used most often in this realm.

Over the past two decades, the authors of this chapter have reviewed a sample of publications on four different occasions to identify the most often used theories (e.g., Glanz et al., 2008; Painter, Borba, Hynes, Mays, & Glanz, 2008). From this review, certain theories or models clearly emerged as the most popular choices. The first three, and by far the most dominant, are social cognitive theory (SCT), the transtheoretical model/stages of change, and the health belief model (HBM). The other leading theories and models are the theory of reasoned action (TRA) and theory of planned behavior (TPB), ecological models/social ecology, stress and coping, community organization, diffusion of innovations, social support and social networks, and patient–provider communication. The three most popular theories and models, along with the representational approach (RA, a recent adaptation that blends psychological and educational theories), are described in more detail later in this chapter.

Our updated review of theory use in published research between 2000 and 2005 revealed that overall, the same theories dominated then as they did in 1999 and 2000 (Painter et al., 2008). Like our previous analyses, this review revealed dozens of theories and models that were used, although only a few of them were used in multiple publications and by multiple authors. Several key constructs cut across the most often cited models for understanding behavior and behavior change: the importance of the individual's view of the world, multiple levels of influence, behavior change as a process, motivation versus intention, intention versus action, and changing behavior versus maintaining behavior change (Glanz & Oldenburg, 2001).

Along with the published observations about which theories are being used, concerns have been raised about how the theories are used (or not used) in research and practice. In the most recent review of theory use, we classified articles that employed health behavior theory along a continuum:

1. *Informed by theory:* A theoretical framework was identified, but there was no or limited application of the theory in specific study components and measures.
2. *Applied theory:* A theoretical framework was specified and several of the constructs were applied in components of the study.
3. *Tested theory:* A theoretical framework was specified and more than half of the theoretical constructs were measured and explicitly tested, or two or more theories were compared to one another in a study.
4. *Building/creating theory:* New or revised/expanded theory was developed using constructs specified, measured, and analyzed in a study.

Of all the theories used in the sample of articles ($n = 69$ articles using 139 theories), 69.1% used theory to inform a study, 17.9% of theories were applied theories, 3.6% were tested, and 9.4% involved building/creating theory (Painter et al., 2008). These findings should encourage researchers and practitioners to strive for more thorough application and testing of health behavior theories to advance science and move the field forward.

Health behavior and health education are concerned with the development and application of knowledge, as well as with approaches to solving health and social problems—in other words, how to bring about change (Glanz et al., 2008). Considerable scholarly and practitioner efforts have been devoted to developing techniques that change behavior. Although these efforts grew out of a desire to produce a better world, techniques that push people to change were experienced by many as manipulative, reducing their freedom of choice and sustaining a balance of power in favor of the change agent (Kipnis, 1994).

A paradigm shift has occurred recently, and most of the behavioral techniques used today (e.g., social support, empowerment, and personal growth) are based on reducing obstacles to change and promoting informed decision making, rather than on pushing people to change.

Advanced practice nurses employ these techniques frequently in caring for patients and their families. This is particularly the case with nurses who provide care to individuals with chronic disorders. They know that merely providing information to patients or telling patients that they need to take their medication, stop smoking, or be more active will not lead to behavior change. Instead, these nurses recognize that their practice needs to be guided by behavior change theories and that teaching needs to be delivered in sessions that are based on mutual collaboration and accompanied by counseling strategies to enlist the individual or patient to consider making changes or adopting a new treatment regimen.

These nurse–patient interactions are guided by several of the strategies that are part of the theories discussed in this chapter. Nurses use elements of SCT in counseling patients about medication adherence (Berg, Dunbar-Jacob, & Sereika, 1997; Burkhart, Rayens, Oakley, Abshire, & Zhang, 2007) and counseling patients with coronary heart disease about reducing risk factors (DeBusk et al., 1994; Haskell et al., 1994). Self-efficacy, derived from SCT, has guided nurse-delivered interventions to improve dietary adherence (Berg, Dunbar-Jacob, & Rohay, 1995; Burke, Dunbar-Jacob, Orchard, & Sereika, 2005) as well as medication adherence (Berg et al., 1995; Burke et al., 2005). The expanded HBM has been used extensively to guide preconception counseling among teens with type 1 diabetes (Charron-Prochownik et al., 2001), while another nurse researcher applied the TPB in her examination of the mediating role of condom self-efficacy between the parent–adolescent relationship and the intention to use condoms (Cha, Kim, & Doswell, 2007). Others have used the transtheoretical theory of behavior change to guide medication adherence among adults taking antidepressants. Finally, a newly derived model, the RA to patient education, has been applied by a group of researchers in four studies: a study of pain management among cancer patients (Ward, Donovan, Gunnarsdottir, Serlin, Shapiro, & Hughes, 2008), symptom management among women with ovarian cancer (Donovan, Ward, Song, Heidrich, Gunnarsdottir, & Phillips, 2007), communication about end-of-life care for patients undergoing cardiac surgery (Song, Kirchhoff, Douglas, Ward, & Hammes, 2005), and a study to improve symptom management and quality of life among women who have survived breast cancer (Donovan et al., 2007; Heidrich et al., 2009). Several of these examples will be described in further detail following the discussion of each of these theories.

## The Health Belief Model

The HBM was one of the first theories of health behavior, and it remains one of the most widely recognized in the field today. This model was developed in the 1950s by a group of U.S. Public Health Service social psychologists who wanted to explain why so few people were participating in programs to prevent and detect disease. For example, the Public Health Service was sending mobile X-ray units out to neighborhoods to offer free chest X-rays as screening for tuberculosis (Hochbaum, 1958). Despite the fact that this service was offered without charge and was available in a variety of convenient locations, the program was of limited success. Not surprisingly, these researchers asked the question, "Why?"

To find an answer, social psychologists examined what was encouraging or discouraging people from participating in the program. They theorized that people's beliefs about whether they were susceptible to disease and their perceptions of the benefits of trying to avoid disease influenced their readiness to act (Glanz & Rimer, 2005).

In ensuing years, researchers expanded upon this theory, eventually concluding that six main constructs influence people's decisions about whether to take action to prevent, screen for, and control illness. They argued that people are ready to act if they meet the following criteria:

1. Believe they are susceptible to the condition (*perceived susceptibility*)
2. Believe the condition has serious consequences (*perceived severity*)
3. Believe taking action would reduce their susceptibility to the condition or its severity (*perceived benefits*)
4. Believe the costs of taking action (*perceived barriers*) are outweighed by the benefits
5. Are exposed to factors that prompt action (e.g., a television ad or a reminder from one's physician to get a mammogram; *cue to action*)
6. Are confident in their ability to successfully perform an action (*self-efficacy*)

Because health motivation is its central focus, the HBM is a good fit for addressing problem behaviors that evoke health concerns (e.g., cancer screening, influenza vaccinations, high-risk sexual behavior and the possibility of contracting human immunodeficiency virus [HIV]). Together, the six constructs of this model provide a useful framework for designing both short-term and long-term behavior change strategies. When applying the HBM to planning health programs, practitioners should ground their efforts in an understanding of how susceptible the patient, his or her family, or the target population feels to the health problem; whether they believe it is serious; and whether they believe action can reduce the threat at an acceptable cost. Changing these factors is rarely as simple as it may appear, however.

Consider high blood pressure screening campaigns, which often identify people who are at high risk for heart disease and stroke that say they have not yet experienced any symptoms. Patient education to promote adherence to medications for hypertension also can encounter this obstacle. Because patients do not feel sick, they may not follow instructions to take prescribed medicine or lose weight. The HBM can be useful for developing strategies to deal with noncompliance in such situations. According to this model, asymptomatic people may not follow a prescribed treatment regimen unless they accept that, even though they may not be experiencing any symptoms, they do actually have hypertension (perceived susceptibility). They must understand that hypertension can lead to heart attacks and strokes (perceived severity). They must believe that taking prescribed medication or following a recommended weight-loss program will reduce the risks (perceived benefits) without negative side effects or excessive difficulty (perceived barriers). Print materials, reminder letters, or pill calendars might encourage people to consistently follow their doctors' recommendations (cues to action). For those who have, in the past, struggled with losing weight or maintaining weight loss, a behavioral contract might help establish achievable, short-term goals to build confidence (self-efficacy).

## Examples of Application of the Health Belief Model

Charron-Prochownik and colleagues (2001) have developed an extensive research program based on the extended health belief model (EHBM) and have used this framework to develop a program of preconceptual counseling for teenagers with type 1 diabetes. One study examined the significant correlates of the variables based on the constructs of this model in relation to an intention to perform or actual performance of behaviors that would prevent an unplanned pregnancy, as well as metabolic control of the diabetes. The findings revealed that most of the 80 teenage participants perceived themselves to be moderately susceptible to severe reproductive problems, but they had little knowledge of diabetes and pregnancy and had moderate self-esteem. The participants' perception was that preconceptual counseling would be beneficial, and they did not envision major barriers to obtaining this type of assistance. The findings also revealed that these same participants did not use effective birth control methods all the time. The correlational analyses demonstrated that there were several significant associations among the individual variables—for example, self-efficacy was significantly associated with other constructs including self-esteem, social support, and stress. The takeaway message of this study was that female adolescents with type 1 diabetes had limited knowledge of reproduction-related complications of diabetes and the role that preconceptual counseling can play in preventing complications; moreover, while participants believed that preconceptual counseling was beneficial, many engaged in unsafe sexual practices.

A later step in this research was the validation of the theory-based instrument to assess preconceptional planning behavior of adolescents with type 1 diabetes. The reproductive health attitudes and behavior (RHAB) instrument drew upon the constructs of the EHBM, the TRA, and SCT, because each theory contributes unique constructs in describing the decision-making processes used by adolescents with diabetes. Overall, the RHAB had good psychometric properties for a newly developed instrument (Charron-Prochownik, Hannan, Sereika, Becker, & Rodgers-Fischl, 2006).

The third phase in this program of research involved the translation of findings from the earlier work into an educational program for teenage girls with diabetes. This program focuses on pregnancy, potential complications among persons with diabetes, and ways to avoid problems. The preconceptual counseling educational program was developed into a CD-ROM that is distributed currently by the American Diabetes Association (Charron-Prochownik et al., 2006). This program of research, from beginning to translation, is based on the EHBM, offering an excellent illustration of how a theoretical framework can guide a body of work.

## The Theory of Reasoned Action, the Theory of Planned Behavior, and the Integrated Behavioral Model

Often people's health decisions are influenced by how they view the actions they are considering and by whether they believe important people such as family members or peers would approve or disapprove of their behavior. The TPB, which evolved from its predecessor, the TRA, focuses on the relationships between behavior and beliefs, attitudes, subjective norms, and intentions (Montano & Kasprzyk, 2008). The concept of perceived behavioral control—which incorporates beliefs about whether one can control his or her performance of a behavior (i.e., individuals may feel motivated if they believe they can do it)—received added attention in TPB. A central assumption of TPB is that behavioral intentions are the most important determinants of behavior (Ajzen, 1991).

TPB has been applied widely to help understand and explain many types of behavior. Both TRA and TPB have been used successfully to predict and explain a wide range of health behaviors and intentions, including smoking, drinking, health services utilization, exercise, sun protection, breastfeeding, substance use, HIV/sexually transmitted infection prevention behaviors and use of contraceptives, mammography, use of safety helmets, and use of seat belts (Montano & Kasprzyk, 2008). As predicted, the core constructs of TPB have been found to predict healthy eating such as fruit and vegetable intake and to explain consumption of low-fat milk (Butterfield-Booth & Reger, 2004). Attitudes and behavioral beliefs about health also have been examined within community interventions in schools and communities and found to mediate outcomes of the interventions (Glanz, 2008). The theoretical constructs help explain why some people change while others do not after they complete health education programs or are exposed to communication campaigns.

Although the idea that behavioral intentions are important is central to TPB, some critics have voiced concern that intentions are too far removed to be good predictors of actual behavior. The concept of implementing intentions involves encouraging patients or people receiving an intervention to be very specific about how they would change (Montano & Kasprzyk, 2008).

In recent years, Fishbein and colleagues (Aizen & Fishbein, 1980; Fishbein & Aizen, 1975) have further expanded TRA and TPB to include components from other major behavioral theories and have proposed the use of an integrated behavioral model (IBM). The IBM can be used as a framework to identify specific belief targets for behavior change interventions in the previously described conceptualization of experiential and instrumental attitudes, injunctive and descriptive norms, and perceived control and self-efficacy being determined by specific underlying beliefs. Interventions built on one model construct may have effects that further affect the same or other model constructs (Montano & Kasprzyk, 2008). While the IBM is a recent expansion of the TPB, it is likely to be more widely used and to have a stronger empirical research base in the coming years.

### Examples of Application of the Theory of Planned Behavior

The TPB provided the framework for a study of male college students in South Korea and their practice of condom use (Cha et al., 2007). A significant relationship had been reported between condom self-efficacy and the intention to use condoms. Cha and colleagues examined the mediating role of condom self-efficacy and the parent–adolescent relationship, as well as the intention to use condoms and actual condom use, to determine if this was a plausible approach for a family-based intervention to improve the sexual health of this young population. A cross-sectional design was used to study the college students and their parents. The mediation analyses revealed that good mother–son communication predicted a higher intention to use condoms and a higher self-efficacy for condom use; in turn, those persons with higher condom self-efficacy had higher intentions to use condoms. After adjusting for condom self-efficacy, however, the quality of the mother–son relationship no longer predicted the intention to use condoms; rather, condom self-efficacy completely mediated the intention to use condoms by mother–son communication.

Interestingly, the quality of the father–son relationship did not predict the intention to use condoms, although a better relationship predicted higher condom self-efficacy for these males. The father–son relationship had an indirect effect on the intention to use condoms.

This study illustrates how different cultural practices in parenting can influence intention and behaviors. The theoretical framework also proved useful during the interpretation of the findings.

## The Transtheoretical Model and the Stages of Change

Long-term behavior change for disease prevention and management involves multiple actions and adaptations over time. For example, some people may not be ready to attempt changes in their diet, whereas others may have already begun implementing dietary modifications. The construct of *stage of change* is a key element of the transtheoretical model of behavior change, which proposes that people are at different stages of readiness to adopt healthful behaviors (Prochaska, Redding, & Evers, 2008). The notion of readiness to change, or stage of change, has been examined in health behavior research on a variety of topics and found useful in explaining and predicting behavior.

Stages of change is a heuristic model that describes a sequence of steps in successful behavior change: *precontemplation* (no recognition of need for or interest in change), *contemplation* (thinking about changing), *preparation* (planning for change), *action* (adopting new habits), and *maintenance* (ongoing practice of new, healthier behavior; Prochaska et al., 2008). People do not always move through the stages of change in a linear manner: They often recycle and repeat certain stages. For example, individuals may relapse and go back to an earlier stage depending on their level of motivation and self-efficacy.

The stages of change model can be used both to explain why patients might not be ready to change their behaviors and to improve the success of patient education or other behavior change interventions. Patients can be classified according to their stage of change by asking a few simple questions. In the case of dietary change, for example, the nurse might ask the following question about each patient: Is he or she interested in trying to change his or her eating patterns, thinking about changing the diet, ready to begin a new eating plan, already making dietary changes, or trying to sustain changes he or she has been following for some time? By identifying the individual's current stage, the nurse can determine how much time to spend with the patient, whether to wait until he or she is more ready to attempt active changes, whether referral for in-depth counseling or case management is warranted, and so on. Knowledge of the patient's current stage of change can lead also to appropriate follow-up questions about past efforts to change, obstacles and challenges, and available strategies for overcoming barriers or obstacles to change.

## Examples of Application of the Transtheoretical Model of Behavior Change

Finnell has applied the transtheoretical model of behavior change to different behaviors in different populations (Finnell, 2003, 2005a, 2005b). Finnell's early work focused on the use of this model to determine whether individuals with co-occurring conditions—mental disorders and substance abuse—undergo change in a similar way to others who have been studied with the use of this model (Finnell, 2003). The presence of several conditions, including impaired decision-making abilities, disordered thought processes, and denial, which can be present with either disorder, may make it difficult for these individuals to recognize that they need assistance and also to ask for it. The findings from a cross-sectional survey that was conducted in this population revealed that individuals with comorbid mental disorders and substance abuse rely on different processes as they adopt new behaviors and may need a different intervention than persons who have only a substance abuse problem (Finnell, 2003).

Finnell is also applying the transtheoretical model of behavior change to the study of medication adherence among patients in a Veterans Administration inpatient facility. The stages of change concept is being used to guide the assessment of patients regarding their readiness to be adherent to antidepressant medication (Finnell, 2005b). Extensive information is provided on various sites on the Web that is dedicated to the use of this theoretical framework, including a video demonstrating the practice of applying the framework.

## Social Cognitive Theory

SCT—the cognitive formulation of social learning theory that has been best articulated by Bandura (1986, 1997)—explains human behavior in terms of a three-way, dynamic, reciprocal model in which personal factors, environmental influences, and behavior continually interact. Because SCT synthesizes concepts and processes from cognitive, behavioristic, and emotional models of behavior change, it can be readily applied to nutritional intervention for disease prevention and management. A basic premise of SCT is that people learn not only through their own experiences, but also by observing the actions of others and the results of those actions. Key constructs of this theory that are relevant to health behavior interventions include *observational learning, reinforcement, self-control,* and *self-efficacy* (McAlister, Perry, & Parcel, 2008).

Principles of behavior modification, which have often been used to promote health behavior change, are derived from SCT. Some elements of behavioral interventions based on SCT constructs of self-control, reinforcement, and self-efficacy include goal setting, self-monitoring, and behavioral contracting (Glanz & Rimer, 2005). For habitual behaviors such as quitting smoking and improving eating patterns, goal setting and self-monitoring seem to be particularly useful components of effective interventions (Glanz, 2008).

Self-efficacy, or a person's confidence in his or her ability to take action and to persist in that action despite encountering obstacles or challenges, seems to be especially important for influencing health behavior change efforts (Bandura, 1997). Health providers can make deliberate efforts to increase patients' self-efficacy using three types of strategies:

1. Setting small, incremental, and achievable goals
2. Using formalized behavioral contracting to establish goals and specify rewards
3. Monitoring and reinforcement, including patient self-monitoring by keeping records (Glanz et al., 2008)

In group programs, it is possible to easily incorporate activities such as problem-solving discussions and self-monitoring that are rooted in SCT.

The key SCT construct of *reciprocal determinism* means that a person can be both an agent for change and a responder to change. Thus changes in the environment, role models, and reinforcements can be used to promote healthier behavior. This core construct is also central to social ecological models and is more important today than ever before.

## Examples of Application of Social Cognitive Theory

The implementation of interventions based on SCT is quite common among advanced practice nurses. Burke and colleagues tested different approaches to self-monitoring diet and physical activity in a behavioral weight-loss study, including use of a paper diary versus use of an electronic diary (personal digital assistant), with and without feedback messages (Burke et al., 2009a). Guided by self-regulation, also derived from SCT, the intervention built on the behavioral change strategy of self-monitoring to increase the individual's awareness of his or her behavior, which serves as a crucial step prior to asking a person to change current behavior. Based on specific goals set with the participant, self-monitoring provides feedback to the person on progress related to those goals. A review of progress made permits self-attribution for the progress and goal achievement. In this study, the delivery of a feedback message via the electronic diary added another element of reinforcement for reported behavior change related to eating behaviors and food selection, as well as physical activity (Burke et al., 2009b).

Other strategies based on SCT include *role modeling*, which can be implemented by having individuals who are successful in changing behavior model the behavior for those who are learning to adopt it. Examples of successful use of this strategy include cardiac rehabilitation programs in which participants who have successfully adopted a physical activity program demonstrate their ability to exercise for individuals who are newly enrolled, as well as having a person who is credible to the patients demonstrate how to prepare a low-fat meal. It is important that the model who demonstrates the skill or behavior be credible and a person with whom the patient can identify.

Sevick and colleagues used SCT to guide the development and implementation of a diabetes self-management intervention for adults with type 2 diabetes. Their intervention included self-monitoring of the person's diet and daily blood glucose levels, use of an electronic diary in the intervention group, group sessions, and cooking demonstrations (Sevick et al., 2008). Goal setting for various components of self-management was part of the intervention; preliminary results indicate that the intervention led to improved self-management behaviors, as well as improved clinical outcomes (Sevick et al., unpublished data).

## Example of Application of Self-Efficacy

Self-efficacy is considered part of SCT and has provided the underpinning for numerous interventions addressing behavior change. Its role in changing behavior has been reported across several behavior domains, including smoking cessation (Gwaltney et al., 2001; Gwaltney et al., 2002; Gwaltney, Shiffman, & Sayette, 2005; Ockene et al., 2000; Warnecke et al., 2001), weight loss (Butler & Mellor, 2006; Clark, Cargill, Medeiros, & Pera, 1996; Clark & King, 2000), and being more physically active (Dallow & Anderson, 2003; Desharnais, Bouillon, & Godin, 1986; Ewart, Stewart, & Gillilan, 1986; Moore, Dolansky, Ruland, Pashkow, & Blackburn, 2003; Pinto, Clark, Cruess, Syzmanski, & Pera, 1999). Self-efficacy is described as the perception of one's capability to mobilize the motivation, cognitive resources, and courses of action required to meet given situational demands (Bandura, 1997).

One example of a self-efficacy–based intervention implemented by a cardiovascular nurse specialist is a study of individuals who were being seen for dyslipidemia and who also reported inadequate dietary adherence (Burke, Dunbar-Jacob, Orchard, & Sereika, 2005). The purpose of the randomized controlled trial was to evaluate the ability of the self-efficacy intervention to improve adherence to a cholesterol-lowering diet. The intervention was delivered as an adjunct to the usual care; the comparison group received only the usual care. The behavioral intervention focused on strategies to improve self-efficacy for following the prescribed diet and included the individual setting short-term, realistic goals for behavior change to improve adherence and self-monitoring in a paper diary (e.g., eliminating high-fat snacks obtained from the vending machine at work).

At each biweekly intervention session, the nurse reviewed with the participant the goal that had been set and the participant reviewed the diary over the phone and practiced self-reinforcement for positive changes. Any progress toward goal achievement was attributed to the individual. As the person experienced success, incremental changes were made in the goals, reinforcing the strategy of *mastery,* which according to the theory is the strongest source for improving self-efficacy.

*Verbal persuasion* was another strategy that was used to increase self-efficacy; it was found to be particularly well suited for the telephone delivery of the intervention. This part of the program entailed the interventionist verbally convincing the participant that she was confident in his ability to perform the new behavior.

At the end of the 14-week intervention, the researchers noted significant improvement in adherence to the recommended intake of dietary cholesterol and total and saturated fat. In addition, a significant improvement in serum low-density lipoprotein cholesterol was seen, with significantly greater improvements occurring in the intervention group (Burke et al., 2005).

## Social Ecological Models

Social ecological models focus on the factors affecting behavior and provide guidance for developing successful programs through social environments. These models emphasize multiple levels of influence (such as individual, interpersonal, organizational, community, and public policy spheres) and the idea that behaviors both shape and are shaped by the social environment (McLeroy, Bibeau, Steckler, & Glanz, 1988; Sallis, Owen, & Fisher, 2008).

The principles of social ecological models are consistent with SCT concepts that suggest initially creating an environment that is conducive to change is important to making it easier to adopt healthy behaviors. Given the widespread problems associated with the unhealthy lifestyles followed by many people today, as well as these lifestyles' role in chronic diseases such as diabetes and lung disease, more attention is being devoted to increasing the health-promoting features of communities and neighborhoods. Examples of environmental change strategies to promote healthful behaviors that are based on social ecological models include reducing exposure to second-hand smoke and the consumption of high-calorie, high-fat foods in large portions. Changing the healthcare system by giving providers such as doctors and nurses reminders and incorporating health counseling into primary care are other examples of the application of social ecological models to health behavior.

# Representational Approach

The theoretical perspective on patient education known as the representational approach was developed by Donovan and Ward and is a patient-centered intervention theory that links existing health psychology and educational theory to specific psycho-educational interventions (Donovan & Ward, 2001; Donovan et al., 2007). Leventhal's common-sense model (CSM) of illness representations (Leventhal, Meyer, & Nerenz, 1980; Leventhal, Nerenz, & Steeler, 1984) provided the centerpiece of this theoretical framework, which also drew upon on educational theory of conceptual change (Hewson & Thorley, 1989; Posner, Strike, Hewson, & Gertzog, 1982).

The RA was developed to increase the probability that individuals will experience conceptual change. It consists of seven elements:

1. Representational assessment
2. Exploring individuals' concerns and misconceptions or any gaps
3. Creating conditions for conceptual change
4. Introducing new information
5. Setting goals and developing management strategies
6. Summarizing
7. Evaluation of strategy evaluation and revision (Donovan & Ward, 2001; Donovan et al., 2007)

These key elements of RA use the CSM to focus on what patients or individuals know and understand about their health problems, which guides the clinician in eliciting these individuals' illness representations. The elements derived from theories of conceptual change center on how patients learn new information and behaviors, which helps ensure that the information is presented in ways that will be not only understood by the individual, but also accommodated and acted on by that person.

The RA requires the provider to elicit and understand the individual's pre-existing representations of illness before he or she provides any new information to the patient. In this way, both the clinician and the patient have the opportunity to recognize voids, misunderstandings, and confusion in the patient's representation. It is also important for the clinician to understand the individual's representations of the health problem so the clinician can give new information in an individualized manner that is specific, highly relevant, and more likely to be accepted by the patient as intelligible, plausible, and fruitful. The efficacy of interventions based on the RA has been supported by evidence from controlled randomized clinical trials conducted by nurse investigators studying other patient populations (Donovan et al., 2007; Heidrich et al., 2009; Song et al., 2005; Song et al., 2009; Ward et al., 2008; Ward et al., 2009).

## Example of Application of the Representational Approach

In one study using the RA, an advanced practice nurse employed a novel delivery mode in a program referred to as the WRITE Symptoms (A *W*ritten *R*epresenta-tional *I*ntervention *T*o *E*ase *S*ymptoms; Donovan et al., 2007). This study evaluated the feasibility and acceptability of delivering the intervention to women with recurrent ovarian cancer via a secure Internet messaging service. It compared the changes in symptom representation, symptom interference with life activities, and quality of life in the group whose members received the WRITE Symptom intervention compared to a group of patients who received usual care. Participants in this study selected several symptoms they wished to address, and the process and content of the intervention session was closely aligned with the seven elements of the RA described earlier in this section.

What was novel about this study was that instead of face-to-face sessions or interviews, the research nurse and study participants communicated through postings on private message boards. This approach permitted each study participant, the researcher, and the clinicians caring for the individual to have more time and greater flexibility to communicate with one another in assisting the participant to manage her symptoms. For example, each participant had a secure bulletin board—a special place where she could go to correspond with the clinicians and work on her symptom management. Use of this approach also permitted the clinician to follow the message thread, review the content, and respond with recommendations when time permitted. Also, because the information exchange could be voluminous and complex, it permitted each party time to process the material; the asynchronous messaging allowed the clinicians time to review the participant's specific concerns and respond with an individualized reply.

In summary, the strength of the RA to patient education is that it was derived from Leventhal's CSM and models of conceptual change in a thoughtful and purposeful evolution. Because it links existing theory and specific interventions, and because it relies on a clear theoretical framework, the RA can be applied to an array of clinical problems. Nurses play a key role in the delivery of patient education; this relatively new approach to patient education provides an organized framework with the seven elements providing sound structure. For the nurse researcher, the framework needs further empirical exploration and testing of the seven elements to determine if all seven are essential for successful outcomes (Donovan et al., 2007).

# Cross-Cutting Concepts

The various theories that can be used for health behavior change interventions are not mutually exclusive. Perhaps not surprisingly, they share several constructs, and common issues cut across multiple theories (Glanz & Oldenburg, 2001). It can be challenging to sort out the key issues in various models. This section focuses on important issues and constructs across models.

## The Patient's View of the World: Perceptions, Cognitions, Emotions, and Habits

The first key point is that successful health behavior change depends on a sound understanding of the patient's (or consumer's) view of the world (Glanz, 2008). For health professionals who work with patients and provide them with advice on health and lifestyle, adherence to treatment is often disappointingly poor, even in response to relatively simple medical advice. Such poor adherence often arises because patients do not have the necessary behavioral skills to make lifestyle changes or to follow a medication regimen. Following a heart attack, for example, patients might well understand the importance of adopting changes to their lifestyle yet be unable to make those changes. In other circumstances, patients might not understand the importance of such changes and may even believe that these changes pose an additional risk to their health. In still other circumstances, a patient might be experiencing depression or anxiety, such that emotional dysfunction will be a major barrier to compliance.

Traditionally, it has been assumed that the relationship between knowledge, attitudes, and behavior is a simple and direct one. In the past, many prevention and patient education programs have been based on the premise that if people understand and believe in the health consequences of a particular behavior, they will modify it accordingly. Research conducted over the past 30 years has revealed a much different finding, however: The relationships between knowledge, awareness of the need to change, intention to change, and an actual change in behavior are very complex, indeed.

Ideally, each patient should be treated as an individual with unique circumstances and health history. Even so, epidemiological research indicates that certain demographic subgroups differ in terms of risk factors and health behaviors. Understanding these population trends can help prepare a provider to work with various types of patients. For example, younger persons may feel invulnerable to coronary events, and older adults may be managing multiple chronic conditions. An active middle-aged professional may place returning to his previous level of activity above important health protective actions. These examples serve as a reminder that the provider must be sensitive to group patterns, yet avoid stereotyping in the absence of first-hand evidence about an individual. Within this general context, various theories and models can guide the search for effective ways to reach and positively motivate patients.

## Behavior Change as a Process

Sustained health behavior change involves multiple actions and adaptations over time. Some people may not be ready to attempt changes, some may be thinking about attempting change, and others may have already begun implementing behavioral modifications. One central issue that has gained wide acceptance in recent years is the simple notion that *behavior change is a process, not an event.* Put simply, it is important to think of the change process as one that occurs in stages. It is not a question of someone deciding one day to stop smoking and the next day becoming a nonsmoker for life. Most people will not be able to make long-term changes in their health behaviors easily.

The idea that behavior change occurs in a number of steps is not particularly new, but it has gained wider recognition in the past few years. Indeed, various multistage theories of behavior change date back more than 50 years to the work of Lewin, McGuire, Weinstein, Marlatt and Gordon, and others (Glanz et al., 2008).

The notion of readiness to change, or stage of change, has been examined in health behavior research and found useful in explaining and predicting a variety of types of behaviors. Prochaska, Velicer, DiClemente, and their colleagues (e.g., 1988) have been leaders in formally identifying the dynamics and structure of change that underlie both self-mediated and clinically facilitated health behavior change. The construct of stages of change described earlier in this chapter is a key element of the transtheoretical model of behavior change; it proposes that people are at different stages of readiness to adopt healthful behaviors (Prochaska et al., 2008).

While the stages of change construct cuts across various circumstances of individuals who need to change or want to change, other theories also address these processes. The remainder of this section looks across various models to illustrate four key concerns in understanding the process of behavior change: (1) motivation versus intention, (2) intention versus action, (3) changing behavior versus maintaining behavior change, and (4) the role of biobehavioral factors.

### *Motivation Versus Intention*

Behavior change is challenging for most people, even if they are highly motivated to change. As noted earlier in this chapter, the relationships between knowledge, awareness of the need to change, intention to change, and an actual change in behavior are very complex. For individuals who are coping with disease and illness, and who are often having to make very significant changes to their lifestyle and other aspects of their lives, this challenge is even greater. According to the transtheoretical model, people in the precontemplation stage are neither motivated nor planning to change, those in the contemplation stage intend to change, and those in the preparation stage are acting on their intentions by taking specific steps toward the action of change (Prochaska et al., 2008). The importance of intentions is emphasized in the TPB (Montano & Kasprzyk, 2008).

# Intention Versus Action

The transtheoretical model makes a clear distinction between the contemplation and preparation stages and the stage in which overt action takes place (Prochaska et al., 2008). A further application of this distinction comes from the TPB (Ajzen, 1991; Montano & Kasprzyk, 2008). Although the TPB proposes that intentions are the best predictor of behavior, researchers are increasingly focusing attention on implementation intentions as being more proximal and even better predictors of behavior and behavior change (Gollwitzer, 1999).

## *Changing Behaviors Versus Maintaining Behavior Change*

Even when there is good initial compliance with a lifestyle change program, such as quitting smoking or changing diet, relapse is very common. It is widely recognized that many overweight persons are able to lose weight initially, only to regain it within a year. Thus it has become clear to researchers and clinicians that undertaking initial behavior changes and maintaining behavior change require different types of strategies. The transtheoretical model's distinction between the action and maintenance stages implicitly addresses this phenomenon (Prochaska et al., 2008). Long-term maintenance of behavior change requires developing self-management and coping strategies, as well as establishing new behavior patterns that emphasize perceived control, environmental management, and improved self-efficacy. These strategies consist of an eclectic mix drawn from SCT (Bandura, 1986), the TPB (Montano & Kasprzyk, 2008), applied behavioral analysis, and the forerunners of the stages of change model.

## *Biobehavioral Factors*

The behavioral and social theories described thus far have some important limitations, many of which are only now beginning to be understood. Notably, for some health behaviors—especially addictive or addiction-like behaviors—there are other important determinants of behavior, which may be physiological or genetically determined. Among the best known are the addictive effects of nicotine, alcohol, and some drugs. Physiological factors increase psychological cravings and create withdrawal syndromes that may impede even highly motivated persons from changing their behaviors (e.g., quitting smoking or not consuming alcoholic beverages). Some behavior changes—for example, weight loss—also affect energy metabolism and make long-term risk factor reduction an even greater challenge than it would be if it depended on cognitive-behavioral factors alone. Research into the psychobiology of appetite, for instance, offers intriguing possibilities for better understanding biobehavioral models of food intake (Glanz, 2008).

## *Control Over Behavior and Health: Control Beliefs and Self-Efficacy*

Sometimes, control beliefs and self-efficacy hold people back from achieving better health. These deterrents to positive health behavior change are commonplace and can be found in several models of health behavior, including SCT and the TPB. One of the most important challenges for these models—and ultimately for the nurses who apply them—is to enhance perceived behavioral control and increase self-efficacy, thereby improving patients' motivation and persistence in the face of obstacles.

## Applications in Nursing and Nursing Research

The examples provided throughout this chapter illustrate how nurses use theory to guide their research and also serve as exemplars of theory application. In selecting a theory to guide one's research, it is important to understand how the framework will shape the entire research process and, where applicable, how it will influence intervention design. It is not sufficient to identify a behavioral theory or model to guide one's conceptual background; the theory needs to guide the variables that will be measured and the measurement tools to assess the variables.

Once the data are collected, the theory should help interpret the findings; in other words, the findings should be placed in the context of the theoretical framework. For example, Charron-Prochownik and colleagues (2001) interpreted girls' reported perceptions of risk for reproductive complications and their limited knowledge related to this issue as part of their study. The findings led to the development of an instrument that was true to the theory and, subsequently, an intervention was developed that was consistent with the HBM framework. Thus a theory is not just a statement but rather a thread or theme that is consistently interwoven throughout a study.

As advanced practice nurses use behavioral change theories as part of their research and practice, they will contribute to the greater understanding and refinement of the constructs that compose the theory. For example, the work by Ward and Donovan and their colleagues is refining an adaptation of the illness representation model. In a similar way, other nurse researchers can make valuable contributions to the theoretical basis of their practice though multiple paths of study.

## Discussion Questions

1. Explain the multiple levels of influence that affect patients' health-related behaviors and the implications for using an ecological perspective in developing health education/promotion programs in outpatient healthcare settings.

2. What are the major differences between *explanatory* theories and *change* theories?

3. The idea of health behavior change as a *process*—not an event—cuts across several behavior change theories. Explain how this idea can be put into action for either adherence with diabetic treatment and self-management regimens or smoking cessation, using constructs from either the stages of change or the TPB.

# References

Ajzen, I. (1991). The theory of planned behavior. *Organizational Behavior and Human Decision Processes, 50*(2), 179–211.

Ajzen, I., & Fishbein, M. (1980). *Belief, attitude, intention, and behavior.* Reading, MA: Addison-Wesley.

Bandura, A. (1986). *Social foundations of thought and action: A social cognitive theory.* Englewood Cliffs, NJ: Prentice Hall.

Bandura, A. (1997). *Self-efficacy: The exercise of control.* New York, NY: W. H. Freeman.

Berg, J., Dunbar-Jacob, J., & Rohay, J. M. (1995). Assessing inhaler medication adherence using an electronic monitoring device: Revisited. *Annals of Behavioral Medicine, 17*(Suppl.), S128 (Abstract).

Berg, J., Dunbar-Jacob, J., & Sereika, S. M. (1997). An evaluation of a self-management program for adults with asthma. *Clinical Nursing Research, 6*(3), 225–238.

Burke, L. E., Dunbar-Jacob, J., Orchard, T. J., & Sereika, S. M. (2005). Improving adherence to a cholesterol-lowering diet: A behavioral intervention study. *Patient Education & Counseling, 57*(1), 134–142.

Burke, L. E., Elci, O. U., Wang, J., Ewing, L. J., Conroy, M. B., Acharya, S. D., & Sereika, S. M. (2009a). Self-monitoring in behavioral weight loss treatment: SMART trial short-term results. *Obesity, 17*(Suppl. 2), 828-P.

Burke, L. E., Styn, M. A., Glanz, K., Ewing, L. J., Elci, O. U., Conroy, M. B., . . . Sevick, M. A. (2009b). SMART trial: A randomized clinical trial of self-monitoring in behavioral weight management-design and baseline findings. *Contemporary Clinical Trials, 30*(6), 540–551.

Burkhart, P. V., Rayens, M. K., Oakley, M. G., Abshire, D. A., & Zhang, M. (2007). Testing an intervention to promote children's adherence to asthma self-management. *Journal of Nursing Scholarship, 39*(2), 133–140.

Butler, P., & Mellor, D. (2006). Role of personal factors in women's self-reported weight management behaviour. *Public Health, 120*(5), 383–392.

Butterfield-Booth, S., & Reger, B. (2004). The message changes belief and the rest is theory: The "1% or less" milk campaign and reasoned action. *Preventive Medicine, 39*(3), 581–588.

Cha, E. S., Kim, K. H., & Doswell, W. M. (2007). Influence of the parent–adolescent relationship on condom use among South Korean male college students. *Nursing & Health Sciences, 9*(4), 277–283.

Charron-Prochownik, D., Hannan, M. F., Sereika, S. M., Becker, D., & Rodgers-Fischl, A. (2006). How to develop CD-ROMs for diabetes education: Exemplar "Reproductive-Health Education and Awareness of Diabetes in Youth for Girls" (READY-Girls). *Diabetes Spectrum, 19*(2), 110–115.

Charron-Prochownik, D., Sereika, S. M., Becker, D., Jacober, S., Mansfield, J., White, N. H., . . . Trail, L. (2001). Reproductive health beliefs and behaviors in teens with diabetes: Application of the expanded health belief model. *Pediatric Diabetes, 2*(1), 30–39.

Clark, M. M., Cargill, B. R., Medeiros, M. L., & Pera, V. (1996). Changes in self-efficacy following obesity treatment. *Obesity Research, 4*(2), 179–181.

Clark, M. M., & King, T. (2000). Eating self-efficacy and weight cycling: A prospective clinical study. *Eating Behaviors, 1*(1), 47–52.

Dallow, C. B., & Anderson, J. (2003). Using self-efficacy and a transtheoretical model to develop a physical activity intervention for obese women. *American Journal of Health Promotion, 17*(6), 373–381.

DeBusk, R., Miller, N. H., Superko, R., Dennis, C., Thomas, R., Lew, H., . . . Gee, D. (1994). A case-management system for coronary risk factor modification after acute myocardial infarction. *Annals of Internal Medicine, 120*(9), 721–729.

Desharnais, R., Bouillon, J., & Godin, G. (1986). Self-efficacy and outcome expectations as determinants of exercise adherence. *Psychological Reports, 59*(3), 1155–1159.

Donovan, H. S., & Ward, S. (2001). A representational approach to patient education. *Journal of Nursing Scholarship, 33*(3), 211–216.

Donovan, H. S., Ward, S. E., Song, M. K., Heidrich, S. M., Gunnarsdottir, S., & Phillips, C. M. (2007). An update on the representational approach to patient education. *Journal of Nursing Scholarship, 39*(3), 259–265.

Ewart, C. K., Stewart, K. J., & Gillilan, R. E. (1986). Usefulness of self-efficacy in predicting overexertion during programmed exercise in coronary artery disease. *American Journal of Cardiology, 57*(8), 557–561.

Finnell, D. S. (2003). Use of the transtheoretical model for individuals with co-occurring disorders. *Community Mental Health Journal, 39*(1), 3–15.

Finnell, D. S. (2005a). Building a program of research based on the transtheoretical model. *Journal of Addictions Nursing, 16*(1–2), 13–21.

Finnell, D. S. (2005b). Promote medication adherence, one stage at a time. *Current Psychiatry, 4*(8), 88.

Fishbein, M., & Ajzen, I. (1975). *Belief, attitude, intention, and behavior: An introduction to theory and research*. Reading, MA: Addison-Wesley.

Glanz, K. (2008). Current theoretical bases for nutrition intervention and their uses. In A. M. Coulston & C. J. Boushey (Eds.), *Nutrition in the prevention and treatment of disease* (2nd ed., pp. 127–138). Amsterdam: Elsevier.

Glanz, K., & Oldenburg, B. (2001). Utilizing theories and constructs across models of behavior change. In R. Patterson (Ed.), *Changing patient behavior: Improving outcomes in health and disease management* (pp. 25–40). San Francisco, CA: Jossey-Bass.

Glanz, K., & Rimer, B. K. (2005). *Theory at a glance: Application to health promotion and health behavior* (2nd ed.). National Cancer Institute, National Institutes of Health, U.S. Department of Health and Human Services (NIH Pub. No. 05-3896). Washington, DC: National Institutes of Health.

Glanz, K., Rimer, B. K., & Viswanath, K. (Eds.). (2008). *Health behavior and health education: Theory, research, and practice* (4th ed.). San Francisco, CA: Jossey-Bass.

Gollwitzer, P. M. (1999). Implementation intentions: Strong effects of simple plans. *American Psychologist, 54*(7), 493–503.

Gwaltney, C., Shiffman, S., Norman, G., Paty, J. A., Kassel, J. D., Gyns, M., . . . Balabanais, M. (2001). Does smoking abstinence self-efficacy vary across situations? Identifying context-specificity within the Relapse Situation Efficacy Questionnaire. *Journal of Consulting & Clinical Psychology, 69*(3), 516–527.

Gwaltney, C. J., Shiffman, S., Paty, J. A., Liu, K. S., Kassel, J. D., Gnys, M., & Hickcox, M. (2002). Using self-efficacy judgments to predict characteristics of lapses to smoking. *Journal of Consulting and Clinical Psychology, 70*(5), 1140–1149.

Gwaltney, C. J., Shiffman, S., & Sayette, M. A. (2005). Situational correlates of abstinence self-efficacy. *Journal of Abnormal Psychology, 114*(4), 649–660.

Haskell, W. L., Alderman, E. L., Fair, J. M., Maron, D. J., Mackey, S. F., Superko, R., . . . Kraus, R. M. (1994). Effects of intensive multiple risk factor reduction on coronary atherosclerosis and clinical cardiac events in men and women with coronary artery disease: The Stanford Coronary Risk Intervention Project (SCRIP). *Circulation, 89*(3), 975–990.

Heidrich, S. M., Brown, R. L., Egan, J. J., Perez, O. A., Phelan, C. H., Yeom, H., & Ward, S. E. (2009). An individualized representational intervention to improve symptom management (IRIS) in older breast cancer survivors: Three pilot studies. *Oncology Nursing Forum, 36*(3), E133–E143.

Hewson, P., & Thorley, N. (1989). The conditions of conceptual change in the classroom. *International Journal of Science Education, 11*(5), 541–553.

Hochbaum, G. M. (1958). *Public participation in medical screening programs: A socio-psychological study.* Washington, DC: U.S. Department of Health, Education, and Welfare.

Kipnis, D. (1994). Accounting for the use of behavior technologies in social psychology. *American Psychologist, 49*(3), 165–172.

Leventhal, H., Meyer, D., & Nerenz, D. (1980). The common-sense representation of illness danger. In S. Rachman (Ed.), *Medical psychology* (Vol. II, pp. 7–30). New York, NY: Pergamon Press.

Leventhal, H., Nerenz, D., & Steeler, D. (1984). Illness representations and coping with health threats. In A. Baum & J. Singer (Eds.), *Handbook of psychology and health* (Vol. IV, pp. 221–252). New York, NY: Erlbaum.

Matarazzo, J. D., Weiss, C. M., Herd, J. A., Miller, N. E., & Weiss, S. M. (Eds.). (1984). *Behavioral health: A handbook of health enhancement and disease prevention.* New York, NY: Wiley.

McAlister, A. L., Perry, C. L., & Parcel, G. S. (2008). How individuals, environments, and health behaviors interact: Social cognitive theory. In K. Glanz, B. K. Rimer, & K. Viswanath (Eds.), *Health behavior and health education: Theory, research, and practice* (4th ed., pp. 169–188). San Francisco, CA: Jossey-Bass.

McLeroy, K., Bibeau, D., Steckler, A., & Glanz, K. (1988). An ecological perspective on health promotion programs. *Health Education Quarterly, 15*(4), 351–377.

Montano, D. E., & Kasprzyk, D. (2008). Theory of reasoned action, theory of planned behavior, and the integrated behavioral model. In K. Glanz, B. K. Rimer, & K. Viswanath (Eds.), *Health behavior and health education: Theory, research, and practice* (4th ed., pp. 68–96). San Francisco, CA: Jossey-Bass.

Moore, S. M., Dolansky, M. A., Ruland, C. M., Pashkow, F. J., & Blackburn, G. G. (2003). Predictors of women's exercise maintenance after cardiac rehabilitation. *Journal of Cardiopulmonary Rehabilitation, 23*(1), 40–49.

Ockene, J. K., Emmons, K. M., Mermelstein, R. J., Perkins, K. A., Bonollo, D. S., Voorhees, C. C., & Hollis, J. F. (2000). Relapse and maintenance issues for smoking cessation. *Health Psychology, 19*(1 Suppl.), 17–31.

Painter, J. E., Borba, C. P., Hynes, M., Mays, D., & Glanz, K. (2008). The use of theory in health behavior research from 2000 to 2005: A systematic review. *Annals of Behavioral Medicine, 35*(3), 358–362.

Pinto, B. M., Clark, M. M., Cruess, D. G., Syzmanski, L., & Pera, V. (1999). Changes in self-efficacy and decisional balance for exercise among obese women in a weight management program. *Obesity Research, 7*(3), 288–292.

Posner, G., Strike, K., Hewson, P., & Gertzog, W. (1982). Accommodation of a scientific conception: Toward a theory of conceptual change. *Science Education, 66*(2), 211–227.

Prochaska, J. O., Redding, C., & Evers, K. (2008). The transtheoretical model of behavior change. In K. Glanz, B. K. Rimer, & K. Viswanath (Eds.), *Health behavior and health education: Theory, research, and practice* (4th ed., pp. 97–121). San Francisco, CA: Jossey-Bass.

Prochaska, J. O., Velicer, W. F., DiClemente, C. C., & Fava, J. (1988). Measuring processes of change: Applications to the cessation of smoking. *Journal of Consulting Clinical Psychology, 56*(4), 520–528.

Sallis, J., Owen, N., & Fisher, E. (2008). Ecological models of health behavior. In K. Glanz, B. K. Rimer, & K. Viswanath (Eds.), *Health behavior and health education: Theory, research, and practice* (4th ed., pp. 465–485). San Francisco, CA: Jossey-Bass.

Sevick, M. A., Stone, R. A., Novak, M., Piraino, B., Snetselaar, L., Marsh, R. M., . . . Burke, L. E. (2008). A PDA-based dietary self-monitoring intervention to reduce sodium intake in an in-center hemodialysis patient. *Patient Preference and Adherence, 2,* 177–184.

Song, M. K., Kirchhoff, K. T., Douglas, J., Ward, S., & Hammes, B. (2005). A randomized, controlled trial to improve advance care planning among patients undergoing cardiac surgery. *Medical Care, 43*(10), 1049–1053.

Song, M. K., Ward, S. E., Happ, M. B., Piraino, B., Donovan, H. S., Shields, A. M., & Connolly, M. C. (2009). Randomized controlled trial of SPIRIT: An effective approach to preparing African-American dialysis patients and families for end of life. *Research in Nursing & Health, 32*(3), 260–273.

Ward, S., Donovan, H., Gunnarsdottir, S., Serlin, R. C., Shapiro, G. R., & Hughes, S. (2008). A randomized trial of a representational intervention to decrease cancer pain (RIDCancerPain). *Health Psychology, 27*(1), 59–67.

Ward, S. E., Serlin, R. C., Donovan, H. S., Ameringer, S. W., Hughes, S., Pe-Romashko, K., & Wang, K. K. (2009). A randomized trial of a representational intervention for cancer pain: Does targeting the dyad make a difference? *Health Psychology, 28*(5), 588–597.

Warnecke, R. B., Morera, O., Turner, L., Mermelstein, R., Johnson, T. P., Parsons, J., . . . Flay, B. (2001). Changes in self-efficacy and readiness for smoking cessation among women with high school or less education. *Journal of Health & Social Behavior, 42*(1), 97–110.

# CHAPTER 12

# Theories Focused on Interpersonal Relationships

*Sandra Nelson*

## Introduction

Several interpersonal nursing theories or conceptual frameworks are discussed in this chapter. The first framework is *interpersonal relations* and focuses on Hildegard Peplau's theory of interpersonal nursing, Ida Jean Orlando's nursing process discipline theory, and Joyce Travelbee's human-to-human relationship model. The second framework is *humanism/caring*, with discussion of Josephine Paterson and Loretta Zderad's humanistic nursing theory. Finally, the *existentialism/phenomenology* framework is addressed through discussion of Jean Watson's theory of human caring, which is also known as the theory of transpersonal caring or transpersonal caring science (Watson & Smith, 2002); Margaret Newman's theory of health as expanding consciousness; and Rosemarie Rizzo Parse's theory of human becoming.

Non-nurse theories are discussed as well. The first is interpersonal relations, through discussion of Harry Stack Sullivan's work. The second is humanism, examined through Carl Rogers' client-centered counseling. Next discussed is existentialism and the work of Viktor Frankl and Rollo May, followed by positive psychology, with contributions from Martin Seligman and Mihaly Csikszentmihalyi, and finally transpersonal psychology.

A new category related to interpersonal care, recovery-oriented care (also known as recovery-oriented systems of care), has emerged and represents a paradigm shift in the nation's behavioral and mental healthcare systems and approaches to health care. It is introduced in this chapter as primarily an interpersonal relationship concept that needs to find a "home" among nursing theories or conceptual frameworks.

Fundamentally, all interpersonal theorists believe that anxiety arises from experiences in relationships with significant others. They emphasize the importance of social forces or what one does in relation to others rather than internal or biological factors. Many of these theorists have asserted that adult mental disorders stem from impaired interpersonal relationships during childhood. Because of the dynamics of interpersonal relationships, understanding these concepts enables nurses to form healthy relationships with their clients at various developmental stages and to influence their patients' ability to adapt to environmental stressors (Antai-Otong, 2008, p. 41).

Interpersonal relationship theories and concepts in health care grew primarily from the research of psychiatrist Harry Stack Sullivan (1892–1949). Moving away from Freudian intrapsychic perspectives of mental illness and research tenets within the positivist period, Sullivan and several other neo-Freudian psychiatrists (Karen Horney, Erik H. Erikson, Erich Fromm, and Frieda Fromm-Reichmann) developed a theory of interpersonal relationships, or interactional relations. Sullivan viewed humans as social beings requiring the support and nurture of their environment, and he saw childhood development as being directly influenced by the interpersonal relations found in a person's social and cultural environment. Essentially, all human processes occur in interrelationships; none occur in isolation.

Hildegard Peplau, one of Sullivan's students and a pioneering psychiatric nurse, developed her theory of interpersonal relations from Sullivan's interpersonal findings. In an expansive discussion, her peer, Margaret Newman (2008) asserted the following:

> In nursing, the emphasis is on relationship: relationships within the client's life and between the nurse and client as being integral to nursing. A relationship may be symmetrical, complementary, or asymmetrical. A *symmetrical* relationship is one in which the action of one part escalates the action of the other, as in competition. *Complementary* relationships tend to move toward equilibrium: the action of one balances the action of another. . . . An *asymmetrical* relationship is one of growth, evolvement, and transcendence. Movement of a symmetrical or complementary relationship to an asymmetrical one requires additional information and new insight, an expansion of consciousness. (p. xv)

## A Sign of the Times: 1800s to 1970s

Nurses writing about nursing between the late 1800s and 1950s addressed all aspects of knowing, perhaps without recognizing it (Chinn & Kramer, 2008, p. 29). Firmly committed to her ideals, Florence Nightingale and subsequent nurse theorists maintained that knowledge developed and used by nursing must be distinct from medical knowledge (Chinn & Kramer, 2008, p. 31). However, throughout most of the first half of the 20th century, the approach to nursing was based largely on medical knowledge. Nurses, taught by physicians, were instructed in what physicians thought they needed to know to carry out the medical regime for the patient. Even the advent of university education did not change the educational approach for nurses as curricula continued to be organized around medical specialty areas (Newman, 1972).

In the 1950s, conceptual frameworks in nursing were based primarily on theories developed from other disciplines. Many of these theories were deemed of value to nursing, but some degree of caution had to be exercised to make certain that the theory used was examined from the perspective of nursing in nursing situations (Walker & Avant, 2004). The shift toward a concept of nursing knowledge as predominantly scientific began in the 1950s and took strong hold in the 1960s (Chinn & Kramer, 2008, p. 45). Throughout the second half of the 20th century, three major trends contributed to evolving directions in the development of nursing knowledge: (1) utilization of theories borrowed from other disciplines, (2) development of conceptual frameworks defining nursing, and (3) the development of middle-range theory linked to practice (Chinn & Kramer, 2008, p. 47).

Conceptual frameworks for nursing education and practice proliferated in the 1960s and 1970s. The movement of psychiatric care into community settings, which followed on the heels of the development of new psychotropic medications, contributed to the theoretical focus on the importance of interpersonal communication—a focus notable in the works of Peplau, Orlando, and Travelbee. Writings in the 1960s and 1970s made significant contributions to the development of theoretical thinking in nursing that not only formed the basis for curricula but also guided research and focused practice. The nursing process also replaced the rule- and principle-oriented approaches that were grounded in a medical model in which the nurse functions as the physician's assistant (Alligood & Tomey, 2010, pp. 48–49).

# Interpersonal Relations

## Hildegard Peplau (1909–1999): The Theory of Interpersonal Nursing

When Peplau's *Interpersonal Relations in Nursing* was published in 1952, nursing was not considered to be a profession, nor was psychiatric nursing (Peplau's chosen specialty practice area) viewed as separate from and independent of medicine and psychiatry (Vandemark, 2006). Indeed, the publication of her book and theory was delayed 4 years because of concern that it was unacceptable for a nurse to publish a book without a physician coauthor (Sills, 1999). In her theory and early writings, Peplau used the term *counseling* to describe the role of the nurse-therapist because the idea of a nurse as therapist was unacceptable (O'Toole & Welt, 1989).

### The Interpersonal Relationship Process

Peplau proposed three phases (orientation, working, and resolution) and six nursing roles in the nurse–patient relationship (stranger, resource person, teacher, leader, surrogate, and counselor). Peplau (1952, 1992) carefully explained that "the nurse–patient relationship has a starting point, proceeds through definable phases, and being time-limited, has an end point" (1952, p. 14). In delineating these roles and phases, Peplau described the mechanisms the nurse uses in facilitating the interpersonal process. The original working phase has two subphases: (1) identification and (2) exploitation. Most current publications list four phases: (1) preorientation or preparation, (2) orientation, (3) working, and (4) termination (resolution). Also, *phases* are often referred to as *stages*.

The core concepts of Peplau's theory were the phases of the nurse–client relationship:

1. *Preorientation:* client data-gathering and "autodiagnosis"
   - Gather health care and other information about the client
   - Nurse engages in autodiagnosis (confront own thoughts and feelings, preconceptions, and attitudes about the particular client or illness/disorder)

2. *Orientation:* problem/issue-defining phase (Peplau, 1997, pp. 163–164)
   - Introductions; nurse and client become acquainted
   - Begin building trust and rapport
   - Asking questions, clarifying issues
   - Nurse and client convey needs, expectations, and limitations to each other
   - Contracting: outcome criteria are established and a plan of care is formulated
   - Time limits for interactions/visits are clarified and agreed upon
   - Termination stage outcomes/behaviors are considered

3. *Working:* major therapeutic activity occurs
   *Identification subphase*
   - Nurse serves as counselor and advocate
   - Specific problems to be addressed are outlined
   - Nurse commits to work on specific problems that require immediate attention
   - Client takes responsibility for behavior and actively works toward change
   *Exploitation subphase*
   - Nurse acts as teacher, advocate, resource person, and leader

- Client takes on new behaviors and tries them out in safe environment(s)
- Identify and use available resources

4. *Resolution:* relationship comes to a close (Peplau, 1997, pp. 163–164)
   - Nurse helps prepare client and situation(s) for termination
   - Nurse and client reduce interaction times; client functions more independently
   - Mutual agreement between nurse and client regarding resolution of issues
   - Needs are met and resolution of issues summarized
   - Follow-up instructions are given
   - Client has health maintenance plan

Peplau developed tasks associated with the stages of personality development as described by Freud and Sullivan. These tasks, which are outlined in **Table 12–1**, had to be learned to achieve a mature personality.

> When psychological tasks are successfully learned at each era of development, biological capacities are used productively and relations with people lead to productive living. When not successfully learned they carry over into adulthood and attempts at learning continue in devious ways, more or less impeded by conventional adaptation that provide a super-structure over the baseline of actual learning. (Peplau, 1991, p. 166)

Peplau's theory development was influenced by Sullivan's research and findings related to anxiety, the self-system, and modes of experiencing (discussed

**TABLE 12–1   Peplau's Stages of Personality Development**

| Age | Stage | Major Developmental Task |
| --- | --- | --- |
| Infancy | Learning to count on others | Learning to communicate in various ways with the primary caregiver in order to have comfort needs fulfilled |
| Toddlerhood | Learning to delay satisfaction | Learning the satisfaction of pleasing others by delaying self-gratification in small ways |
| Early childhood | Identifying oneself | Learning appropriate roles and behaviors by acquiring the ability to perceive the expectations of others |
| Late childhood | Developing skills in participation | Learning the skills to compromise, compete, and cooperate with others; establishment of a more realistic view of the world and a feeling of one's place in it |

in more detail later in the chapter). She also drew upon concepts in learning theory and developmental psychology, as well as the ideas of such humanistic psychologists as Carl Rogers, Abraham Maslow, and Rollo May (Peplau, 1952, 1992, 1997).

Peplau's contribution to nursing's history and practice is immeasurable.

She was the first nurse to initiate a significant move from an intrapsychic, Freudian emphasis within psychiatric mental health nursing and a dominant focus on physical care within general nursing to an interpersonal focus on both. She was also the first nurse to synthesize nursing theory from other scientific fields, such as Sullivan's theory. Peplau's theory emerged largely from clinical observations, is inductive, and is derived from the phenomenological domain of nursing practice. She regarded the nurse as a professional with "particular expertise" (Fawcett, 2005, p. 531) and sought to have nursing identified as a profession with a unique focus. She differentiated the nursing profession from other healthcare professions—especially physicians.

Peplau was also instrumental in guiding the development of the definition of nursing that was to be permanently represented in nursing's declaration of a social contract with society, the American Nurses Association's (ANA) *Nursing: A Social Policy Statement* (ANA, 1980, 2003).

- "Nursing is the diagnosis and treatment of human responses to actual or potential health problems" (ANA, 1980, p. 4).
- "Nursing is the protection, promotion and optimization of health and abilities, prevention of illness and injury, alleviation of suffering through *the diagnosis and treatment of human response*, and advocacy in the care of individuals, families, communities and populations" (ANA, 2003, p. 5).

In addition, Peplau was the first nurse to suggest the essential relationship between therapeutic use of self and the outcome of patient well-being (Haber, 2000, p. 60). She emphasized the treatment milieu as it affects clients' mental health and nursing's role in milieu therapy. She was instrumental in designing the first *Statement on Psychiatric-Mental Health Nursing Practice* (ANA, 1967) that preceded the development of other specialty area scope of practice statements.

She was a harbinger of the nursing process, as indicated by her statement: "Nursing is a significant, therapeutic interpersonal process. It functions cooperatively with other human processes that make health possible for individuals in communities" (Peplau, 1952, p. 16). She developed a theory that is adaptable to any area of nursing (practice, education, and research) and any nursing specialty area where the end purpose is meeting patients' needs.

According to Fawcett (2005, p. 531), Peplau did not devote much attention to the environment but noted the importance of culture on the formation of personality and increasing multi-ethnicity as a contemporary world factor that nurses should include in their information gathering, especially when it is about cultures other than one's own (Peplau, 1997, p. 162)

Peplau seriously influenced the ANA's (1980) report, *Nursing: A Social Policy Statement*. Sills (2000) celebrated Peplau's "influence in the evolutionary processes of increasing professionalization of nursing in America: ". . . The social policy statement for the first time in nursing's history states the phenomenological focus of nursing" (p. 33).

## Peplau on Nursing Education

> The central task of the basic professional school of nursing is viewed as the fullest development of the nurse as a person who is aware of how she functions in a situation. (Peplau, 1952, p. xii)

The purpose of Peplau's book on interpersonal relations in nursing was to promote recognition of the importance of the nurse's personality in this context. She stated that "the basic task of nursing education should not be concern for the patient but rather development of each nurse as a person who wants to nurse patients in a helpful way" (p. xii). Thus, the direction for this development is maturity (Vandemark, 2006).

## Peplau on Nursing Practice

> The nurse–patient relationship is the primary human contact that is central in a fundamental way to providing nursing care. (Peplau, 1997, p. 163)

The one-to-one nurse–client relationship, also known as the therapeutic nurse–client relationship, is the situation in which clients can accomplish developmental tasks such as learning to trust and collaborate, and practicing healthy communication and behaviors. Peplau's teachings are still relevant to practice in understanding and guiding decisions in the one-to-one relationship and individual counseling. In the relationship, the nurse uses theoretical understandings, personal attributes, and appropriate clinical techniques to provide opportunities for a corrective emotional experience for clients (Kneisl & Trigoboff, 2009, p. 775). The goal transcends any particular nursing specialty. Analysis of Peplau's works illuminates a scholarship of nursing practice that remains relevant today (Reed, 1996, p. 29).

## Peplau on Nursing Research

Peplau's interpersonal relationship in nursing theory was originally identified as a conceptual framework. Peplau also referred to it as a middle-range theory or a partial theory. She proposed that her theory is useful as an interpersonal process applicable to all nurses' practice (Peplau, 1991, p. 261). McCamant (2006) asked "Is Peplau's model still relevant today?" (p. 336). In response she insisted, "Peplau's theory was predicated on the recognition that nurses have more actual direct patient contact than any other healthcare professional. . . . The theory occurs precisely in the expected order, despite abbreviated interactive time between nurse and patient" (p. 336). "Some say that these phases are ancestors of the nursing process (Kniesl & Trigoboff, 2009, p. 25). Peplau's work on nurse–patient relationships is so well known globally that it continues to influence how nursing practice is viewed and evaluated (Johnson & Webber, 2010). Moreover, the interpersonal process is no longer limited to nursing.

Critique of Peplau's theory, similar to critiques of Sullivan's theory, suggests that her theory has not been supported by sufficient empirical investigation and has not yet been tested in terms of its relevance for multidisciplinary, or interprofessional, practice. For the theory to gain credibility within the dynamics of the multidisciplinary team, it must be tested through a robust research design involving various diagnostic groups and practice settings. Until then, the theory's utility remains questionable (Mohr, 2008).

## Ida Jean Orlando Pelletier (1926–2007): Nursing Process Discipline Theory

Orlando Pelletier's study grew out of her dissatisfaction with the possibility that nursing care was governed by organizational rules rather than attention to clients' needs and her desire to offer nursing students a theory of effective nursing practice. In her first book, *The Dynamic Nurse Patient Relationship: Function, Process and Principles* (Orlando, 1961), she identified her work as a theory of effective nursing practice; however, in the preface to her 1990 reprint, she wrote:

> If I had been more courageous in 1961, when this book was first written, I would have proposed it as "nursing process theory" instead of as a "theory of effective nursing practice." A "deliberative" process was presented as a guide for nurses to practice "effectively." Conversely, an "automatic" process was shown to be "ineffective." "Effectiveness" was conceptualized and illustrated as "improvement" in the patient's behavior. The "improvement" stemmed from the fact that the deliberative process made it possible for the nurse to identify and meet the patient's *need for help*. (p. vii)

In answering questions about the elements of effective care and nursing actions, she conducted a study to evaluate what is good and bad nursing practice. From an analysis of approximately 2,000 recorded nurse–patient interactions, Orlando identified three areas of concern for nursing: (1) nurse–patient relations, (2) the nurse's professional role, and (3) the identity and development of knowledge that is distinctly nursing (Orlando, 1961; Tyra, 2008). She also was able to link effective nursing care to the nurse's knowledge of patient needs that are validated by patient response (Johnson & Webber, 2010). In 1972, Orlando wrote *The Discipline and Teaching of Nursing Process (An Evaluative Study)*, in which she renamed her deliberative nursing process as a nursing process discipline, emphasizing the importance of deliberative nursing actions—a process that assists the nurse to consciously identify and respond to patient needs based on the meanings that are validated between nurse and client (Kniesl & Trigoboff, 2009)—to the need for every student nurse to receive special training in the deliberative nursing process. The purpose of the training "is to change the responsiveness of the nurse from the one described as personal and automatic to one [that] is disciplined and professional" (p. 33).

Orlando then published the final version of her theory, the nursing process discipline theory. According to Johnson and Webber (2010), although Orlando's theory of nursing process discipline resembles the nursing process used in practice, it is not the same. Her theory not only requires more comprehensive interaction and involvement between nurse and patient, but her process is also "reflexive and circular, occurring during encounters with patients, not the linear process taught in nursing education" (Rittman, 2001, p. 12).

Orlando believed that nursing is an interpersonal process involving a nurse's interaction with an ill individual to meet an immediate need. The nursing situation was identified as consisting of (1) the person's behavior, (2) the nurse's reaction, and (3) nursing actions appropriate to the person's need. Essential nursing activities include an automatic nursing process and a deliberative nursing process. The automatic nursing process involves several nursing process activities that are "without discipline" (Orlando Pelletier, 1990, p. vii), meaning that "some automatic activities are ordered by the doctor; others are concerned with routines of caring for patients, and still others are based on principles pertinent to protecting and fostering the health of people in general" (1990, p. 60). This nursing process, even if correct, does not meet the patient's need for help.

The deliberative nursing process comprises nursing process activities that are "with discipline" (Orlando Pelletier, 1990, p. vii), meaning nurse-initiated process activities done to ascertain how the patient is affected by what she says or does (Orlando, 1961, p. 67). These activities include instructions, suggestions, directions, explanations, information, requests, and questions directed toward the client; making decisions for the client; and shaping the client's immediate environment. For Orlando Pelletier (1990), only "deliberation is needed to determine whether the activity actually achieves its intended purpose and whether the patient is helped by it (p. 60).

Fundamentally, Orlando believed that nursing is unique and that licensure gives nurses the authority to work independently from medicine. Thus, the nurse is accountable directly to the individual receiving care (Chinn & Kramer, 2008; Johnson & Webber, 2010). According to Schmieding (n.d.),

> Orlando was one of the first to use field methodology to develop her theoretical perspectives long before it was accepted as appropriate. From participant-observer notes, she derived an ingenious conception of the elements and relationships involved as the nurse determines the meaning of the patient's immediate behavior. (p. viii)

Her contribution to nursing practice helped nurses focus on the whole patient rather than on diseases or institutional demands, improved nurses' decision-making skills, provided for more effective resolution of staff and staff–physician conflicts, and promoted a more positive nursing identity and unity (Tyra, 2008). Her ideas continue to be useful today and current research supports her model (Boyd, 2008; Potter & Bockenhauer, 2000).

## Joyce Travelbee (1926–1973): The Human-to-Human Relationship Model

While Peplau drew upon the works of neo-Freudian psychiatrists, Travelbee credited discussions with existential psychologists and philosophers such as Viktor Frankl and Rollo May as significantly influencing her thinking and allowing her to bring an existential perspective to nursing (Meleis, 2007).

As a result of psychiatric nursing experiences in a Catholic charity hospital, Travelbee came to believe that the care given in these types of institutions lacked compassion. She argued that nursing needed a "humanistic revolution" and a renewed focus on caring as central to nursing. It was her belief that unless nurses became more aware of the value of caring as the basic goal of the nursing profession, consumers of nursing would demand the services of a new and different kind of healthcare worker (Moses, 1994; Travelbee, 1966).

She proposed that the caring goal of nursing was to assist an individual, family, or community to prevent or cope with the experiences of illness and suffering and, if necessary, find meaning in these experiences, with the ultimate goal being the presence of hope (Travelbee, 1966, 1971). The concept of hope was defined as a mental state characterized by the desire to gain an end or accomplish a goal combined with some degree of expectation that what is desired or sought is attainable. Her original conceptualization of hope was directed toward clients with psychiatric illness, but she later expanded her concept to long-term physical illnesses.

Travelbee (1969) described understanding as acknowledging the uniqueness of the ill person. She contended that understanding was "a force which can provide the ill person with the necessary endurance and courage to face the inevitable problems which lie before him" (p. 81). Focusing her attention on individuals who must learn to live with chronic illness, she believed that the nurse's spiritual values and philosophical beliefs about suffering would determine the extent to which the nurse could help ill people find meaning in these situations (Boyd, 2008).

Similar to Peplau and Orlando, Travelbee (1966, 1971) emphasized the importance of communication in the phases of the nurse–client relationship and described the instrument for delivery of the process of one-to-one nursing as the therapeutic use of self. However, as Travelbee focused on the *meaning* in nurse–client interactions, "her unique synthesis of their ideas differentiated her work from theirs in terms of the therapeutic human-to-human relationship between nurse and patient" (Alligood & Tomey, 2010, p. 61; Kniesl & Trigoboff, 2009). She insisted that nursing is defined and accomplished through the relatedness found in the human-to-human relationship and successfully working through the phases of initial encounter, emerging identity, empathy, sympathy, and rapport (Moses, 1994, p. 200).

## Travelbee's Phases of the Nurse–Client Relationship

*Original encounter.*    Emotional knowledge colors the impressions and perceptions of both nurse and patient during initial encounters. The task is to "break the bond of categorization in order to perceive the human being in the patient and vice versa" (Travelbee, 1966, p. 133).

*Emerging identities.*    Both nurse and patient begin to transcend their respective roles and perceive uniqueness in each other. Tasks include separating oneself and one's experiences from others and avoiding "using oneself as a yardstick" by which to evaluate others. Barriers to such tasks may be caused by role envy, lack of interest in others, inability to transcend the self, or refusal to initiate emotional investment (Travelbee, 1966, p. 139).

*Developing feelings of empathy.*    Empathy means sharing another's psychological state but standing apart and not sharing another's feelings; it is characterized by "the ability to predict the behavior of another." When empathizing, the warmth and urge to action are not present (Travelbee, 1966, p. 143).

*Developing feelings of sympathy.*    This means sharing, feeling, and experiencing what others are feeling and experiencing. This phase demonstrated emotional involvement and discredits objectivity as dehumanizing. The task of the nurse is to translate sympathy into helpful nursing actions (Travelbee, 1964, p. 70.) Sympathy "implies a desire, almost an urge to help or aid an individual in order to relieve his distress" (Rich, 2003, p. 202; Travelbee, 1964, p. 68 ).

*Rapport.*    All previous phases culminate into rapport, defined as all those experiences, thoughts, feeling, and attitudes that both nurse and the client undergo and are able to perceive, share, and communicate (Travelbee, 1964, 1966, pp. 133–162).

## The Empathy Versus Sympathy Disagreement

Travelbee believed that it was as important for the nurse to sympathize as it was to empathize if the nurse and patient were to develop a human-to-human relationship. In 1964, Travelbee, in an article titled, "What's Wrong with Sympathy?" expressed dismay that nursing, as a profession, was losing its value of sympathy and compassion in response to comments by nurses that "they were too busy to be sympathetic" (p. 68).

According to Rich (2003), Travelbee believed that nursing students should be encouraged to experience sympathy when caring for patients; sympathy and compassion are at the heart of nursing. Sympathy, to Travelbee, involves an act of courage on the part of the nurse because he or she is risking pain (p. 203). Travelbee outlined several dangers of sympathy that nurses are cautioned about: becoming too soft-hearted; overidentifying with patients; developing a distorted sense of pity; causing harm to the patient; or having their will become paralyzed (Rich, 2003).

Of current interest is the continuing acceptance of empathy as a teachable skill and crucial helping component in therapeutic nurse–patient interactions and the "demise" of sympathy as influential (Ancel, 2006; Reynolds & Scott, 1999). While there are a number of definitions of empathy and approaches to implementation, the most commonly cited and used, even among nurses, is drawn from the works of the humanistic psychologist Carl Rogers (discussed later; Reynolds & Scott, 2000); there is little reference to Travelbee's theory, her phases of the nurse–client relationship, or sympathy as a critical component in interpersonal relationships. Rich (2003), revisited Travelbee's question and wrote,

> In an age of technology, where many people feel the impact of individual isolation and existential aloneness, it is worth revisiting Travelbee's reasons why nurses may avoid feelings of sympathy. A focus on compassion may be a similar and acceptable alternative. (p. 202)

With regard to updating Travelbee's perspective on compassion, Rich stated that, ". . . we may find the Eastern philosophy idea of compassion may be more acceptable to the nursing profession" (p. 203).

Unfortunately, Travelbee's model was never subjected to empirical testing, and, because her investigations were based on direct observations, interviews, and documented analysis, it is not possible to summarize the wealth of her empirical findings. Nonetheless, her reports presented clear descriptive statements that illustrated her human-to-human theory (Moses, 1994). Her use of the interpersonal process in nursing intervention and her focus on suffering and illness helped to define areas of concern for psychiatric mental health nurses (Kneisl & Trigoboff, 2009, p. 38). She also is credited with greatly influencing the hospice movement and being far ahead of her time when, in 1949, she called for natural childbirth, prenatal instruction, father participation in birth process, and rooming-in. While her view of humanity, uniqueness, existential encounters, and nursing is highly congruent with values in psychiatric-mental health nursing, Travelbee (1969) believed that the human-to-human relationship process is central to all nursing.

## A Sign of the Times: 1970s to the Present

In the 1970s and 1980s, there was a noticeable shift to themes and patterns that characterize the essence of caring in nursing practice. Frameworks changed from reflecting functional nursing roles to unfolding the essence of what nursing is. The common, significant thread is the primacy of human interaction in creating human health and wholeness (Chinn & Kramer, 2008, pp. 52–55).

Nursing frameworks began to be influenced by nurse scientists who benefited from early funding of doctoral education and received training in anthropology and sociology. This education is reflected in the works of Rogers, Parse, and Newman, whose theoretical perspectives are linked to developments in modern physics that moved beyond earlier system concepts of equilibrium (Chinn & Kramer, 2008, p. 49). The progression of nursing research and theory development has been influenced by two philosophies: *modernism* and *postmodernism*. "Put simply, whereas the focus in modernism was on proving theory, the focus of postmodernism was on the development of new theory through the discovery of meaning without empirical evidence" (Johnson & Webber, 2010, p. 239). Of particular significance, the postmodern view represents an epistemological shift in nursing theory development to include the modernistic search for the truth and validity of empirical findings but also the exploration of phenomenological findings unique to human beings and their experiences (Johnson & Webber, 2010, pp. 239–240).

## Humanism/Caring

### Josephine Paterson (1924–Present) and Loretta Zderad (1925–Present): Humanistic Nursing Theory (1976)

Out of necessity nursing, as a profession, reflects the qualities of the culture in which it exists. In our culture for the past quarter of a century nursing has been assailed with rapid economic, technological, shortage-abundance, changing scenes' vicissitudes. In the individual nurse these arouse turmoil and uncertainty. These cultural stirrings inflame that part of the nurse's spirit capable of chaotic conflict and doubt. Often she questions her professional identity. "Just what is a nurse?" Her nurse colleagues, other professionals, and nonprofessionals freely, directly and indirectly on television, in the theater, through the news media and the literature, pummel her with their multitudinous varied views. As searching, wondering, reflecting, relating microcosms within this perplexing health nursing world for longer than a quarter of a century, we present this book. Descriptively we view the chapters as hard-wrung, philosophical foundations, synthesized extracts from our lived experiences. (Paterson & Zderad, 1976, p. ix)

In 1960, Paterson and Zderad were not impressed with the objective nature of empirical science that represented human beings as predictable objects. They believed that understanding how people experience their existence could facilitate their nursing work. The humanistic approach has its roots in existentialist thought, and both philosophies (humanism and existentialism) assert a broad view of human beings and their potential. Thus they selected humanistic-existential philosophy to inform their developing theory.

In 1976, Paterson and Zderad proposed that nurses consciously and deliberately approach nursing as an existential experience. They suggested that the science of nursing would be built over time by compilation and complementary synthesis of phenomenological descriptions of experiences in the nursing situation. They spoke of humanistic nursing as a framework that recognizes the uniqueness of each human being and "a quality of being that is expressed in the doing" (Paterson & Zderad, 1978, p. 13).

The term *humanistic nursing* was selected thoughtfully to designate the theoretical pursuit to reaffirm and floodlight this responsible characteristic as fundamentally inherent to all artful-scientific nursing. Humanistic nursing embraces more than a benevolent technically competent subject–object one-way relationship guided by a nurse on behalf of another. Rather, it dictates that nursing is a responsible searching, transactional relationship whose meaningfulness demands conceptualization founded in a nurse's existential awareness of self and of the other. "Nursing is an experience lived between human beings" (Paterson & Zderad, 1988, p. 3). Humanistic nursing, then, is neither a break with nor a repetition of nursing's past. It is neither a rejection of nor a satisfaction with nursing's present state. Rather it is an awakening to the possibilities of shaping our nursing world here and now and for the future (Paterson & Zderad, 1976, preface).

Within the construct of humanistic theory, the act of nursing is understood in terms of both the nurse and patient—often experienced and described as a "call and response" relationship (Decker-Brown, 2003, para. 14). The client calls for nursing care with an expectation that care will be provided or an unmet need will be satisfied. The nurse responds with the intention of providing the care or satisfying the unmet need. The nurse is concerned with the client's unique expression of the body related to its position in time and space (Paterson & Zderad, 1988, p. 29). Authentic presence is expressed when the nurse goes beyond being an object within the perceptual field of the client.

The goal of humanistic nursing is not attainment of mere health or *well-being*, but rather attainment of a state of dynamic *more-being* (Praeger & Hogarth, 1985). The object is for the nurse to assist the client to become *more*, to realize a potential not yet attained in the present moment of their interaction. Health is conceptualized as a process of becoming whatever is possible for the human being. Nursing phenomena are those things that nurses think are important and to which they must pay close attention, are experienced as nurturing, being nurtured, or the process between these two reference points. While humanistic nursing focuses on the intersubjectivity experience, the most important activity for the nurse to engage in may be the use of self, or presence, with the client (Frisch & Frisch, 2011). Paterson and Zderad (1988) outlined 12 behaviors for providing comfort to a client. (See **Box 12–1.**)

According to Kniesl and Trigoboff (2009), Paterson and Zderad (1976, 1988) were a decade ahead of their time in rejecting a mechanistic cause and effect view of nursing science and urging instead that observations of the experiences of nurses in practice should be the basis of any useful nursing theory. Theirs is a highly abstract theory with a major focus on the process of interaction or dialogue between nurse and client (Kniesl & Trigoboff, 2009, p. 26).

# Box 12–1 Twelve Humanistic Nursing Behaviors for Providing Comfort

1. The nurse introduces herself to the client by name, which supports the client's dignity, worth, and individual identity and is essential for an authentic subject–subject relationship.

2. The nurse provides information about the client's situation as the client seeks it or when the nurse perceives the client is puzzled about what is happening. The nurse's action is based on the existential belief that the client has the right to know and make choices about his own life, and such choices are shaped by honest information.

3. The nurse accepts the client's expression of feelings by verbalizing this acceptance when appropriate. This validates clients' right to feelings and can help them learn appropriate ways to express feelings.

4. The nurse accepts the client's expression of feeling by staying with him or doing something for the client when a verbal expression of acceptance by the nurse is not appropriate. The message conveyed is that the patient's feelings are valid but a better method of expressing the feeling is socially desirable. By remaining with the client, the nurse validates the feeling and may model a more appropriate behavioral expression.

5. The nurse expresses authentic positive feelings for the client when appropriate. The purpose of this action is to refute negative self-concepts that the client may hold.

6. The nurse supports the client's rights to have loving relationships with family members, staff, and other clients.

7. The nurse shows respect for clients as persons who have rights to make choices as their capabilities permit.

8. The nurse helps clients consider current expression of feelings and behaviors in the light of previous life experiences. This behavior enables clients to formulate self-understanding by recognition of patterns that may be helpful or unhelpful to their healing.

9. The nurse encourages clients to express themselves openly so that the nurse can respond in a helpful and therapeutic manner.

10. The nurse verifies the intuitive grasp of how the client experiences events by asking questions and making comments to the client, and then observing the client's response.

11. The nurse encourages realistic (not false) hope through discussing the positive outcomes that might occur if the client were to engage in a therapeutic opportunity.

12. The nurse supports the client's self-image with concrete examples.

Adapted with permission of the National League for Nursing, Washington, DC from Paterson, J. G., & Zderad, L. T. (1988). *Humanistic nursing.* New York, NY: National League for Nursing.

# Existentialism

## Jean Watson (1940–Present): Theory of Human Caring

Watson wrote *Nursing: Philosophy and Science of Caring* in 1979. In 1996, Watson stated that she had continued to refine her original theory "until this moment in history" (p. 141). It is clear that, over a decade later, she is still refining her theory. In exploring the progression of "refining" over the years, a relationship in her theory and publications can be traced to many of her revealed personal life situations. Her classic work is in the process of being updated (Watson, 2007).

Watson credited Jungian psychology, feminist theory, and Maslow's psychological concept of self-actualization as influencing her early theory development. Carl Rogers received credit for much of her thinking on therapeutic relationships and communication through his work in identifying congruency, empathy, and warmth as foundational to a caring relationship that conveys authenticity and genuineness and facilitates the client's expression of emotions. More recently, Watson acknowledged drawing heavily on the sciences, humanities, Buddhism, and Eastern philosophies that provide a phenomenological-existential and spiritual orientation to theory development (Watson, 1995, 1999, 2005). Influential nurse theorists were Peplau, Henderson, Leininger, Rogers, Newman, and, especially Nightingale (Watson, 1985, 1997, 2005).

Watson (1996) claimed that her theory of human caring is metaphysical, "it goes beyond the rapidly emerging existential-phenomenological approaches in nursing, to perhaps a higher level of abstraction and sense of personhood incorporating the concept of the soul and transcendence" (p. 141). Clearly, the life events of the theorists discussed in this chapter have been influential in outlining and clarifying their various philosophical or conceptual approaches; Watson's personal journey in particular has been a significant influence on the development and directions of her theory. She indicated that the building blocks of her theory and concepts were "derived from clinically inducted, empirical experiences, combined with my philosophical, intellectual and experiential background; thus, my earlier work emerged from my own values, beliefs, and perceptions about personhood, life, health, and healing (Watson, 1997, p. 49). Initially Watson (1979, 1988) differentiated nursing and medicine by stating that *curing* is the domain of medicine, and *caring* is the domain of nursing. From her original discussion of holistic human caring, her thoughts have evolved to a model of the transpersonal caring relationship (Watson, 1999, 2002, 2005).

Watson (1996) indicated that the transpersonal caring relationship depends on a moral commitment to human dignity, wholeness, caring, and healing. It also depends on the nurse's (1) orientation to affirming the significance of the person; (2) ability to realize, detect, and connect with the spirit of another; (3) ability to realize the other's state of being in the world and to feel a union with that other; and (4) caring, healing modalities to potentiate comfort, wholeness, and harmony, including promoting inner healing and own life history and ability to care for self.

Caring-healing within her theory is based on kindness, concern, love of self and others, and the ecology of the earth and involves what she terms *carative* factors: a humanistic-altruistic value system, faith-hope, and sensitivity to self and others (Watson, 1999). Her theory emphasizes sensitivity to self and values clarification regarding personal and cultural beliefs that might pose barriers to transpersonal caring. Establishing a helping and trusting human care relationship is pivotal to her theory. In 2003, Watson expanded self-care to include the ability to forgive self and others, to be grateful for life and its blessings, and to surrender and let go of ego, accepting experiences without seeking control.

In her recent work (Watson, 2005), she developed the notion of spiritual environment and the interconnectedness of all things, including the connection between natural healing approaches, self-knowledge, self-control, self-caring, self-healing potential, and caring, healing relationships with self and others. Her theory is philosophically congruent with contemporary global approaches to health and health promotion (Falk-Rafael, 2000; Pilkington, 2007).

While Watson's emphasis on caring is not unique, the strength of her emphasis on the embodied spirit is. She set a very high standard for nurses to follow and has brought a number of important concepts into her theoretical work. Her curative approach is deeply aligned with spiritual as well as existential and phenomenological philosophical concepts and subjects more abstract than many nurses wish to pursue. However, Watson's theory continues to evolve and to attract the attention of many, as nurses are drawn to the holistic and spiritual nature of the theory (Kneisl & Trigoboff, 2009, p. 26).

According to Boyd (2008):

> Watson's theory is especially applicable to the care of those who seek help for mental illness. This model emphasizes the importance of sensitivity to self and others, the development of helping and trusting relations, the promotion of interpersonal teaching and learning, and provision for a supportive, protective and corrective mental, physical, sociocultural and spiritual environment. (p. 71)

Frisch and Frisch (2011), however, cautioned, "Despite the strong therapeutic potential of nursing intervention based on caring, the withdrawn, angry, suspicious, and depressed person may be very slow to enter into this kind of mutuality. The nurse . . . must be willing to persevere, to consult with colleagues and mentors . . . to carefully examine her own feelings and responses, and . . . consider a switch in theory and approach" (p. 309).

The basic premises of transpersonal caring are outlined here:

1. Being human is more than a physical body; it includes an embodied spirit; a consciousness that supports sharing between and beyond persons; a unity of mind, body and spirit, expressed as *mindbodyspirit*; and a connected oneness of the person, nature, and the universe.
2. There is a human–environment energy field that includes caring-healing consciousness.

3. Consciousness is energy; forgiveness and surrender are the highest level of consciousness.
4. Modalities that arise from caring-healing involve the mind, the hands, the heart, and the soul.
5. The process and relationships linking caring-healing are sacred, and the nurse can provide a sacred healing environment.
6. Viewing the connectedness of all (subject, object, environment, person, and all living things) is unitary consciousness; unbroken wholeness is the ultimate form of healing, and transcendence is love (Frisch & Frisch, 2011, p. 32).

Watson adapted her 10 carative factors from Yalom's 11 curative factors. She later enhanced the factors to include clinical caritas processes that offered ways in which the 10 factors could be implemented in the clinical setting. *Caritas* is a Latin word meaning to "cherish, appreciate, or, give special attention to" (Alligood & Tomey, 2010, p. 97).

## Margaret Newman (1933–Present): Theory of Health as Expanding Consciousness

Every person in every situation, no matter how disorganized and hopeless it may seem, is part of the universal process of expanding consciousness. (Newman, 1992, p. 45)

Newman began developing her theory of expanding consciousness as a result of caring for her mother throughout a long period of illness. During this period and years of learning in undergraduate and graduate school, she came to realize that "long term illness can be dealt with if a person's consciousness is expanding"—essentially gaining a deeper appreciation for life and having more meaningful relationships (Newman, 1992, p. 45). In 1994, Newman wrote:

Basic among these learnings was that illness reflected the life pattern of the person. And that what was needed was the recognition of the pattern and acceptance of it for what it meant to that person. Years later I came to the conclusion that health is the expansion of consciousness. It frightens me to think that I might have missed that revelation, it is so important to me now. But even my fear is unwarranted because the gist of all that I am saying is that one can trust the evolving pattern, that it is a pattern of evolving, expanding consciousness *regardless* of what form or direction it may take. This realization is such that illness and disease have lost their demoralizing power. (p. xxiii)

Newman's (1990) major theoretical concepts are health, pattern/pattern recognition, consciousness, expanding consciousness, and movement-space-time. "Patterning of persons in interaction with the environment is basic to my view that consciousness is a manifestation of an evolving pattern of person-environment interaction" (p. 38). Newman's theory is derived from Rogers' (1970) life process model, now known as the science of unitary human beings (1994): "Rogers's insistence that health and illness are simply manifestations of rhythmic fluctuations of the life process led me to view health and illness as a unitary process moving through variations of order-disorder" (Newman, 1990, p. 38).

Newman (1994) realized that her theory was "a radical departure from traditional concepts of health" and that "the essence of the theory required a 180-degree turn in thinking about health" (p. xv). In her theory, health is a synthesis of the fusion of disease and nondisease—being well and being ill. Disease and nondisease are each reflections of a larger wholeness that takes on a new and different form that is not diminished by illness and thus creates a new concept of health. Health and the evolving pattern of consciousness are the same and viewed as "a transformative process to more inclusive consciousness" (Newman, 2008, p. 16).

Newman (2008) specified five major assumptions (stated in part here):

1. Health encompasses conditions heretofore described as illness or, in medical terms, pathology.
2. These pathological conditions can be considered a manifestation of the total pattern of the individual.
3. The pattern of the individual that eventually manifests itself as pathology is primary and exists prior to structural or functional changes.
4. Removal of the pathology in itself will not change the pattern of the individual.
5. If becoming "ill" is the only way an individual's pattern can manifest itself, then that is health for that person.

In Newman's view, the focus of nursing is on the nurse–client relationship. Clients get in touch with the meaning of their lives through identification of meanings in the process of their evolving patterns of relating. "The emphasis of the process is on knowing/caring through pattern recognition" (Newman, 2008, p. 10). The nurse facilitates pattern recognition by forming relationships with clients at critical points in their lives and connecting with them in authentic ways. According to Newman, pattern recognition is the essence of practice and the task of intervention. "The more expanded the consciousness of the nurses, the more readily they [are] able to enter into a transformative relationship with clients" (Newman, 1994, p. 18). Expanding consciousness is described as insight and the recognition of patterns. Newman suggested that nurses will be transformed by nursing theory and, thereby, will become transforming partners with clients (Vandemark, 2006, p. 606).

For Newman, research is praxis or practice. In 2003, she wrote, "Nursing praxis integrates theory, research, and practice. It is art, science and practice" (p. 242). Theory, practice, and research are viewed as a process rather than as separate nursing domains. Newman called for a specific curriculum and focus of education for nurses using the theory. The new curriculum must reflect the shift in worldview from the traditional views of health and illness to the transformative expectation of pattern recognition. "Attention to the nature of transformative learning will help to establish the priorities of the discipline" (Newman, 2008, p. 73). Newman espoused the professional doctorate degree as a requirement for professional practice, one that "requires a strong arts and sciences background as pre-professional education . . . and brings students with added personal maturity" (p. 127).

Vandemark (2006) cautioned that for advanced practice (psychiatric) nurses providing psychotherapy to clients, the need for self-awareness is more acute and more specific to their practice. The development of insight and self-awareness vis-à-vis the practice of psychotherapy is a significant responsibility for professional schools of nursing to leave to the individual nurse. Although the role of the psychiatric advanced practice nurse includes individual and family therapy, many existing psychiatric nurse practitioner programs have no courses or practicum experiences in patient-centered psychotherapy (Wheeler & Haber, 2004). While psychiatric clinical nurse specialist programs often do include course work in individual and group or family therapy and accompanying clinical supervision, this mentorship is, as Peplau counseled, focused on the content of the nurse's interaction with the patient, not the interpersonal dynamics of the nurse.

## Rosemarie Rizzo Parse (Year of birth unknown–Present): Humanbecoming Theory

Parse's theory of human becoming (1992) was originally introduced as the man-living-health theory (1981). Parse developed her theory of human becoming with tenets from existential-phenomenological philosophers, primarily Heidegger, Sartre, and Merleau-Ponty (Parse, 1981, 1998) and the work of Martha Rogers (1970). Although Parse initially labeled her work a theory, in 1998, to extend Rogers' work and add greater density to the philosophical underpinning, she changed her label from a theory to a *school of thought*. Although it is "consistent with Rogers' principles and postulates about unitary human beings and it is consistent with major tenets and concepts from existential-phenomenological thought, it is a new product, a different conceptual system" (Parse, 1998, p. 135).

The theory was originally guided by three principles incorporating the central ideas of meaning, rhythmicity, and transcendence (Parse, 1981, 1995, 1998). Recently, and within the context of rapidly changing technological developments and cost efficiencies in health care, she has further emphasized the idea of indivisible co-creation by joining the word "human" and "becoming" to form the term *humanbecoming* (Parse, 2007). The wording of the three principles has changed slightly for clarification, but the meanings remain unchanged. The three principles are (1) structuring meaning, (2) configuring rhythmical patterns of relating, and (3) co-transcending with possibles (Parse, 2007). Underlying the three principles are the postulates of illimitability, "indivisible unbounded knowing extended to infinity (Parse, 2007, p. 308), paradox, "lived rhythms" (p. 308); freedom, "contextually construed liberation," and mystery, "the unexplainable" (p. 308).

Parse's (1998) first set of nine assumptions about humans and becoming were later synthesized into three assumptions related to humanbecoming (2007). These three assumptions are:

1. *Humanbecoming* is freely choosing personal meaning with situation, intersubjectively living value priorities.
2. *Humanbecoming* is configuring rhythmical patterns of relating with *humanuniverse*.
3. *Humanbecoming* is co-transcending illimitably with emerging possibilities.

Although Parse did not include nursing in her metaparadigm, she challenged the traditional medical view of nursing and has distinguished the discipline of nursing as a unique, basic science focused on human lived experience. Nursing's goal consists of being with or in the presence of mutual nurse–client processes to understand and value the meaning of the client's lived experience and assimilate preferences and beliefs that influence healthcare choices and preference (Parse, 1998). The nurse also uses a nonjudgmental approach and reveres the client's expertise in knowing what is best for him or her within the nurse–client relationship. The nurse uses her true presence with the client to establish mutual processes and ensure shared decision making with the client to assess behavior, identify treatment choices, develop a client-centered treatment plan, and observe changing health patterns. Exhibiting true presence by the nurse involves mindfulness to the client.

Parse views health as inseparable and irreducible from both human and universe. Health is humanbecoming. It is structuring meaning, configuring rhythmical patterns of relating, and co-transcending with possibles (Parse, 2007). Humans are intentional beings and by nature live a seamless symphony throughout the life span. People are involved with the universe in directing their personal becoming through relationships with others. Individuals live in the moment within the presence of mutual processes with the universe structures that are multidimensional. Mutual processes enable persons to manage their lives and health through the freedom and right to make choices and live their lives as they choose (Parse, 1998, 2002). Environment includes the universe and mutual processes. Humans are in mutual process with the universe structure or with others who are with the individual.

## Quality of Life Versus Health

Quality of life is explicit in Parse's theory (1994). Quality of life is "the indivisible human's view on living moment to moment as the changing patterns of shifting perspectives weave the fabric of life through the human-universe interconnectedness" (p. 17). It is a subjective, global perception of the meaning of one's lived experiences in the moment. It fluctuates moment to moment in co-creation with the universe (Parse, 1994). Parse has used words such as *shifting*, *changing*, and *in-the-moment* in reference to quality of life. The personal nuances of the nurse–person process enhance quality of life (Parse, 1994).

The concept has been well-developed through extensive research. Parse and colleagues have explicitly described quality of life to inform understanding as it is constituted in different contexts. Understanding promotes nurses' ability to be with people in ways that honor their lived experiences. Parse's contribution to quality of life has pragmatic utility for the discipline of nursing because it articulates the goal of nursing practice.

Fawcett (2005) explained that the term *metaparadigm* is the result of Masterman pointing out that Kuhn's use of the term *paradigm* had multiple meanings and "one reflected a metaphysical rather than scientific notion or entity. The metaparadigm is the most abstract set of central concepts for the discipline of nursing (i.e. human beings, environment, health and nursing)" (p. 4). In relating contemporary practice needs to nursing's current metaparadigm, Phillips (1995) stated,

> A clear definition of quality of life is important to nursing knowledge development because it guides the art of practice. Defining quality of life from a holistic perspective is also important to nursing because it reflects contemporary practice and it helps nurses to understand the inherent indivisibility of life and its qualities. (pp. 100–101)

Plummer and Molzahn (2009) conducted a critical review and comparison of the concept, quality of life, as it is conceptualized in the contemporary nursing theories of Peplau, Rogers, Leininger, King, and Parse. The goal of the study was twofold: (1) to enhance clarity of the concept from a nursing perspective and (2) to assess the usefulness of the concept to nursing science. Each theoretical "perspective was compared to the others in order to identify commonalities, similar themes, and differences" (p. 135). According to Plummer and Molzahn (2009), the findings "contributed to the understanding of the interconnectedness of the person, relationships, and environment with quality of life" (p. 140). Thus, Plummer and Molzahn (2009) summarized, "Given the breadth of nursing practice and the value of the concept for nursing . . . it is appropriate to consider replacing health as a metaparadigm concept with quality of life" (p. 140).

# Non-Nursing Theories Focused on Interpersonal Relationships

## Interpersonal Relations Theory

Interpersonal philosophy defines personality as behavior that can be observed within interpersonal relationships. Interpersonal theorists emphasize the socialization of humans throughout their developmental stages. Failure to proceed through these stages satisfactorily lays the foundation for later maladaptive behavior. Supporters believe that unsatisfactory interpersonal relations are the primary cause of maladaptive behaviors. The interpersonal perspective also is concerned with the anxiety-arousing aspects of interpersonal relationships. At present, no systemic view of human nature and behavior is based entirely on interpersonal theory or the social context in which people live and work. The closest approximation may be the viewpoint developed by the neo-Freudian psychologist Harry Stack Sullivan. Several nursing theories also can be classified as interpersonal relations theory (see Table 12–2).

## Harry Stack Sullivan (1892–1949): Theory of Interpersonal Relations

Sullivan believed that all human processes occur in interrelationships; none occur in isolation. His research and practice broke with Freudian theories and research

### TABLE 12–2    Interpersonal Theories and Theorists

| Theory/Discipline | Theorist | Therapeutic Process |
|---|---|---|
| Interpersonal (Psychiatry) | Sullivan, Harry Stack | The purpose of all behavior is to get needs met through interpersonal interactions, not personality reconstruction as in psychodynamic theories. He coined the terms *participant observer* and *security* operations. |
| Nurse–Patient Relationship (Nursing) | Peplau, Hildegard | Influenced by Sullivan's theory. First nurse theorist to describe the nurse–client relationship as the foundation for the professional practice of psychiatric nursing. Used the technique of process recording to facilitate communication and interpersonal skill building. Synonymous with the concept of helping relationship as used in counseling. |
| Nursing Process Theory (Nursing) | Orlando, Ida Jean | Study grew out of her dissatisfaction with the possibility that nursing care was governed by organizational rules rather than attention to client needs and her desire to offer nursing students a theory of effective nursing practice. She was also able to link effective nursing care to the nurse's knowledge of patient needs that are validated by patient response(s). |
| Human-to-Human Relationship Model (Nursing) | Travelbee, Joyce | Focuses on meaning in the nurse–client relationship and the relief of client suffering through the use of communication skills within the phases of the nurse–client relationship. |

in that he based his primary work on direct and verifiable observations. In his words, one must pay attention to the "interactional," not the "intrapsychic" (Sullivan, 1953, p. 3). Sullivan's approach laid the groundwork for understanding the specific social context, environment, and relationship(s) in which an individual interacts/interacted with other human beings.

In addition, Sullivan (1953) outlined a stage theory of interpersonal development that is comprised of life processes. Each stage prepares an individual for the next stage; failure to successfully navigate a stage could severely limit personality development and a person's potential for a successful life (Table 12–3). Sullivan believed that cultural environment greatly shapes personality and that personality development does not end at 5 years of age, as espoused by Freud, but continues until young adulthood. In essence, Sullivan emphasized the pervasive interaction between the organism and the environment as well as the tasks of personality development.

**TABLE 12–3  Sullivan's Stages of Interpersonal Development**

| Age | Stage | Task/Key Concept |
|-----|-------|------------------|
| Birth to 18 months (to appearance of speech) | Infancy | Experiences anxiety in interaction with mother figure; learns to use maternal tenderness to gain security and avoid anxiety. Major task is gratification of needs. |
| 18 months to 6 years (first speech to need for playmates) | Childhood | Learns to delay gratification in response to interpersonal demands; uses language and action to avoid anxiety. |
| 6–9 years | Juvenile | Develops peer relationships; uses environment outside the family to shape self. Learns competition, cooperation, and compromise. |
| 9–12 years | Preadolescence | Develops caring relationship with same-sex peer, chum relationships, and the ability to collaborate with another person. |
| 12–14 years | Early adolescence | Develops interest in and satisfactory relationships with persons of opposite-sex; develops a sense of identity that is separate and independent from parents. |
| 14–21 years | Late adolescence | Establishes a self-identity. Has satisfying relationships; direct sexual impulses. |
| 21+ years | Adulthood | Achieves independence within society. Establishes a love relationship. |

Sullivan introduced several new terms and concepts that became influential to the care of individuals and nursing. One concept critical to the organization of behavior is the *self system*, a construct that includes three components: the *good me*, the *bad me,* and the *not me.* The self system is built from the child's experience and provides tools that enable people to deal with the tasks of avoiding anxiety and establishing security. Sullivan emphasized the development of the self-system *personification* that includes all related attitudes, feelings, and concepts about oneself or another acquired from extensive experience. Other major concepts introduced into psychiatric literature include interpersonal security and the term *significant other* (Antai-Otong, 2008, p. 41).

Sullivan (1953, p. 25) believed that poor relationships cause anxiety and serve as the basis for all emotional problems:

> One of the greatest mysteries of human life, [is] how some unfortunate people carry on in the face of apparently overwhelming difficulties, whereas other people are crushed by comparatively insignificant events, contemplate suicide, perhaps actually attempt it. This is to be understood on the basis not of the particular "objective" events which bring about the circumstance of success under great hardship or self-destruction; it is to be understood on the basis of the self system, the organization of experience reflected to one from the significant people around one—which determines the personal characteristics of those events. In no other fashion can we explain the enormous discrepancy between people's reaction to comparable life situations. (Sullivan, 1947, p. 11)

Haber, Krainovich-Miller, McMahon, and Hoskins (1997, p. 94) caution nurses that Sullivan's interpersonal theory remains empirically unverified and nurses should take care when generalizing from his theory to the client.

## Humanistic Theory

Humanistic philosophy/psychology focuses on the personal worth of the individual and the essential role of human values. The person is a "work in progress." Humanistic psychology took root in the United States in the Cold War era. Humanistic psychology has been described as a broad spectrum of approaches to treatment that arose as a spirited challenge to the rival orthodoxies of Freudian theory.

### Carl Rogers (1902–1987): Humanistic Psychology and Client-Centered Therapy

> Rogers' greatest contribution has not been in giving us a technique to fix people, but in creating a new form, a new definition of relationship in which people can function more fully and be more self-determining. (Farson, 2001, p. 201)

Carl Rogers, along with Abraham Maslow and Rollo May, was a forerunner in the identification of humanistic psychology as a person-centered approach involving specific values that emphasize the individual, choice, responsibility, and creativity (Rogers, 1980). However, Maslow and May eventually went on to carry the banner of humanistic psychology and focus on ideas of self-actualization rather than Rogers' emphasis on the treatment of sick persons.

The five fundamental building blocks of humanistic psychology can be identified as follows:

1. Actualizing human potentialities for creativity and growth
2. Regarding the person in the here and now
3. Emphasizing the centrality of self
4. Placing significance of experience as well as behavior
5. No assumptions of disease process, unconscious motivation, or developmental history.

Carl Rogers is now best known for his contributions to experience-oriented therapy, which focuses on the client's experiences as an agent for producing change. This therapy engages the client in new interactions and ways of being within the therapeutic situation. His therapy was originally called nondirective, was later renamed client-centered, and is now known as Rogerian therapy; even so, the terms *nondirective* and *client-centered* are still commonly used.

In Rogerian therapy the client is viewed as the expert about himself; "It is *client* who knows what hurts, what directions to go, what problems are crucial, what experiences have been deeply buried" (Rogers, 1962, p. 422). As such, the therapist serves as a supportive facilitator. Rogers (1962) stated:

> [C]onstructive personality growth and change comes about only when the client perceives and experiences a certain psychological climate in the relationship. The conditions which constitute this climate . . . are feelings or attitudes which must be experienced by the counselor and perceived by the client if they are to be effective. Those I have singled out as being essential are: a sensitive empathic understanding of the client's feelings and personal meanings; a warm, acceptant prizing of the client; and unconditionality in this positive regard. (p. 422)

Rogers' healthy person is "fully-functioning" and possesses the following qualities: (1) openness to experience, (2) existential living, (3) organismic trusting, (4) experiential freedom, and (5) creativity.

According to Farson (2001), Rogers has given us a way to be with one another, an ethical basis for human interaction, guidelines for important considerations in assessing not just the outcome but the process of a relationship, a different way in which we think about human relationships, the expectations we have about intimate personal contact, the nature of interpersonal and organizational behavior, and the right to self-determination. Professionals from education, religion, counseling, nursing, medicine, psychiatry, law enforcement, race relations, and social work, to mention only a few disciplines, have taken his humanistic theory and client-centered techniques more seriously than those in psychology. Unfortunately, in spite of its demonstrated impact, Rogers' work has been corrupted over the years by practitioners who have discovered the technique but not the philosophy.

> His is essentially a linear theory, as opposed to a curvilinear one; maximizing rather than optimizing. His concepts, like most in humanistic psychology, are based on the idea of 'the more the better' as opposed to 'there can too much of a good thing'. Rogers would have you believe that the more congruence, the more honesty, the more intimacy, the more closeness, the more empathy, the better. Sounds good, but with most linear thinking, it fails in the extreme . . . For a revolutionary, Rogers has paid precious little attention to role, power, status, culture, politics, history, systems, technology, and perhaps most significantly, the paradoxical quality of human experience. (Farson, 2001, pp. 200–201)

There are several commonalities in humanistic psychology and existential psychotherapy:

- Suffering might have a redemptive function, pointing the person toward a more authentic, integrated existence, rather than being a mere nuisance to be eliminated so he can get on with the *real* business of living.
- The role of self-authorship or self-determination in the formation our character and conduct; namely, we are never entirely determined by our experiences. Personal choice plays a significant role in who we are and what we become.
- To varying degrees, and in different ways, both humanistic psychology and existential psychotherapy draw on an older, European tradition of literary and philosophical humanism (Burston, 2003, p. 314). (See **Table 12–4**.)

## Existentialism/Phenomenology

Existential philosophy seeks meaning of life or of human experience. It is based on the doctrine that existence takes precedence over essence; humans are totally free to act and responsible for their acts. What counts are acts performed. Decision making is not based on knowledge; instead, knowledge is the result of decision making. These theories claim that physical laws are not enough to explain the complexities of human behavior. Existentialists are more subjective than other theorists. Creativity, individual initiative, and self-fulfillment are important personality factors. *Phenomenology*, the study of one's subjective experiences/perceptions, is one aspect of existential thought.

### *Viktor Frankl (1905–1997): Logotherapy*

Frankl was a Viennese psychiatrist and neurologist who developed his own existential philosophy and therapeutic technique known as logotherapy, which

**TABLE 12–4   Humanistic and Existential Philosophies and Theories**

| Therapy | Therapist | Therapeutic Process |
| --- | --- | --- |
| Rational Emotive | Ellis, Albert | A cognitive therapy using confrontation of "irrational beliefs" that prevents the individual from accepting responsibility for self and behavior. |
| Logotheraphy | Frankl, Viktor | A therapy designed to help individuals assume personal responsibility. The search for meaning (*logos*) in life is a central theme and the magnitude of love—*the salvation of man is through love and in love* (1963, pp. 58–59). |
| Reality | Glasser, William | The need for identity through responsible behavior is the therapeutic focus. Individuals are challenged to examine ways in which their behavior thwarts their attempts to achieve life goals. |
| Gestalt | Perls, Frederick "Fritz" | Therapy focuses on the overall general meanings of client situations and behavior. Identification of feelings in the "here and now" leads to self-acceptance. |
| Positive Psychology | Seligman, M. E. P. & Csikszentmihalyi, M. | This theory focuses on prevention. It is a new approach to improving health that focuses on "health strengths," instead of the traditional emphasis on diagnosis, treatment and prevention of disease. The premise is that Positive Health is a buffer against physical and mental illness. |
| Transpersonal Psychology | Maslow, Abraham Grof, Stanislav Sutich, Anthony | The concern is with the "study of humanity's highest potential, and the recognition, understanding, and realization of unitive, spiritual, and transcendent states of consciousness" (Lajoie & Shapiro, 1992, p. 231). Issues considered in transpersonal psychology include spiritual *self-development, peak experiences, mystical experiences, systemic trance* and other *occult* experiences of living. |

involves an application of the principles of existential philosophy to clinical practice. It is the term *meaning* that framed Frankl's therapeutic work. Logotherapy postulates a *will to meaning*; it proceeds *from* the spiritual, whereas existential analysis proceeds *toward* the spiritual. When comparing his therapy to Freud and Adler's therapies, Frankl suggested that Freud essentially postulated a *will to pleasure* as the root of all human motivation and Adler a *will to power*.

Frankl's theory and therapy grew out of his experiences in Nazi death camps. Watching who did and did not survive (given an opportunity to survive!), he concluded that the philosopher Friedrich Nietzsche (1961) was right: "He who has a *why to live for* can bear with almost any *how*" (p. 121). Frankl saw that people who had hopes of being reunited with loved ones, or who had projects they needed to complete, or who had great faith, tended to have better chances of survival than those who had lost all hope. Frankl's first book was published in 1946 in German and translated into English in 1959 under the title *From Death Camp to Existentialism*. In 1963 this book was revised to include the basic concepts of logotherapy and redistributed under the title *Man's Search for Meaning*.

For Frankl, the essence of human motivation is the *will to meaning* (*Der zum Sinn*). When meaning is not found, the individual becomes "existentially frustrated." This may or may not lead to clinical pathology. *Logotherapy*, (from the Greek word "logos," meaning study, word, spirit, God, or meaning) is the method of psychotherapy for treating what Frankl termed an *existential vacuum*, which manifests itself mainly in a state of boredom. Frankl identified two types of symptoms for treatment: one he called *noogenic neurosis* ("noos" meaning "of the spirit or mind), which emerges from conflicts involving existential problems. The other chief dynamic of the existential vacuum is *existential frustration*, which arises from failures and disappointments related to the will to meaning.

### Rollo May (1909–1994): Existentialism

I have described the human dilemma as the capacity of man to view himself as object and as subject. My point is that both are necessary—necessary for psychological science, for effective therapy, and for meaningful living. I am also proposing that in the dialectical process between these two poles lie the development, and the deepening and widening, of human consciousness. (May, 1967, p. 20)

. . . Existentialism . . . is the endeavor to understand man by cutting below the cleavage between subject and object which has bedeviled Western thought and science since shortly after the Renaissance. (May, 1967, p. 11)

Rollo May was an American psychologist who, although a Congregationalist minister, preferred psychology. He introduced existential perspectives into the

United States and is credited with being one of the editors of *Existence*, the first U.S. book on existential psychology, published in 1958, which highly influenced the emergence of American humanistic psychology.

While he accepted many Freudian psychodynamic principles (such as neurosis, repression, and defense), May believed that individuals only could be understood in terms of their subjective sense of self. He was influenced by American humanism theory and was interested in reconciling existential psychology with other approaches, especially Freud's. May believed that abnormal behavior is often just a stratagem for protecting the *center*, the subjective sense of self, against perceived threats. Persons may give up on self-growth if they perceive that their center is threatened and retreat to the secure, known center. As May put it in 1967, this is "a way of accepting nonbeing . . . in order that some little being may be preserved" (p. 75). May also was concerned with people's loss of faith in values. If we lose our commitment to a set of values, we will feel lonely and empty. Life will be meaningless. Ultimately we need to take responsibility for ourselves and find meaning in our lives.

May identified four stages of development: (1) innocence, (2) rebellion, (3) ordinary, and (4) creative. *Innocence* is the pre-self-conscious stage of the infant. An innocent does have a degree of will in the sense of a drive to fulfill his or her needs. *Rebellion* is the childhood and adolescent stage of developing one's ego or self-consciousness. The rebellious person wants freedom but does not yet have full understanding of the responsibility that goes with it. Teenagers may want to spend their allowance in any way they choose, yet they still expect the parent to provide the money and will complain about unfairness if they do not get it. *Ordinary* is the normal adult ego. Adults have learned responsibility but find it too demanding and so seek refuge in conformity and traditional values. The *creative* stage is the authentic adult, the existential stage, beyond ego and self-actualizing.

May believed that knowing we will die gives life meaning. It reminds us that we must do something now, or never do anything. He also believed that anxiety is a force that could be channeled within the individual, thereby enabling the person to achieve and live a meaningful life. This knowledge was tested when, after surviving tuberculosis, he decided that struggling against the disease had been the key to remaining alive. His perpetual anxiety and fear of dying had been helpful, he determined, because it kept him from becoming resigned to death.

May wrote about this experience in his first major book, *The Meaning of Anxiety* (1950), and continued to express his philosophical and therapeutic approaches in a number of subsequent books between 1953 and 1981.

## Positive Psychology

Positive psychology was founded on the belief that people want more than an end to suffering. People want to lead meaningful and fulfilling lives, to cultivate what is best within themselves, and to enhance their experiences of love, work, and play. The aim of positive psychology is to begin to catalyze a change in the focus of psychology—that is, to move away from a preoccupation with only repairing the worst things in life and toward building positive qualities. At the subjective level, the field of positive psychology is about valued subjective experiences: well-being, contentment, and satisfaction (in the past); hope and optimism (for the future); and flow and happiness (for the present). At the individual level, it is about positive individual traits: the capacity for love and vocation, courage and interpersonal skill, aesthetic sensibility, perseverance, forgiveness, originality, future-mindedness, spirituality, high talent, and wisdom. At the group level, it is about the civic virtues and the institutions that move individuals toward better citizenship: nurturance, altruism, civility, moderation, tolerance, and work ethic. At the forefront of this approach is the issue of prevention (Seligman, 2002).

Three pillars undergird the three central concerns of positive psychology: (1) positive experiences, (2) positive individual traits, and (3) positive institutions. Understanding positive emotions entails the study of contentment with the past, happiness in the present, and hope for the future. Understanding positive individual traits consists of the study of the strengths and virtues: the capacity for love and work, courage, compassion, resilience, creativity, curiosity, integrity, self-knowledge, moderation, self-control, and wisdom. Understanding positive institutions entails the study of the strengths that foster better communities, such as justice, responsibility, civility, parenting, nurturance, work ethic, leadership, teamwork, purpose, and tolerance.

According to Seligman and Csikszentmihalyi (2000, p. 5), the major psychological theories have changed to undergird a new science of strength and resilience. No longer do the dominant theories view the individual as a passive vessel responding to stimuli; rather, individuals are now seen as decision makers, with choices, preferences, and the possibility of becoming masterful, officious, or in malignant circumstances, helpless and hopeless (p. 8).

Seligman prodded psychologists to study life's joys and, in 2002, he wrote a book outlining his theory of authentic happiness, which posited that happiness could be analyzed into three different elements that one chooses for their own sake: *positive emotion, engagement,* and *meaning.*

Since its inception, the science of positive psychology has moved into areas of practice and research that ensures "human beings are seen as possessing essential freedom, or psychological determinism," in any sort of situation (Seligman, 2002, p. 10). Positive psychology theory and initiatives have been applied across a number of healthcare domains. However, as research proceeded, Dr. Seligman (2008) began seeing certain limitations to the concept of happiness as a positive emotion. People did not find joy or happiness in succeeding or in accomplishment. "They wanted to win for its own sake, even if it brought no positive emotion," says Dr. Seligman. Thus, in 2011, Seligman announced that authentic happiness as a theory was overrated; happiness actually had certain limitations and he regretted creating the "authentic happiness" title. Essentially people did not find aesthetic satisfaction, or meaning, in an accomplishment. "They wanted to win for its own sake, even if it brought no positive emotion" (p. 8).

In 2011, Seligman announced the creation of a new theory of positive psychology, "well-being" or "flourishing, which not only measures one's mood at the moment but also relationships with others and the sense that something worthwhile is being accomplished. Seligman also created PERMA, an acronym for what he defines as the five crucial elements of well-being: *P*ositive emotion, *E*ngagement (the feeling of being lost in a task), *R*elationships, *M*eaning, and *A*ccomplishment—each pursued for its own sake (pp. 16–18). "Well-being cannot exist just in your own head," he writes, "Well-being is a combination of feeling good as well as actually having meaning, good relationships and accomplishment" (p. 16).

> If we just wanted positive emotions, our species would have died out a long time ago. . . . We have children to pursue other elements of well-being. We want meaning in life. We want relationships. . . . My view of positive psychology is that it describes rather than prescribes what human beings do. . . . I don't want to mess with people's values. I'm not saying it's a good or a bad thing to want to win for its own sake. I'm just describing what lots of people do. One's job as a therapist is not to change what people value, but given what they value, to make them better at it. (Seligman, 2011, p. 26)

## Transpersonal Psychology

Transpersonal psychology is an academic discipline, not a religious or spiritual movement, developed from earlier schools of psychology, including psychoanalysis, behaviorism, and humanistic psychology. There is a strong connection between the transpersonal and the humanistic approaches to psychology. This is not surprising, according to Aanstoos, Serlin, and Greening (2000), given that transpersonal psychology started off within humanistic psychology (pp. 23–24).

Lajoie and Shapiro (1992) suggested that transpersonal psychology "is concerned with the study of humanity's highest potential, and with the recognition, understanding, and realization of unitive, spiritual, and transcendent states of consciousness" (p. 231). Issues considered in transpersonal psychology include spiritual self-development, peak experiences, mystical experiences, systemic trance, and other occult experiences of living. Transpersonal psychology was developed in an attempt to describe and integrate the experience of mysticism within modern psychological theory. Types of mystical experience examined vary greatly but include religious conversion, altered states of consciousness, trance and other spiritual practices. Although Carl Jung and others explored aspects of the spiritual and transpersonal in their work, Miller (1998, pp. 541–542) notes that Western psychology has had a tendency to ignore the spiritual dimension of the human psyche.

Transpersonal psychology is associated with New Age beliefs (Friedman, 2000). Although the transpersonal perspective has many overlapping interests with theories and thinkers associated with the term *New Age*, it is still problematic to place transpersonal psychology within such a framework. Indeed, associations between transpersonal psychology and the New Age movement have probably contributed to the failure in the United States to win formal recognition of transpersonal psychology by its national professional body, the American Psychological Association (APA). A significant breakthrough in this area was the successful establishment of a Transpersonal Psychology Section within the British Psychological Society (the U.K.'s professional body equivalent to the APA) in 1996, co-founded by David Fontana, Ingrid Slack, and Martin Treacy, the first section of its kind.

Today transpersonal psychology also includes approaches to health, social sciences, and practical arts such as process art. Transpersonal perspectives are being applied to such diverse fields as psychology, psychiatry, anthropology, sociology, pharmacology (Scotton, Chinen & Battista, 1996), and social work theory (Cowley & Derezotes, 1994). Transpersonal therapies are included in many therapeutic practices.

Criticisms of transpersonal psychology have come from several commentators. For example, Rollo May, discussed earlier in the chapter, disputed the conceptual foundations of transpersonal psychology (Aanstoos et al., 2000, p. 25). Albert Ellis (1989), the cognitive psychologist and humanist, questioned transpersonal psychology's scientific status and its relationship to religion and mysticism. Friedman (2000) criticized the field of transpersonal psychology for being underdeveloped as a field of science, placing it at the intersection between the broader domain of inquiry known as transpersonal studies (which may include a number of unscientific approaches) and the scientific discipline of psychology.

## Recovery-Oriented Systems of Care

### "Change is enviable; Growth is optional"

Personal communication: Tavis Smiley (May 2013).

> The goal of recovery is not to become normal. The goal is to embrace the human vocation of becoming more deeply, more fully human. (Deegan, 1996)

### Background

Within the literature, *recovery*, as a term, has been described by a number of professional disciplines and used to mean an approach, a model, a philosophy, a paradigm, a movement, a vision, and a myth (Roberts & Wolfson, 2004; Whitwell, 1999). As a health care concept, recovery is also not new. In health care, substance use and mental disorders treatment as well as "lived recovery" have been identified and discussed for decades. Yet now, the push toward recovery-oriented care lies at the core of the Substance Abuse and Mental Health Services Administration's (SAMHSA's) mission, and fostering development of recovery-oriented systems of care and services is a Center for Substance Abuse Treatment priority. Allott, Loganathan, and Fulford (2003) insist that the present claims of the recovery movement being a new paradigm are "probably exaggerated, as it represents a rediscovery of practices initiated more than 200 years ago" (p. 41).

Nevertheless, the public is admonished in SAMHSA's *Welcome to Recovery to Practice* statement (2010): "Recovery should not be mistaken for a passing fad. . . . As its reintroduction is intended to bring about a fundamental transformation of behavioral health care . . . [recovery] should not become simply a new word to be used in describing current practices" (2010).

In the U.S. healthcare system, recovery indicates a normal adaptation process of healing, improvement, or mending, to mention a few meanings. Globally, interest in recovery has been a focus for mental health services in the United Kingdom and New Zealand for several decades. Anthologies of personal stories of recovery have been used by governments and professionals as a means of combating stigma and reasserting a focus on *personal* perspectives (Lapsley, Waimarie, & Black, 2002; Leibrich, 1999). New Zealand's mental health services have been based on a recovery-centered blueprint, "which has led them to become a wellspring of ideas and guidance on recovery-based practice" (O'Hagen, 2001; Roberts & Wolfson, 2004).

In 1999, the U.S. Surgeon General set recovery as the focus of mental health policy (Ralph, Lambert, & Kidder, 2002; U.S. Department of Health and Human Services, 1999). Recovery-oriented care was originally envisioned as "the most important aim of behavioral health [meaning substance use and alcohol] services" (President's New Freedom Commission, 2003). In 2005, O'Connell, Tondora, Croog, Evans, and Davidson identified the elements of a recovery-oriented environment among alcohol and substance users. At that time, SAMHSA maintained separate definitions for mental disorders and substance use disorders. Noticeable disparity in care services and opportunities available caused considerable disagreement between the two areas. Mental health clients, practitioners, and other stakeholders confronted SAMHSA administrators about the limitation in scope of transformation services designation.

After several conferences held between SAMHSA administrators and mental health participants, O'Connell and colleagues (2005) identified the elements of a recovery-oriented environment as follows (see **Box 12–2**).

According to Roberts and Wolfson (2004), "Recovery is usually taken as broadly equivalent to 'getting back to normal' or 'cure,' and by these standards few people with severe mental illness recover" (p. 37). The goal of the discussions with SAMHSA was to achieve inclusion for the mentally ill and a redefinition of what recovery means to those with severe mental health problems. The redefinition, then, identified recovery as "a process of *personal* discovery, of how to live (and to live well) with enduring symptoms and vulnerabilities [which] opens the possibility of recovery to all. The 'recovery movement' argues that this reconceptualisation is personally empowering, and raises realistic hope for a better life alongside whatever remains of illness and vulnerability" (p. 37).

In a 2007 article, Gagne, White, and Anthony described the vision and values of recovery-oriented care that intersect the addiction and mental health fields, as shown in **Box 12–3**, and concluded that recovery should serve as the organizing construct for service provision and for systems improvement.

## Box 12-2 The Elements of Recovery-Oriented Environments

Encourages individuality;

Promotes accurate and positive portrayals of psychiatric disability while fighting discrimination;

Focuses on strengths;

Uses a language of hope and possibility;

Offers a variety of options for treatment, rehabilitation, and support;

Supports risk-taking, even when failure is a possibility;

Actively involves service users, family members, and other natural supports in the development and implementation of programs and services;

Encourages user participation in advocacy activities;

Helps develop connections with communities; and

Helps people develop valued social roles, interests and hobbies, and other meaningful activities.

*Source:* O'Connell, M., Tondora, J., Croog, G., Evans, A., & Davidson, L. (2005). From rhetoric to routine: Assessing perceptions of recovery-oriented practices in a state mental health and addiction system. *Psychiatric Rehabilitation Journal, 28*(4), 378–386. Reprinted with permission.

## Box 12-3 The Vision and Values of Recovery-Oriented Care

Recovery is a personal and individualized process of growth that unfolds along a continuum, and there are multiple pathways to recovery.

People in recovery are active agents of change in their lives and not passive recipients of services.

People in recovery from mental illness and/or addiction disorders often note the important role of family and peer support in making the difference in their recovery.

The values of recovery-oriented mental health and addictions systems are based on the recognition that each person is the agent of his or her own recovery and all services can be organized to support recovery.

Person-centered services offer choice, honor each person's potential for growth, focus on a person's strengths, and attend to the overall health and wellness of a person with mental illness and/or addiction.

*Source:* Gagne, C. A., White, W., & Anthony, W. A. (2007). Recovery: A common vision for the fields of mental health and addictions. *Psychiatric Rehabilitation Journal, 31*(1), 32–37. Published by The American Psychological Association. Reprinted with permission.

Finally, SAMHSA published the *Working Definition of Recovery from Mental Disorders and/or Substance Use Disorders,* which provided a unified working definition of recovery and set of recovery principles (see **Box 12–4**) designed to "help advance recovery opportunities for all Americans and help to clarify these concepts for peers, families, funders, providers, and others."

## Box 12–4 Working Definition of Recovery

A process of change through which individuals improve their health and wellness, live a self-directed life, and strive to reach their full potential.

### Four Major Dimensions Supporting a Life in Recovery

- *Health:* overcoming or managing one's disease(s) as well as living in a physically and emotionally healthy way;
- *Home:* a stable and safe place to live;
- *Purpose:* meaningful daily activities, such as a job, school, volunteerism, family caretaking, or creative endeavors, and the independence, income and resources to participate in society; and
- *Community:* relationships and social networks that provide support, friendship, love, and hope

### 10 Guiding Principles of Recovery

*Recovery emerges from hope:* The belief that recovery is real provides the essential and motivating message of a better future–that people can and do overcome the internal and external challenges, barriers, and obstacles that confront them.

*Recovery is person-driven:* Self-determination and self-direction are the foundations for recovery as individuals define their own life goals and design their unique path(s).

*Recovery occurs via many pathways:* Individuals are unique with distinct needs, strengths, preferences, goals, culture, and backgrounds including trauma experiences that affect and determine their pathway(s) to recovery. Recovery is built on the multiple capacities, strengths, talents, coping abilities, resources, and inherent value of each individual. Recovery pathways are highly personalized. They may include professional clinical treatment; use of medications; support from families and in schools; faith-based approaches; peer support; and other approaches. Recovery is non-linear, characterized by continual growth and improved functioning that may involve setbacks. Because setbacks are a natural, though not inevitable, part of the recovery process, it is essential to foster resilience for all individuals and families. Abstinence from the use of alcohol, illicit drugs, and non-prescribed medications is the goal for those with addictions. Use of tobacco and non-prescribed or illicit drugs is not safe for anyone. In some cases, recovery pathways can be enabled by creating a supportive environment. This is especially true for children, who may not have the legal or developmental capacity to set their own course.

*Recovery is holistic:* Recovery encompasses an individual's whole life, including mind, body, spirit, and community. The array of services and supports available should be integrated and coordinated.

*Recovery is supported by peers and allies:* Mutual support and mutual aid groups, including the sharing of experiential knowledge and skills, as well as social learning, play an invaluable role in recovery.

*Recovery is supported through relationship and social networks:* An important factor in the recovery process is the presence and involvement of people who believe in the person's ability to recover; who offer hope, support, and encouragement; and who also suggest strategies and resources for change.

*Recovery is culturally based and influenced:* Culture and cultural background in all of its diverse representations including values, traditions, and beliefs are keys in determining a person's journey and unique pathway to recovery. Services should be culturally grounded, attuned, sensitive, congruent, and competent, as well as personalized to meet each individual's unique needs.

*Recovery is supported by addressing trauma:* Services and supports should be trauma-informed to foster safety (physical and emotional) and trust, as well as promote choice, empowerment, and collaboration.

*Recovery involves individual, family, and community strengths and responsibility:* Individuals, families, and communities have strengths and resources that serve as a foundation for recovery.

*Recovery is based on respect:* Community, systems, and societal acceptance and appreciation for people affected by mental health and substance use problems–including protecting their rights and eliminating discrimination–are crucial in achieving recovery.

> For further detailed information about the new working recovery definition or the *gui*ding principles of recovery please visit: http://www.samhsa.gov/recovery/

*Source:* SAMHSA's Blog. (2012a). *SAMHSA's working definition of recovery.* Retrieved from http://store.samhsa.gov/shin/content/PEP12-RECDEF/PEP12-RECDEF.pdf

### Recovery and Trauma-Informed Care

Another reality emerged among the care and service considerations for persons with behavioral and mental health needs—trauma as a near universal experience of individuals with behavioral and mental health problems. Greater than 90% of people served in public and mental health settings have histories of repeated exposure to trauma and violence—many patients reported a history of trauma and abuse most commonly having occurred in childhood (National Council for Behavioral Health (2012). Individuals with histories of physical and sexual abuse and other types of trauma-inducing events often experience mental health and co-occurring disorders such as chronic health conditions, substance abuse, eating disorders, and HIV/AIDS, as well as contact with the criminal justice system. According to SAMHSA (2012b), "Although exact prevalence estimates vary, there is a consensus in the field that most consumers of mental health services are trauma survivors and that their trauma experiences help shape their responses to outreach and services." When expanding the recovery construct to other inclusive concepts, the generalizability of the recovery framework to include trauma emerges. Yet Ragins (2010) states, "Ultimately to recover one must achieve some meaningful role apart from the destruction [trauma]. . . . Becoming a [trauma] victim is not a recovered role, and frankly, neither is [trauma] survivor. After achieving increased hopefulness, inner strength and self-responsibility, these traits are applied to meaningful roles apart from the [trauma]" (p. 3).

Despite Ragins' (2010) statement, Trauma-informed Care, by definition, is a strength-based framework that is grounded in an understanding of the responsiveness to the *impact of trauma*; emphasizes physical, psychological, and emotional safety for both providers and survivors; and creates opportunities for survivors to rebuild a sense of control and empowerment. It is an approach *made by providers* to engaging people with histories of trauma that recognizes the presence of trauma symptoms and acknowledges the role that trauma has played in their lives.

---

Trauma-specific interventions are designed to address the consequences of trauma in the individual and to facilitate healing. Treatment programs generally recognize the following:

- The survivor's need to be respected, informed, connected, and hopeful regarding their own recovery
- The interrelation between trauma and symptoms of trauma (e.g., substance abuse, eating disorders, depression, and anxiety)
- The need to work in a collaborative way with survivors, family and friends of the survivor, and other human services agencies in a manner that will empower survivors and consumers

*Source:* Substance Abuse and Mental Health Services Administration (2012b). *Welcome to the National Center for Trauma-Informed Care.* Washington, DC: SAMHSA Retrieved: http://www.samhsa.gov/nctic/

In all of these environments, the goal of care is to change the paradigm from one that asks, "What's wrong with you?" to one that asks, "What has happened to you?"

According to SAMHSA (2012b), "When a human service program takes the step to become trauma-informed, every part of its organization, management, and service delivery system is assessed and potentially modified to include a basic understanding of how trauma affects the life of an individual seeking services. Trauma-informed organizations, programs, and services are based on an understanding of the vulnerabilities or triggers of trauma survivors that traditional service delivery approaches may exacerbate, so that these services and programs can be more supportive and avoid re-traumatization." Thus, a *recovery-oriented system* now describes and coordinates the delivery of care for individuals with substance use *and* mental disorders *and* trauma-related issues.

## Conclusions about the Recovery-Oriented System of Care

As healthcare continues to change rapidly, the need for change in our traditional nursing roles has never been more apparent. Traditional models of healthcare have focused on curing illness. Right now, recovery is primarily viewed as a cross-cutting framework unifying mental health and substance use disorder treatments. However, recovery should be envisioned as an overarching framework for practice development and focus for all healthcare treatment. It has been suggested that practitioners need to change their practice in a number of ways; to mention a few: 1) we need to get out of the "treatment box" and accept that treatment is only one part of recovery; we must implement value-based approaches to care; 2) language use has to change to facilitate the value-based focus of recovery. To this end, Jensen et al. (2013) champion the use of person-first language; 3) we must view and approach the expected change as a process, with starts and stops, not a destination; and remember, the purpose of recovery is *hope*—a movement from hopelessness to hopefulness. Again, change is inevitable, growth is optional.

## Building a Framework for Recovery-Oriented and Trauma-Informed Nursing Care

Quality of life is "the indivisible human's view on living moment to moment as the changing patterns of shifting perspectives weave the fabric of life through the human-universe interconnectedness." It is a subjective, global perception of the meaning of one's lived experiences in the moment. It fluctuates moment to moment in co-creation with the universe. (Parse, 1994, p. 17)

Today, health care must be client (person)-driven. Nurses must always be at the forefront of changes that provides quality, cost-effective care for the betterment of the client, family, and community. Evidence of effective recovery-oriented, trauma-informed interventions or best practices in nursing is limited. Effectiveness of existing recovery-oriented interventions, programs, or models of care needs to be evaluated (Sheedy & Whitter, 2009).

Munhall (2011) states, "the sands of science itself are shifting as more and more scientists including nurse scientists, realize that science cannot be a field of absolute and final truth but is an endeavor focused on *illuminating an ever-changing body of ideas* . . . some consider this shift a 'grievous loss' while others consider it 'exhilarating and liberating'" (pp. 12–13).

Preparation for the inevitable paradigm change in nursing science and practice, as outlined by Whall (2005), is more a matter of what Munhall (2011, p. 46) called a *"perspective development* than an anticipation of a specific occurrence."

Recovery is about the lived experience and understanding the lived experience. It is not what is wrong with a person, but rather what has happened to them; in essence, as a lived experience, the only way out is to go through it (Anthony, 2008; Beck, 2011). Clinicians must remember "recovery is not a step-by-step process but rather is viewed as nonlinear, a growth experience with setbacks." Instead of focusing on the illness, the focus is on the recovery process—which is strength based. The patient and clinician in partnership facilitate recovery by managing the illness, strengthening coping abilities, and building resilience for life's challenges" (Boyd, 2012, p. 17).

As the opening statement to this section offers—change is inevitable; *growth* is optional. While the immediate national push to integrate recovery-oriented systems of care is focused on, or seemingly limited to, being a framework for transforming mental and behavioral health, exciting implications for nursing and advanced practice nurses emerge to identify and expand recovery-oriented, trauma-informed nursing care in all areas of practice, not just psychiatric mental health and substance use practice. This push is well within nursing's capacity to exert considerable influence to broaden the scope of needed services.

According to Moller and McLoughlin (2013), "One could argue that the American Nurses Association's (ANA) definition of general nursing epitomizes the recovery philosophy but has not been recognized as so . . ." (p. 114). Dual diagnosis patients can also have comorbid diseases. Advanced practice nurses representing any specialty practice area or population group can use recovery-oriented, trauma-informed focused care approaches with any patients, not just those with behavioral and/or mental health problems.

Oftentimes in finding new ways of thinking about transforming care practices to meet emerging social trends and discipline needs, a reassessment of one's philosophy of nursing, theory of nursing, and tenets of nursing practice is required. "The future of nursing knowledge development requires nurses to blend philosophical aspects with the emerging social trends and needs in the discipline (Munhall, 2011, p. 46). "Human science," as explained by Polifroni (2011) in outlining the Continental Philosophy of Science,

... deals with persons and their connectedness to the world in which they live and the lived experiences of their life. ... the continental philosophy of science ... is concerned with the connection of an idea to the world around the idea and its historical context. [This philosophy] ... is not about theories or truths, but rather about relationships among people, ideas, meanings, and their historical connectedness. [Like patient assessment, it] requires an examination of historical context as much as it does what is happening in the present time. [One's belief] is not cause and effect, but rather in connectedness and the often used adage, "Past is prologue." (p. 14)

Zuzelo (2011, p. 538) states, "nursing practice is ... built upon the premise that experiences are individual and unique. ... As a result, nursing requires a pluralistic, multimethod approach to its knowledge-building endeavors." Newman (2008) insists, "The link between nursing science [postmodernism, neomodernism], theory [interpersonal theory], and what is seen [patient-driven data focused on one's lived experience] makes important differences in practice" (p. 45). Aligning nursing science, interpersonal theory, and recovery care seems to be an attainable goal at all levels of nursing, particularly advanced practice specialties. Any successful alignment ought to be highly generalizable across all practice areas.

It is common to find nursing theories or conceptual frameworks classified in a number of ways. Today, although research and practice still are not always connected, there is absolute awareness that nursing practice is also a process of knowledge development. The goal of recovery-oriented nursing care transcends any particular disagreement.

In attempting to provide a cursory outline for building a framework for recovery-oriented research and practice using SAMHSA's principles and guidelines and reference to Polifroni's (2011 phrase, "the past is prologue" leads to a review of the works of such previously mentioned influential interpersonal nurse theorists as Joyce Travelbee (human-to-human relationship model), Margaret Newman (theory of health as expanding consciousness), and especially Rosemarie Rizzo Parse (humanbecoming theory) who states, "Nursing's goal consists of being with or in the presence within mutual nurse-client processes to understand and value the meaning of the client's lived experience and assimilate preferences and beliefs that influence health care choices and preference" (Parse, 1998, p.14 ).

Travelbee (1966, 1971) proposed that the caring goal of nursing is to assist an individual, family, or community to prevent or cope with the experiences of illness and suffering and, if necessary, find meaning in these experiences, with the ultimate goal being *to instill hope*. The concept of hope is defined as *a mental state characterized by the desire to gain an end or accomplish a goal combined with some degree of expectation that what is desired or sought is attainable.* Her original conceptualization of hope was directed toward patients with psychiatric illness, but she later expanded her concept to include patients with long-term physical illnesses. Because Travelbee focused on *meaning* in nurse–client interactions, "her unique synthesis of [other theorists'] ideas differentiated her work from theirs in terms of the therapeutic human-to-human relationship between nurse and patient" (Alligood & Tomey, 2010, p. 61; Kneisl & Trigoboff, 2009). She insisted that nursing is defined and accomplished through the relatedness found in the human-to-human relationship and successfully working through the phases of the initial encounter, emerging identity, empathy, sympathy, and rapport (Moses, 1994, p. 200).

Parse views health as inseparable and irreducible from both human and universe. Humans are intentional beings and, by their very nature, live a seamless symphony throughout the life span. People are involved with the universe in directing their personal becoming through their relationships with others. Individuals live in the moment within the presence of mutual processes with the universe structures that are multidimensional. In turn, these mutual processes enable persons to manage their lives and health through the freedom and right to make choices and live their lives as they choose (Parse, 1998, 2002). The environment includes the universe and mutual processes. Humans are engaged in mutual processes with the universe structure or with others who are with the individual. Thus, Plummer and Molzahn summarized, "Given the breadth of nursing practice and the value of the concept for nursing . . . it is appropriate to consider replacing health as a metaparadigm concept with quality of life" (p. 140).

These interpersonal theories continue to provide integrative theoretical perspectives that are important for advanced nursing practice and *should* drive or actually undergird nursing research as new knowledge continues to evolve.

## Back to the Future

*When they see me, when they seriously meet and relate to me, then I exist as a person.*

—Gaillard, Shattell, & Thomas, 2009, p. 192

There's an old adage, "Unless you know the history you're doomed to repeat it." According to Whall (2002), nurses in the United States "did not focus on (or perhaps understand) the nature and importance of a paradigm shift that occurred just a few decades ago" (p. 72). Whall (2005) further offered:

When nursing in the past was not clear concerning its meta-theoretical stance, practicing nurses at times assumed the practice values of other disciplines. The result might be described as analogous to a 'rudderless ship,' greatly influenced by the winds of the day and not by specific values of nursing. (p. 1)

Nursing's focus on interpersonal relations in the 1950s, has been replaced by a focus on existentialism. Arguments abound as to where we are philosophically.

Philosophical and paradigmatic issues foundational to nursing have gone through a shift from positivism to postmodernism and increasingly to neomodernism.

Given the thrusts to move nursing research away from mechanistic models for explaining human activity, the opportunities for healthcare system growth found in recovery-oriented and trauma-informed care seem poised to foster new directions not only for nursing knowledge, research, and practice but also to the nation's health and well-being.

## Discussion Questions

1. According to Kneisl & Trigoboff (2009), "Approaches associated with two or more different theories are often used in combination" (p. 26). Discuss the possibility of the Recovery-oriented and Trauma-informed Care frameworks being universal care concepts generalizable across all practice areas, appropriate to any nursing specialty, and a fit with your practice.

2. Because the future of nursing practice is being transformed by multiple complex factors and given the pervasiveness of substance use and mental health issues present in our society, discuss the concept that aligning nursing science, Interpersonal theory or theories, and Recovery and trauma-informed care principles would be an attainable goal, if not an expectation of practice, for all levels of nursing, particularly *all* advanced practice specialties.

3. Given the focus offered in Item #2, select an Interpersonal Relationship theory; then discuss the *fit* of your selected theory with the recovery-oriented and/or trauma-informed goals and principles in your work setting; specifically would it fit? What would be required to make it fit?

4. Discuss the concept of envisioning Recovery as an overarching framework for practice development and focus for all healthcare treatment.

5. Rich (2003), in an article that revisited a question raised by Travelbee (1964) asked, What's Wrong with Sympathy? Discuss whether or not Travelbee's (1964) belief that it is as important for you (the nurse) to sympathize as it is to empathize with a patient in order to develop a human-to-human relationship would influence your practice.

## References

Aanstoos, C., Serlin, I., & Greening, T. (2000). History of division 32 (humanistic psychology) of the American Psychological Association. In D. Dewsbury (Ed.), *Unification through division: Histories of the divisions of the American Psychological Association, Vol. V.* Washington, DC: American Psychological Association.

Alligood, M. R., & Tomey, A. M. (2010). *Nursing theorists and their work* (7th ed.). Maryland Heights, MO: Mosby.

Allott, P., Loganathan, L., & Fulford, K. W. M. (2003). Discovering hope for recovery from a British perspective. In S. Lurie, M. McCubbin, & B. Dallaire (Eds.), International innovations in community mental health (special issue). *Canadian Journal of Community Mental Health, 21*(3).

American Nurses Association. (1967). *Statement on psychiatric-mental health nursing practice* (Publication No. S-85). New York, NY: Author.

American Nurses Association. (1980). *Nursing: A social policy statement.* Kansas City, MO: Author.

American Nurses Association. (2003). *Nursing: A social policy statement* (2nd ed.). Washington, DC: American Nurses Publishing.

Ancel, G. (2006). Developing empathy in nurses: An inservice training program. *Archives of Psychiatric Nursing, 20*(6), 249–257.

Antai-Otong, D. (2008). *Psychiatric nursing: Biological & behavioral concepts* (2nd ed.). Philadelphia, PA: F. A. Davis.

Anthony, K. H. (2008). Helping partnerships that facilitate recovery from severe mental illness. *Journal of Psychosocial Nursing, 46*(7), 25–53.

Beck, C. T. (2011). Exemplar: Teetering on the edge: A second grounded theory modification In P. L. Munhall (Ed.), *Nursing research: A qualitative perspective* (5th ed., pp. 257–281). Sudbury, MA: Jones & Bartlett Learning.

Boyd, M. A. (2008). *Psychiatric nursing: Contemporary practice* (4th ed.). Philadelphia, PA: Lippincott Williams & Wilkins.

Boyd, M. A. (2012). *Psychiatric nursing: Contemporary practice* (5th ed.). Philadelphia, PA: Lippincott Williams & Wilkins.

Burton, D. (2003). Existentialism, humanism, and psychology. *Existential Analysis, 14*(2), 309–319.

Chinn, P. L., & Kramer, M. K. (2008). *Integrated theory and knowledge development in nursing.* (7th ed.). St. Louis, MO: Mosby.

Cowley, A. S., & Derezotes, D. (1994). Transpersonal psychology and social work education. *Journal of Social Work Education, 30*(1), 100.

Decker-Brown, K. (2003). Humanistic theory information website, Retrieved: from: HYPERLINK "http://www.humanisticnursingtheory.com" www.humanisticnursingtheory.com

Deegan, P. (1996). Recovery as a journey of the heart. *Psychiatric Rehabilitation Journal, 19,* 19–97.

Ellis, A. (1989, February). Dangers of transpersonal psychology: A reply to Ken Wilber. *Journal of Counseling & Development, 67*(6), 336.

Falk-Rafael, R. A. (2000). Watson's philosophy, science and theory of human caring as a conceptual framework for guiding community health nursing. *Advances in Nursing Science, 23*(2), 34–49.

Farson, R. (2001). Carl Rogers, quiet revolutionary. *Education, 95*(2), 197–203.

Fawcett, J. (2005). *Contemporary nursing knowledge: Analysis and evaluation of nursing models and theories* (2nd ed.). Philadelphia, PA: F. A. Davis.

Frankl, V. E. (1963). (I. Lasch, Trans.). *Man's search for meaning: An introduction to logotherapy.* New York, NY: Washington Square Press. (Earlier title, 1959: *From death-camp to existentialism.* Originally published in 1946 as Ein Psycholog erlebt das Konzentrationslager).

Friedman, H. (2000). *Toward developing transpersonal psychology as a scientific field.* Paper presented at Old Saybrook 2 Conference, May 11–14, 2000, State University of West Georgia.

Frisch, N. C., & Frisch, L. E. (2011). *Psychiatric mental health nursing* (4th ed.). Clifton Park, NY: Delmar.

Gagne, C. A., White, W., & Anthony, W. A. (2007). Recovery: A common vision for the fields of mental health and addictions. *Psychiatric Rehabilitation Journal, 31,* 32–37.

Gaillard, L. M., Shattell, M. M., & Thomas, S. P. (2009). Mental health patients' experiences of being misunderstood. *Journal of the American Psychiatric Nurses Association, 15,* 191–199.

Haber, J. (2000). Hildegard Peplau: The psychiatric nursing legacy of a legend. *Journal of the American Psychiatric Nurses Association, 6*(2), 56–62.

Haber, J., Krainovich-Miller, B., McMahon, A. L., & Hoskins, P. P. (1997). *Comprehensive psychiatric nursing* (5th ed.). St. Louis, MO: Mosby.

Jensen, M. E., Pease, E. A., Lambert, K., Hickman, D. R., Robinson, O., McCoy, K. T., . . . King, J. K. (2013). Championing person-first language: A call to psychiatric mental health nurses. *Journal of the American Psychiatric Nurses Association, 19*(3), 146–151.

Johnson, B. M., & Webber, P. B. (2010). *An introduction to theory and reasoning in nursing* (3rd ed.). Philadelphia, PA: Lippincott Williams & Wilkins.

Kneisl, C. R., & Trigoboff, E. (2009). *Contemporary psychiatric-mental health nursing* (2nd ed.). Upper Saddle River, NJ: Pearson.

Lajoie, D. H., & Shapiro, S. I. (1992). Definitions of transpersonal psychology: The first twenty-three years. *Journal of Transpersonal Psychology, 24,* 230–241.

Lapsley, H., Waimarie, L. N., & Black, R. (2002). *Kia Mauri Tau! Narratives of recovery from disabling mental health problems.* Wellington: Mental Health Commission.

Leibrich, J. (1999). *A gift of stories: How to deal with mental health illness.* Dunedin: University of Otago Press.

May, R. (1950). *The Meaning of Anxiety.* New York, NY: W.W. Norton. (rev. ed.).

May, R. (1967). *Psychology and the human dilemma.* New York, NY: W. W. Norton.

McCamant, K. L. (2006, October). Humanistic nursing, interpersonal relations theory, and the empathy-altruism hypothesis. *Nursing Science Quarterly, 19*(4), 334–338.

Meleis, A. I. (2007). *Theoretical nursing: Development and progress* (4th ed.). Philadelphia, PA: Lippincott Williams & Wilkins.

Miller, J. J. (1998). Book review: Textbook of transpersonal psychiatry and psychology. *Psychiatric Services, 49,* 541–542.

Mohr, W. K. (2008). *Psychiatric mental health nursing: Evidence-based concepts, skills, and practices* (7th ed.). Philadelphia, PA: Lippincott Williams & Wilkins.

Moller, M. D., & McLoughlin, K. A. (2013). Integrating recovery practices into psychiatric nursing: Where are we in 2013? *Journal of the American Psychiatric Nurses Association, 9*(3), 113–116.

Moses, M. M. (1994). Caring incidents: A gift to the present. *Journal of Holistic Nursing, 12,* 193–203.

Munhall, P. L. (2011). *Nursing research: A qualitative perspective* (5th ed.). Sudbury, MA: Jones & Bartlett Learning.

National Council for Behavioral Health. (2012). Trauma-informed care. Retrieved from http://www.thenationalcouncil.org/topics/trauma-informed-care/

Newman, M. A. (1972). Time estimation in relation to gait tempo. *Perceptual and Motor Skills, 34,* 359–366.

Newman, M. A. (1990). Newman's theory of health as praxis. *Nursing Science Quarterly, 3,* 37–41.

Newman, M. A. (1992). Nightingale's vision of nursing theory and health. In F. Nightingale, *Notes on nursing: What it is and what it is not* (commemorative edition, pp. 44–47). Philadelphia, PA: Lippincott.

Newman, M. A. (1994). *Health as expanding consciousness* (2nd ed.). New York, NY: National League for Nursing.

Newman, M. A. (2003). The world on no boundaries. *ANS Advances in Nursing Science, 26*(4), 240–245.

Newman, M. A. (2008). *Transforming presence: The difference that nursing makes.* Philadelphia, PA: F. A. Davis.

Nietzsche, F. W. (1961). *Thus spoke Zarathustra: A book for everyone and no one.* London, UK: Penguin Group.

O'Connell, M., Tondora, J., Croog, G., Evans, A., & Davidson, L. (2005). From rhetoric to routine: Assessing perceptions of recovery-oriented practices in a state mental health and addiction system. *Psychiatric Rehabilitation Journal, 28*(4), 378–386.

O'Hagan, M. (2001). Recovery Competencies for New Zealand Mental Health Workers. Wellington: Mental Health Commission. http://www.mhc.govt.nz/publications/2001/Recovery_Competencies.pdf

Orlando, J. J. (1961). *The dynamic nurse patient relationship: Function, process and principles.* New York, NY: G. P. Putnam's Sons.

Orlando, J. J. (1972). *The discipline and teaching of nursing process (an evaluative study).* New York, NY: G. P. Putnam's Sons.

Orlando Pelletier, J. J. (1990). Preface to the NLN edition. In J. J. Orlando, *The dynamic nurse patient relationship: Function, process and principles* (pp. vii–viii). New York, NY: National League for Nursing.

O'Toole, A. W., & Welt, S. R. (Eds.). (1989). *Interpersonal theory in nursing practice: Selected works of Hildegard E. Peplau.* New York, NY: Springer.

Parse, R. R. (1981). *Man-living-health: A theory of nursing.* New York, NY: Wiley.

Parse, R. R. (1992). Human becoming: Parse's theory of nursing. *Nursing Science Quarterly, 5,* 35–42.

Parse, R. R. (1994). Quality of life: Sciencing and living the art of human becoming. *Nursing Science Quarterly, 7*(1), 16–21.

Parse, R. R. (1995). Nursing theories and frameworks: The essence of advanced practice nursing. *Nursing Science Quarterly, 8*(1), 1.

Parse, R. R. (1998). Moving on. *Nursing Science Quarterly, 11*(4), 135.

Parse, R. R. (2002). Transforming health care with a unitary view of human. *Nursing Science Quarterly, 15,* 46–50.

Parse, R. R. (2007). The humanbecoming school of thought in 2050. *Nursing Science Quarterly, 20,* 308.

Paterson, J. G., & Zderad, L. T. (1976). *Humanistic nursing.* New York, NY: Wiley.

Paterson, J. G., & Zderad, L. T. (1978). *The tortuous way toward nursing theory* (National League for Nursing Publication No. 15-1708). New York, NY: National League for Nursing.

Paterson, J. G., & Zderad, L. T. (1988). *Humanistic nursing.* New York: National League for Nursing.

Peplau, H. (1952). *Interpersonal relations in nursing*. New York, NY: G. P. Putnam's Sons.

Peplau, H. (1991, re-issued). *Interpersonal relations in nursing: A conceptual frame of reference for psychodynamic nursing*. New York, NY: Springer.

Peplau, H. (1992). Interpersonal relations: A theoretical framework for application in nursing practice. *Nursing Science Quarterly, 5*, 13–18.

Peplau, H. (1997). Peplau's theory of interpersonal relations. *Nursing Science Quarterly, 10*(4), 162–167.

Phillips, J. R. (1995). Quality of life research: Its increasing importance. *Nursing Science Quarterly, 8*, 100–101.

Pilkington, F. B. (2007). Envisioning nursing in 2050 through the eyes of nurse theorists: Leininger and Watson. *Nursing Science Quarterly, 20*(1), 8.

Plummer, M., & Molzahn, A. E. (2009, December). Quality of life in contemporary nursing theory: A concept analysis. *Nursing Science Quarterly, 22*, 134–140.

Polifroni, E. C. (2011). Philosophy of science: An introduction. In J. B. Butts & K. L. Rich. *Philosophies and Theories for Advanced Nursing Practice* (pp. 3–18). Sudbury, MA: Jones & Bartlett Learning.

Potter, M. L., & Bockenhauer, B. J. (2000). Implementing Orlando's nursing theory. *Journal of Psychosocial Nursing and Mental Health Services, 38*(13), 14–21.

Praeger, S. G., & Hogarth, C. R. (1985). Josephine E. Paterson and Loretta T. Zderad. In J. B. George (Ed.), *Nursing theories* (2nd ed., pp. 287–299). Englewood Cliffs, NJ: Prentice Hall.

President's New Freedom Commission, Mental Health. (2003). Achieving the promise: Transforming mental health care in America—final report (DHHS Publication No. SMA- 03-3832).

Ragins, M. (2010). Four Levels of Recovery Practice. Development Services Group, Inc.: Bethesda, MD.

Ralph, R. O., Lambert, D., & Kidder, K. A. (2002). The Recovery Perspective and Evidence-Based Practice for People with Serious Mental Illness: A Guideline Developed for The Behavioural Health Recovery Management Project. http://bhrm.org/guidelines/Ralph%20Recovery.pdf

Reed, P. G. (1996). Transforming practice knowledge into nursing knowledge—A revisionist analysis of Peplau. *Journal of Nursing Scholarship, 28*(1), 29–33.

Reynolds, W. J., & Scott, B. (1999). Empathy: A crucial component of the helping relationship. *Journal of Psychiatric and Mental Health Nursing, 6*, 363–379.

Reynolds, W. J., & Scott, B. (2000). Do nurses and other professional helpers normally display much empathy? *Journal of Advanced Nursing, 31*, 226–234.

Rich, K. (2003). Revisiting Joyce Travelbee's question: What's wrong with sympathy? *Journal of the American Psychiatric Association, 9*(6), 202–204.

Rittman, M. R. (2001). Ida Jean Orlando: The dynamic nurse-patient relationship. In M. E. Parker (Ed.), *Nursing theories and nursing practice*. Philadelphia, PA: F. A. Davis.

Roberts, G., & Wolfson, P. (2004). The rediscovery of recovery: Open to all. *Advances in Psychiatric Treatment, 10*, 37–48. doi: 10.1192/apt.10.1.37

Rogers, C. (1962). The interpersonal relationship: The core of guidance. *Harvard Educational Review, 32*(4), 422.

Rogers, C. (1980). *A way of being*. Boston, MA: Houghton Mifflin.

Rogers, M. E. (1970). *An introduction to the theoretical basis of nursing.* Philadelphia, PA: F. A. Davis.

Rogers, M. E. (1994). Science of unitary human beings. Current perspectives. *Nursing Science Quarterly, 7,* 33–35.

Schmieding, N. J. (n.d.). *Ida Jean Orlando's nursing process theory.* Retrieved from www.uri.edu/nursing/schmieing/orlando

Scotton, B. W., Chinen, A. B., & Battista, J. R. (Eds.). (1996). *Textbook of transpersonal psychiatry and psychology.* New York, NY: Basic Books.

Seligman, M. E. P. (2002). *Authentic happiness: Using the new positive psychology to realize your potential for lasting fulfillment.* New York, NY: Free Press (Simon & Schuster).

Seligman, M. E. P. (2008). Positive health. *Applied Psychology: An International Review, 57,* 3–18. doi: 10.1111/j.1464-0597.2008.00351.x

Seligman, M. E. P. (2011). *Flourish: A visionary new understanding of happiness and well-being.* New York, NY: Free Press (Simon & Schuster).

Seligman, M. E. P., & Csikszentmihalyi, M. (2000, January). Positive psychology: An introduction. *American Psychologist, 55*(1), 5–15.

Sheedy, C. K., & Whitter, M. (2009). Guiding Principles and Elements of Recovery-Oriented Systems of Care: What Do We Know From the Research? HHS Publication No. (SMA) 09-4439. Rockville, MD: Center for Substance Abuse Treatment, Substance Abuse and Mental Health Services Administration. Retrieved from http://www.samhsa.gov/shin

Sills, G. M. (1999). Hildegard E. Peplau, RN: Ed.D; FAAN: Nurse scholar, educator, leader. *Nursing Science Quarterly, 12*(3), 188–189.

Sills, G. M. (2000). Peplau and professionalism: The emergence of the paradigm of professionalism. *Journal of the American Psychiatric Nurses Association, 6*(1), 29–34.

Stevens, B. J. (1984). *Nursing theory: Analysis, application, evaluation* (2nd ed.). Boston, MA: Little, Brown.

Substance Abuse and Mental Health Services Administration. (2012a). *SAMHSA's working definition of recovery.* Washington, DC: Retrieved from http://store.samhsa.gov/shin/content/PEP12-RECDEF/PEP12-RECDEF.pdf

Substance Abuse and Mental Health Services Administration. (2012b). *Welcome to the National Center for Trauma-Informed Care.* Washington, DC: SAMHSA. Retrieved from http://www.samhsa.gov/nctic/

Sullivan, H. S. (1947). *Conceptions of modern psychiatry* (2nd ed.). Washington, DC: William Alanson White Psychiatric Foundation.

Sullivan, H. S. (1953). *The interpersonal theory of psychiatry.* New York, NY: W. W. Norton.

Travelbee, J. (1964). What's wrong with sympathy? *The American Journal of Nursing, 6*(1), 68–71.

Travelbee, J. (1966). *Interpersonal aspects of nursing.* Philadelphia, PA: F. A. Davis.

Travelbee, J. (1969). *Intervention in psychiatric nursing: Process in the one-to-one relationship.* Philadelphia, PA: F. A. Davis.

Travelbee, J. (1971). *Interpersonal aspects of nursing* (2nd ed.). Philadelphia, PA: F. A. Davis.

Tyra, P. A. (2008). In memoriam: Ida Jean Orlando Pelletier. *American Psychiatric Nurses Association, 14*(3), 231–232.

U.S. Department of Health and Human Services. (1999). Mental health: A report of the Surgeon General. Rockville, MD: Author. Retrieved from http://profilesnlm.nih.gov/ps/access/NNBBHS.pdf

Vandemark, L. M. (2006). Awareness of self and expanding consciousness: Using nursing theories to prepare theories to prepare nurse-therapist. *Issues in Mental Health Nursing, 27,* 605–615.

Walker, L. O., & Avant, K. C. (2004). *Strategies for theory construction nursing* (4th ed.). Upper Saddle River, NJ: Prentice Hall.

Watson, J. (1979). *Nursing: Philosophy and science of caring.* Boston, MA: Little, Brown.

Watson, J. (1985). *Nursing: Human science and human care—A theory of nursing.* Norwalk, CT: Appleton & Lange.

Watson, J. (1988). *Nursing: Human science and human care—A theory of nursing.* New York, NY: National League for Nursing.

Watson, J. (1995). Post modernism and knowledge development in nursing. *Nursing Science Quarterly, 8*(2), 60–64.

Watson, J. (1996). Watson's theory of transpersonal caring. In P. J. Walker & B. Neuman (Eds.), *Blueprint for the use of nursing models: Education research, practice, and administration* (pp. 141–184). New York, NY: National League for Nursing Press.

Watson, J. (1997). The theory of human caring: Retrospective and beyond. *Nursing Science Quarterly, 10*(1), 49–52.

Watson, J. (1999). *Postmodern nursing and beyond.* Edinburgh: Churchill Livingstone.

Watson, J. (2002). *Instruments for assessing and measuring caring in nursing and health sciences.* New York, NY: Springer.

Watson, J. (2003). Love and caring: Ethics of face and hand. *Nursing Administration Quarterly, 27*(3), 197–202.

Watson, J. (2005). *Caring science as sacred science.* Philadelphia, PA: F. A. Davis.

Watson, J. (2007). Theory evolution. Retrieved from http//www2.uchs.edu/son/caring/content/evolution.asp

Watson, J., & Smith, M. (2002). Transpersonal caring science and the science of unitary human beings: A transtheoretical discourse for nursing knowledge development. *International Journal of Advanced Nursing, 37*(5), 452–461.

Whall, A. L. (2002). The unrecognized paradigm shift in nursing: Implications, problems, and possibilities. *Nursing Outlook, 50*(2), 72–76.

Whall, A. L. (2005, January/February). "Lest we forget": An issue concerning the doctorate in nursing practice (DNP). *Nursing Outlook, 53*(1), 1.

Wheeler, K., & Haber, J. (2004). Development of psychiatric mental health nurse practitioner competencies: Opportunities for the 21st century. *Journal of the American Psychiatric Nurses Association, 10*(3), 129–138.

Whitwell, D. (1999). The myth of recovery from mental illness. *Psychiatric Bulletin, 23,* 621–622.

Zuzelo, P. R. (2011). Evidence-based nursing and qualitative research: A partnership imperative for real-world practice. In P. L. Munhall (Ed.), *Nursing research: A qualitative perspective* (5th ed., pp. 533–552). Sudbury, MA: Jones & Bartlett Learning.

# CHAPTER 13

# Environmental Philosophy and Theories

*Steven J. Vanderheiden*

---

## Introduction

Environmental theories fall into one of two distinct but related categories: explanatory and normative. *Explanatory* environmental theories offer an account of the nature of various environmental phenomena, their relationship to human life, and the causal connections between the two. Anthropogenic climate change, for example, is a phenomenon that depends on an explanatory theory that posits climatic changes are a result of human activities and affect human welfare. This theory seeks to explain the role that various human activities play in causing and being affected by climate change, although in its strictly explanatory sense it prescribes no particular response to the phenomenon. *Normative* environmental theories are, by contrast, prescriptive, in that they posit some set of values and recommend action on the basis of those values. Arguments in favor of endangered species protection laws made on grounds of the important value of biodiversity offer an example of the application of normative environmental theory, at least insofar as theory-based reasons are offered on behalf of biodiversity.

While explanatory environmental theories are primarily based on facts and normative environmental theories primarily on values, these two kinds of theories are often dependent on each other, because most explanatory theories contain at least some implicit or explicit normative elements and all normative theories depend on at least some explanatory theories. People who defend anticruelty laws to protect nonhuman animals, for example, typically invoke explanatory claims concerning animal cognition and sentience, asserting that animals actually do suffer when treated in certain ways. Those working on primarily explanatory questions concerning animal cognition and sentience often do so with the recognition that normative judgments about how animals should be treated follow directly from their empirical theoretical research. Without the explanatory theories, there would be no grounds for believing that people could do anything to cause nonhuman animals to experience something qualitatively similar to human suffering, which is both a physical and psychological response to some loss or injury. Without the normative theories, there would be no grounds for calling this avoidable suffering wrong or unjust.

When fact-based claims aimed primarily at explanation are bundled together with normative value judgments in a coherent theoretical system, they produce environmental discourses (Dryzek, 1997). These discourses characterize problems in certain ways, focusing attention on particular attributes of some phenomena at the expense of others, and generating support for one or another prescription as the appropriate way to address the problem at hand. Some problems are described quite differently by competing environmental discourses, with divergent remedial prescriptions issuing from the distinct conceptual lens through which different discourses shed light on the problem.

For example, the problems of natural resources depletion and pollution engender a range of environmental discourses that offer various diagnoses of the root causes of these problems or, conversely, dispute their status as problems in the first place. These diagnoses of the causes or nature of environmental problems prompt recommendations for various courses of action that presumably follow from the combination of facts and values they posit.

Notably, some people find the problems of pollution and depletion to be the inevitable result of a human population that has grown too large for the carrying capacity of the planet; according to this perspective, pollution and resource depletion may be viewed as the symptoms of an overtaxed habitat, akin to the way that other animals overshoot their optimal populations and in so doing create environmental problems that threaten some of their members. Based on this discourse, which depends crucially on the idea of ecological limits to growth for its explanatory theory, the appropriate response to such problems is to limit or reduce the human population.

Other people see these problems as being caused primarily by overconsumption of resources by the affluent; to relieve these pressures, they counsel that big consumers scale back their consumption activities. Still other discourses lead to a diagnosis of problems such as those resulting from market failures, where resources are depleted because they are underpriced or heavily subsidized and pollution results from environmental externality. Yet others deny that resources are, in fact, being depleted or that pollution represents any serious threat to human health or welfare. Driving these various judgments are different explanatory theories and value systems, which together work to capture the essence of a problem and identify its proper solution.

While environmental theories are typically applied to ethics (i.e., the distinction between right and wrong actions undertaken by individual persons in the way that each of us interacts with the environment) and to politics (i.e., the just or legitimate rules or courses of action for public institutions and collective action as these relate to the environment), the interaction between facts and values within environmental theories is also instructive for many healthcare decisions. An ethical question that depends on environmental theories might concern the moral permissibility of eating tuna caught with drift nets that also snare and drown dolphins; in such a case, consumer demand for the tuna that is not "dolphin safe" endangers an intelligent aquatic mammal that many think deserves some of the same protections that are afforded to humans by virtue of its similarity to us. A question for political theory might concern the limits on the allowable release into the air or water of known toxins such as sulfur dioxide or mercury, to be enforced by regulatory agencies like the Environmental Protection Agency, or the justice problems associated with locating toxic waste facilities near minority communities. Traditionally, ethical questions have been considered the provenance of environmental ethicists working in philosophy departments, while political questions have been addressed by political theorists working in political science departments. More recently, however, these disciplinary boundaries have been challenged by theorists on both sides, who often contend that ethics and politics are so intimately intertwined that such jurisdictional distinctions between them are increasingly irrelevant. If some action is morally wrong, they assert, this is relevant to politics, and vice versa.

This chapter introduces and briefly discusses several families of environmental theories, along with the implications of each family for ethical and political theories. Where relevant, implications of these environmental theories for policy making are considered. After surveying theories based on ecological limits, environmental value, holistic analysis, and distributive justice, current developments in environmental theories and their application to contemporary problems are briefly considered.

## Ecological Limits Theories

The first generation of normative environmental theories called attention to the finite stock of natural resources and capacity of the environment to assimilate pollution, drawing inferences for humans from laws of nature that were seen as applying to all species in similar ways. In one of the first works of this kind, Rachel Carson's (1962) largely explanatory work on pesticides and bird mortality called attention to the widespread dissemination of toxins within the environment and the often deadly consequences of human attempts to control aspects of the natural world.

Even more notably, Paul Ehrlich's (1968) population analysis and the "limits of growth" thesis proposed by the Club of Rome, a nonprofit international organization (Meadows, Meadows, Randers, & Behrens, 1972), established the idea of *carrying capacity* as a scientific concept with profound normative implications. According to this notion, ecological systems have the capacity to support a finite population of any given species, but beyond this threshold further growth in population is accompanied by ecological stress, decline in support capacity, ecological collapse, and the dying off of populations that "overshoot" the carrying capacity of their natural habitats. According to Ehrlich (1968), just as deer populations tend to expand beyond carrying capacity when their natural predators are eradicated, only to die back as available food becomes insufficient to support a growing population, so humans may also face ecological crises if population growth rates remained unchecked. The Club of Rome expanded this analysis through a sophisticated computer model that demonstrated increasing scarcity in a wide range of natural resources and ecological services, predicting future calamity if current trends were not corrected.

Garrett Hardin's (1968) analysis of "the tragedy of the commons" emerged from this limits literature, defending draconian intrusions into reproductive freedoms as the only solution to the population problem, which he characterized as a collective action problem that results from the absence of ownership in the environmental commons. More recent contributions to ecological limits theory include analyses of individual and group environmental impacts through the ecological footprint, which measures the resource use and waste production of a person or group based on the amount of land that would be needed to support that person's or group's consumption habits (Wackernagel & Rees, 1998). As with the first generation of ecological limits scholarship, the empirical analysis of ecological footprints—which scholars have calculated for most nations based on aggregate consumption and pollution patterns, and which several online calculators estimate for individual persons—implies specific moral judgments about permissible shares of resource production and waste assimilation capacity for each and posits that insidious harm ensues when those shares are exceeded. Recognizing an ecological limit may involve empirical measurement and projection from current trends, but it also contains a moral judgment about how persons or groups ought to control their behavior.

Ehrlich's work contains a strong prescription for sustainable population sizes, and the Club of Rome's analysis does so for sustainable consumption patterns. Ecological footprint analysis updates the role of ecological limits in setting the moral constraints on human action by noting the footprint size that is sustainable for a given population and then implicitly condemning environmental impacts that exceed this threshold. As environmental theory, then, ecological limits approaches derive implicit norms from observable facts combined with a concern for the future consequences of continuing trends, drawing their normative force from this tight connection between facts and values. If people want to avoid outcomes that all agree would be calamitous (e.g., famine, intensified conflicts over increasingly scarce resources), they suggest that patterns of behavior that the environment cannot support indefinitely must be altered. Scientific study of ecology yields the insights necessary for sustainable human living on the planet, but it also reveals the extent to which many current human activities are unsustainable and predicts dire future consequences of imprudent current action. Such theories, therefore, contribute to a discourse of environmental concern that Dryzek (1997) termed "survivalist" because of its focus on the necessary conditions for continued human survival on earth.

## Environmental Value Theories

The second generation of environmental theories developed accounts of value that encompass nonhumans or the environment itself as morally considerable or worthy of respect (Attfield, 1987; Taylor, 1986), giving rise to the academic field of *environmental ethics*. Value theory lies at the root of any normative claim about what ought to be done in personal or political life: It offers an account of what is genuinely important and why, of interests that must be taken into account in decision making, and of how various things or states of affairs figure into a larger hierarchy of value. Theories of environmental value aim to extend the moral value that is commonly attributed only to human beings and their experiences beyond humanity to other entities, typically supposing that the root cause of environmentally destructive behavior is a failure to adequately recognize the harm to valuable nature that such action causes. Thus these theories bring previously excluded entities into the domain of ethics, decrying as wrong environmentally harmful actions that might previously have been condemned as imprudent but not immoral, and conferring moral status on nonhumans of various sorts, depending on the approach.

While utilitarian ethics has long held all sentient creatures to be morally valuable by virtue of their ability to experience pain, most moral and political philosophy prior to the advent of such approaches simply denied that nonhumans have any morally relevant interests. This conventional approach, now termed *anthropocentrism* for its assumption that only humans and their experiences have intrinsic value, was challenged by the hedonistic utilitarianism of Jeremy Bentham (1879/2007) more than two centuries ago, but the project of expanding ethics beyond human interests remained obscure until the latter half of the 20th century. Bentham's expanded moral community included the higher mammals with sufficiently advanced nervous systems that could feel pain; other approaches to environmental value theory expanded that community even further to include all or nearly all animals (Regan, 1983), all living things (Taylor, 1986), or whole ecosystems (Callicott, 1989; Leopold, 1949). In so doing, these new environmental theories challenged anthropocentrism in ethics, either on the basis of ontological claims about what constitutes a relevant difference between humans and other animals (Singer, 1975) or on the basis of empirical evidence concerning the experiences of other beings.

At the center of this challenge was a contested concept—*intrinsic* value, which nonanthropocentric environmental theories posited is at the core component of all normative judgment. Intrinsic value can, therefore, be contrasted with *instrumental* value. Things can be valuable in the latter sense when a person subjectively values them for some purpose that presumably reduces to human welfare;

in contrast, things that are valuable in the former sense need no further referent to a human who values them for their service to human welfare because they are valuable in themselves. Proponents of anthropocentric value theories admit that land or nonhuman animals can have value, but they insist that this value is only instrumental to human welfare or that the capacity to confer value (a cognitive and subjective process through which estimates of worth are made) is attributable only to humans. For example, it might be seen as wrong under anthropocentric ethical theories to kill someone's dog or despoil a person's property, in that these nonhuman things are seen as having some value that would be lost through such actions, but their owners—rather than the dog or land itself—are the ones wronged by such actions. According to this view, a person can have moral duties *with respect to* nonhumans (e.g., to refrain from destroying), but cannot have duties *to* those nonhumans, because they lack intrinsic value and, therefore, do not have moral status.

According to anthropocentric value theories, nonhuman nature (including individual plants or animals or whole ecosystems) has no morally relevant interests or good of its own, although persons may have interests in nature. It might be wrong to clear-cut a forest if this practice destroys someone's aesthetic appreciation of a striking landscape, because human aesthetic experience can have moral value; even so, the forest has no value of its own, independent of this experience. Also, the wrongness of clearing a forest would depend on other sources of instrumental human value, such as that provided by the lumber and wood products yielded by timber harvests. Needless to say, the negative impacts of deforestation on other species would not be considered morally relevant by these accounts, except insofar as some lost species might in some way affect some human welfare interests.

Some environmental ethicists and political theorists have identified these kinds of anthropocentric value theories as the root cause of environmental degradation, suggesting that the failure to recognize intrinsic value in nature leads humans to exploit rather than conserve it. Things other than humans can be of intrinsic value, they argue, and, therefore, can be the object of moral obligations or political responsibilities, apart from any effect that they might have on humans or their welfare (Goodin, 1992). Sometimes the opposing value theory to anthropocentrism is termed *ecocentrism* (for being ecosystem centered) and sometimes it is called *biocentrism* (life centered); both notions expand the notion of intrinsic value beyond humanity. Baird Callicott (1984) goes so far as to identify nonanthropocentrism with the scholarly field of environmental ethics, rejecting humanistic ethics as incompatible with ecological analysis and environmental protection. Robyn Eckersley (1992) subtitled her seminal book on environmental political theory "Toward an Ecocentric Approach" in recognition of her critique that anthropocentric political theories could not be reconciled with strong environmental protection.

Merely asserting that things other than humans contain intrinsic value does not by itself provide much guidance for environmental decision making, unless different kinds or sources of value can be meaningfully compared. For example, the construction of a hydroelectric dam that brings a new source of inexpensive electricity to a city but causes the extinction of an endangered species may not necessarily be wrong simply because that species is recognized as intrinsically valuable. The judgment made ultimately depends, instead, on how the value of cheap power for humans compares with the value of the threatened species.

Although few theorists had made serious attempts to develop a taxonomy of value that could make these kinds of comparisons feasible, Peter Singer (1975) argued that the life of a dog does have moral value, but less than that of a typical human life. Employing an updated version of Bentham's utilitarian ethics that treats pleasure as valuable and pain as bad, such that all sentient creatures have a moral interest in maximizing pleasure and minimizing pain, Singer claims that it would be morally permissible to kill a dog rather than a human if one or the other must die (if, for example, starving people and dogs on a lifeboat could be saved if they were to eat one from among their number), given the additional disutility that a human person would suffer in anticipation of his or her killing and the additional sorrow that this fate would cause for the person's family and friends. In this kind of analysis, the respective moral worth of persons and dogs depends on facts about their cognitive capacities and neural transmitters. Such facts assist in determining which of two valuable beings is more valuable than the other, which in turn dictates how ethical dilemmas are resolved.

Environmental value theories have been successful in critiquing anthropocentric biases in conventional ethical and political theories and calling attention to the pressing need to inform decision making with values that recognize the importance of human reliance on the natural world. In doing so, such approaches have spawned the scholarly fields of environmental ethics and political theory, and debates over value theory continue unabated in the scholarly journals from both fields. More recent work in both fields has turned from primarily ontological and meta-theoretical questions about value theory to the applied ethics and political theory topics through which such theories make their critical analyses. This shift in focus has been partly pragmatic and largely a result of the success of earlier scholarly work on value theory. Many philosophers now accept that nonhumans have noninstrumental value or interests that cannot be reduced to human welfare but wonder how such an account of value might inform potential solutions to current environmental problems.

## Holistic Theories

Individualistic environmental value theories constitute one approach to environmental theory, in that they aim to challenge the common presumption that things other than humans can be of intrinsic value and have moral worth. Their influence can be seen in the social movement for animal rights, for example, which asserts this sort of intrinsic value on behalf of nonhuman animals that are used in scientific research or raised on factory farms.

A subset of such theories goes even further in challenging the conventional individualistic basis of ethics by claiming that groups or whole ecosystems can have value of their own, beyond the sum of their constituent individual parts. For example, advocates of this position claim that an entire species is more valuable than all of its individual members, particularly when that species is threatened with extinction. To invoke a widely discussed case, the loss of a single snail darter may not be significant enough to halt a major construction project near its habitat, presuming that the project confers benefits to humans that outweigh any such loss, and as long as the entire species of snail darters is not threatened with extinction. When that individual snail darter is the last of its kind, however, the loss is often thought to be greater, perhaps trumping the project's economic value. Hence, legislation such as the U.S. Endangered Species Act confers no particular value on individual members of unthreatened species but places very high value on threatened or endangered species taken as a whole. Because an entire species represents an evolutionary line that cannot be replaced if it disappears, in the same way that an individual member of that species can be replaced by another member if one dies, its loss is viewed as more serious and weighty according to holistic environmental theories.

Perhaps the most famous of holistic environmental theories is Aldo Leopold's (1949) land ethic, which places ultimate moral value on whole ecosystems rather than on particular species or individual plants or animals. According to Leopold's core moral principle, "a thing is right if it tends to preserve the stability, integrity, and beauty of the biotic community. It is wrong if it tends otherwise" (p. 272). In contrast with individualistic ethics, where right and wrong are defined in terms of effects on individuals, Leopold's holism assumes that the whole "biotic community" is the relevant unit of analysis. Thus something might be right in that it is good for the whole system yet bad for one or more individual members of that community. For example, Gary Varner (1998) defends the "therapeutic hunting" of "management species" such as deer populations as bad for the individual deer that are culled in management efforts but good for the larger population of deer of which these individuals are part and also for the ecosystem on which that population depends. To the extent that Leopold's holistic value theory assumes the welfare of entire ecosystems to be more important than the welfare of their constituent members, as Callicott argues that it should, it is "holistic with a vengeance" (Callicott, 1989, p. 87).

Holistic theories need not necessarily posit that the interests of whole systems trump those of their individual members, and so they may avoid this call for sacrifice of individuals on behalf of whole systems that Callicott endorses. One might instead interpret Leopold's land ethic as asserting the moral considerability of ecosystems without in any way diminishing the moral importance of each system's individual members (Warren, 2000), much as Christopher Stone's (1974) assertion of the moral considerability of trees did not undermine the moral importance of the persons who might use those trees as resources.

Ultimately, however, such attempts to resolve the tension between holistic and individualistic value theories undermine the ability of ethical systems built with such value theories as their foundation to resolve hard cases where individual and systemic interests conflict. While still popular in some circles, such as among those philosophers embracing "deep ecology" (Devall & Sessions, 2001), holistic environmental theories have been significantly tempered by their former supporters in response to charges of advocating "environmental fascism." Today, they are more ecumenically structured, but less action guiding, in their effort to balance the sometimes competing interests of individuals and whole systems.

## Justice Theories

Whereas the previously mentioned approaches to environmental theory aim primarily to revise conventional ethics in order to take account of nonhumans in moral decision making, several other approaches to environmental theory apply to the domain of political theory and employ anthropocentric value theories when approaching environmental problems. Rather than invoking ethics on behalf of environmental protection, they work within concepts in political theory such as justice, understood in its distributive sense. *Distributive justice* theories take the distribution of "goods" and "bads" among persons to be the primary subject matter for justice, articulating principles for how those "goods" and "bads" should be distributed. For example, John Rawls's (1971) well-known account states that social goods such as income and wealth should be distributed so that inequalities in shares held by various individuals are justified only insofar as this inequality benefits society's least advantaged. Others (Anderson, 1999; Miller, 2001; Walzer 1984) working in the distributive justice tradition claim that justice requires that a basic minimum of important social goods be available to all, or that inequalities of one kind of goods (e.g., wealth) not lead to inequalities in other kinds of goods (e.g., health). Regardless, these approaches assume that justice is an attribute of relationships between and among human persons and communities, rather than attempting to extend the concept to nonhumans.

Early efforts to theorize environmental problems through concepts of justice arose from Murray Bookchin's (1982) school of social ecology, which concentrated on the way that class divisions were often reflected in environmental problems and which saw sustainability as a component of social justice. Like social ecologists, ecofeminists (Plumwood, 1993; Warren, 2000) theorize that the root causes of environmental degradation are based in domination, whether toward women by men, toward developing countries by industrialized ones, or toward nature by industrial societies. Such theories avoid an explicitly distributive conception of justice, however.

Working within distributive justice theory, some environmental theorists have more recently seized upon the apparent injustice of the way that important environmental goods and hazards have been distributed among persons and groups of people. Robert Bullard (1990) coined the term *environmental racism* to describe the way in which hazardous waste facilities in the United States have been disproportionately located in poor neighborhoods largely populated by people of color, implicitly accusing the site selection decisions for such facilities of being unjust and giving rise to the *environmental justice* social movement. This movement later expanded the justice frame to include analysis of inequities in group recognition and participation, as well as injustice in distribution (Schlosberg, 2007), but remained primarily concerned with equity issues among human communities.

Justice-based environmental theories have been particularly prominent in areas related to the allocation of natural resources or the production of pollution, where those theories are able to specify what is unjust about certain patterns of resource use or pollution. Besides environmental justice concerns about connections between race and toxic waste, for example, justice-based environmental theories have been applied to the distribution of costs in global climate policy (Vanderheiden, 2008) and variability in the ecological footprints of nations and individual persons (Dobson, 1990). Social movements invoking the goals of "climate justice" or "environmental justice" demonstrate power or justice-based environmental discourses and the theories on which they have been constructed. Although most such theories do not explicitly posit environmental values that are distinct from human concerns for justice, often they do endorse a program whereby environmental harm is avoided and nonhuman interests accommodated, even if the latter are not recognized as intrinsically valuable. Because they rely upon normative theories that were originally developed to articulate justified relationships among human persons and communities rather than between humans and nature, they can be more accurately called theories *for* the environment rather than *of* the environment. Nonetheless, they are action guiding and are regarded as a useful basis on which to theorize obligations with respect to the environment, and from which to design the institutions of a sustainable society.

## Summary

By the nature of professionalization within the scholarly fields of environmental ethics and political theory, a wide variety of apparently competing normative theories have been developed over the past four decades. Most such theories can be grouped into one of the categories described in this chapter, although proponents of competing theories within each of those categories continue to subject the validity of this taxonomy to debate. From the outside, it appears that scholars are deeply divided on questions of environmental theory and that no consensus on what constitutes the most plausible contemporary view exists. Within the field, however, there is considerable consensus on judgments concerning what are considered environmental problems and even rough agreement on how to solve those problems (Norton, 1991), even if scholars continue to disagree about why such issues are problems and what the best philosophical approach to theorizing those problems might be.

Nearly all scholars currently working within environmental ethics and political theory agree that the manner in which people understand value affects their behavior. Given this understanding, they seek to enlighten people about the nonhuman things that are, in fact, valuable to them, if not also intrinsically so. Most people agree on the critical need for reforming unsustainable practices, viewing sustainability as constitutive of right action and a just society, even as they disagree about the best way to incorporate such concerns into contemporary ethical and political theories. All environmental philosophers agree that environmental decision making should be more reflexive when it affects the environment, whether such decisions are personal or social and institutional, because narrowly instrumental action is widely viewed as responsible for most, if not all, current environmental problems.

Environmental theories of various kinds, like all normative theories, are designed to guide action and to bring our facts in line with our values and our values in line with facts. In this sense, they are consonant with other efforts to bring abstract knowledge to bear on practical problems in the world, and to resolve those problems in light of rationality and concern for others.

## Discussion Questions

1. How are facts and values related in environmental theories, and how might this relationship parallel decision making in healthcare ethics or allocation issues?

2. To what extent are environmental issues also issues of human health, and vice versa? Is environmental protection an aspect of public health?

3. Caring for the natural world is like caring for ill patients in some respects but different in others. Physicians and nurses often can know the wishes of the patients whom they treat, but can humans know how the natural world prefers to be treated? Insofar as we must hypothesize about the latter, does the way that we think about the best interests of patients who are unable to communicate their wishes resemble the way that nature's interests are considered?

## References

Anderson, E. (1999). What's the point of equality? *Ethics, 109*, 287–337.

Attfield, R. (1987). *A theory of value and obligation.* London, UK: Croom Helm.

Bentham, J. (2007). *An introduction to the principles of morals and legislation.* Mineola, NY: Dover. (Original work published 1879.)

Bookchin, M. (1982). *The ecology of freedom: The emergence and dissolution of hierarchy*. Palo Alto, CA: Cheshire Books.

Bullard, R. (1990). *Dumping in Dixie: Race, class, and environmental quality*. Boulder, CO: Westview Press.

Callicott, J. B. (1984). Non-anthropocentric value theory and environmental ethics. *American Philosophical Quarterly, 21*(4), 299–309.

Callicott, J. B. (1989). *In defense of the land ethic: Essays in environmental philosophy*. Albany, NY: SUNY Press.

Carson, R. (1962). *Silent spring*. London, UK: Hamish Hamilton; New York, NY: Fawcett Crest.

Devall, B., and Sessions, G. (2001). *Deep ecology: Living as if nature mattered*. Layton, UT: Gibbs Smith.

Dobson, A. (1990). *Green political thought*. London, UK: HarperCollins.

Dryzek, J. S. (1997). *The politics of the earth: Environmental discourses*. New York, NY: Oxford University Press.

Eckersley, R. (1992). *Environmentalism and political theory: Toward an ecocentric approach*. London, UK: UCL Press.

Ehrlich, P. R. (1968). *The population bomb*. New York, NY: Ballantine Books.

Goodin, R. (1992). *Green political theory*. Oxford, UK: Blackwell.

Hardin, G. (1968). The tragedy of the commons. *Science, 162*, 1243–1248.

Leopold, A. (1949). *A Sand County almanac*. New York, NY: Oxford University Press.

Meadows, D. H., Meadows, D. L., Randers, J., & Behrens, W. W. (1972). *The limits to growth*. New York, NY: New American Library.

Miller, D. (2001). *Principles of social justice*. Cambridge, MA: Harvard University Press.

Norton, B. (1991). *Toward unity among environmentalists*. New York, NY: Oxford University Press.

Plumwood, V. (1993). *Feminism and the mastery of nature*. London, UK: Routledge.

Rawls, J. (1971). *A theory of justice*. Cambridge, MA: Belknap Press.

Regan, T. (1983). *The case for animal rights*. London, UK: Routledge & Kegan Paul.

Schlosberg, D. (2007). *Defining environmental justice: Theories, movements, nature*. New York, NY: Oxford University Press.

Singer, P. (1975). *Animal liberation*. New York, NY: Random House.

Stone, C. D. (1974). *Should trees have standing?* Los Angeles, CA: Kaufmann.

Taylor, P. (1986). *Respect for nature*. Princeton, NJ: Princeton University Press.

Vanderheiden, S. (2008). *Atmospheric justice: A political theory of climate change*. New York, NY: Oxford University Press.

Varner, G. E. (1998). *In nature's interests? Interests, animals rights, and environmental ethics*. New York, NY: Oxford University Press.

Wackernagel, M., & Rees, W. (1998). *Our ecological footprint: Reducing human impact on the earth*. Vancouver, BC: New Society.

Walzer, M. (1984). *Spheres of justice: A defense of pluralism and equality*. New York, NY: Basic Books.

Warren, K. (2000). *Ecofeminist philosophy: A Western perspective of what it is and why it matters*. Lanham, MD: Rowman & Littlefield.

# Economic Theories

*Sherry Hartman*

## Introduction

"It is an exciting time to be writing this chapter. The public debate over health-care reform is raging." This was the opening statement of this chapter in the first edition of this text, and it still holds true with this second edition. Since the publication of the first edition, Congress has passed historical legislation with the enactment of the Patient Protection and Affordable Care Act, commonly called the Affordable Care Act (ACA) or Obamacare. Throughout the political and public debate, differing economic philosophies and theories held by the policy makers were evident, and they were often at odds with one another. Controversy and resistance were pervasive and led to a Supreme Court ruling on the legislation. It was deemed constitutional and implementation continues amid both support and opposition. Both before and after passage of the ACA, the public paid more attention to and became more aware of and concerned with healthcare delivery in our country. However, commentaries continue to indicate, first, that the general public misunderstands the U.S. healthcare system, and second, that little is known about health economics and health care as a unique market situation. Having faced many classrooms of "citizens" aspiring to be nurses, I struggled often to create some enthusiasm among undergraduate nursing students for economic ways of thinking about health care and nursing. It was not so long ago that two nurse theorists expressed concern about a "disconnection between corporate executives as economic decision makers and practicing nurses as providers of human care" (Turkel & Ray, 2000, p. 308).

The climate of the last few years has made it easier to persuade nurses that they have a stake in the public decisions being made and that they need to understand the economic arguments put forth either to justify or oppose the enacted reform, its continuing implementation, and new proposals. Advanced practice nurses, especially, beyond worrying about basic clinical skills and becoming licensed, have the professional experience to see that economic concerns and mandates shape their practice every day and affect the lives of their patients. They have to join the conversation. A favorite quip to my students was that they cannot join an ongoing conversation and say anything meaningful unless they have knowledge of what was said before they arrived. In this chapter, I attempt to lay the groundwork for taking part in the conversations based on economic theory.

Economic theory of market competition increasingly has been a major topic in the healthcare conversation, following on the heels of a general trend in the United States to view the market as efficient and government as inefficient. One economist has described this circumstance as a cyclical American romance with "utopian laissez-faire" (Kuttner, 1997, p. 4). Any discussion of the situation of health care begins with the process of collecting data on soaring costs, calling into question whether higher costs are related to higher quality, and making dire predictions of the consequences of failing to control costs. Some analysts and policy makers claim the competitive market as the superior option to bring efficiency to the system, as well as greater social welfare. The Reagan presidency was noted for early reforms relying on managed competition. Evidence in the 1990s indicated that increased competition did slow the growth of costs but had an ambiguous effect on efficiency, with concerns being voiced that consumers and the public were not receiving quality for their money spent and about the corporatization of health care. The numbers of uninsured and underinsured continued to increase, accompanied by claims that this increase is partially related to increased competition among insurance providers. The deep recession of the latter years of the first decade of the 2000s worsened the statistics and created a more urgent need to make decisions about healthcare resources in the United States. Implementation of the ACA addresses increased coverage, but there are conflicting claims about its effect on costs. A disappointment for many during the reform struggles was the failure to achieve universal coverage or a single-payer system. The involvement of employers and reliance on the competitive market of insurers and providers remain the mainstays of our delivery system.

Economics is considered both a social science and a foundational form of knowledge. All financial management is ultimately built on economics. In fact, accounting and finance are applied areas of microeconomics. Economic theory and research also guide policy makers, yet policy is but one familiar application of economic theory. Because it is a science of human behavior, it serves as a framework for exploring diverse phenomena. For example, Wagoner (2012) interestingly used previous economic theory to explore the generation of economic theory. Exploring the relationships between economic theory and nursing administration research, Jones and Yoder (2010) found that economic theory is useful in the study of allocation of scarce nursing resources in acute care hospitals. In this chapter, I aim to provide advanced practice nurses with broad and general understandings of the lens through which such varied application occurs. Using Fawcett's (1998) definitions, the chapter will look at how economists approach and examine phenomena of interest, conceptual models, and grand theories. It will also introduce the area of economic analysis, which is an application of economic concepts considered increasingly necessary in healthcare cost analysis and control, included in parts of the ACA, and thus, of interest to nursing.

The steps in theory analysis provided by nurse theorists (e.g., Fawcett, 2005; Parse, 2005) were inspiration for the discussion sequence in this chapter. Theories are best understood when attention is paid to their history and assumptions before turning to the concepts and relationships that make up the theory content. I cannot hope to present a comprehensive evaluation and critique of economic theory in this brief chapter, but I believe this is a helpful starting point.

Some healthcare economists raise serious objections to the prospect of relying on competition in health care, as economic theory would prescribe. It is especially important for advanced practice nurses to be aware of the potential problems with market competition. Rice (1998) is one economist widely referenced for his arguments showing the misunderstanding of economic theory as it applies to health. He stated, "It is vitally important that we get our theory right when applying economics to health—and the key to this understanding is the validity of the assumptions" (p. 6). After identifying assumptions and presenting the major concepts, several core assumptions that support concepts, relationships, and principles of marketplace competition are critiqued and then rationale is given for why they are invalid, often making specific reference to the case of health services.

# The History and Beginnings of Mainstream Economics

Although humankind has long engaged in reflection related to commerce and market exchange, modern economic thought developed only as society became increasingly industrialized. The move away from agrarian relationships to an industrial economy resulted in more socially interdependent relationships. Economics sought to understand the exchange of resources, which were assumed to be limited. Scarcity of resources is a basic assumption of economics. *Scarcity* is the concept of finite resources and infinite wants. Broadly, it means not having enough resources to satisfy all the needs or wants of humankind. Scarcity also means that resources have alternative uses. What is not spent on health care can be spent on food, education, recreation, and the like. Scarcity leads to rationing or competition for the limited resources.

Without scarcity, the science of economics would not exist. When people freely have all they want and need, there are no choices or exchanges to make, and no trade-offs among possible alternatives, and, therefore, no economic problem. The healthcare debate occurring today would not be necessary if there was no scarcity of health resources and no unmet needs for health care.

The phenomenon of interest for economics is human behavior in the choices and interactions taken to overcome the problem of scarce resources with alternative uses. Interestingly, one nurse scholar has grasped the assumption of scarcity itself as a problem and urges the use of quantum physics theory to assume abundance instead; with this perspective, we would see the human situation differently (Dunham-Taylor, 2005). For the most part, economists do not question that the assumption of scarcity is valid, although abundance economics is not unheard of in the field and has even been considered discussion worthy at Harvard University (Heskett, 2006). Mainstream scarcity economics is addressed in this chapter.

Contemporary economics consists of many schools and branches, with variants existing within even orthodox economics. A significant amount of work in mainstream economics is applied economics using simple theoretical concepts. However, both applied and theoretical economics can be identified as microeconomics or macroeconomics. As implied, the difference between the two fields lies in the scale of focus.

- *Microeconomics* explains the behavior of individual markets and small economic units, such as individual household consumers, firms that produce goods or services, or governmental agencies, to see how they behave within a market. Individual behaviors often are considered in the aggregate. Areas examined could include human capital, competition policy, problems of industry, and the role of government in resource allocation. For example, microeconomic study of firms in the market underlies financial concepts such as normal profit, fixed costs, and variable costs.
- *Macroeconomics* allows economists to look at the "big picture" market, considering the aggregate functions of all the markets within the larger focus. Such issues as growth, unemployment, monetary policy, deficits, and inflation are of concern in macroeconomics.

Economic theory as it is known today is derived from schools of thought from the last few centuries that have become the building blocks for today's economic thinking. Ideas have been revised and some discarded, only to be revived later. **Table 14-1** offers an abbreviated look at these benchmarks in history. Current thought is commonly called *neoclassical economics*, which builds on the ideas of Keynesian theory and the work of classic thinkers. It is also often called *mainstream economics*. The concepts and principles presented in this chapter come from mainstream economics.

In the history of economics, the specialty of *healthcare economics* is a recently developed field. The origins of this field are credited to Nobel Prize–winning economist Kenneth Arrow (1963) based on his article published in *The American Economic Review* (Peterson, 2001; Savedoff, 2004). Arrow clarified the conceptual distinctions between health and other goals. Those factors

**TABLE 14–1    Major Schools of Thought in Economic Theory**

| | |
|---|---|
| 16th to 17th century: Mercantilism | Accumulation of gold and silver made a nation wealthy, and those who did not have these items naturally could obtain them only by selling more than they bought from abroad. Leaders intervened in the market with tariffs and subsidies to regulate trade and commercial activities. Promoted a materialist perspective. |
| 18th century: Physiocratic | Reaction against the many trade regulations. French theorists opposed promoting trade, saw agriculture as the source of economic wealth, and advocated a laissez-faire policy (minimal government interference). |
| 1776: Classical | Adam Smith publishes *The Wealth of Nations* in 1776. Land, labor, and capital are identified as factors of production contributing to a nation's wealth. The ideal economy is a self-regulating market guided by an "invisible hand," which leads self-interested individuals to produce the greatest good for society. The classical view adopted a laissez-faire policy but disagreed that only agriculture was productive. |
| | David Ricardo focused on income distribution among landowners, workers, and capitalists. Landowners conflict with labor and capital. Population and capital growth pushing against a fixed land supply raises rents and lowers wages and profits. |
| | Thomas Robert Malthus explained low living standards with the idea of diminishing returns. Rapid population growth against limited land meant diminishing returns to labor. Chronic low wages kept the standard of living from rising above the subsistence level for most of the population. Malthus questioned whether a market economy would tend to produce full employment. Unemployment is caused by too much saving, rather than too little spending in the economy. |
| | John Stuart Mill opposed earlier classical thinking that income from the market is necessarily distributed by the market and noted the differences between the two roles of the market. The market is efficient at allocating resources but not at distributing income. Society must intervene in the distribution of income. |

*(continues)*

**TABLE 14-1  Major Schools of Thought in Economic Theory (*Continued*)**

| | |
|---|---|
| 1960s to late 1900s: Marginalists | Added demand as a factor in determining price to the classicists' theory that production costs determine price. Demand depends on satisfaction gained from goods and services. Marginalists offered the basic analytical tools of demand, supply, and utility and developed a framework to use these tools. In a free market, the factors of production receive returns equal to their contribution—an idea used to justify distribution of income: People earn what their labor or property contribute to production. |
| Mid-19th century: Marxists | Capitalism is a phase of development, which will eventually destroy itself. At that point, private property will not exist. All production belongs to labor; workers are exploited by capitalist owners, who deny them a fair share of production. Competition for profit leads to adoption of more machinery. The resulting unemployed will rise up and seize the means of production. |
| Mid-19th century: Institutionalists | Individual behavior reflects a larger social context influenced by cultures. Economic self-interest is rejected as a primary motivation. Institutionalists argued against laissez-faire policy and advocated more equitable income distribution via government intervention and social reform. |
| Mid-19th century: Keynesians | John Maynard Keynes broke with convention with his *General Theory of Employment, Interest and Money* (1936). The Keynesian view argues against the classical view that falling wages and prices in a recession will eventually restore full employment. Instead, low prices and wages are seen as depressing income and preventing spending. Government should intervene in a recession to increase total spending. The Keynesian view remains the core of macroeconomic analysis. |

*Source:* Adapted from SNBCHF. (2013). Major schools of economic theory. Retrieved from http://snbchf.com/economic-theory/major-schools-of-economics/

that differentiate health economics from other areas include amount of government intervention, intractable uncertainty in many areas, asymmetrical information, and externalities. Among his many contributions, Arrow is especially well known for his theoretical insights on the economics of uncertainty. He argued that uncertainties in the incidence of disease and the efficacy of treatments lead to inefficient allocation of resources, which force nonmarket institutions to compensate for these inequalities. Hammer, Haas-Wilson, and Sage (2001) claimed that even decades after the publication of Arrow's seminal article and the introduction of more competitive forces as means to control costs, the same questions remain:

> What is the proper role of markets in delivering health care services? Can we base our health care system exclusively on private competition? What place should be reserved for government or for social mechanisms such as professionalism, nonprofit status or trust? Do these "non-market institutions" help markets overcome uncertainty, or do they replace markets that have failed because of information asymmetry? How does one define the proper boundary between market and non-market institutions? (p. 836)

Such questions fall within the realm of *normative economics*, which advocates for what ought to be and then judges how well the performance of a market or outcome of economic policies conforms to those values. The field of *welfare economics* deals with issues that are considered normative economics. *Positive economics,* in contrast, describes "facts" or "what is." Rice (1998) pointed out that unlike other social sciences, which predominately study and describe how people behave, prescription is more prevalent in positive economics such that "in economics one commonly sees the word 'ought' (e.g., people ought to maximize their utility otherwise they are being 'irrational'; to maximize social welfare a society 'ought' to depend on a competitive marketplace)" (p. 38).

In summary, early classical economists developed a full explanation of abstract, general laws or principles of the operation, functioning, and process of the liberal economy. That economy was a system consisting of free "private" producers, consuming households, and competitive markets. The neoclassical economists developed superior analysis of the economy with fuller solutions to many of the problems. Branches of specialized areas of economics exist, and healthcare economics is a relatively new specialized application of economic thought. However, a consensus that market forces, as theorized by traditional economics, are appropriate for healthcare services delivery is yet to be attained.

## Assumptions of Economic Theory

Advanced practice nurses in select fields are likely to have used clinical applications of some of the assumptions of classical economic theory in the form of social exchange theory. In *social exchange theory*, assumptions that were held about individuals in economic exchange relationships have been adapted to explain human interactions in all social contexts (Bielkiewicz, 2002). In addition to scarcity, as discussed in the previous section, several assumptions are held in economics. Rational behavior is a major assumption. Aspects of assumed rational behavior and other assumptions relevant to health care are summarized in **Table 14–2**. These assumptions will be revisited in the discussion of the concept of market failure, introduced in the following section.

---

**TABLE 14–2    Twelve Assumptions of Economic Theories**

1. There are no externalities of consumption.
2. Individuals know what is best for themselves.
3. Individuals use reason to determine a balance in their choices.
   - They have the cognitive ability.
   - They have the time.
4. Individuals seek to maximize benefits and minimize costs of alternative choices (the most useful product or greatest reward for the lowest price).
5. Individual preferences are revealed by choices.
6. Individual preferences can be ranked.
7. Preferences are determined and stable over time.
8. Consumers have full and perfect information with which to make good choices.
9. Consumers know, with certainty, the results that will follow their choices.
10. Supply and demand are independently determined.
11. No one firm dominates the marketplace.
12. Firms seek to maximize profits.

*Source:* Adapted from Rice, T. (1998). *The economics of health reconsidered.* Chicago, IL: Health Administration Press.

---

# Concepts, Relationships, and Principles in Economic Theories

## Markets

Markets are the means by which buyers and sellers engage in trade. A market economy is based on private ownership of scarce resources. The market facilitates the efficient allocation of scarce resources through interactions of individual buyers and businesses that produce and sell goods or services.

Within the market, consumers seek to maximize their *utility*, which is determined by the bundle of goods they possess. They purchase their ideal bundle of goods based on preferences, the price, and their available resources. Consumers must make *trade-offs*, giving up some of one thing they like to get another thing. When they have reached their maximum utility given their resources, they quit trading.

Producers in the market seek to *maximize profits,* just as consumers seek to maximize utility. The profit motive drives producers' decisions. They purchase inputs and turn them into outputs through a production process. Firms seek to produce as much as they can by using the least costly mix of inputs. The two most important classes of inputs are *labor* and *capital*. Thus, production theory indicates that firms will try to use their inputs in the most efficient way and make output choices to maximize profits. Their actions are also socially desirable in conserving inputs and producing only what consumers will use.

Competition in the marketplace is the mechanism for setting price and quality. Producers compete for buyers of their products. Marketplaces that operate most efficiently will flourish; those that do not have satisfied consumers will close down. Price is the most common basis for competition, but competition can also be based on technical quality, amenities, access, and other factors if prices are stable.

*Efficiency* is an important concept related to production in the market. Efficiency refers to the practice of maximizing the production of goods or services while minimizing the resources required for their production (Penner, 2004). *Technical efficiency* is attained when a firm produces a maximum output with a given amount of inputs. *Economic efficiency* (production efficiency) occurs when the mix of inputs used to produce maximum output is the least costly possibility. Alternatively, given a certain cost for inputs, the outputs are maximized. *Allocative efficiency* entails minimizing the amount and thus the costs of inputs or using a set amount of inputs to produce outputs of greater value. At the level of the economy as a whole, allocative efficiency is a state of the market rather than a firm.

Eventually, an economy could reach the point where it is impossible to make someone better off (better welfare) without making someone else worse off; this is referred to as *Pareto optimality*. According to economic theory of the market, under ideal conditions a free or competitive market will reach a *competitive equilibrium* that is Pareto optimal. However, a Pareto optimal competitive equilibrium ensures only allocative efficiency, not equity. Equilibrium could occur in which one person has nearly all the output, while another has almost no output. Society may be better off with an inefficient use of resources and a better distribution of income (output).

## The Production Possibility Curve

Economic analysis often is carried out under the assumption of economic efficiency. The *production possibility curve* measures the quantities of two goods that have the potential to produce with currently available resources and technology. It is a graphic representation of the trade-offs between the two goods. Points on the curve represent alternative combinations of inputs that will produce the maximum output. Points that lie above the curve are impossible production; points that lie inside the curve represent inefficient production. The production possibility curve depicts possibilities with fixed amounts of resources and technology. If either increases as the result of economic growth, the curve would shift outward to the right, indicating the potential for producing greater amounts of both products.

*Opportunity cost* is a concept related to the trade-offs that are made in the marketplace and made evident on the production possibility curve. A consequence of scarcity is that when resources are used to buy or produce one product, they are not available for other goods. Opportunity cost is the value of the forgone alternative service or product.

## Demand

*Demand* is the force that drives market competition. Demand is the quantity a buyer is willing to purchase at various prices. The amount of a commodity that is produced is determined by the demand for it. In addition, in economic theory, demand forms the basis for evaluating economic welfare. The things people demand are, by definition, those goods and services that allow for their highest level of welfare given their available resources. If all individuals act and choose to maximize their utilities within their incomes, then society as a whole will also be at a welfare maximum.

Demand is represented by a demand schedule of the quantities a buyer is willing to purchase at different prices. When plotted on a graph, these data form a *demand curve*. According to the *law of demand*, as the price goes up, the quantity demanded goes down—an inverse relationship. Two kinds of changes can be depicted with the graph of a demand curve. A *change in the quantity* demanded is a movement *along the demand curve*. If a price changes from $2.00 to $4.00, for example, the quantity demanded moves to the left (down) along the curve, a decrease. A *change in demand* is represented by a *shift in the demand curve*: The quantity demanded will have changed at all prices. A shift of the curve to the *left* will mean that at all possible prices, the quantity demanded is *less*. A *right*ward shift means that at all possible prices, the quantity demanded is *greater*. It is important to keep these differences clear. Only one thing will change the quantity demanded (change along the curve): a change in price. There are several reasons why demand could change and shift.

### Reasons for Demand to Shift

*Shifters* are factors other than price that influence the quantity demanded. Income has a powerful influence: Greater income equals greater demand at all prices. Goods for which changes in demand vary directly with income are called *normal goods*. If an increase in income is related to a decrease in quantity demanded, then the product is labeled as an *inferior good*. Similar to the effect seen with increases in income, insurance increases the quantity of covered services demanded because they are largely paid for by the insurer.

The price of related goods is another demand shifter. A *substitute* is any good that satisfies the same needs as the original product. If the price of a good rises and a substitute is available, demand will decrease for the original good as it is replaced with the substitute. A good can also be related as a *complement*, a good closely related to a specific good or service. If the price goes up for one product, the demand curve for its complement will shift to the left (less demand), and vice versa.

Changes in preferences can shift demand, such as decreased demand for cigarettes as more consumers quit smoking. A shift may also occur from circumstances that change expectations; for example, a recession and fear of unemployment will shift the demand curve for goods with long-term payments to the left. Illness would make a person's demand curve shift to the right, as his or her demand for health care rises at all price levels.

## Utility

*Utility* is a term used by economists to describe the pleasure or satisfaction that a consumer obtains from consumption of goods or services. This subjective measure is dependent on the consumer's tastes, preferences, beliefs, culture, and values. Although the concept of utility is derived from classical utilitarianism, modern economists reject the utilitarian assumption that utility can be measured or that one person's utility can be compared to another's.

The utility received from consuming a particular amount of a good is a consumer's total utility. *Marginal utility* is the addition to total utility that consuming just one more unit of the good or service brings to the individual. The *law of diminishing marginal utility* states that as consumption increases, marginal utility will decrease. Once an individual is saturated, additional consumption adds no additional utility. Eyeglasses are an example. One set provides a certain utility and a second set used as a spare will have a good deal of utility, but a fourth or fifth pair will be of much less use, and a tenth one would hold no utility at all. The notion of marginal utility can also be illustrated with this example. If you have three apples, you have a total utility (enjoyment) from eating all of them. But the third will not be quite as "good" because you are already full—so whatever enjoyment you get is less than others receive. The third apple, then, contributes less to total enjoyment (utility). Marginal utility is what the last (unit) apple added to the total—always the smallest amount of all units (usually—never say "always," because there is always some exception case!).

## Supply

*Supply* is the quantity of a good or service that producers are able and willing to sell at a particular price. Like demand, supply determines market price and quantities. The *law of supply* states that there is a direct relationship between the price of goods and the amount supplied: As price increases, the quantity supplied will increase.

Similar to consumer demand, a seller's quantity supplied can be depicted with a supply schedule and a graph. A change in the quantity supplied is a *movement along the supply curve* because of a change in the price. A change in demand is represented by a *shift of the supply curve*. A shift of an original supply curve to a new curve located to the left results in a reduced supply at all prices. A shift to the right indicates an increased supply at all prices.

### Reasons for Supply to Shift

Several factors can cause a shift in the supply curve. Two notable ones are changes in the prices of inputs and technology. Prices for inputs of labor, materials, and services from facilities can increase the costs of production. If inputs became cheaper, the supply curve would shift to the right and a greater quantity would be supplied at all prices. Conversely, higher prices for supplies would increase costs of production, so the supply curve would shift to the left, indicating less quantity supplied. Cost is highly important to producers. Producers are interested in total costs—the costs of all inputs needed to produce a given level of output, and they are interested in average costs—the total costs of production in a time period divided by the quantity produced in the same period. *Marginal cost* is the increase in total costs given one more unit of output. The *law of increasing costs* maintains that marginal costs increase with increased output, so total costs increase at an increasing rate as production increases. The corollary is the law of diminishing returns.

Technology-related changes can also cause a shift in the supply curve. For example, a technological breakthrough could lower the cost of production, shifting the curve outward to the right. Technology in health care can also be used to increase well-being and comfort, but not to reduce costs of production.

If there is a change in the number of suppliers of a product or if existing suppliers increase their capacity, total supply will increase and shift the supply curve to the right. For any single supplier of several products, if prices for one product fall and it becomes less profitable, the supplier will produce more of the profitable goods, thereby increasing the available supply of those goods and moving the supply curve to the right.

## Equilibrium

Although demand and supply can be analyzed separately, in the market decisions of producers interact with decisions of consumers. Supply and demand set the prices paid by consumers and the quantities of the goods and services delivered to them. When the demand for a product equals the supply for a product, the market is considered to be in *equilibrium*.

A simple narrative of what economists depict with graphs and equations is presented here. To demonstrate equilibrium, the supply and demand curves are plotted on one graph. Equilibrium is the point at which the two curves intersect. The intersection marks a point of equilibrium price and equilibrium quantity supplied. If a demand or supply shift occurs (for any of the reasons discussed previously), the appropriate curve will shift; along with the increase or decrease in either demand or supply, the equilibrium point will change to indicate a higher or lower price and higher or lower quantity demanded, as necessary. The relationships described and often shown on graphs allow economists to gather data and describe and make predictions about market activity. They can answer questions such as these: How has the price of a product changed? What caused it to change? What are the resource allocation implications of the changes?

Disequilibrium occurs when the quantities supplied and demanded do not balance. A *surplus* occurs when there is an excess of quantity supplied or a drop in the quantity demanded. A *shortage* is a market situation in which quantity demanded is greater than quantity supplied. In either of these instances of disequilibrium, market forces are put in play. The automatic actions of buyers and sellers, acting independently of one another, move the market price toward equilibrium. In a shortage, consumers are willing to pay more and then prices rise; in response to these higher prices, suppliers increase the quantity produced. In a surplus, producers lower the price, consumers buy more, and the market moves back to equilibrium.

## Elasticity

In addition to theorizing about how equilibrium prices change as supply and demand change, economists have developed explanations of how demand and supply change in response to changes in prices and incomes. Such responsiveness is measured by *elasticity* of demand or supply. Both can be calculated by formulas:

Price elasticity of demand =
Percent change in quantity demanded ÷ Percent change in price

Price elasticity =
Percent change in quantity supplied ÷ Percent change in price

When the price elasticity of the demand ratio is greater than 1 (the percent change in quantity demanded is greater than the percent change in price), demand is said to be price elastic, meaning that it is very responsive to price changes. If the change in quantity demanded is smaller than the price change, the ratio is less than 1 and demand is price inelastic, or not very responsive to price. The same relationships hold for supply elasticity.

The same formulas can be used to determine income elasticity. To calculate the ratio, one would replace "change in price" with "change in income." Elasticity of demand for income is positive for a normal good: As income rises, demand rises. It is negative for an inferior good: With greater income, there is less demand for the good.

# Market Failure

Economists who advocate the superiority of competitive marketplaces base their preferences on what would happen in an ideal, pure market. Based on the concepts and principles that have been described so far, in an ideal market the following occurs: On the demand side, consumers have a variety of choices for goods and services to purchase. For individual consumers in the health marketplace, these include choices among doctors, hospitals, home health agencies, pharmacies, medical equipment suppliers, and so on. Consumers maximize their satisfaction through self-motivated behavior and pick the quality they want for the price they are willing to pay. Income, tastes, preferences, and information about the product are all factors that influence their choices.

Consumers' choices reveal to suppliers whether their products are priced correctly and are of appropriate quality. Suppliers then adjust the price and quality of their goods to satisfy consumers. For suppliers in a competitive industry, there are strong incentives to minimize the costs of making their products and services. They can then be priced competitively to sell in the marketplace. Suppliers must be innovative and respond to customers' perceptions of quality.

These two behaviors—*benefit-maximizing behaviors of consumers* and *profit-maximizing behaviors of suppliers*—through the mechanism of the market produce the best patterns of production and consumption for society. Because each individual has attained the best outcome that can be personally reached, the welfare of all is socially optimal (Hartman, 2009).

For the market to work in the manner described here, the assumptions listed in Table 14–2 must hold. Economic theorists recognize that the realities of the market often are not in accordance with the assumptions, creating *market failure*. In a failed market, the necessary competition does not occur as it should. Consumers and producers fail to take necessary actions and to make optimal choices. Market mechanisms fail to produce the best outcomes for achieving the best use of resources. Fair allocation, quality and cost control, and setting of social priorities that enhance social welfare—all of which are posited to be the gains associated with an effective market—are not realized. In practice, economic theory does not operate in the pure form; such markets do not exist.

## Assessing Assumptions for Validity

Externalities, addressed in the first assumption in Table 14–2, represent uncompensated consequences to the utility of others when an individual produces or consumes some goods and services (Penner, 2004). The example of vaccinations is cited often to illustrate a positive externality. A consumer who gets a flu shot benefits other members of society who are less likely to get the flu when more people are vaccinated. Public consumption of tobacco creates a negative externality by creating a harmful environment for others.

Rice (1998) presented two more examples of externalities found in the market: one positive, one negative. Through an argument too long to summarize here, he showed that status concerns relative to others create demand in the market, thereby causing an overproduction of goods and services that convey status. Such increased production, however, does not encourage redistribution of wealth such that society is better off. The case of a positive externality is concern about others: An individual wants to help others. The problem with giving, which increases the individual's utility, is that if many individuals want to help others, soon too many people are tempted to become *free riders*. In a competitive market where caring for the poor and giving are voluntary, it will seem to people that their relatively small portion of caring/giving does not have an impact, so they will cease to care/give. As more people follow this path, too little money is redistributed. Rice discussed how taxes and subsidies could be a remedy in this case, but the point made here is the market operates inefficiently because of an externality: One person's desire to give has consequences for others' willingness to do so.

There are several challenges to the assumptions about individual actors in the market system. Assumptions 2 to 4 in Table 14–2 can be considered problems with rational decision making and perfect information. There are reasons to doubt that individuals do know what is best for themselves (Rice, 1998). It takes considerable time to work through Rice's carefully constructed evidence; just a sampling is summarized here with reasons why Assumptions 2, 3, 4, 8, and 9 are not met.

For Assumption 2, being the best to judge one's own welfare, Rice maintained that the many rules of society intended to hinder individual choice demonstrate that we make many public choices for other people for two reasons: (1) we believe that some individuals will not choose wisely on their own and (2) in some cases, there are experts who know more. Some people do not choose wisely because they make decisions to enhance their status; others need protection from their obviously foolish waste of money.

Regarding Assumption 8, having full and perfect information, Rice included these points: (1) authors in journal articles frequently call for more consumer education; (2) studies indicate that patients do not act as consumers by becoming aware of costs, seeking information, and shopping around for services; and (3) little evidence shows that consumers understand concepts of managed care and reimbursement.

On knowing the consequences of consumption decisions, Assumption 9, Rice pointed out that for individuals to determine they made the right choices, they must answer many counterfactual questions, such as "Would the result have been different if I had seen a different physician than the one I sought?" (p. 73). Knowing what is best for themselves and having adequate information about options does not mean that individuals act rationally on that knowledge, as Assumption 3 would indicate. Rice cited several examples, such as informed smokers who continue to smoke, concluding, "When cognitive dissonance is important there is little reason to suppose that people will act in a rational manner" (p. 77). Regarding the expectation that patients are capable of using cognitive skills, Penner (2004) noted some physical and psychological barriers that can exist. In addition, emergency needs do not allow time for reasoned action. Consumers who are not knowledgeable or informed cannot make rational decisions and thus cannot act on their own behalf to maximize their utility, as Assumption 4 indicates.

Another consideration here is the notion of *preferences*. To analyze this issue, Rice (1998) turned to both game theory and the concept of commitment. *Game theory* illustrates the importance of interdependencies between people, making the point that behavior that will make two individuals better off in their real preferences is not the behavior that will reveal those preferences (p. 79). *Commitment* can compel individuals to choose something they are committed to over an alternative that yields a higher welfare such that true preference is not evident. Assumptions 5, 6, and 7 in Table 14–2 are not met.

Assumption 10 brings up the problem of supplier-induced demand. In economic theory, it is assumed that supply and demand are independent of one another. Power lies with the consumer but, in reality, physician suppliers are often viewed as agents acting on behalf of their clients. Thus consumer demand is subject to artificial demand, commonly called *supplier-induced demand*

(Shi & Singh, 2011). In some cases, physicians own laboratories and invest in healthcare organizations, which can affect their impartiality in recommending the use of those resources. This problem, according to Rice (1998), is one of the most studied in all of health economics. He drew the conclusion that in spite of the difficulty of testing for demand inducement, sufficient evidence exists to doubt the independence of demand and supply curves in the physician's market. It is questionable whether Assumption 10 is valid.

For the market to work, Assumption 9 must be true or else market power will lead to market failure (Penner, 2004). A monopoly occurs when there are only a few competitors in the market, which cooperate to control production and service. Some monopolies are natural, such as when a rural hospital is the only community provider of acute care. In contrast, consolidation among healthcare networks of hospitals and multispecialty group practices gives large market shares to these groups. Mergers such as these create massive local market leverage. Rice (1998) dealt briefly with monopoly power, saying that it has been studied thoroughly and clearly: In health services, firms do have monopoly power. Assumption 11 is strongly refuted.

Do firms seek to maximize profits, as Assumption 12 declares? Notably, many providers in the healthcare arena operate on a nonprofit basis. (Again, there is a vast literature collection on this subject.) Managers in health, like their counterparts in other sectors, often seek to fulfill their firm's goals and objectives rather than maximizing the firm's overall profit. Even if owners of a healthcare firm do want to maximize profits, they typically hire others as their agents to accomplish this task but, for differing reasons, some agents are not motivated, efficient, or trustworthy enough to meet those expectations. Assumption 12 is another strongly refuted assumption.

## Economic Analysis of Clinical and Managerial Interventions

So far the chapter has reviewed the following topics: (1) the history of economic theory development, (2) the identification of assumptions that form the foundations for economic theory, (3) the major concepts and principles from mainstream economics, and (4) an assessment of the validity of some of the key assumptions. The chapter next addresses an important area of application of economic theory—economic analysis of interventions.

The startling increases in healthcare costs in recent decades and the many efforts to control them have dramatically increased the relevance of economic analysis of clinical interventions. In the ACA health reform bill passed by Congress in early 2010, considerable resources were designated for increased funding of cost-effectiveness research in health care. Money is at stake. Achievement of the same outcomes accompanied by smaller cost increases saves money for payers and increases profits for providers. In capitated systems, where keeping enrollees healthy is key to profitability, discovering strategies to increase disease prevention, self-care, or adherence to clinically beneficial treatments can also have payoffs. Economics, the field that was born out of the problem of scarcity, has developed methods to assist society in using scarce resources more wisely.

Healthcare administrators are finding that those methods for production and labor cost identification and measurement used successfully by business firms in the private sector now need to be adopted by or adapted in the healthcare arena. An analysis of interventions is designed to support decision makers, but not to make decisions. *Analysis* provides the framework for understanding data and information.

Four types of cost analysis are common, each with its own strengths and weaknesses. The individuals conducting the analysis need to know what each type of analysis accomplishes and what the relative advantages and disadvantages of each are so that they can choose the most appropriate approach. It is also important as a clinician to be able to interpret, and make decisions based on, study findings.

## Cost Analysis

A major contribution of economics to analysis is *cost analysis*. There are three tasks in measuring: (1) clarifying the perspective taken, (2) identifying the resources used, and (3) identifying the opportunity costs of those resources. Which costs are relevant depends on the stakeholder involved. Customers, managers, boards, clinicians, and a healthcare system will all identify costs from their perspective. The authority for conducting such studies in the United States is the Panel on Cost Effectiveness in Health and Medicine, which was convened in 1993 by the U.S. Public Health Services (Chang, Price, & Pfoutz, 2001). This panel first recommended assuming the broadest perspective—society as a whole. This approach recognizes all costs, no matter where or to whom they accrue.

Costs equal the volume of resources used for an intervention multiplied by the opportunity costs of those resources (Lee, 2009). To capture all costs, construction of a clinical pathway and developing a good clinical understanding of an intervention itself are helpful. Opportunity cost usually is equivalent to what was paid for a resource, but if it is old or no longer available, valuation of its best alternative use has to be filled in as a substitute. Costs include both *direct costs* and *indirect costs*. For health services, three categories of costs are included: (1) the cost of an intervention, (2) costs borne by patients and their families, and (3) external costs borne by the rest of society. Some costs must be *discounted*. In economics, in recognition of the "time value of money," a dollar today is more valuable than a dollar in the future. Thus, any expenditures or costs incurred in the future must be discounted back to a *present value* using a *discount rate*.

*Cost of illness studies* estimate the total monetary effects of a specific disease or condition. This information is used for public planning and to estimate the costs of health care and the financial burden of disease and illness.

*Cost minimization analysis* is the simplest comparison analysis. Only two steps are needed: (1) identifying the expected costs for each option and (2) showing that the lowest-cost option has outcomes at least equal to the outcomes for the alternative. It can be difficult sometimes to show evidence that the outcomes are comparable or that the lowest-cost option is superior or at least equal.

*Cost–benefit analysis* is a method used to compare benefits in terms of disease prevention with the costs of a program. In this analysis, benefits are measured in monetary terms. Cost–benefit analysis is the principal method used to evaluate decisions involving public expenditures. Decisions are biased toward alternatives providing the greatest net benefit, which is the greatest level of economic efficiency. One of the drawbacks of using this method in health care is the difficulty of placing a dollar value on outcomes, such as pain or loss of life. Methods developed by economists in this regard are quite controversial (Lee, 2009).

In conducting a *cost-effectiveness analysis*, which is sometimes considered a more acceptable alternative for health care, a ratio is calculated in which health outcome is measured in health-related units, such as number of infections avoided or years of life saved. The cost for the treatment or intervention is measured in dollars, so results are presented on the basis of cost per case prevented or cost per life saved. The point is to compare the relative value of different interventions in creating better health or longer life. Costs of alternative interventions are compared based on a single nonmonetary outcome.

# Conclusion

Healthcare professionals who become familiar with the content of this chapter will experience a sense of comfort when they enter into a conversation with others about economics and health care. Although this attempt at an orderly presentation could seem to confine economics to a static set of beliefs, it is a mistake to think that the real-world conversation will be confined to a narrow or orthodox set of ideas. Any explanation of core ideas tends to be a backward look, but, as is the case with nursing theory, at any point in time a successful discipline will have hundreds of new ideas being tried and tested.

Collander, Holt, and Rosser (2004) stated almost 10 years ago that they expected new ideas to change the way economics is done. Their interviews with "cutting-edge" economists provided evidence that the orthodoxy of economic thought—rationality, greed, and equilibrium—was being challenged by another set of assumptions—purposeful behavior, enlightened self-interest, and sustainability. According to these authors, theories and ideas from a "new economics" are already recognizable to other professionals and the lay public. The popular press is discussing behavioral economics, agent-based models, evolutionary game theory, and experimental economics. It is exciting to consider how the specialized field of healthcare economics will be influenced by insights brought by new and revised theories. Equally encouraging is the availability of large data sets and dramatic growth in computing power in recent years that allows researchers in economic analysis to make greater sense of economic information (Jones, Rice, d'Uva, & Balia, 2012). We remain hopeful that we will apply new knowledge wisely to achieve society's goals, or at least to achieve improved efficiency and equity in health care.

## Discussion Questions

1. One of the assumptions of economic theory is that producers of products and consumers of products act independently of one another, without influencing one another. Is this assumption valid in health care? How do providers and consumers act? Are they independent? Is there any incursion of the provider into the consumer role? Of the consumer into the production role? Think about economic theory and how well the "production of health" conforms to the theory.

2. In theory derivation, one can shift terminology or structure from one theoretical field or context to another. Which concepts or principles from economic theory could be useful to conceptualize phenomena of interest to nursing?

3. From the individual's point of view, what are the conditions that determine the optimal resource allocation between health and other goods?

4. Can the often volatile pattern of behavior ("Sinning against health as long as health is good; sacrificing everything for health when health is bad") be brought into line with rationality? Or are individual preferences inconsistent, implying that medical experts should perhaps determine the appropriate amount of preventive behaviors?

5. Can the economic concept of substitution be applied to health production even though situations can easily be envisioned in which only medical services (rather than one's own health-enhancing efforts) offer the prospect of improvement?

6. Is there a research question from your practice that could be situated in an economic framework for study? Which sorts of nursing questions can you imaginatively explore using economic concepts and analysis?

## References

Arrow, K. (1963). Uncertainty and the welfare economics of medical care. *The American Economic Review, 53,* 941–973.

Bielkiewicz, G. M. (2002). Theories from the sociological sciences. In M. McEwen & E. M. Wills (Eds.), *Theoretical basis for nursing* (pp. 229–249). Philadelphia, PA: Lippincott Williams and Wilkins.

Chang, C. F., Price, S. A., & Pfoutz, S. K. (2001). *Economics and nursing: Critical professional issues.* Philadelphia, PA: F. A. Davis.

Collander, D. E., Holt, R. P. F., & Rosser, J. B. (2004). *The changing face of economics: Conversations with cutting edge economists.* Ann Arbor, MI: University of Michigan Press.

Dunham-Taylor, J. (2005). *Health care financial management for nurse managers.* Sudbury, MA: Jones and Bartlett.

Fawcett, J. (1998). *The relationship of theory and research* (3rd ed.). Philadelphia, PA: F. A. Davis.

Fawcett, J. (2005). *Contemporary nursing knowledge: Analysis and evaluation of nursing models* (2nd ed.). Philadelphia, PA: F. A. Davis.

Hammer, P. J., Haas-Wilson, D., & Sage, W. M. (2001). Kenneth Arrow and the changing economics of health care. Why Arrow? Why now? *Journal of Health Policy, Politics, and Law, 26,* 835–849.

Hartman, S. (2009). Economics of health care. In K. S. Lundy & S. Janes (Eds.), *Nursing in the community: Caring for the public's health* (2nd ed., pp. 157–185). Sudbury, MA: Jones and Bartlett.

Heskett, J. (2006). What happens when the economics of scarcity meets the economics of abundance? *Working knowledge: A first look at faculty research.* Harvard Business School. Retrieved from http://hbswk.hbs.edu/item/5469.html#original

Jones, A. M., Rice, N., d'Uva, T. B., & Balia, S. (2012). *Applied health economics* (2nd ed.). London and New York: Routledge Taylor and Francis Group.

Jones, T. L., & Yoder, L. (2010). Economic theory and nursing research: Is this a good combination? *Nursing Forum, 45,* 40–53.

Kuttner, R. (1997). *Everything for sale: The virtues and limits of markets.* New York, NY: Alfred A. Knopf.

Lee, R. H. (2009). *Economics for healthcare managers* (2nd ed.). Chicago, IL: Health Administration Press.

Parse, R. R. (2005). Parse's criteria for evaluation of theory with a comparison of Fawcett's and Parse's approaches. *Nursing Science Quarterly, 18,* 135–137.

Penner, S. (2004). *Introduction to health care economics and financial management.* Philadelphia, PA: Lippincott Williams & Wilkins.

Peterson, M. A. (2001). Editor's note: Kenneth Arrow and the changing economics of health care. *Journal of Health Policy, Politics, and Law, 26,* 823–828.

Rice, T. (1998). *The economics of health reconsidered.* Chicago, IL: Health Administration Press.

Savedoff, W. D. (2004). Kenneth Arrow and the birth of health economics. *Bulletin of the World Health Organization, 82.* Retrieved from http://www.scielosp.org/scielo.php?pid=S0042-96862004000200012&script=sci_arttext

Shi, L., & Singh, D. A. (2011). *Delivering health care in America. A systems approach* (5th ed.). Sudbury, MA: Jones & Bartlett Learning.

SNBCHF. (2013). Major schools of economic theory. Retrieved from http://snbchf.com/economic-theory/major-schools-of-economics/

Turkel, M. C., & Ray, M. A. (2000). Relational complexity: A theory of the nurse-patient relationship within an economic context. *Nursing Science Quarterly, 13,* 307–313.

Wagoner, R. E. (2012). The social construction of theoretical landscapes: Some economics of economic theories. *American Journal of Economics and Sociology, 71,* 1186–1204.

# Theories of Organizational Behavior and Leadership

*Sandra Bishop*

## Introduction

> Theories are used in management not to mirror reality but to help explain it. They may do so deductively by helping us to slot the behavior of organizations into categories, but they must also do so inductively by providing the concepts through which we can see new things, and so make better diagnoses. (Mintzberg, 1989)

Theories of organizational behavior "are important because they continue to influence the assumptions people in organizations make" (Daft & Noe, 2001, p. 6). Theories of organizational behavior and leadership have an interesting history, and the unique principles and processes of each theory have remained substantially consistent in application over time. Although the earlier organizational behavior theories are not as popular as they were in times past, they remain the foundation for more contemporary theories. This chapter provides an overview of the classical, neoclassical, and modern organizational theories.

## Classical Organization Theory

History reveals that thinking about organizations began in the ancient civilizations, such as with the Sumerians (Sullivan & Decker, 2005). Organizational thinking continued sporadically but remained mostly unfamiliar until the Industrial Revolution, when the school of thought evolved to one of organizational structure and

> ### Box 15–1 Classical Theory
>
> Classical theorists pioneered ideas related to organizational behavior and leadership. As their theories were conceived, a merger of the concepts of scientific management, administrative theory, and bureaucratic theory began to occur. Considering these concepts, answer the following questions:
>
> 1. Are the principles of scientific management useful today in the healthcare industry? If so, where and how? If not, explain why.
> 2. Is a bureaucracy necessary to minimize chaos in today's healthcare organizations? Defend your answer.

efficiency where individuals functioned with extremely defined tasks to accomplish the main purpose of the organization (see **Box 15–1**).

## Frederick Winslow Taylor: Principles of Scientific Management

> The determination of the best method of performing all of our daily acts will, in the future, be the work of experts who first analyze and then accurately time while they watch the various ways of doing each piece of work and who finally know from exact knowledge—and not from anyone's opinion—which method will accomplish the results with the least effort and in the quickest time. (Taylor, cited in Crainer, 2003, p. 49)

Frederick Winslow Taylor first addressed his views of management in the classic book written in 1911, titled *The Principles of Scientific Management*. Taylor conducted extensive studies of steel workers and analyzed each worker's task in relation to the tools used, the design of the tools, how the worker held and used the tools, and so on. Taylor theorized that there was one best way to accomplish each step in the production of work, and he applied the scientific method to discover that best way. Taylor believed that managers should be as detailed with the assignment of tasks and supervising workers as workers should be with the structure of task performance. In his view, increased productivity, rewards, and salaries should be tied to production. The manager's responsibility, then, is to scientifically determine the best way to do a job, to select the best employee for the job, to train the employee, and to share the responsibility for results with the workers. This stepwise management practice became known as *Taylorism*.

At the time when Taylor was developing his ideas, workers and managers generally were considered to have opposing ideals and values. Moreover, managers did not take responsibility for the work of their subordinates. Taylor contended, however, that workers and managers shared the responsibility for production. Taylor's systemized methods for dividing work for workers and managers into the smallest elements and standardizing assignments were intended to maximize efficiency.

When scientific management first became popular in the early 20th century, its methods replaced rule-of-thumb standards and traditional methods. Unfortunately, Taylor's methods had an unintended effect: Many jobs were changed into a succession of dull tasks, and many people believed that such methods diminished the role of the manager. Some workers disliked Taylor's approach because it standardized procedures and thus prohibited creativity in much of their daily work. Taylor's critics argued that scientific management dehumanized workers and placed people second to production. Other people supported his work and believed that his methods greatly improved the working conditions of the era (Johnson, 2009). Whether Taylor's methods were appreciated or not, he certainly changed the way organizational leaders viewed workers and managers.

Taylor also is credited with being the first theorist to contribute to the organization and technology of the factory system, such as through the introduction of assembly lines (Nelson, 1980). Taylor's management principles continue to be translated into today's workplace in the form of employee education, goal setting, and performance incentives (McShane & Von Glinow, 2005).

## Henri Fayol: General Principles of Administration

> Management . . . is neither an exclusive privilege nor particular responsibility of the head or senior members of the business; it is an activity spread, like all other activities, between head and members of the body corporate. (Fayol, as cited in Parker & Ritson, 2005, p. 182)

Henri Fayol is considered to be the first author to develop a complete administrative theory. In the early 1900s, Fayol suggested that management consists of 14 basic but flexible universal principles: (1) specialization and division; (2) formal authority based on the job, not the person; (3) discipline; (4) unity of command, one boss per person; (5) unity of direction, orders coming from one boss; (6) group interests over individual interests; (7) fair and equitable pay; (8) centralizing communication and authority; (9) scalar chain; (10) an orderly work environment; (11) equity; (12) stability of personnel; (13) individual initiative; and (14) esprit de corps—harmony and unity in the organization (Johnson, 2009).

Fayol recognized that management is universal, no matter what the industry. In particular, Fayol considered administration to be the "art of managing people" (Breeze, 1981, p. 102), and in his theory he stressed the concepts of coordination and specialization. He also included the concepts of organizing, planning, controlling, and coordinating in his theory of management. The 14 principles, along with these concepts, were the foundation for his approach to organizational design, chain of command, and span of control (Brunsson, 2008).

Although Fayol's principles were based on his own experiences rather than on empirical research, he offered a language to communicate management theory. As a consequence, he is credited with initiating a move toward management thought that focuses on management of the total organization. Unlike Taylor and his followers, who prescribed sets of all-encompassing principles, Fayol hoped to arouse debate from which a substantial theory of management might emerge (Parker & Ritson, 2005).

## Max Weber: Bureaucratic Theory

> Bureaucratic and patriarchal structures are antagonistic in many ways, yet they have in common the most important peculiarity: permanence. (Weber, as cited in Eisenstadt, 1968, p. 3)

During roughly the same era that Taylor and Fayol were developing scientific management and principles for management, Max Weber was developing a theory of bureaucracy. Weber's bureaucratic theory extended Taylor's theory and emphasized the need to reduce ambiguity and diversity in organizations. Weber believed in the value of a hierarchical structure and recognized the significance of specialization and the necessity of division of labor. In addition, he endorsed the idea of promotion based on merit and impersonal rules. Three forms of legitimate authority were identified in his theory: (1) rational or legal authority, (2) traditional authority, and (3) charismatic authority. Weber believed that having rational or traditional authority is most stable for administrators (Johnson, 2009). He considered bureaucracies to be suitable settings in which administrators could use rational authority because bureaucratic organizations are bound to analyzable rules (Eisenstadt, 1968).

As one of the founders of social science, Weber defined bureaucracy as "the means of carrying 'community action' over into rationally ordered 'societal action'" (Weber, cited in Eisenstadt, 1968, p. 75). Bureaucracy, in his view, was considered a tool or power instrument. In a bureaucracy, he suggested, the importance of individuals is not emphasized, but rather the rules and offices of the organization are valued. The established offices and policies remain part of the organization, even if individuals holding offices are not. According to Weber, a good bureaucrat worries about the means, not the ends (Hargreaves, 2006). Thus, in contrast to a process of aristocratic ascendancy, bureaucrats should be selected for office based on their skills, not on their ancestry (Sager & Rosser, 2009). Weber believed that the masses cannot rule without chaos; once it is well established, a bureaucracy is seen as a tool to combat chaos that is difficult to destroy. Over the years, Weber's work has been criticized for not distinguishing between position or line authority and staff or expert authority.

# Neoclassical Organization Theories

## Human Resource Theory: The Hawthorne Experiments

> The point of view which gradually emerged from these studies is one from which an industrial organization is regarded as a social system. (Roethlisberger & Dickson, 1967, p. 551)

One of the more powerful movements in the development of human relations theory stemmed from a study conducted at the Western Electric plant in Hawthorne, Illinois, a city bordering Chicago. Serendipitously, though the study was begun under the auspices of interest in worker efficiency and output, the data from the Hawthorne study bridged scientific management and human relations theories. The large Western Electric organization covered a wide range of occupations and amassed a huge array of equipment. In 1924, researchers working in conjunction with the National Research Council of the National Academy of Sciences undertook a study at the Hawthorne plant with the purpose of determining the "relation of quality and quantity of illumination to efficiency in industry" (Roethlisberger & Dickson, 1967, p. 14). Essentially, the initial research question guiding the study was "Does increased lighting intensity increase productivity?" Careful attention was given to the selection of workrooms and types of illumination used. The study was done experimentally with test and control groups and produced surprising results—high intensity, low intensity, or no change in intensity of lighting seemed to have no relationship to the workers' output. However, the researchers believed that something "screwy" was happening with the experiments. They wondered if the unexpected results were related to the researchers, the workers, or the data. Rather than being discontinued, the research was continued for more than 10 years. Study methods such as observation and interviews were added to the experimental methods to learn about the thoughts and feelings of the workers.

From the results of the study emerged a new view of organizations as large social systems. Two major functions of the organization were identified: the production of a product and satisfaction among the individual workers in the organization. From these functions, researchers identified two facets of the overall organization: a technical organization (e.g., products, tools, materials) and a human organization (satisfied workers; Roethlisberger & Dickson, 1967).

Critics of the Hawthorne study concluded that the Industrial Revolution had caused workers to lose a sense of work-related security and camaraderie. Although researchers originally planned to manipulate the esthetics of the work environment and determine how such changes affected quality and productivity, they soon discovered that *any* change that involved increased attention to employees was sufficient to improve productivity. In other words, it was the attention to employees and the study itself that made the difference—a phenomenon now known as the *Hawthorne effect* (Johnson, 2009). "Perhaps the most lasting contribution of the Hawthorne studies themselves was their emphasis on the proposition that a human problem to be brought to a human solution requires human data and human tools" (Filley & House, 1969, p. 23).

## The Economy of Incentives

Careful inspection of the observable actions of human beings in our society—their movements, their speech, and the thought and emotions evident from their action and speech—shows that many and sometimes most of them are determined or directed by their connection with formal organizations. (Barnard, 1938, p. 3)

Chester Barnard (1938) also studied and theorized about individuals and their relationships in organizations. Like the Hawthorne researchers, Barnard came to view workers as having social, behavioral, and psychological dimensions. Barnard introduced one of the first neoclassical theories by defining an organization as "a system of consciously coordinated personal activities or forces" (p. 72). Coordinated activities, he suggested, include the physical environment, the social environment, individuals, and other variables. Barnard argued that organizations cannot operate if individuals do not communicate and are not willing to contribute to common goals (Hellriegel & Slocum, 1976). He viewed organizations as systems that should be treated as a whole because all of their parts are related in a significant way. In addition, Barnard viewed organizations as hierarchies with defined authority and clear communication linkages. The success of each organization was linked to the leader's ability to generate a cohesive environment.

Other aspects of Barnard's work focused on fair treatment of workers and humane leadership. His work informed much later research on job design, participative decision making, worker satisfaction, culture, behavior, supervision, and groups, to name a few areas. Barnard is considered a transitional theorist, because his theory contains elements drawn from both classical and neoclassical methods (Barnard, 1938).

## The Proverbs of Administration

The anatomy of the organization is to be found in the distribution and allocation of decision-making functions. The physiology of the organization is to be found in the processes whereby the organization influences the decisions of each of its members—supplying these decisions with their premises. (Simon, 1976, p. 220)

When Herbert Simon dissected the administrative principles proposed by Taylor and Fayol, he decided that they were contradictory. In developing his own theory, Simon considered a description of administrative situations and the weight of administrative criteria. He viewed the primary administrative situations to be allocation of functions and formal structures of authority. After investigating the science of administration, Simon proposed that administrative science can be theoretical and practical. He viewed the behaviors of human beings in organized groups as the sociology of administration. Thus, Simon proposed that the practical science of administration "consists of propositions as to how men would behave if they wished their activity to result in the greatest attainment of administrative objectives with scarce means" (Simon, 1976, p. 253).

Simon (1976) believed that "the hierarchy of means and ends is as characteristic of the behavior of organizations as it is of individuals" (p. 63). In other words, the work at one level in the organization serves as the means to accomplish

## Box 15–2 Neoclassical Theory

Neoclassical theorists focused on the behavior of workers, speaking to the issues intrinsic to classical theory, such as rigidity and structured work environments. Classical theory squelched workers' growth and creativity, whereas neoclassical theory exhibited a concern for workers. Based on these points, answer the following questions:

1. Are the results of the Hawthorne study relevant to advanced nursing practice today? Explain your answer.
2. How are authority and leadership differentiated? What subconcepts can be used to characterize each of these broad concepts?
3. Do nurses today respond more positively to authority or leadership?
4. Identify and discuss examples of healthcare organizations and departments that use the principles of neoclassical theory.

the end purpose of the level above it in the organizational hierarchy. These hierarchal relationships are seen as guiding decision making from the bottom up. In his work, Simon (1976) defined the means–end chain sequence of related elements, from behavior to resulting values.

Whereas Taylor and Simon were attentive to workers, Weber and Fayol focused on the organization. All of these theorists believed that the role of administration is to maintain balance within the organization. Consequently, they emphasized managers' ability to manipulate workers and their environments.

The neoclassical theorists viewed hierarchies, principles, authority, rules, and goals as important concepts. These theorists focused on the behavior of workers (see **Box 15–2**).

# Modern Organization Theories

## Contingency Theory

The most successful organizations tended to maintain states of differentiation and integration consistent with the diversity of the parts of the environment and the required interdependence of these parts. (Lawrence & Lorsch, cited in Filley & House, 1969, p. 97)

The classical and neoclassical theorists' position was that conflict should be avoided because it causes an imbalance in the organization. In contrast, contingency theorists consider conflict to be an inescapable occurrence and believe that it should be actively managed. They suggested that the environment in which conflict exists complements organizational performance. Environment, according to this view, includes the influences of objects, people, and ideas outside of the organization.

## Paul Lawrence and Jay Lorsch

In 1967, Lawrence and Lorsch considered organizations as social systems. As such, they viewed contingency theory to be a fit between individual predispositions, internal characteristics, and external conditions, including environmental uncertainty. Lawrence and Lorsch asserted that there is no best way to organize; instead, each organization's environment determines the structure that results in best performance. The environmental variables or contingencies affecting this determination include such determinants as size, geography, technology, and uncertainty. The organizational structures that are considered to be contingent on these variables are differentiation, decentralization, the degree of formalization, and integration (Johnson, 2009; Sullivan & Decker, 2009). Integration includes the internal relationships of organizational members and is influenced by "the nature of the task being performed, the form of relationships, rewards, and controls, and the existing ideas within the organization about how a well-accepted member should behave" (Filley & House, 1969, p. 95). Integration also incorporates the quality of collaboration. The formality of departments and between organizations may be differentiated, based on how members of each department utilize different interests and viewpoints; because of their differences, they often find it difficult to reach consensus (Filley & House, 1969).

To Lawrence and Lorsch, "the environment of the organization determines both the character and degree of differentiation and the mode of integration" (Filley & House, 1967, p. 96). They foresaw that competitive demand and environmental uncertainty have an effect on each organization's differentiation and integration in terms of its interpersonal orientation, goals, and perception of time. In their research conducted at a group of plastics factories, Lawrence and Lorsch found that "the state of differentiation in the effective organization was consistent with the diversity of the parts of the environment, while the state of integration achieved was consistent with the environmental demands for interdependence" (p. 98).

## Fred Fiedler

> Leadership performance depends then as much on the organization as it depends upon the leader's own attributes. (Fiedler, 1967, p. 281)

Fred Fiedler's contingency model proposed that group performance was based on a balance between the leader's style and his or her level of control. To measure leadership style, Fiedler developed an instrument called the least preferred coworker (LPC) questionnaire. After assessing their leadership style, Fiedler matched leaders with situations. Three contingency dimensions were identified that determined leadership effectiveness: (1) leader–member relations, (2) task structure, and (3) position power. The results of Fiedler's research showed that the better the relationship between the leader and the member, the more structured the job and the stronger the position power or leader control. In other words, the best leadership style depends on situational control. From this evidence, Fiedler developed a model to match leaders with situations. Advocates of Fiedler's findings contended that there was sufficient evidence to support Fiedler's model, although the LPC scores were not stable and the questionnaire was not well understood (Robbins & Judge, 2007).

## Organizational Configuration Framework

> Large politicized organizations are increasingly allowed to sustain themselves by political means, threatening the destruction, not of the single spent organization, but of the whole society of organizations instead. (Mintzberg, 1989, p. 367)

Henry Mintzberg began his research in 1966 in an attempt to describe what managers do, with the goal of using different words and concepts than those presented by Fayol. During his research, Mintzberg observed chief executives, from both medium and large organizations, for 1-week periods. Based on his findings, he presented two sets of conclusions: characteristics of managerial work and the basic content of the manager's work. Six characteristics were deemed to be significant skills needed by managers to enable them to administer in a complex organization:

1. The manager performs a great quantity of work at an unrelenting pace.
2. Managerial activity is characterized by variety, fragmentation, and brevity.
3. Managers prefer issues that are current, specific, and ad hoc.
4. The manager sits between his or her organization and a network of contacts.
5. The manager demonstrates a strong preference for verbal media.
6. Despite the preponderance of obligations, the manager appears to be able to control his or her own affairs (Mintzberg, 1971, pp. B102–B103).

Managers were considered to function in three distinct roles: (1) interpersonal roles (figurehead, leader, liaison), (2) informational roles (nerve center, spokesperson, disseminator), and (3) decision-making roles (entrepreneur, resource allocator, disturbance handler, negotiator).

Mintzberg (1971) questioned whether management should be considered a profession or a science. To be defined as a profession, there should be an associated body of knowledge or science. Mintzberg did not believe that his research proved that a science of management exists, as managers "do not work according to procedures that have been prescribed by scientific analysis" (p. B107). Consequently, he recommended greater and more refined definition and study of managerial roles as the first step toward the development of a scientific base for management.

Mintzberg (1989) also sought to classify types of organizational structure and power: "We can no more talk of *the* organization than we can talk of *the* mammal, no more prescribe one best way to run all organizations than prescribe one pair of glasses for all people" (p. 93). He noted that organizational theory was not dependent on recognition of strict boundaries, but rather often shifted to reflect organizational power struggles. Mintzberg contended that the organization is the total of all the ways labor is coordinated, while divided into distinct tasks. The six coordinating mechanisms were identified as (1) mutual adjustment, (2) standardization of work processes, (3) direct supervision, (4) standardized work outputs, (5) standardized labor skills, and (6) standardized labor norms. As part of his work, Mintzberg developed a model of organizational structures that considers combinations of environmental complexity and stability. The four broad categories on his matrix are (1) decentralized bureaucratic, (2) centralized bureaucratic, (3) decentralized organic, and (4) centralized organic. The horizontal axis of the model contrasted organic and bureaucratic structures: Bureaucratic structures represent more stable environments, and organic structures represent more dynamic environments (Matheson, 2009).

One of the more innovative organizations described by Mintzberg is the *adhocracy*: a high-technology organization characterized by a basic orientation of entrepreneurship (indicating dependence on a variety of workers to achieve strategic initiatives). Adhocracy was described as a structure appropriate for the current (information) age, albeit one that is difficult for the machine bureaucracy to comprehend.

For an organization to be innovative, one of two basic forms of adhocracy must be engaged: *operating adhocracy* or *administrative adhocracy*. "The operating adhocracy innovates and solves problems directly on behalf of its clients. . . . For every operating adhocracy, there is a corresponding professional bureaucracy, one that does similar work but with a narrower orientation" (Mintzberg, 1989, p. 201). In contrast, administrative adhocracy takes on projects to serve itself, "to bring new facilities or activities on line, as in the administrative structure of a highly automated company" (Mintzberg, 1989, p. 203). The administrative adhocracy, unlike the operating adhocracy, creates an apparent distinction between its operating core and administrative component.

## General Systems Theory

> The only meaningful way to study an organization is to study it as a
> system. (von Bertalanffy, 1969a, p. 9)

Ludwig von Bertalanffy introduced general systems theory in the late 1950s. According to von Bertalanffy, when the theoretical frameworks for various scientific disciplines become isolated from one another, communication between them becomes difficult. He suggested that, in fact, a common element in all frameworks can be found crossing the periphery of physics, biology, sociology, psychology, and so on—namely, systems. The central theme in his work is that nonlinear relationships may exist between variables. As a consequence, a small change in one variable may cause a significant change in another. The nonlinear concept introduced by von Bertalanffy added to the complexity of understanding organizations (Johnson, 2009).

Von Bertalanffy believed the task of biology is to determine the laws of biological science, which in turn requires an understanding of all levels of an organism. This systems theory of the organism, called organismic biology, later was understood as general systems theory. In outlining systems theory, von Bertalanffy "gave mathematical descriptions of system properties (such as wholeness, sum, growth, competition, allometry, mechanization, centralization, finality, and equifinality), derived from the system description by simultaneous differential equations" (von Bertalanffy, 1969b, p. 412). As a practicing biologist, von Bertalanffy sought to develop a theory of open systems. According to Drack (2009), his definition of the open system is one that maintains itself "through a continuous flux of matter and energy, by assimilation and dissimilation, and is distant from true equilibrium, and able to supply work" (p. 566). Von Bertalanffy also described the principle of ontogenesis, which was later recognized as a key concept underlying hierarchy or progressive organization.

Von Bertalanffy (1969a) defined an organization as an "alien to the mechanistic world" and noted that characteristics of organizations "are notions like those of wholeness, growth, differentiation, hierarchical order, dominance, control, competition, etc." (p. 47). Unlike biological theories, which can be quantitatively measured, organizations lend themselves to more qualitative review, according to von Bertalanffy. He discussed general systems theory as it relates to individuals, education, and science. His general systems theory propelled organizational theory into the era of open systems thinking, where the environment plays a major role.

## Change Theory
### Kurt Lewin

> To be stable, a cultural change has to penetrate all aspects of a
> nation's life. The change must, in short, be a change in the cultural
> atmosphere, not merely a change of a single item. (Lewin, cited in
> Burnes, 2004, p. 980)

Kurt Lewin, a behavioral scientist, outlined a model for change used by industry in the 1940s. His force field model included the steps of unfreezing, moving, and refreezing. In this model, change is described as a dynamic force within the organization that moves in opposing directions. A driving force pushes participants toward change, while participants use a restraining force to push back the change being directed their way. Lewin viewed change as a dynamic balance of these forces, not an event. *Unfreezing* is the act of destabilizing old behaviors and is a necessity for old behaviors to be unlearned or discarded. Once this step is accomplished, the manager may consider the method that will result in the least resistance in moving a change forward. *Moving* enables individuals and groups to switch to more acceptable behaviors. *Refreezing* involves a return of the dynamic force field and a new quasi-stationary state of equilibrium (Hellriegel & Slocum, 1976; Sullivan & Decker, 2009).

Lewin had a strong, ethical belief in democratic values in society and democratic institutions. His pioneering work set the standard for behavioral science and group issues in organizations.

### Peter Drucker

> One cannot manage change. One can only be ahead of it. (Drucker, 1999, p. 73)

Peter Drucker (1999) addressed change process and theory in his book, titled *Management Challenges for the 21st Century*. Because he considered change to be unavoidable, Drucker was convinced that organizations that do not embrace change will not survive. A *change leader* knows how to look for change, can find the right change, and understands the effects of change, both internal and external to the organization.

The first step in the process identified by Drucker is to establish change policies that will enable the organization to abandon yesterday and know how to act on abandonment. The second step is to create change through a policy of systematic innovation. This step facilitates looking for windows of opportunity. The third step focuses on piloting—that is, the use of pilot studies to test the reality of the change. The final step is change and continuity: "Change and continuity are thus poles rather than opposites" (p. 90). To successfully adopt the role of change leader, an organization needs to establish internal and external continuity and find the right balance between rapid change and continuity.

## Theories X, Y, and Z

> The normal science of management is long since in need of a new paradigm. (Ouchi, 1981, p. 220)

### Douglas McGregor: Theory X and Theory Y

The social psychologist Douglas McGregor criticized both classical and human relations theories as being insufficient to address workplace realities. He developed a general characterization of their principles in a theory that he dubbed theory X. Theory X is based on beliefs that the average person dislikes work and tries to avoid it; most people have to be coerced or threatened to do a job; and the average person wishes to avoid responsibility, yet wants security. McGregor distinguished theory X from propositions that he named theory Y, which is based on the following assumptions regarding human nature:

- The expenditure of effort at work is as natural as rest and play.
- Humans do have a measure of self-control and self-direction, and coercion is not the only means to bring about effort.
- A direct product of effort is the satisfaction of ego and meeting of self-actualization needs.
- The average person can seek and accept responsibility under proper conditions.

- There are significant variations in individuals' degree of ingenuity, creativity, and imagination.
- The average person's potential is not utilized in modern industrial life.

People who accept McGregor's analysis also essentially accept Maslow's hierarchy of needs. Theory X includes the assumption that lower-order needs in Maslow's hierarchy govern behavior, and theory Y includes the assumption that human behavior is governed by higher-order needs. Unfortunately, there was no evidence to confirm either theory (Filley & House, 1969; Robbins & Judge, 2007).

### William Ouchi: Theory Z

While theory X and theory Y were developed as a criticism of the work of classical organizational theorists, theory Z was derived by William Ouchi in the 1970s from his work comparing the work ethic and industry in the United States to the work ethic and industry in Japan. Trust, loyalty, and commitment are key employee elements in theory Z. Companies that adhere to theory Z principles, like their Japanese counterparts, have long-term employees; establish evaluation and promotion policies based on complex, subtle, and intimate peer evaluation; and allow for unique career path development. In these companies, decision making is consensual and participative. Such companies also have a holistic orientation and an egalitarian atmosphere, where relationships tend to be informal and emphasize that "whole people deal with one another at work, rather than just managers with workers and clerks with machinists" (Ouchi, 1981, p. 79). Theory Z organizations are considered to be clans rather than bureaucracies, given the ongoing interchange between employees' social and work life. Ouchi proposed 13 steps as necessary to become a theory Z organization:

1. Understand roles in the type Z organization. Read, discuss, and have open discussions about the substance of theory Z.
2. Audit the company's philosophy. The company philosophy expresses the values to live and work by.
3. Involve company leadership in the design of desired management philosophy. Organizational change cannot occur without support of the hierarchy.
4. Implement the chosen philosophy by constructing incentives and structures. The structure should be a guide to cooperation and subtlety.
5. Support interpersonal skills development. Recognize problem-solving and decision-making patterns of interaction.
6. Test the system. Internal and external testing of the organization is not easy but is necessary to measure success.
7. Allow for union involvement. If there is a union involved, the union must have an understanding of the emerging work relationships and organizational structure.
8. Stabilize employment. This step is a direct result of policy. Slow evaluation and promotion are pivotal factors in stabilization of employees.

9. Develop a system for slow evaluation and promotion. Employees will learn that promotions and salary increases are based on performance over time.
10. Expand career path development. A mingling of expertise benefits everyone and allows for a program of career circulation.
11. Plan for implementation at the first level—management first, and then lower-level employees. Change cannot take place unless those who rate higher in the hierarchy offer an invitation to lower-level employees to do so.
12. Seek areas for implementation. Utilize areas that have shown commitment and productivity.
13. Allow for the development of holistic relationships. These relationships are a consequence of organizational integration (Ouchi, 1981).

Modern theorists of organizational behavior recognized that conflict, change, and structure are inherent in all organizations. They considered organizations as systems and cultures working in an environment of certain mingled with uncertainty (see **Box 15–3**).

The logic of these steps is seen as the equivalent of going from A to Z and reaching every worker in the organization. This process encourages greater productivity and efficiency, which will thrive unless the process is thwarted intentionally by top managers or a union that is threatened. Critics of theory Z, however, suggest that this philosophy may make organizations more sexist or racist (based on Japanese philosophy), the proposed changes may be difficult given certain aspects of U.S. culture, and a decline in professionalism by employees may occur.

---

### Box 15–3  Modern Theories of Organizational Behavior

With the ideas of the modern theories of organizational behavior in mind, answer the following questions:

1. Describe a healthcare organization from a systems perspective.
2. Research change theory in scholarly literature and on the Internet. Evaluate how change occurs within the organization where you work. Does change occur according to a theory of change?
3. Can change be static or is it always dynamic? In other words, are the terms *static* and *change* contradictory?
4. Give personal examples of organizational change and explain how the involved organizations managed change.
5. Compare and contrast concepts and propositional statements that can be drawn from theories X, Y, and Z. Which of these theories is mostly closely aligned with your worldview? Defend your position. Which of these theories do you believe is most useful to advanced nursing practice? Explain.

Although they are not composed of a homogeneous group of people, organizations should find innovations that balance integration and freedom (Shafritz, Ott, & Jang, 2005).

## Summary

The discussion in this chapter only touches the tip of the iceberg of organizational behavior and leadership. Each organization has its own culture, structure, and environment (internal and external) in which it operates. Is there a theory that fits all situations? Certainly not. What has been learned over the years of theory development is that both products and people are of equal importance and that organizations must plan and operate with both in mind.

## References

Barnard, C. I. (1938). *The functions of the executive*. Cambridge, MA: Harvard University Press.

Breeze, J. D. (1981). Henry Fayol's basic tools of administration. *Proceedings of the 41st Annual Meeting of the Academy of Management, 101*, 101–105.

Brunsson, K. H. (2008). Some effects of Fayolism. *International Studies of Management and Organization, 38*(1), 30–47.

Burnes, B. (2004). Kurt Lewin and the planned approach to change: A re-appraisal. *Journal of Management Studies, 41*(6), 977–1002.

Crainer, S. (2003). One hundred years of management. *Business Strategy Review, 14*(2), 41–49.

Daft, R. L., & Noe, R. A. (2001). The scope of organizational behavior. In *Organizational behavior* (pp. 1–36). Fort Worth, TX: Harcourt College Publishers.

Drack, M. (2009). Ludwig von Bertalanffy's early system approach. *Systems Research and Behavioral Science, 26*, 563–572.

Drucker, P. F. (1999). *Management challenges for the 21st century*. New York, NY: HarperCollins.

Eisenstadt, S. N. (Ed.). (1968). *Max Weber: On charisma and institution building*. Chicago, IL: University of Chicago Press.

Fiedler, F. E. (1967). *The theory of leadership effectiveness*. New York, NY: McGraw-Hill.

Filley, A. C., & House, R. J. (1969). *Managerial process and organizational behavior*. Englewood Cliffs, NJ: Prentice Hall.

Hargreaves, S. (2006). Latham, Weber and compassion. *IPA Review, 58*(1), 20–21.

Hellriegel, D., & Slocum, J. W. (1976). *Organizational behavior* (2nd ed.). St. Paul, MN: West.

Johnson, J. A. (2009). *Health organizations: Theory, behavior, and development*. Sudbury, MA: Jones and Bartlett.

Matheson, C. (2009). Understanding the policy process: The work of Henry Mintzberg. *Public Administration Review, 69*(6), 1148–1161.

McShane, S. L., & Von Glinow, M. A. (2005). *Organizational behavior: Emerging realities for the workplace revolution* (3rd ed.). New York, NY: McGraw-Hill/Irwin.

Mintzberg, H. (1971). Managerial work: Analysis from observation. *Management Science, 18*(3), B97–B110.

Mintzberg, H. (1989). *Mintzberg on management: Inside our strange world of organizations.* New York, NY: Free Press.

Nelson, D. (1980). *Frederick W. Taylor and the rise of scientific management.* Madison, WI: University of Wisconsin Press.

Ouchi, W. (1981). *Theory Z: How American business can meet the Japanese challenge.* Reading, MA: Addison-Wesley.

Parker, L. D., & Ritson, P. A. (2005). Revisiting Fayol: Anticipating contemporary management. *British Journal of Management, 16,* 175–194.

Robbins, S. P., & Judge, T. A. (2007). *Organizational behavior* (12th ed.). Upper Saddle River, NJ: Pearson/Prentice Hall.

Roethlisberger, F. J., & Dickson, W. J. (1967). *Management and the worker: An account of a research program conducted by Western Electric Company, Hawthorne Works, Chicago.* Cambridge, MA: Harvard University Press.

Sager, F., & Rosser, C. (2009). Weber, Wilson, and Hegel: Theories of modern bureaucracy. *Public Administration Review, 69*(6), 1136–1147.

Shafritz, J. M., Ott, J. S., & Jang, Y. S. (2005). *Classics of organization theory.* Independence, KY: Cengage Learning.

Simon, H. A. (1976). *Administrative behavior* (3rd ed.). New York, NY: Macmillan.

Sullivan, E. J., & Decker, P. J. (2005). How organizations are designed. In *Effective leadership and management in nursing* (6th ed.). Upper Saddle River, NJ: Pearson/Prentice Hall.

Sullivan, E. J., & Decker, P. J. (2009). *Effective leadership and management in nursing* (7th ed.). Upper Saddle River, NJ: Pearson/Prentice Hall.

Taylor, F. W. (1911). *The principles of scientific management.* New York, NY: Harper & Brothers.

von Bertalanffy, L. (1969a). *General system theory: Foundations, development, applications.* New York, NY: George Braziller.

von Bertalanffy, L. (1969b). The history and status of general systems theory. *Academy of Management Journal, 15*(4), 407–426. Reprinted from Klir, G. J. (1972). *Trends in general systems theory.* New York, NY: Wiley-Interscience.

# Theoretical Approaches to Quality Improvement

# 16

*Patsy Anderson*

## Introduction

Numerous theories about how to improve the quality and performance of organizations have emerged over the last 50 years. Today there is so much information available about quality theory and measurement that users of this information are becoming confused. One of the *Essentials* in the American Association of Colleges of Nursing's (AACN, 2006) *The Essentials of Doctoral Education for Advanced Nursing Practice* is "Organizational and Systems Leadership for Quality Improvement and Systems Thinking" (p. 10). As part of their responsibilities, advanced practice nurses now need to understand total quality management, methods for process improvement, quality process tools and techniques, and performance measurement systems. These elements can be divided into quality theories and methods for measuring quality. This chapter provides an overview and the historical context for quality theories that are useful for leadership, management, and practice.

Nurses know that concepts used in theories need to be defined. If 20 people were asked to define quality, they probably would give 20 different answers. This is not surprising given that, for many years, even experts in quality improvement have differed in their conceptualization of quality and the ways in which it can be improved. According to Crosby (1984), quality is "conformance to requirements" (p. 60). Deming (2000) never specifically defined quality but noted that "quality should be aimed at the needs of the consumer, present and future" and that quality "begins with the intent, which is fixed by management" (p. 5). Florence Nightingale viewed quality from an absence of perspective. An interesting aside is that Pirsig (1974/1999), in his cult classic *Zen and the Art of Motorcycle Maintenance: An Inquiry into Values,* described how the indefinable nature of quality quite literally contributed to driving him mad.

Nightingale was one of the first persons who should be credited with developing a theoretical approach to quality improvement. She was followed in this endeavor by Ernest Codman and Avedis Donabedian, both of whom developed methods to study quality in health care. Healthcare industry leaders, particularly The Joint Commission, have based much of their quality improvement initiatives on the work of Codman and Donabedian, as well as on the work of leaders who focused on developing quality initiatives in the manufacturing industry, such as W. Edwards Deming, Joseph M. Juran, and Philip B. Crosby. This chapter focuses on the work of these pioneers in the field of quality improvement and management.

## Florence Nightingale

Florence Nightingale (1820–1910) was born into a rich, upper-class British family and became known worldwide as a nurse and as a statistician. One of her well-known contributions to health care occurred during the Crimean War (1853–1856). Nightingale left for Scutari, Turkey, on October 21, 1854, along with her Uncle Sam Smith and her nurses. Once she arrived in Turkey, she found deplorable conditions in the hospitals (General Hospital and Barack Hospital). The Barack Hospital was situated over a network of blocked cesspools, and privies overflowed into the hallways. Nightingale began to suspect that more soldiers were dying of disease than were being killed during battle. In January 1855, conditions were so poor that 1,000 out of 1,174 men died (Dossey, 1999).

As part of her assessment of hospital conditions, Nightingale began keeping detailed records of wounds, diseases, and deaths. In her records, deaths were divided by causes, such as contaminated food and water, lack of supplies, and organizational problems. In March 1855, the British Sanitation Commission and Nightingale began to work on improving the quality of sanitation and environmental conditions at the hospital.

During the 4 months prior to initiating her joint work with the Sanitation Commission, Nightingale had begun organizing the nurses and improving hospital supplies, general cleanliness, and the soldiers' welfare. Within 3 months, she and her associates were able to reduce wounded soldiers' death rates from 43 deaths per 1,000 to 2 per 1,000 (Dossey, 1999).

After she left Turkey in 1856, Nightingale began to work tirelessly toward implementing hospital reform in England. During the Crimean War, she had used new statistical analysis techniques to identify problems and to plan improvements. These tools and techniques essentially represented one of the first attempts to measure the quality of patient care. Later, Nightingale used her experiences in the Crimea as a basis for her reform work in England. Six months after he met with Nightingale in 1856, Lord Panmure, the British Secretary of State for War, formally requested that she submit a report about her observations related to the sanitary requirements of the army and the medical care and treatment of the sick and wounded in the Crimea. This report became an 830-page document entitled "Notes on Matters Affecting the Health, Efficiency, and Hospital Administration of the British Army" (Small, 1999). It was during this same time period that Nightingale developed her polar diagram, which was used to document the number of soldiers' deaths caused by battle compared to the number of soldiers who died from iatrogenic hospital causes. Pie charts similar to Nightingale's polar diagram remain important tools used in quality management today.

Nightingale revolutionized quality management by demonstrating the value of objectively measuring and mathematically analyzing mortality data so that the results could be used to improve patient outcomes. Quality care for Nightingale was the absence of factors that hinder the reparative process of disease. These hindrances were identified as mostly environmental things such as lack of fresh air, lack of light, and inappropriate room temperature (Nightingale, 1969/1860). In addition, for Nightingale, the environment included nurses' behaviors, such as chattering and wearing petticoats that rustled. She focused on eliminating those irritating environmental factors that often went unnoticed by nurses, but bothered patients. These environmental irritants needed to be eliminated, she suggested, so that patients would be in the best condition for healing to occur.

# Ernest Codman

Ernest Codman (1869–1940), a physician and surgeon, is known for his work in hospital reform and outcomes management in patient care. Codman was trained at Harvard Medical School and Massachusetts General Hospital; while at the hospital, he began what is believed to be the first morbidity and mortality conferences. He left the hospital after he and members of the Boston medical community were unable to reach agreement about his idea for evaluating surgeon competency.

In 1890, Codman proposed the end-result system of hospital standardization. Under this system, hospital staff tracked every patient treated at a hospital to determine whether the treatment was effective. The system required a determination of the appropriate time frame for tracking. If the treatment was not effective, the staff would then attempt to determine why, so that similar patient cases could be treated successfully in the future. Using this method from 1900 to 1910, Codman reviewed 600 abdominal surgery cases treated at Massachusetts General Hospital—not by diagnosis, but by physician. The benefits of having these results were so convincing that the medical staff agreed to conduct research and to improve their surgical skills and share the results with others.

In 1914, in protest of the surgical seniority system, Codman resigned from Massachusetts General Hospital. He believed that patient outcomes—not seniority—should be the basis for a surgeon's promotion. He continued to anger his fellow surgeons by advocating that the quality of surgical operations should be evaluated based on patient outcomes. In his system, indicators were identified and classified based on whether problems were related to organizational factors, clinician factors, or patient factors. Codman tracked the occurrence frequency for each factor and used the data to target an evaluation and correction of variables so that preventable problems did not reoccur. His system was not exactly "high tech." All of the data were recorded on 3 × 5 index cards.

Because of this controversial work and criticism he received from the Boston Medical Society during a conference on hospital efficiency, members of the medical community eventually ostracized Codman. In 1911, Codman opened his own hospital called The End Result. During a visit to England in 1912, he was appointed chair of the Committee for the Standardization of Hospitals of the American Colleges of Surgeons. This committee monitored and developed hospital quality standards. The committee continued to function until 1950, at which time the American Medical Association and the American Hospital Association renamed the committee The Joint Commission (originally The Joint Commission on Accreditation of Healthcare Organizations). In 1996, The Joint Commission established the Codman Award, which is given to a healthcare organization or professional person for achievement in the use of process and outcome measures to improve organizational performance and, ultimately, the quality and safety of care provided to the public (Joint Commission, 1996).

## Avedis Donabedian

Another 20th-century healthcare professional who had an important impact on the development of quality improvement theory and practice was Avedis Donabedian (1919–2000). Donabedian was born in Beirut, Lebanon. He came to the United States and received a master's degree in public health from Harvard University in 1955. He subsequently taught epidemiology and social medicine at New York Medical College. Later, Donabedian went to the University of Michigan School of Public Health, where he taught the principles of quality measurement.

Donabedian was one of the first people to concentrate on quality issues as they pertain to the healthcare industry. He focused on total quality management using an approach similar to the one used by Joseph Juran in his work outside the healthcare industry (discussed later in the chapter). Donabedian believed that quality in health care is defined by structure, process, and outcomes. In his work, structure was conceived as the environment in which services are provided and includes material and human resources. Process was described as the steps involved in the provision of medical services, and outcomes were measured by various criteria according to the particular study in progress. According to Donabedian (1988), these factors were all affected by the ambiguities of cost, public expectations, and resource limitations.

Donabedian's quality improvement process accounts for the difficulty of standardizing care-caused variances in populations of patients and among healthcare providers. He also recognized that different clinical practices could achieve the same outcome. The role of the quality manager in health care, he suggested, is to find the most efficient and legitimate processes to arrive at the greatest benefit at the least cost for the patient (Donabedian, 1990). Donabedian was the first recipient of the Codman Award from The Joint Commission. The National Database of Nursing Quality Indicators (American Nurses Association, 2013) is based on Donabedian's model.

## W. Edwards Deming

W. Edwards Deming (1900–1993) was a formidable figure in the field of quality improvement. Notably, he was the primary quality consultant credited with revolutionizing Japanese industry after World War II and helping Japanese companies achieve an unprecedented level of quality in their products and productivity.

Deming was educated as a physicist, obtaining a doctorate at Yale University in 1928. As a result of his work at the U.S. Department of Agriculture and his statistical expertise, he was sent to Japan in 1946 immediately after the war ended to study agricultural production and related problems. Deming was able not only to help Japanese businesses with statistical methods for quality improvement but also to improve the Japanese people's level of confidence in their products. He convinced the Japanese industrial leaders and workers that if they used his methods, in 5 years they would be able to capture the world market (Walton, 1986). Prior to his work with the Japanese, their products were considered cheap and of low quality.

When he returned from Japan, Deming tried to convince U.S. industrial leaders to implement the same theories and tools that he had implemented in Japan. However, it took much longer for Americans to appreciate his methods than it did to convince the Japanese. In contrast to the priorities established by Japanese industries after World War II, U.S. industries at that time focused on goals related to quantity rather than quality. In the late 1970s, competition from the Japanese automobile industry, especially Toyota, began to capture the attention of U.S. industry leaders. Deming became nationally known when he was featured in an NBC White Paper and television broadcast called "If Japan Can, Why Can't We?"

Deming stressed that focusing on the process is more important than focusing on the product. He found that inspection, reprocessing, and customer complaints were more costly than ensuring that a process is done correctly the first time (Walton, 1986). The Deming system is based on continuous improvement and statistical methods that must be embraced by top executives and implemented throughout an organization. Deming's theory of quality is encapsulated in his famous 14 points for management that he thought would be the basis for

## Box 16-1 Deming's 14 Points for Management

1. Create constancy of purpose for improvement of product or service.
2. Adopt the new philosophy.
3. Cease dependence on mass inspection.
4. End the practice of awarding business on the basis of price tag alone.
5. Improve constantly and forever the system of production and service.
6. Institute training and retraining.
7. Institute leadership.
8. Drive out fear.
9. Break down barriers between staff areas.
10. Eliminate slogans, exhortations, and targets for the workforce.
11. Eliminate numerical quotas.
12. Remove barriers to pride of workmanship.
13. Institute a rigorous program of education and retraining.
14. Take action to accomplish the transformation.

*Source:* Deming, W. E. (2000). *Out of the crisis.* Cambridge, MA: MIT Press.

transforming U.S. industry (see **Box 16–1**). These 14 points were developed to be widely applicable to organizations of all sizes and missions, both service and manufacturing. A discussion of each of the 14 points based on Deming's (2000) work follows.

*Point 1: Create constancy of purpose for improvement of product or service.* To fulfill this aim, organizations, while not ignoring the problems of today such as budget, employment, and public relations, must deal with the more challenging problems of tomorrow. Coping with future problems requires constancy of purpose. This constancy of purpose entails not allowing the desire for immediate profit to hurt the organization's long-term improvement and competitiveness. For long-term improvement to occur, management must innovate by allocating resources for long-term planning, by using resources for research and education, and by continually improving the design of its products and services. Regarding constant improvement, Deming reminded managers that their obligation never stops. These actions are as essential in the healthcare field as they are in any other industry.

*Point 2: Adopt the new philosophy.* The "new philosophy" to which Deming referred is quality improvement as it was being practiced in Japan after World War II. Adopting this philosophy meant stopping the bad practices that American industry had adopted. Deming believed that leaders in U.S. organizations and companies should no longer accept the level of mistakes, defects, and ineffective supervision and management that were being tolerated. Deming did not limit this challenge to management but rather stated that government must remove obstacles to U.S. industry's competitive position as well.

*Point 3: Cease dependence on mass inspection.* Using a system based on mass inspection leads to a need for rework. It implies that defects are expected to occur and will need to be fixed or in some way repaired. Although inspection may be necessary for safety and accuracy, especially in certain very complex processes and products, reliance on inspection means that attention is not focused on improvements that would make the outcome right the first time.

*Point 4: End the practice of awarding business on the basis of price tag alone.* Price does not indicate quality. When an item purchased is not of high quality, high costs may result from its use. Deming suggested that long-term relationships with single vendors will elicit loyalty, trust, and, in the long run, lower costs. Even if an organization uses a single vendor, however, unwanted variations may still be introduced into the products and services.

*Point 5: Improve constantly and forever the system of production and service.* One way to explain this point is to discuss what it does not mean. It does not mean solving immediate problems as they arise. Rather, it means making an ongoing commitment to ensure that quality is built in at the development stage and that all existing processes are continually studied and revised to improve their outputs. Deming argued that improvement does not occur simply by allocating money for quality; rather, knowledge is the key. The better the understanding that managers and others have about the processes employed, the more effective change will be. Using reliable statistical methods to study processes is also necessary.

*Point 6: Institute training and retraining.* Deming stressed two kinds of training. First, managers must be trained in the complete functioning of the organization and in the concepts of quality improvement, especially focusing on reducing variations rather than on meeting specifications. Second, appropriate training and placement of staff members will ensure that their rich talents are not squandered. Appropriate training for staff members and managers includes (1) ensuring that there is training, (2) making sure that the means of training is effective, and (3) ending the practice of having staff trained by other staff who may themselves have acquired bad habits because of poor training. Training should be ongoing while evidence indicates that it is still helpful, and training should occur when circumstances require it. Continuing education is a part of the culture in health care. This education should include the tenets of quality improvement and statistical control.

*Point 7: Institute leadership.* Managers must, Deming said, not supervise but lead. To do this, managers must remove barriers that make it difficult for workers to take pride in their work. Managers also must know how to do the work that they supervise. To lead, managers must not treat every problem as a fire to be put out, but rather must look toward making systems improvements. Finally, leaders should not accept numerical fallacies, especially the notion that all workers should meet the average. In fact, not everyone can be average; some people will always be below average. This is demonstrated in statistical normal distribution.

*Point 8: Drive out fear.* Fear is inherent in the bad apple approach to quality and in the perception that quality is something imposed by outside forces peering over the shoulder of each member of the organization. In health care, there tends to be under-reporting of medication and medical errors because of the fear of retaliation from organization leaders and managers. This, in turn, can lead to unintended consequences for both patients and organizations.

*Point 9: Break down barriers between staff areas.* The structure of an organization can work against quality improvement; lack of communication between people in various departments and services can impede improvement and cause problems. In health care, this is especially true. The coordination of, for example, nursing, anesthesia, surgery, and post-anesthesia care is crucial for any surgical procedure. As another example, communication between professional and administrative staff is essential when contemplating equipment purchases or changes in procedures. In addition, the process by which systems are studied and improved requires close cooperation of all involved parties, regardless of their work department or service area. Removing such barriers can mean a change in the culture of an organization.

*Point 10: Eliminate slogans, exhortations, and targets for the workforce.* Deming emphasized that such tactics are meaningless without a plan to back them up. Also, they generate frustration by asking workers to improve without providing the necessary means to make such improvements.

*Point 11: Eliminate numerical quotas.* Organizational managers typically set rates of production for the average worker. If one considers the normal distribution curve, it is evident why this pattern occurs. Setting production levels, however, can result in undesired outcomes, such as various types of loss, disorganization, dissatisfaction, and turnover. In some organizations, the production rates are set based on the work of the overachiever, which puts even greater stress on workers and creates organizational problems. Quotas for managers are equally problematic, such as those engendered by the practice of management by objectives. Often these goals are not accompanied by plans, and if the system itself is not stable, a goal is meaningless.

*Point 12: Remove barriers to pride of workmanship.* Deming listed several specific barriers. For example, a system in which an annual performance evaluation is linked to a pay increase for salaried workers focuses on the end product, and the end of the stream—not on leadership to help people. The resultant effect is fear and self-preservation, rather than action to improve the organization. Barriers to staff having a sense of pride arise when staff members are treated as if they are commodities, they are powerless to communicate their ideas and knowledge to management, and when they do not know what is expected of them. "Quick fix" solutions to mitigate these barriers do not work. Instead, managers must demonstrate over a period of time that action will be taken to improve systems, that there is no continuing hunt for bad apples, and that there is a commitment to the long-term survival and improvement of the organization.

*Point 13: Institute a rigorous program of education and retraining.* As stated under Point 6, ongoing education of the sort practiced in the healthcare field is essential for people to fully develop and effectively use their talents. In addition, as the organization changes because of quality improvement activities, re-education becomes necessary to help people adapt to the changing environment.

*Point 14: Take action to accomplish the transformation.* Deming believed that managers would struggle in trying to comply with all of the previous 13 points. To deal with this problem, he suggested that managers organize as a team to meet the challenges. Every employee and manager of an organization should be taught how to improve quality continually, and this initiative must come from the top down.

In addition to proposing these 14 points, Deming also identified seven deadly diseases that afflict many organizations and prevent their transformation toward quality improvement. He thought that the cure of these diseases would require a complete change in the Western style of management. These seven deadly diseases include issues such as an emphasis on short-term profits, frequent mobility of managers, and excessive medical costs (Walton, 1986).

Deming identified several statistical processes that could be used to implement his theory. Among those statistical methods are flow diagrams to identify work processes; cause and effect diagrams that display all factors that contribute to a problem and their relationships to outcomes; statistical process control, which is used to evaluate special and common causes of process outcomes; and the Shewhart cycle, more commonly known today as the plan–do–check–act (PDCA) cycle (Deming, 2000).

The Shewhart cycle—named for Walter A. Shewhart, who developed it in the 1920s—is the most widely used planning and improvement process in the field of quality management. It was introduced in Japan by Deming, which explains why it is sometimes called the Deming cycle. The PDCA (Shewhart) cycle provides a quality improvement framework to carry out ongoing processes focused on assessing, planning, acting, monitoring and evaluating, reassessing, and acting again (Deming, 2000).

## Joseph M. Juran

Joseph M. Juran (1904–2008) was another consultant credited with leading the quality revolution in Japan. Through the Juran Institute, he conducted public and in-house seminars for managers throughout the world. Juran's legacy continues to be carried out by the Juran Institute.

Juran promoted ideas relating to the integration of quality improvement into corporate plans, with quality being defined as fitness for purpose rather than conformance to specification, teamwork, delighting customers, and problem solving. Juran suggested that quality has a dual meaning. In one sense, quality refers to freedom from deficiencies or, put in more realistic terms, the error rate. In another sense, quality refers to product features. Juran identified freedom from deficiencies as reduced rework, reduced need for inspection, and reduced customer dissatisfaction. Reduced deficiencies, he noted, tend to lower costs. Product features, by comparison, are intended to meet customers' needs and produce customer satisfaction. Higher quality, in terms of product features, makes products more appealing to consumers, increases sales, increases competitiveness, and often increases costs. This distinction is especially applicable to health care (Juran, 1989). According to Juran, these two aspects of quality are not polar opposites. Rather, to satisfy customers, a product must both have the features they desire and be as free from deficiencies as possible. One or the other aspects, by itself, does not constitute high quality.

The primary foundation of Juran's quality process is the Juran trilogy (Juran, 1989). The Juran trilogy consists of three components: (1) quality planning, (2) quality control, and (3) quality improvement. The starting point is quality planning, which entails developing a process that will meet established goals and current operating conditions. *Quality planning* involves building quality—in terms of both freedom from deficiencies and increased desirability of product features—into processes and products. *Quality control* is focused on maintaining the status quo, that is, to reduce variation in processes and products. To help evaluate quality control, quality control limits should be established; Juran advocated using a feedback loop in the control process. *Quality improvement* is the purposeful action taken by upper management to introduce new processes into the system (Juran, 1992). **Box 16–2** provides a synopsis of Juran's primary concepts.

# Philip B. Crosby

Philip B. Crosby (1926–2001) rose from line inspector at International Telephone and Telegraph to corporate vice president, giving him a unique understanding of quality from various points of view. In 1979, Crosby's book *Quality Is Free* was published and became a best seller in the field of quality management. Like Deming, Crosby emphasized the importance of systems knowledge and improvement, the pitfalls of inspection, and the need for statistical quality control.

Crosby defined quality in simple and absolute terms. The principal strength of Crosby's theory is the attention it gives to transforming the quality culture of an organization. As Crosby (1992) wrote in his book, *Completeness: Quality for the 21st Century*, "The problem with quality has always been management's lack of understanding of their responsibility for causing a culture of prevention in their company" (p. xi). He believed that quality is a matter of philosophy, rather than just being based on techniques and statistics. Quality, he suggested, should not be delegated from leaders to another group. It is the job of leadership to have quality actually become part of the fabric of the organization.

Crosby thought that quality means conformance to carefully determined requirements and not to goodness. By stressing individual conformance to requirements, he involved everyone in the organization in his process. While working on his theory,

## Box 16–2 The Juran Trilogy

| Quality Planning | Quality Control | Quality Improvement |
|---|---|---|
| Identify the customers (internal and external) | Choose control subjects | Prove the need for improvement |
| Determine customer needs | Choose units of measurement | Identify specific projects for improvement |
| Develop product features that respond to customer needs, both products and services | Establish measurement | Organize to guide the projects |
| Establish quality goals that meet customers' and suppliers' needs at minimum cost | Establish standards of performance | Organize for diagnosis—for discovery of causes |
| Develop processes that can produce the needed product features | Interpret the difference (actual versus standard) | Diagnose to find the causes |
| Improve process capability—the ability of the process to meet the quality goals under operating conditions | Take action on the difference | Prove remedies |
| | | Prove that the remedies are effective under operating conditions |
| | | Provide for control to hold the gains |

Source: Stephens, K. S., & Juran, J. M. (2004). *Quality and a century of improvement*. Milwaukee, WI: ASQ Quality Press. No further distribution allowed without permission.

Crosby observed that organizations that are determined to improve their processes but fail to accomplish this have five common characteristics:

1. They called their effort a program instead of a process.
2. They aimed most of their quality efforts toward the lower operational levels.
3. They employed quality control staff who were cynical.
4. They used training materials that sometimes perpetuated an error or had a detrimental effect on quality.
5. They were impatient for results (Crosby, 1984).

Crosby began his theory with four basic concepts or absolutes of a quality improvement process. These absolutes answer four questions: (1) What is quality?, (2) What kind of system is needed to cause quality?, (3) Which performance standard should be used?, and (4) What kind of measurement system is required? (Crosby, 1984, p. 58).

The first absolute is that "the definition of quality is conformance to requirements" (p. 59). In regard to their work, Crosby argued that everyone should "do it right the first time" (DIRFT) (p. 59). For this first absolute, he believed that management has the basic tasks of establishing the requirements that employees are asked to meet, supplying the resources for the employees to meet the requirements, and spending time encouraging and helping the employees meet the requirements. His contention was that when it is evident that the management supports DIRFT, then everyone will DIRFT.

The second absolute is that "the system of quality is prevention" (p. 66). Crosby asserted that checking for goodness after the fact is a waste of resources and that prevention is successful if everyone understands key processes. The ideal system for producing quality, he suggested, focuses on prevention, not appraisal. The service industry, which includes healthcare organizations, was found to have greater difficulty with prevention than the manufacturing industry because it is more challenging to identify organization-wide problems. For service industries, Crosby advocated the use of a statistical quality control process. This process requires that each variable of the process be identified and measured. When a variable begins to move out of control, it can then be adjusted back. Such a process consists of a measurement technique relying on charts that identify the upper and lower control limits, with the section between the limits being defined as the tolerance level for the process (Crosby, 1984).

The third absolute is that "the performance standard is zero defects" (p. 74). According to Crosby, "a company is an organism with millions of little seemingly insignificant actions that make it all happen. Each and every little action has to be done just as planned in order to make everything come out right" (p. 74). He argued that when a company does not encourage everyone to DIRFT, deviation from performance standards will occur, and these deviations ultimately become acceptable practices. Organizations of all kinds, he suggested, help their employees fail to meet performance standards by allowing or overlooking percentages of errors in certain tasks. For example, in hospitals today, certain levels of medication errors are expected to occur. Leaders or quality managers are satisfied when errors do not reach a pre-identified error limit. Crosby noted that it is interesting that people seem willing to accept a certain percentage of errors in some areas of an organization, but not in the areas of finance and payroll. In regard to finance and payroll, the expectation is that error rates will be zero (Crosby, 1984).

The fourth absolute is "the measurement of quality is the price of nonconformance" (p. 83). Crosby divided the cost of quality into two parts: the price of nonconformance (PONC) and the price of conformance (POC). The PONC includes the expenses involved in doing things wrong. He found that this PONC usually represents 20% or more in manufacturing companies and 35% or more in service organizations. The POC is what is spent for quality outcomes; it includes professional quality functions, all preventive measures, and quality education. According to Crosby, the POC represents 3% to 4% in a well-managed organization. Crosby encouraged individuals to keep track of the cost of quality, because this is a persuasive way to measure quality and to demonstrate the value of quality improvement.

Beyond these four absolutes, Crosby proposed a vaccine to provide "antibodies that will prevent hassle" (p. 6). This quality vaccine is a clear picture of the characteristics of an organization that fulfills the principles of quality improvement. To administer this vaccine, managers must be determined to implement quality improvement, must educate all employees in quality improvement, and must be dedicated to a long-term process of implementing quality improvement rather than looking for a quick or easy fix. The vaccination consists of a combination of certain key ingredients divided into the five categories of integrity, systems, communications, operations, and policies (Crosby, 1984). **Box 16–3** provides details of the Crosby vaccination.

---

### Box 16–3  The Crosby Vaccination Serum Ingredients

**Integrity**
- The CEO is dedicated to having the customer receive what is promised, believes that the company will prosper only when all employees feel the same way, and is determined that neither customers nor employees will be hassled.
- The COO believes that management performance is a complete function requiring that quality be "first among equals"—including schedule and cost.
- The senior executives who report to the CEO and the COO take requirements so seriously that they cannot stand deviations.
- The managers who work for the senior executives know that the future rests with their ability to get things done through people—right the first time.
- The professional employees know that the accuracy and completeness of their work determines the effectiveness of the entire workforce.
- The employees as a whole recognize that their individual commitment to the integrity of requirements is what makes the organization sound.

**Systems**
- The quality management functions are dedicated to measuring conformance to requirements and reporting any differences accurately.
- The quality education system ensures that all employees of the organization have a common language of quality and understand their personal roles in causing quality to be a routine part of the organization's operations.

*(Continues)*

## Box 16–3 The Crosby Vaccination Serum Ingredients (*Continued*)

- The financial method of measuring nonconformance and conformance costs is used to evaluate processes.
- The use of the organization's services or products by customers is measured and reported in a manner that causes corrective action to occur.
- The organization-wide emphasis on defect prevention serves as a base for continual review and planning that utilizes current and past experience to keep the past from repeating itself.

**Communications**
- Information about the progress of quality improvement and achievement actions is continually supplied to all employees.
- Recognition programs applicable to all levels of responsibility are a part of normal operations.
- Each person in the organization can, with very little effort, identify error, waste, opportunity, or any other concern to top management quickly—and receive an immediate answer.
- Each management status meeting begins with a factual and financial review of quality.

**Operations**
- Suppliers are educated and supported to ensure that they will deliver services and products that are dependable and on time.
- Procedures, products, and systems are qualified and proven prior to implementation and then continually examined and officially modified when the opportunity for improvement is seen.
- Training is a routine activity for all tasks and is particularly integrated into new processes and procedures.

**Policies**
- The policies on quality are clear and unambiguous.
- The quality function reports on the same level as those functions that are being measured and has complete freedom of activity.
- Advertising and all external communications are completely in compliance with the same requirements that the products and services must meet.

*Source:* Crosby, P. (1995). *Quality without tears: The art of hassle-free management.* New York, NY: McGraw-Hill.

# Summary

The quest for quality in health care will continue. As the United States seeks to provide quality health care to all of its citizens, the U.S. healthcare industry and the federal government are developing outcomes measurement systems, practice standards, and reimbursement based on performance. While quality improvement experts differ somewhat in their approaches, their theories share several common characteristics.

## Quality Is Driven by Organization Leaders

Experts agree that leaders must be committed to quality improvement if an organization-wide program is to be successful. Leaders must embody the principles of quality improvement if they expect staff to commit themselves to the desired cultural shift. The manager's job is to remove barriers that prevent staff from providing quality services all of the time.

## Customer-Mindedness Permeates the Organization

A new definition of the customer must be articulated throughout the organization. According to Deming (2000), each organization has both internal and external customers. External customers for healthcare organizations, for example, include patients, physicians, and insurance companies. Internal customers include people such as the staff who work in the organization, as well as the departments receiving services from other departments within the organization.

## An Emphasis on Process Improvement

At the heart of quality improvement is a body of knowledge and tools referred to as *systems thinking* that emerged over the last half-century. Systems thinking is a framework for seeing inter-relationships rather than discrete things, for seeing patterns of change rather than static snapshots (Senge, 1990). By taking a systematic view, the many processes and factors that affect outcomes become clear—for example, protocols, guidelines, and management systems. Adopting a quality improvement philosophy involves rejecting the idea that people are the problem and, instead, shifts the focus toward looking at the organization's systems.

Deming believed that most employees want to do the best job they can, but the systems they work in often prevent them from doing so. He concluded that 85% of the problems detected are systems based and only 15% can be traced to the worker (Deming, 2000). Organizations that implement quality improvement, when necessary, form teams composed of members across functional or departmental lines to examine and reexamine clinical and administrative processes and to analyze how these processes might be improved. However, all process improvements do not necessarily require the formation of a team. Juran, for instance, believed that teams sometimes are vulnerable to *groupthink,* a phenomenon that can hinder effective work on issues of quality improvement. A sign that quality improvement is beginning to infiltrate an organization is when management and staff begin to use the concepts in their everyday activities.

## Formal Process Improvement Methods and Tools

To guide process improvement efforts, organizations use time-tested scientific methods and statistical tools. When improvement is needed, staff measure and analyze the current process to determine the root cause or primary reason that the process is inadequate; they then take action toward improvement based on that analysis. Organizations use a variety of tools for quality improvement purposes, such as flowcharts, cause and effect diagrams, and control charts.

## Involvement of All Employees

Quality improvement is a cultural transformation that begins with a slow change in attitudes, which is then gradually realized in improved outcomes, staff morale, and patient care. It requires a commitment from everyone in the organization, from the housekeeper to the chief executive officer. A quality improvement department or a subcommittee cannot shoulder all of the responsibility for the institution's ultimate survival. One way in which this wide-scale, shared involvement is most visible is in the makeup and dynamics of teams. Quality improvement empowers staff by providing them with the methods and structure to approach their jobs, and empowered employees are better prepared to participate in quality improvement activities.

# Resources

In today's ever-changing healthcare industry, quality improvement remains highly relevant. All healthcare organizations need to evaluate the quality of their services for their own improvement or for external reviewers and payers. Listed here are accreditation organizations that evaluate the quality of care provided by healthcare organizations:

Accreditation Association for Ambulatory Health Care (AAAHC)
http://www.aaahc.org
*AAAHC is an American organization that accredits ambulatory healthcare organizations, including ambulatory surgery centers, office-based surgery centers, endoscopy centers, and college student health centers, as well as health plans, such as health maintenance organizations and preferred provider organizations.*

Accreditation Commission for Health Care (ACHC)
http://www.achc.org
*ACHC is a U.S. nonprofit accrediting organization. Home care health providers established it to create an accreditation option that was more focused on the needs of small providers.*

Centers for Medicare & Medicaid Services
http://www.cms.gov
*CMS is a federal agency within the U.S. Department of Health and Human Services that administers the Medicare program and works in partnership with state governments to administer Medicaid, the State Children's Health Insurance Program, and health insurance portability standards.*

Community Health Accreditation Program (CHAP)
http://www.chapinc.org
*CHAP is a U.S. nonprofit accrediting body for community-based healthcare organizations.*

DNV Healthcare
http://dnvaccreditation.com
*DNV Healthcare, Inc. is a leading provider of international hospital accreditation, infection risk management, and standards development. The company was approved in 2008 by the U.S. Centers for Medicare & Medicaid Services (CMS) to accredit acute care hospitals in the United States and since then has also been granted CMS deeming authority for critical access hospitals. It is part of the larger multinational group Stiftelsen Det Norske Veritas (DNV).*

Healthcare Facilities Accreditation Program (HFAP)
http://www.hfap.org
*HFAP is a U.S. nonprofit organization that provides accreditation programs for hospitals, clinical laboratories, ambulatory surgical centers/office-based surgery, and critical access hospitals. In addition, HFAP accredits mental health and physical rehabilitation facilities and provides certification for primary stroke centers.*

Healthcare Quality Association on Accreditation
http://www.hqaa.org
*HQAA is a U.S. nonprofit healthcare accrediting body that provides an accreditation option specifically designed for DME companies. These company types include DME, infusion and compounding pharmacies, medical practice, facility base ventilator units, and third-party billing.*

National Committee for Quality Assurance (NCQA)
http://www.ncqa.org
*NCQA is a U.S. nonprofit organization designed to improve healthcare quality. NCQA manages voluntary accreditation programs for individual physicians, health plans, and medical groups.*

The Compliance Team
http://www.thecomplianceteam.org
*The Compliance Team Inc. is a U.S. for-profit organization that runs the "Exemplary Provider" accreditation programs. The Compliance Team accredits all types of*

*durable medical equipment (DME), including respiratory, mobility, wound care, orthopedic, prosthetics, orthotics, diabetic, ostomy, and incontinence supplies, as well as DME point-of-service providers including pharmacy, home care, podiatrists, and orthopedic surgeons. The Compliance Team has accredited approximately 5,000 DME providers in the United States and Puerto Rico.*

The Joint Commission
http://www.jointcommission.org
*The Joint Commission is a U.S.-based nonprofit organization that accredits more than 19,000 healthcare organizations and programs. It accredits ambulatory care, behavioral care, critical access hospital, home care, hospitals, laboratory services, nursing and rehabilitation centers, and international organizations.*

## Discussion Questions

1. What does the concept of quality mean?
2. How is quality defined in nursing literature?
3. Does mass inspection improve the quality of care delivered by people working in the healthcare industry? Support your answer.
4. Is the goal of zero defects realistic in health care? Support your answer.
5. How are evidence-based practice and quality management related?

## References

American Association of Colleges of Nursing. (2006). *The essentials of doctoral education for advanced nursing practice.* Washington, DC: Author.

American Nurses Association. (2013). NDNQI data. Retrieved from http://www.nursingquality.org/data

Crosby, P. (1979). *Quality is free.* New York, NY: McGraw-Hill.

Crosby, P. (1984). *Quality without tears: The art of hassle-free management.* New York, NY: McGraw-Hill.

Crosby, P. (1992). *Completeness: Quality for the 21st century.* New York, NY: Penguin Books.

Deming, W. E. (2000). *Out of the crisis.* Cambridge, MA: MIT Press.

Donabedian, A. (1988). The quality of care: How can it be assessed? *Journal of the American Medical Association, 260,* 1743–1748.

Donabedian, A. (1990). The seven pillars of quality. *Archives of Pathology and Laboratory Medicine, 114,* 1115–1118.

Dossey, B. M. (1999). *Florence Nightingale.* Springhouse, PA: Springhouse.

The Joint Commission. (1996). *A study in hospital efficiency as demonstrated by the case report of the first five years of a private hospital.* Oakbrook Terrace, IL: Author.

Juran, J. M. (1989). *Juran on leadership for quality.* New York, NY: Free Press.

Juran, J. M. (1992). *Juran on Quality by Design.* New York, NY: Free Press.

Nightingale, F. (1969/1860). *Notes on nursing: What it is, and what it is not.* New York, NY: Dover Publications.

Pirsig, R. M. (1999). *Zen and the art of motorcycle maintenance: An inquiry into values* (25th anniversary ed.). New York, NY: Vintage. (Originally published in 1974).

Senge, P. M. (1990). *The fifth discipline: The art and practice of the learning organization.* New York, NY: Doubleday.

Small, H. (1999). *Florence Nightingale: Avenging angel.* New York, NY: Palgrave Macmillan.

Stephens, K. S., & Juran, J. M. (2004). *Quality and a century of improvement.* Milwaukee, WI: ASQ Quality Press.

Walton, M. (1986). *The Deming management method.* New York, NY: Putnam.

# PART 4

# Select Nursing Models and Theories

# CHAPTER 17

# Models and Theories Focused on Nursing Goals and Functions

*Kathleen Masters*

## Introduction

There are numerous perspectives from which nursing models and theories may be viewed and subsequently classified. This chapter examines nursing models and theories that may be categorized as focusing on goals and functions. From the standpoint of each model or theory, it will address the roles and functions of advanced practice nurses (APNs) and the goals of nursing care. Four of the most prominent nursing models and theories in this category include Florence Nightingale's environmental model of nursing, Virginia Henderson's 14 components of basic nursing care, Dorothy Johnson's behavioral system model, and Nola J. Pender's health promotion model.

While neither Nightingale nor Henderson defined her work as a theory of nursing, it is evident from the current vantage point that the work of these nursing pioneers provided the theoretical foundation for the practice discipline of nursing. Johnson was also a pioneer in the world of nursing theory. While influenced by the thinking of Nightingale, Johnson also incorporated theories from other disciplines and pushed theoretical thinking in nursing to a higher conceptual level with the development of the behavioral system model. While these three works were general in nature, more recently Pender has contributed to the theoretical basis for nursing practice with the introduction of a model that, while still allowing for generalization across populations, is specific to health promotion. In this chapter, the work of these nurse theorists will be presented in chronological order, beginning with background information and followed by a discussion of each theory.

# The Environmental Model of Nursing: Florence Nightingale

## Background

Florence Nightingale was born on May 12, 1820, in Florence, Italy, the second child of an affluent British family. As a youngster, she displayed exceptional intellectual ability and was well educated for a female in the Victorian era, having been tutored by her father in math, philosophy, languages, and religion. Nightingale was active in aristocratic society but believed that her life could be more useful. She was obsessed with the poverty, disease, and suffering of the masses; to the dismay of her family, she believed that she was called by God to be a nurse (Woodham-Smith, 1951). At the age of 25, Nightingale expressed a desire to become a nurse, but her parents refused her request. Over the next 7 years, she continued her study of math, science, hospitals, and public health while she made repeated attempts to change the minds of her parents (Dietz & Lehozky, 1963).

During a trip to Egypt with family and friends in 1849, Nightingale spent time with the Sisters of Charity of St. Vincent de Paul, where her conviction to study nursing was reinforced (Tooley, 1910). The next year, Nightingale traveled to the Kaiserwerth Institute in Germany. She spent only 2 weeks at Kaiserwerth but vowed that she would return to study nursing. In 1851, Nightingale announced to her family that she planned to return to Germany to study nursing. Finally, at the age of 31 Nightingale was permitted to travel back to Kaiserwerth, where she learned about the care of the sick and the importance of discipline and commitment to God (Donahue, 1985).

In 1853, after receiving an endowment from her father, Nightingale moved to London, where she became superintendent of the Hospital for Invalid Gentlewomen, thereby realizing her goal of working as a nurse (Cook, 1913). During the Crimean War, Nightingale traveled to Üsküdar (called Scutari in Nightingale's era), Turkey, along with 38 other nurses. When they arrived, the women were faced with the prospect of overcrowded barracks and atrocious sanitary conditions. Nightingale focused her efforts on organizing nursing services and eliminating sanitation problems in the hospital; ultimately, she proved successful in decreasing the mortality rate in the Crimean War. Upon her return home to London, she eventually established the Nightingale School of Nursing at St. Thomas's Hospital, which was the beginning of professional nursing (Donahue, 1985).

Nightingale expressed her views about nursing in many formats. She wrote letters, pamphlets, and government reports. In addition, in 1859, Nightingale published *Notes on Nursing: What It Is and What It Is Not*, a book that represented her first effort at putting her philosophy and description of nursing into one document (Reed & Zurakowski, 1989).

During the last 50 years of her life, although Nightingale suffered from poor health, she spent significant time writing letters, books, reports, and meeting with friends and colleagues from within the confines of her home. She died in London on August 13, 1910, at the age of 91.

## Nightingale's 13 Canons Central to the Environmental Model of Nursing

In her writings, Nightingale did not plan to develop a theory, but rather sought to describe nursing and delineate general rules for nursing practice, thereby making her model both descriptive and practical. Nursing care using Nightingale's model is centered on her 13 canons, which include the following precepts (Nightingale, 1860/1969):

1. *Ventilation and warmth:* The interventions subsumed in this canon include keeping the patient and the patient's room warm and keeping the patient's room well ventilated and free of odors. Specific instructions included to "keep the air within as pure as the air without" (p. 10).
2. *Health of houses:* This canon includes the five essentials of pure air, pure water, efficient drainage, cleanliness, and light.
3. *Petty management:* Continuity of care for the patient when the nurse is absent is the essence of this canon.
4. *Noise:* Instructions include the avoidance of sudden noises that startle or awaken patients and keeping noise in general to a minimum.
5. *Variety:* This canon refers to an attempt to provide variety in the patient's room in order to avoid boredom and depression.
6. *Food intake:* Interventions include the documentation of the amount of food and liquids that the patient ingested.
7. *Food:* Instructions include trying to include patient food preferences.
8. *Bed and bedding:* The interventions in this canon include comfort measures related to keeping the bed dry and wrinkle free.
9. *Light:* The instructions contained in this canon relate to adequate light in the patient's room.
10. *Cleanliness of rooms and walls:* This canon focuses on keeping the environment clean.
11. *Personal cleanliness:* This canon includes measures such as keeping the patient clean and dry.
12. *Chattering hopes and advice:* Instructions in this canon include the avoidance of talking without reason or giving advice that is not supported by fact.
13. *Observation of the sick:* This canon includes instructions related to making observations and documenting observations.

When they incorporate Nightingale's 13 canons into their caregiving, APNs include questioning and observation in their nursing assessments of patients. Questions the nurse asks relate to food preferences, as well as food and fluid intake. Nursing observations are focused on environmental influences on patients—for example, the effects of noise, light, and nutrition on patients. The Nightingale model involves nurses manipulating environmental factors that affect the patient's health status, including noise, light, cleanliness, bedding, and ventilation. Evaluation is based on the effect of changes in the environment on the patient's health. Observation is the primary method of data collection and evaluation of

## Box 17-1  Case Study Utilizing Nightingale's Environmental Model

Mrs. Little, who is age 78 and a Caucasian, visits your primary care clinic. She recently underwent coronary artery bypass graft surgery. This morning at the clinic, Mrs. Little complains that she has not been able to sleep since she was hospitalized. She lives with her daughter's family, which includes two teenagers. Mrs. Little has not eaten much recently.

Nursing care for Mrs. Little using the Nightingale environmental model begins with an assessment of environmental factors that are impacting the patient—in this case, manipulation of the environment is needed to promote sleep and nutrition. This manipulation of the environment might include educating Mrs. Little and her daughter about eliminating noise and unnecessary light during the hours when Mrs. Little normally sleeps. Inquiry related to the patient's food preferences is conducted in the presence of Mrs. Little's daughter. In addition, teaching might include information about comfort and relaxation measures such as clean, wrinkle-free linens and maintenance of room temperature conducive to sleeping. Evaluation will be based on the quantity and quality of sleep and the nutritional intake of Mrs. Little, as well as her subsequent restoration of health.

outcomes (Nightingale, 1860/1969). A case illustrating care and treatment administered by APNs using Nightingale's environmental model of nursing appears in **Box 17-1**.

The 13 canons are central to Nightingale's model, but they are not all-inclusive. Nightingale believed that nursing is a calling and that the recipients of nursing care are holistic individuals with a spiritual dimension; thus, under her model, the nurse is expected to care for the spiritual needs of patients in spiritual distress. (What are some ways that modern-day APNs might provide holistic care with a spiritual dimension?) Nightingale also believed that nurses should be involved in health promotion and health teaching both with patients who are sick and with those who are well (Bolton, 2006).

## Major Concepts of the Environmental Model of Nursing According to Nightingale

Nightingale's environmental model of nursing represented a landmark in the development of nursing science and provided the foundation for the discipline's four metaparadigm concepts of (1) person, (2) environment, (3) health, and (4) nursing. Her model, however, focuses primarily on the patient and the environment. In other words, the primary function of the nurse in Nightingale's view is to manipulate the physical and social factors that affect health and illness in order to enhance patient recovery.

## Person

While not specifically defined, the person in Nightingale's environmental model is quite simply the recipient of nursing care. The person is viewed in relation to the environment and the impact of the environment on the person's health status.

## Environment

The physical environment was stressed in Nightingale's model, although she did acknowledge the potential impact of the social environment on the health of the patient. Components of the environment discussed by Nightingale include aspects of both the external environment (temperature, bedding, ventilation) and the internal environment (food, water, and medications).

## Health

Nightingale did not specifically define the concept of health, but she believed that nature alone could cure disease. She described health as "not only to be well, but to be able to use well every power we have to use" (Nightingale, 1860/1969, p. 24).

## Nursing

Nursing to Nightingale was, above all, "service to God in the relief of man" (Nightingale, 1858, p. 2). The nurse's function, according to Nightingale, is to alter or manage the environment to put patients in the best possible situation for the natural laws of health to act upon them (Johnson & Webber, 2010); thus the ultimate goal of nursing activities is patient health. Nightingale also believed that nurses should provide care for both healthy and ill people and discussed health promotion activities as part of the role of the nurse (Lobo, 2002).

## Analysis of Nightingale's Environmental Model of Nursing

The analysis and critique of Nightingale's environmental model of nursing presented here will consist of an examination of assumptions and propositions, as well as the analysis of clarity, simplicity, generality, empirical precision, and derivable consequences of this model.

### Assumptions of Nightingale's Environmental Model of Nursing

While Nightingale did not explicitly state any theoretical assumptions, a number of assumptions can be extracted from her work. Philosophical assumptions that can be extracted include the following: (1) nursing is a calling; (2) nursing is an art and a science; (3) persons can control the outcomes of their lives and, therefore, can pursue perfect health; (4) nursing requires a specific educational base; and (5) nursing is distinct and separate from medicine (Selanders, 1995). The following assumptions also may be inferred from Nightingale's work: (1) maintaining a clean room, bedding, and clothes aids in patient recovery; (2) noise can be harmful to patients; and (3) managing the environment improves the health of the patient (Johnson & Webber, 2010).

### Propositions of Nightingale's Environmental Model of Nursing

The primary relationship statements that APNs can derive from the writings of Nightingale include (1) the person is desirous of health, so the nurse, nature, and the person will cooperate in order for all reparative processes to occur and (2) the nurse's role is to prevent the reparative process from being interrupted and to provide conditions that optimize the reparative process (Pfettscher, 2010). The APN reader of this chapter might imagine scenarios where these two propositions are included in advanced practice.

### Analysis: Clarity, Simplicity, Generality, Empirical Precision, and Derivable Consequences

The analysis of Nightingale's environmental model presented here is based on the theory evaluation criteria of clarity, simplicity, generality, empirical precision, and derivable consequences as suggested by Chinn and Kramer (2008).

Nightingale's model places an emphasis on relationships not regarded as revolutionary or complex by current standards. At the same time, it provides a broad framework for organizing observations about a large number of nursing phenomena, thereby making the model broad in scope and giving it generality (Reed & Zurakowski, 1989). The components of the model are clearly articulated. The model is a simple one, with only three major relationships specified—(1) environment to patient, (2) nurse to environment, and (3) nurse to patient—yet attempts to provide guidelines for all nurses in all situations. While some of the specific directives may no longer be applicable, the general concepts, including the relationships between the nurse, the patient, and the environment, remain highly relevant to modern-day practitioners (Pfettscher, 2010).

Nightingale's environmental model of nursing was developed inductively, with the proposed laws of health and nursing being derived from Nightingale's observations and many of the principles originating from the observations made during her wartime experiences (Pfettscher, 2010). The major concepts are clearly defined, and the relationships among the concepts flow logically based on the definitions of the concepts, giving the model internal consistency (Reed & Zurakowski, 1989). The concepts and relationships are presented as truths, rather than testable statements, however (Pfettscher, 2010).

Nightingale's writings remain important to the profession of nursing at all levels of nursing practice. The basic principles of environmental manipulation and psychological patient care are applied in modern nursing practice situations (Pfettscher, 2010).

## Discussion

Nightingale probably would not have described her work as theoretical, but today it is recognized as a scholarly effort that continues to give credibility to basic ideas related to nursing theory. Nightingale's model was developed long ago in response to a need for environmental reform. Although some of Nightingale's rationales have been modified or disproved by advances in medicine and science, many of the concepts in her theory have not only endured, but they have been used as general guidelines for nurses for more than 150 years (Pfettscher, 2010). In particular, her work in relation to illness prevention and health restoration remains highly relevant to current nursing practice (Johnson & Webber, 2010) in both the acute care and community health settings, and in both the domestic and global healthcare arenas.

# Fourteen Components of Basic Nursing Care: Virginia Henderson

## Background

Virginia Avenel Henderson was born on March 19, 1897, in Kansas City, Missouri, and died on November 30, 1996, at the age of 98. During her lifetime and over the course of her more than 60-year career as a nurse, teacher, author, and researcher, Henderson made such significant contributions to the discipline of nursing that she has been referred to by some as "the Florence Nightingale of the twentieth century" (Tomey, 2006).

Henderson's interest in nursing began during World War I and stemmed from her desire to help the sick and wounded in the military. Henderson graduated from the Army School of Nursing in 1921 and began practice at the Henry Street Visiting Nurse Service in New York City. In 1926, she returned to school at Columbia University Teachers College in New York City, where she would complete her bachelor's of science and master's of arts in nursing education. Henderson taught nursing at Teachers College and Yale University. In her faculty role, Henderson worked with Harmer on the revision of *Textbook of the Principles and Practice of Nursing* (1939). In the next edition, published in 1955, Henderson introduced her now famous definition of nursing. Some of Henderson's other scholarly endeavors included the *Nursing Studies Index Project* (four volumes) (1959–1971); *Basic Principles of Nursing Care* (1960, 1997), which was translated into more than 20 languages; *The Nature of Nursing* (1966); and *The Nature of Nursing: Reflections After 25 years* (1991). At the age of 75, Henderson began to focus on international teaching and speaking.

Henderson authored one of the most accurate definitions of nursing, promoted nursing research as the basis for nursing knowledge, advocated for humane and holistic care for patients internationally, and represented nursing with dignity, honor, and grace throughout her career, which spanned most of the 20th century. Henderson was awarded 12 honorary doctoral degrees, as well as the International Council of Nursing's prestigious Christiane Reimann Prize during her exemplary career (American Nurses Association, n.d.).

## Henderson's 14 Components of Nursing Care

Henderson elaborated on her definition of nursing by identifying 14 basic needs on which nursing care is based. Eight of these needs pertain directly to bodily functions; the remaining six relate to safety and finding meaning in life (Shelly &

Miller, 2006). It follows that the fundamentals of nursing (i.e., the 14 components of nursing care) include helping others provide for their 14 basic needs:

1. To breathe normally
2. To eat and drink adequately
3. To eliminate bodily wastes
4. To move and maintain desirable postures
5. To sleep and rest
6. To select suitable clothes; dress and undress
7. To maintain body temperature within normal range by adjusting clothing and modifying the environment
8. To keep the body clean and well groomed and protect the integument
9. To avoid dangers in the environment and avoid injuring others
10. To communicate with others in expressing emotions, needs, fears, or opinions
11. To worship according to one's faith
12. To work in such a way that there is a sense of accomplishment
13. To play or participate in various forms of recreation
14. To learn, discover, or satisfy the curiosity that leads to normal development and health and use the available health facilities (Henderson, 1966, 1991)

## Nursing Care and Henderson's 14 Components of Nursing

Delivering nursing care based on the 14 basic needs and the corresponding 14 components of nursing care identified by Henderson is not difficult to conceptualize because Henderson and Nite used the 14 components as a framework for the 1978 edition of their textbook, *Principles and Practice of Nursing*. Advanced nursing practice and care utilizing Henderson's theory revolves around meeting patient needs in the areas of respiration, nutrition, elimination, body mechanics, rest and sleep, keeping clean and well groomed, controlling the environment, communication, human relations, work, play, and worship.

Henderson and Nite (1978) offered specific details for administering nursing care. APNs can apply these same interventions in advanced nursing care. For example, meeting basic needs involving patient respiration includes caregiving related to the following areas:

- Pulmonary ventilation
- Diffusion and transport of gases
- Regulation of respiration
- Factors affecting normal respiration (i.e., smoking, age, obesity, emotions, environmental pollution, anesthesia, and surgery)

Providing advanced nursing care to meet basic needs involving nutrition will include caregiving related to these areas:

- Nutrition and quality of life
- Dietary essentials

- Fluid balance
- Food selection and the optimal diet
- Conditions that favor digestion and assimilation
- Diet in sickness
- Nursing measures in oral feedings

Advanced nursing care to meet basic needs involving elimination covers the following areas:

- Elimination of waste from the intestines
- Elimination of waste from the kidneys
- Elimination of waste by the skin and lungs
- Measuring and recording elimination

Meeting basic needs involving patient movement and posture focuses on the following areas:

- Body mechanics and posture
- Exercise in health and sickness
- Helping the sick and handicapped to move
- Transportation in illness and traveling with patients
- Prevention and treatment of pressure ulcers

Meeting basic needs involving patient rest and sleep requires the APN to focus on two areas:

- Rest in health and illness
- Inducing sleep

Providing advanced nursing care to meet a patient's basic needs involves educating caregivers about keeping the patient clean and well groomed and maintaining temperature. This education includes caregiving related to the following areas:

- Personal cleanliness and morning care (care of skin and nails; shaving; care of the mouth, teeth, and dentures; care of the nose; hygiene of the eyes; care of the hair; making the patient's bed)
- Providing the patient with suitable clothing and conditions to maintain body temperature

Advanced nursing practice involved in controlling the environment will meet the patient's basic needs related to the following issues:

- Lighting (natural light, artificial light, psychology of lighting)
- Atmospheric conditions (humidity, temperature, purity of air, air pressure, altitude)
- Water supply and waste disposal
- Esthetics
- Controlling pests (insects and rodents)
- Preventing mechanical injury, burns, poisoning, and electric shock
- Providing and maintaining a sanitary environment

- Providing and maintaining a sanitary food service and maintaining a sanitary laundry service
- Disinfection and sterilization
- Preventing and controlling infection

Advanced nursing care involved in basic needs of communication, human relations, and learning includes factors associated with the following areas:

- Ways of communication (being as communication, use of the senses in communication, speech and language, nonlanguage communication, and communication technology)
- Communication: strengthening bonds and reducing barriers (mental states and sensory defects as barriers; language, culture, age-related, and gender-related communication bonds and barriers, and hospitalization and illness effects upon communication)
- Therapeutic communication and relationships (nurse–patient interaction; family and groups; communication through touch, music, art, role-playing, reading and writing; and creating a therapeutic environment)
- Learning and perception through the life cycle
- Health goals (national and international health goals, individual health goals, health education for health promotion and prevention of illness) and health guidance or health teaching

Advanced nursing care also involves basic needs of work and play:

- The meaning and nature of work and leisure
- Retirement and leisure time
- Adult play and recreation
- Children's play
- The nurse's role in providing an opportunity for work and play

Providing advanced nursing care to meet basic needs involving worship will cover the following areas:

- The search for meaning in life
- Knowledge of major living religions
- Religious leaders as members of health teams
- Ways in which nurses help those they serve meet their spiritual needs

For the assessment phase of the nursing process using Henderson's theory, APNs will assess the needs of the patient based on the 14 basic needs. Specifically, the APN will assess the patient's respiratory status, nutritional status, elimination, movement, activities of daily living, sleep, maintenance of body temperature, hygiene, environment, ability to communicate, needs related to work, recreation and learning, and spiritual needs. Based on the assessment data and considering the strength, will, and knowledge of the patient, the APN will determine whether the patient requires assistance to meet his or her basic needs. If assistance is required in any area, a plan will be designed so that the necessary nursing care can be provided.

The goal of the planning phase of the nursing process is to design a plan to meet patient needs based on any deficits identified in the assessment phase of the process, while simultaneously helping the patient gain independence as rapidly as possible so that the nurse becomes dispensable rather than indispensable. The implementation phase focuses on assisting the patient with the performance of activities that contribute to the maintenance of health, recovery from illness, or peaceful death. Interventions in this phase of the nursing process are based on physiological principles, as well as individual characteristics such as age; culture; and physical, intellectual, and emotional capabilities. Evaluation is based on the ability of patients to meet their basic human needs without or with decreasing assistance of the nurse.

## Major Concepts of Nursing According to Henderson

Henderson did not consider her work to be a theory of nursing and did not explicitly define all of the domains of nursing. It is possible, however, to identify and describe the metaparadigm concepts of nursing from her publications (Furukawa & Howe, 2002).

### Person

Henderson viewed the person as the patient who is composed of biological, psychological, sociological, and spiritual components (although these components are inseparable), but who requires assistance to achieve independence in relation to the 14 basic needs that correspond to the 14 identified components of nursing care. The patient and family are viewed as a unit (Henderson, 1964).

### Environment

Henderson broadly defined environment as "the aggregate of all the external conditions and influences affecting the life and development of an organism," using a definition taken from the 1961 edition of *Webster's New Collegiate Dictionary* (Henderson & Nite, 1978). She considered the environment to be composed of three components—biological, physical, and behavioral. Biological components of the environment include all living things, such as plants, animals, and microorganisms. Physical components of the environment comprise sunlight, water, oxygen, carbon dioxide, organic compounds, and the nutrients used by plants for growth and provide a sphere "in which all living things operate" (Henderson & Nite, 1978, p. 829). According to Henderson, these biological and physical components come together to form an ecosystem characterized by a delicate balance; thus, an interdependent relationship exists between living organisms and their surroundings, such that changes in one component result in changes in other parts of the ecosystem.

A third environmental component also exists. This behavioral component comprises the way in which human beings are engaged in social interactions, customs, and economic, legal, political, and religious systems, all of which influence human health (Henderson & Nite, 1978).

## *Health*

While Henderson did not explicitly state a definition of health, she implied that health is equivalent to independence. The level of health is directly related to the patient's ability to independently meet the 14 basic needs (Henderson & Nite, 1978).

## *Nursing*

Henderson is perhaps best known for her definition of nursing, first published in 1955 (Harmer & Henderson, 1955), and presented again in 1966 with minor revisions. According to Henderson:

> [T]he unique function of the nurse is to assist the individual, sick or well, in the performance of those activities contributing to health or its recovery (or to a peaceful death) that he would perform unaided if he had the necessary strength, will, or knowledge and to do this in such a way as to help him gain independence as rapidly as possible. (Henderson, 1966, p. 15)

While Henderson defined nursing in functional terms, she emphasized the art of nursing, as well as the need for empathetic understanding, stating that the nurse must "get inside the skin of each of her patients in order to know what he needs" (Henderson, 1964, p. 63). She believed that "the beauty of . . . nursing is the combination of your heart, your head and your hands and where you separate them, you diminish them" (McBride, 1997, as cited by Gordon, 2001).

Henderson went on to say, "[T]he nurse is, and should be an independent practitioner and able to make independent judgments as long as he, or she, is not diagnosing, prescribing treatment for disease, or making a prognosis, for these are the physician's functions. But the nurse is viewed as the authority on basic nursing care" (Henderson, 1991). Over the last 40 years, however, advanced nursing practice has evolved to include many of the independent functions previously described by Henderson as functions reserved only for physicians. Today's APNs promote a comprehensive approach to health care, which includes making advanced practice judgments, diagnosing, prescribing, and emphasizing the overall health and wellness of their patients. Henderson's definition of nursing and her 14 components of nursing are completely viable for advanced nursing practice today.

## Analysis of Henderson's Definition of Nursing and 14 Components of Nursing

The analysis and critique of Henderson's work presented here encompass an examination of her assumptions and propositions, as well as an analysis of the clarity, simplicity, generality, empirical precision, and derivable consequences of the definition of nursing and 14 components of nursing as proposed by Henderson.

## Assumptions of Henderson's Definition and 14 Components of Nursing Care

Henderson did not explicitly state assumptions. Even so, it is possible to extrapolate 17 primary assumptions from her publications:

1. The nurse has a unique function to help well or sick persons.
2. The nurse functions as a member of the medical team, but independently of the physician.
3. The patient's needs are covered by the 14 components of nursing.
4. The 14 components of nursing care encompass all possible functions of nursing.
5. The nurse and patient are always working toward a goal, whether it is patient independence or a peaceful death.
6. Health promotion is an important goal of the nurse.
7. The patient and the family are a unit.
8. The mind and the body of the person are inseparable.
9. The patient requires assistance toward independence.
10. The person must maintain physiological and emotional balance.
11. Health is basic to human functioning.
12. Health requires independence and interdependence.
13. Persons will achieve or maintain health if they have the strength, will, and knowledge to do so.
14. Illness may interfere with the ability of persons to control their environment.
15. Nurses should protect persons from environmental injury.
16. Nurses should know about social customs and religious practices.
17. Professional practice is generated from research-based knowledge (Henderson, 1966, 1991; Runk & Muth Quillin, 1989; Tomey, 2002, p. 102).

## Propositions of Henderson's Definition and 14 Components of Nursing Care

The primary relationship statements gleaned from Henderson's work are related to the nurse–patient relationship: (1) the nurse as a substitute for the patient, (2) the nurse as a helper to the patient, and (3) the nurse as a partner with the patient (Tomey, 2002). In times of serious illness, the nurse is seen as the substitute for what the patient is missing owing to lack of strength, will, or knowledge. Henderson reflected this view when she stated that the nurse "is temporarily the consciousness of the unconscious, the love of life for the suicidal, the leg of the amputee, the eyes of the newly blind, a means of locomotion for the infant, knowledge and confidence for the young mother, and the mouthpiece for those too weak or withdrawn to speak and so on" (1966, p. 16; 1991, p. 22).

During the patient's convalescence, the nurse assists the patient in regaining his or her independence. Working as partners, the nurse and the patient together formulate the plan of care. Henderson asserts that the "nurse must get inside the skin" of each patient to know what the patient needs and then the identified needs must be validated with the patient (Henderson, 1966, p. 16; Henderson, 1991, p. 22; Tomey, 2002).

### Analysis: Clarity, Simplicity, Generality, Empirical Precision, and Derivable Consequences

Henderson seems to have used deduction to develop her definition of nursing and 14 needs from physiological and psychological principles. The assumptions of Henderson's definition are logical and have a high level of agreement with literature and research conclusions of scientists in other fields. For example, the 14 basic needs correspond closely to Maslow's hierarchy of human needs, even though Henderson had no knowledge of Maslow's work at the time she identified these needs in her work (Tomey, 2002).

Henderson's definition of nursing and the basic needs are simply stated and clear, yet broad enough in scope to include the function of nurses at all levels of practice caring for all types of patients. Her work is of sufficient scope to affect nursing theory and practice. Moreover, Henderson's definition of nursing has the potential to include the whole person, even though the definition is derived primarily from the physiological perception (Runk & Muth Quillin, 1989).

The concept of nursing in Henderson's work contains many variables and relationships, and the 14 needs, although they appear simple, can become complex when an alteration in need occurs and all of the parameters relating to the need are considered. Even with this level of complexity, the conceptual definitions and relationships demonstrate internal consistency (Tomey, 2002).

Because Henderson did not intend to develop a theory of nursing, she did not develop the interrelated theoretical statements or operational definitions necessary to provide theory testability. As Tomey (2002) pointed out, however, this extension is possible. Henderson's work has been influential in nursing curriculum development, in clinical nursing practice, and in the promotion of clinical nursing research.

### Discussion

Henderson's work is viewed as a philosophy of the purpose and function of nursing (Pokorny, 2010). Her textbook *Principles and Practice of Nursing*, in which the definition of nursing and 14 nursing functions were explicated, was widely used in schools of nursing for several decades; thus, her definition of nursing has significantly influenced the practice of multiple generations of nurses. Henderson's definition of nursing and 14 nursing functions were aimed at explaining the totality of nursing behavior rather than laying the foundation for the development of a nursing theory; however, her ideas have continued to be useful in promoting further conceptual development among nurse theorists. In addition, Henderson's philosophy that nursing care should be based on evidence rather than tradition, an idea that was novel at the time, is currently foundational to the discipline of nursing, including advanced practice nursing.

# The Behavioral System Model: Dorothy Johnson

## Background

Dorothy E. Johnson was born in 1919 in Savannah, Georgia. She graduated from nursing school in 1938, earned a bachelor's of science in nursing from Vanderbilt University in 1942, and received a master's of public health from Harvard University in 1948.

Johnson served as faculty at both Vanderbilt University School of Nursing and the University of California in Los Angeles. Over the course of her career, she published more than 30 articles, 4 books, and many reports, and she was presented with numerous honors. She died in 1999 at the age of 80.

According to Johnson, her behavioral system model was in the process of development for nearly the entire course of her professional life (Johnson, 1990). Through a comprehensive analysis, Fawcett (2005) identified Johnson's behavioral system model as one of the seven conceptual models of nursing. The model's roots can be traced back to the work of behavioral scientists in psychology, sociology, and ethnology, with heavy reliance on systems theory (Loveland-Cherry & Wilkerson, 1989). Johnson's theory was also influenced by Nightingale's work—especially her belief that nursing's goal is to help individuals prevent or recover from disease or injury with a focus on the patient rather than the specific disease (Johnson, 1990). Johnson's initial work began with an effort to develop content for nursing courses in the basic curriculum by focusing on common human needs and using care and comfort as organizing principles, and then moved to stress tension reduction. Through reasoning, Johnson began to theorize that nursing's specific contribution to patient welfare was the fostering of efficient and effective behavioral functioning. That perspective led her to accept the theoretical view of the person as a behavioral system, similar to the way that physicians accept the person as a biological system (Fawcett, 2005; Johnson, 1990).

## Johnson's Behavioral System Model

The goals of nursing in Johnson's behavioral system model are to maintain or restore behavioral system balance. Her model for nursing presents the patient as a living open system, comprising a collection of behavioral subsystems that interrelate to form a behavioral system. Because the subsystems are linked and open, a disturbance in one subsystem will likely have an effect on the other subsystems (Johnson, 1980). The seven subsystems of behavior proposed by Johnson include the (1) achievement, (2) affiliative, (3) aggressive, (4) dependence, (5) sexual, (6) eliminative, and (7) ingestive subsystems.

Subsystems include four structural components:

1. The drive or goal of the subsystem reflects the motivation or reasons for the behaviors of the subsystem. Motivational drives directing the activities or behaviors of the subsystems may vary from strong to weak and are constantly changing because of maturation, experience, and learning.

2. The set is the ordinary or normal behaviors that the patient prefers to use to meet the goal of a subsystem.
3. The choice represents the options that are available to patients to meet their subsystem goals. This structural component is influenced by variables such as gender, age, culture, socioeconomic status, and health status.
4. The action or behavior emanates as a consequence of the previous three structural components. The question of concern in relation to the structural component of behavior is whether the behavior is efficient and effective in relation to subsystem goal attainment. This is the only structural component that can be directly observed (Johnson, 1980).

Each of the seven subsystems has a function. The achievement subsystem functions to control or master an aspect of self or environment to achieve a standard. This subsystem encompasses intellectual, physical, creative, mechanical, and social skills. The affiliative or attachment subsystem forms the basis for social organization. Its consequences include social inclusion, intimacy, and the formation and maintenance of strong social bonds. The aggressive or protective subsystem functions to protect and preserve the system. The dependency subsystem promotes helping or nurturing behaviors. Its consequences include approval, recognition, and physical assistance. The sexual subsystem has the function of procreation and gratification and includes development of gender-role identity and gender-role behaviors. The eliminative subsystem addresses "when, how, and under what conditions we eliminate," whereas the ingestive subsystem "has to do with when, how, what, how much, and under what conditions we eat" (Johnson, 1980, p. 213).

Johnson asserted that each of these subsystems, as well as the system as a whole, has certain functional requirements that must be met through the effort of the individual or through outside assistance for continued growth, development, and viability. These functional requirements include (1) protection from noxious influences with which the system cannot cope, (2) nurturing through input of supplies from the environment (examples include food, friendship, and caring), and (3) stimulation by experiences, events, and behavior that would enhance growth and prevent stagnation (Johnson, 1980, p. 212).

The nursing process for the behavioral system model is Johnson's nursing diagnostic and treatment process. The components of this process include determination of the existence of a problem, diagnostic classification of problems, management of nursing problems, and evaluation of behavioral system balance and stability.

When nurses use Johnson's conceptual model as part of advanced practice, the focus of the assessment process is obtaining information to evaluate current behavior in terms of past patterns, determining the effects of the current illness on behavioral patterns, and establishing the maximum level of health. The assessment specifically focuses on gathering information related to the structure and function of the seven behavioral subsystems, as well as the environmental factors that influence the behavioral subsystems (Holaday, 2006). During the assessment phase, APNs obtain data about the nature of the behavioral functioning related to goal attainment—specifically, whether the patient's behavior is purposeful, orderly, and predictable. APNs need to interview the patient and family also to assess the condition of the subsystem structural components and evaluate the patient's behavior for behavioral system balance and stability. From the data collected, APNs make inferences and independent judgments related to the organization, interaction, and integration of the subsystems (Fawcett, 2005).

Within Johnson's conceptual model, problems may be classified as internal subsystem problems or intersystem problems. Internal subsystem problems include situations when functional requirements are not met, there is inconsistency or disharmony among components of the subsystem, or behavior is not appropriate for the culture. Intersystem problems include situations when the behavioral system is dominated by one or two subsystems or a conflict exists between two or more subsystems (Fawcett, 2005).

The goals of the management of nursing problems for APNs and other nurses are to restore, maintain, or attain the patient's behavioral system balance and stability and to help the patient achieve an optimal level of balance and functioning. The goals of management could be accomplished through the temporary imposition of external regulatory or control mechanisms, the repair of damaged subsystem structural components, or the fulfillment of subsystem functional requirements (Johnson, 1980). For example, APNs may temporarily impose external regulatory or control mechanisms by setting limits for behavior, inhibiting ineffective behavioral responses, assisting the patient to develop new responses, and reinforcing appropriate behaviors. Repair of damaged structural components includes interventions that modify the drive or motivation, or redirect goals. Interventions can also attempt to alter set behaviors through instruction or counseling and add choices through teaching new skills. In addition, the nurse can intervene to fulfill functional requirements by protecting the patient from overwhelming negative influences that exceed the patient's coping ability, by nurturing the patient through input of adequate essential supplies, and by providing stimulation to enhance growth and prevent stagnation (Fawcett, 2005; Johnson, 1980).

Evaluation is based on the attainment of the goal of balance in the identified subsystems. Evaluation of behavioral system balance and stability is accomplished as the APN compares the patient's behavior after treatment to indices of behavioral system balance and stability (Fawcett, 2005; Johnson, 1980). A case involving advanced nursing practice that illustrates the use of Johnson's behavioral system model appears in **Box 17–2**.

## Major Concepts of Nursing According to Johnson
### Person

Within the behavioral system model, the person is viewed as a behavioral being— that is, a behavioral system with seven subsystems of behavior. Under the original

## Box 17–2 Case Study Utilizing Johnson's Behavioral System Model

Mrs. Akins is the primary caregiver for her husband, who has been diagnosed with Alzheimer's disease. Nursing care begins with the assessment phase of Johnson's nursing diagnostic and treatment process and includes an assessment of each of the subsystems.

Assessment of the aggressive or protective subsystem reveals that Mrs. Akins is frustrated and is struggling to cope with the increasing burden of caring for her husband, who often does not recognize her. Assessment of the dependency subsystem reveals that Mrs. Akins feels isolated socially and emotionally, because she has no time for socialization while caring for her husband; in addition, few friends or family members understand what is happening to Mr. Akins. Assessment of the achievement subsystem reveals that Mrs. Akins not only struggles with the question of why this is happening to her, but she is trying also to remain self-sufficient and thus has not asked friends and family members for help. Affiliative or attachment subsystem assessment reveals that Mrs. Akins's relationships with family and friends have been adversely affected because she has no time or energy left to socialize while constantly caring for Mr. Akins.

Assessment of the ingestive and eliminative subsystems reveals Mrs. Akins to be slightly overweight but with no bowel function abnormalities. She admits that she does not have time to cook as much as she did before Mr. Akins became sick. In response to sexual subsystem assessment, Mrs. Akins states that she is often tired, depressed, and overwhelmed with caring for her husband and finds intimacy difficult with a person who often cannot remember who she is.

Structural component assessment includes the assessment of drive, set, choice, and action. Next, the problems are diagnostically classified. Nursing management of the problems is then initiated.

Nursing management of Mrs. Akins's problems should include attention to the issues identified in the aggressive, dependency, affiliative, and achievement subsystems. The nurse encourages Mrs. Akins to express her feelings of frustration and to ask for assistance from family members. The nurse provides information related to professional services and community resources, including support groups and respite care services. The nurse facilitates education of family members and provides informational materials related to Alzheimer's disease. Evaluation includes an assessment of behavioral system balance.

model, the role of medicine was to focus on the biological system and the role of nursing was to focus on the behavioral system. Today's APNs, however, focus on both biological and behavioral systems.

### Environment

In the behavioral system model, the environment includes both the internal environment and the external environment; the latter is not a part of the individual's behavioral system, but it nevertheless influences the system. Strong environmental forces can disturb the balance of the behavioral system and threaten stability of the system (Loveland-Cherry & Wilkerson, 1989).

### Health

Johnson referred to two types of health: physical health and social health (Johnson, 1980). According to Johnson, health is determined by the interaction of various psychological, social, biological, and physiological factors. Efficient and effective functioning of the system, which results in behavioral system balance and stability, is equivalent to a state of health. Illness can be defined then as behavioral system imbalance and instability.

### Nursing

According to Johnson's behavioral system, nursing is an external regulatory force that acts to preserve the organization and integrity of the patient's behavior at an optimal level under those conditions in which the behavior constitutes a threat to physical or social health or in which illness is found. This force operates through the imposition of external regulatory or control mechanisms, through attempts to change structural units in desirable directions, or through the fulfillment of the functional requirements of the subsystems. Under Johnson's behavioral system, the purpose of nursing practice is "to facilitate restoration, maintenance, or attainment of behavioral system balance and stability" (Johnson, 1980, p. 214). These goals are accomplished through the use of Johnson's nursing diagnostic and treatment process, which is a pragmatic method for APNs. Today's APNs using Johnson's behavioral system model would consider the balance and stability of the biological system in attempting to accomplish these goals. During the nursing era when Johnson developed her behavioral system with her specifications and language, nurses did not take on these responsibilities; thus, she did not account for today's role of the APN. Even so, because of its relevance, her nursing diagnostic and treatment process can be translated easily to advanced practice.

## Analysis of the Behavioral System Model

The analysis and critique presented here consist of an examination of assumptions and propositions, as well as an analysis of the clarity, simplicity, generality, empirical precision, and derivable consequences of the behavioral system model as proposed by Johnson.

### Assumptions of the Behavioral System Model

Johnson based her theory on four explicit and implicit assumptions:

1. Behavior is the sum total of physical, biological, and social factors.
2. A person is a system of behavior characterized by repetitive, predictable, and goal-directed behaviors that always strive toward balance.
3. There are different levels of balance and stabilization, and levels are different during different time periods.
4. Persons expend large amounts of energy attempting to maintain or reestablish behavioral system balance in response to imbalance caused by persistent excessive forces (Holaday, 2010; Meleis, 2007, p. 281).

### Propositions of the Health Behavior Model

Primary relationships are seen in the behavioral system model between the person and the environment; the person, health, and the environment; and the person, nursing, and health. Primary relationships of the behavioral system model include the following notions: (1) the behavioral system manages its relationship with the environment, which is self-maintaining as long as conditions remain orderly; (2) balance is essential for effective and efficient functions of the person, and a lack of balance in the structural or functional requirements of the subsystems leads to poor health; and (3) nursing is an external regulatory force that acts to restore balance to the behavioral system (Holaday, 2010; Johnson, 1980).

### Analysis: Clarity, Simplicity, Generality, Empirical Precision, and Derivable Consequences

Johnson developed the behavioral system model using inductive reasoning that was based on her observations during many years of nursing practice, as well as on nursing literature and research. The model is fairly simple in terms of the number of concepts, and the concepts of nursing and behavioral system are described in detail. Johnson's model has nearly unlimited applicability with ill persons; however, it has not yet been used as extensively with well persons (Holaday, 2010). Regarding the criticism that her model did not allow for a focus on prevention, Johnson stated, "[P]reventive nursing is not possible until problems in the behavioral system are explicated. To the extent that any problem that might arise can be anticipated . . . preventive action is in order" (1990, p. 31).

The concepts within the behavioral system model are clearly and consistently defined (Loveland-Cherry & Wilkerson, 1989), and the comprehensiveness of this conceptual model has proven to be adequate for providing direction for nursing research, education, administration, and practice (Fawcett, 2005). Some adaptations of Johnson's model have appeared in the literature as the model has been used by others, including the addition of an eighth subsystem dealing with restorative behavior and some alternative interpretations of the functions of subsystems (Fawcett, 2005). In response to these additions and alterations, Johnson stated,

"[T]hese changes are such that they alter the fundamental nature of the behavioral system as originally proposed, and I do not agree with them" (1990, p. 27).

## Discussion

Johnson's behavioral system model makes an important contribution to nursing knowledge by directing attention to the person's behavior rather than the disease state. Johnson used that distinction to clarify the different foci of the disciplines of nursing and medicine (Fawcett, 2005). At the time when she undertook her work, there was no delineated theoretical framework for the discipline of nursing. Thus Johnson began her work in earnest related to the conceptualization of nursing and the other components of the behavioral system model; according to this pioneer, it was only when these elements were defined and specific goals were articulated that professionals would be able to begin to speak of a "science of nursing" (Johnson, 1959).

# The Health Promotion Model: Nola J. Pender

## Background

Nola J. Pender was born in 1941 in Lansing, Michigan. She graduated in 1962 with a diploma in nursing. In 1964, Pender completed a bachelor's of science in nursing at Michigan State University. By 1969, she had completed a doctor of philosophy in psychology and education. During this time in her career, Pender began looking at health and nursing in a broad way, including defining the goal of nursing care as optimal health.

In 1975, Pender published a model for preventive health behavior; her health promotion model first appeared in the first edition of the text *Health Promotion in Nursing Practice* in 1982. Pender's health promotion model has its foundation in Albert Bandura's (1977) social learning theory (which postulates that cognitive processes affect behavior change) and is influenced by Fishbein's (1967) theory of reasoned action (which asserts that personal attitudes and social norms affect behavior).

## Pender's Health Promotion Model

McCullagh (2009) labeled Pender's health promotion model as a middle-range integrative theory, and rightly so. Fawcett (2005) decisively presented the difference between a conceptual model for nursing and a model for middle-range theory. A model for middle-range theory is usually a graphic representation or schematic diagram of a middle-range theory. McCullagh's (2009) rationale for labeling Pender's model a middle-range integrative theory is that it portrays the multidimensionality of persons interacting with their interpersonal and physical environments as they pursue health while integrating constructs from expectancy-value theory and social cognitive theory with a nursing perspective of holistic human functioning (Pender, 1996). With the third edition of *Health Promotion in Nursing Practice* (1996), Pender revised the health promotion model significantly. This revised model is the subject of the discussion in this chapter.

Pender's health promotion model includes three major categories: (1) individual characteristics and experiences, (2) behavior-specific cognitions and affect, and (3) behavioral outcome. Each of these categories will be considered here separately.

The first category includes each person's unique personal characteristics and experiences, which affect that individual's actions. Significant components within this category are prior related behavior and personal factors. Prior related behavior is important in influencing future behavior. Pender proposed that prior behavior has both direct and indirect effects on the likelihood of engaging in health-promoting behaviors. In particular, past behavior has a direct effect on the current health-promoting behavior through habit formation: Habit strength increases each time a behavior occurs. Prior behavior is proposed to indirectly influence health-promoting behavior through perceptions of self-efficacy, benefits, barriers, and activity-related affect or emotions (Pender, Murdaugh, & Parsons, 2006). Personal factors include biological factors such as age, body mass index, pubertal status, menopausal status, aerobic capacity, strength, agility, or balance; psychological factors include self-esteem, self-motivation, and perceived health status; and sociocultural factors include race, ethnicity, acculturation, education, and socioeconomic status. Some personal factors are amenable to change, whereas others are immutable (Pender et al., 2006).

The second category encompasses behavior-specific cognitions and affect, which serve as behavior-specific variables within the health promotion model. Behavior-specific variables are considered to have motivational significance. In the health promotion model, nursing interventions target these variables because they are amenable to change. The behavior-specific cognitions and affect identified in the health promotion model include (1) perceived benefits of action, (2) perceived barriers to action, (3) perceived self-efficacy, and (4) activity-related affect. Other cognitions fall into the category of interpersonal influences and situational influences. Sources of interpersonal influences on health-promoting behaviors include family, peers, and healthcare providers. Interpersonal influences include norms, social support, and modeling; they shape the person's tendency to participate in health-promoting behaviors. Situational influences on health-promoting behavior include perceptions of available options, demand characteristics, and aesthetic features of the environment. Within Pender's model, nursing plans are tailored to meet the needs of diverse patients based on assessment of prior behavior, behavior-specific cognitions and affect, interpersonal factors, and situational factors (Pender et al., 2006, pp. 54–56).

The third category within Pender's model is the behavioral outcome. Commitment to a plan of action marks the beginning of a behavioral event. This commitment propels the person into the behavior unless that action is confounded by a competing demand that cannot be avoided or a competing preference that is not resisted. Interventions in the health promotion model focus on raising consciousness related to health-promoting behaviors, promoting self-efficacy, enhancing the benefits of change, controlling the environment to support behavior change, and managing the barriers to change. Health-promoting behavior, which is ultimately directed toward attaining positive health outcomes, is the product of the health promotion model (Pender et al., 2006, pp. 56–63).

## Major Concepts of Nursing According to Pender
### Person
The person in the health promotion model refers to the individual who is the primary focus of the model. In Pender's model, each person has unique personal characteristics and experiences that affect subsequent actions. It is recognized that individuals learn health behaviors within the context of the family and the community, which explains why the model for assessment includes components and interventions at the family and community levels, as well as the individual level (Pender, Murdaugh, & Parsons, 2002, 2006). This is taken a step further in the latest edition (Pender, Murdaugh, & Parsons, 2011), in which the term client refers to individuals, families, and communities who are all viewed as active participants in health promotion.

### Environment
In the health promotion model, the environment encompasses the physical, interpersonal, and economic circumstances in which persons live. The quality of the environment depends on the absence of toxic substances, the availability of restorative experiences, and the accessibility of human and economic resources needed for healthful living. Socioeconomic conditions such as unemployment, poverty, crime, and prejudice have adverse effects on health, whereas environmental wellness is manifested by balance between human beings and their surroundings (Pender et al., 2006, p. 9; Pender et al., 2011, p. 8).

### Health
Health is viewed as a positive high-level state. According to Pender, the person's definition of health for himself or herself is more important than any general definition of health (Pender et al., 2006; Sakraida, 2010). Health is viewed in the context of health promotion and disease prevention. Health promotion is behavior that is motivated by a desire to increase well-being and optimize human health potential, whereas disease prevention or health protection is behavior motivated by a desire to actively avoid illness, detect illness early, or maintain functioning within the constraints of illness (Pender et al., 2011, p. 5). Health promotion is viewed as a multidimensional concept that includes the dimensions of the individual, the family, the community, socioeconomic status, cultural factors, and environmental factors (Pender et al., 2011, pp. 6–8).

### Nursing

The role of the nurse in the health promotion model revolves around raising consciousness related to health-promoting behaviors, promoting self-efficacy, enhancing the benefits of change, controlling the environment to support behavior change, and managing the barriers to change (Pender et al., 2006, pp. 57–63). A major function of the APN role is the focus on health promotion. This model serves as a significantly pragmatic process for APNs to use to encourage health-promoting behaviors by patients and to address the benefits of change.

## Analysis of the Health Promotion Model

The analysis and critique presented here comprise an examination of assumptions and propositions, as well as the analysis of clarity, simplicity, generality, empirical precision, and derivable consequences of Pender's health promotion model.

### Assumptions of the Health Promotion Model

Assumptions of the health promotion model reflect both nursing and behavioral science perspectives. The seven major assumptions emphasize the active role of the patient in shaping and maintaining health behaviors and in modifying the environmental context for health behaviors:

1. Persons seek to create conditions of living through which they can express their unique human potential.
2. Persons have the capacity for reflective self-awareness, including assessment of their own competencies.
3. Persons value growth in directions viewed as positive and attempt to achieve a personally acceptable balance between change and stability.
4. Persons seek to actively regulate their own behavior.
5. Persons in all their biopsychosocial complexity interact with the environment, both progressively transforming the environment and being transformed over time.
6. Health professionals constitute a part of the interpersonal environment, which influences persons throughout their life span.
7. Self-initiated reconfiguration of person–environment interactive patterns is essential for behavior change (Pender et al., 2002, p. 63).

### Propositions of the Health Promotion Model

The health promotion model is based upon 14 theoretical propositions. These theoretical relationship statements provide a basis for research related to health behaviors:

1. Prior behavior and inherited and acquired characteristics influence health beliefs, affect, and enactment of health-promoting behavior.
2. Persons commit to engaging in behaviors from which they anticipate deriving personally valued benefits.

3. Perceived barriers can constrain commitment to action (a mediator of behavior), as well as actual behavior.

4. Perceived competence or self-efficacy to execute a given behavior increases the likelihood of commitment to action and actual performance of behavior.

5. Greater perceived self-efficacy results in fewer perceived barriers to a specific health behavior.

6. Positive affect toward a behavior results in greater perceived self-efficacy, which can, in turn, result in increased positive affect.

7. When positive emotions or affect are associated with a behavior, the probability of commitment and action are increased.

8. Persons are more likely to commit to and engage in health-promoting behaviors when significant others model the behavior, expect the behavior to occur, and provide assistance and support to enable the behavior.

9. Family, peers, and healthcare providers are important sources of interpersonal influence who can increase or decrease commitment to and engagement in health-promoting behavior.

10. Situational influences in the external environment can increase or decrease commitment to or participation in health-promoting behavior.

11. The greater the commitment to a specific plan of action, the more likely health-promoting behaviors will be maintained over time.

12. Commitment to a plan of action is less likely to result in the desired behavior when competing demands over which persons have little control require immediate attention.

13. Commitment to a plan of action is less likely to result in the desired behavior when other actions are more attractive and thus preferred over the target behavior.

14. Persons can modify cognitions, affect, and the interpersonal and physical environments to create incentives for health actions (Pender et al., 2002, pp. 63–64).

### Analysis: Clarity, Simplicity, Generality, Empirical Precision, and Derivable Consequences

Pender's health promotion model was formulated using inductive reasoning with existing research, which is a common approach to the building of middle-range theories. The research used to derive the model was based on adult samples that included male, female, young, old, well, and ill populations; this design allows the model to be generalized easily to adult populations (Sakraida, 2010).

The health promotion model is simple to understand, because it uses language familiar to nurses. The concept of health promotion is also popular in nursing practice and, therefore, is a practical principle for APNs' use. The relationships among the factors are linked, and relationships are identified and consistently defined. Considering all of these factors, it is not difficult to see why Pender's model is popular with practicing nurses and is frequently used as a tool in research. Nevertheless, it has not been used extensively in nursing education, where the emphasis is on illness care in acute care settings (Sakraida, 2010).

## Discussion

Pender identified health promotion as a key global goal for the 21st century (Pender et al., 2011) and, through development of the health promotion model, has assisted in the delineation of the role of nursing in meeting that goal. Although Pender has now retired, her work on the health promotion model continues. Pender views the nurse's role in health promotion as more important than ever considering existing health disparities and the challenges of our current healthcare system (Pender et al., 2011). The current scenario of increasing costs for health care associated with episodic illness treatment increases in chronic, preventable conditions within the population, and the focus on managing healthcare costs provide ample incentive to further explore the concepts of the health promotion model as APNs strive to improve health outcomes in patient populations.

## Summary

Although the four nursing models described in this chapter were conceived by four very different nurses whose careers spanned more than a century, they share a common thread: All place emphasis on the function of nursing practice in relation to health outcomes. For Nightingale, the function of nursing is to alter the environment to allow for action on the person by natural laws of health; for Henderson, the function of nursing is to assist the person to perform activities to gain independence; for Johnson, the function of the nurse is to impose external regulatory mechanisms in order to facilitate restoration of system balance; and for Pender, the nurse functions to raise consciousness, promote self-efficacy, and control the environment to allow for behavior change resulting in high-level health. All four of these nursing models also conceptualize the goal of nursing care as a restoration of the health of the patient, however differently the concept of health—or, for that matter, the concept of the patient—may be defined in their respective theories.

## Discussion Questions

1. Nightingale and Henderson considered the discipline of nursing to be both an art and a science. Esthetic patterns of knowing and empirical patterns of knowing both constitute complex yet divergent ways of thinking. How can the APN perform simultaneously from an esthetic perspective and a perspective based on empiricism?

2. Johnson's behavioral system model has been used in practice and research; as a result, multiple adaptations of this model have appeared in the literature. In response to these additions and alterations, Johnson (1990, p. 27)

stated, "[T]hese changes are such that they alter the fundamental nature of the behavioral system as originally proposed, and I do not agree with them." Does a theory belong to the nurse theorist or to the discipline of nursing? Who has the right to add to or alter a theory? Should a theory be altered based on research evidence even if the original nurse theorist is not in agreement, or should the theory be maintained intact as a historical record?

3. Considering a patient scenario from advanced nursing practice and using a middle-range theory such as the health promotion model, demonstrate the connection and reciprocal relationship between theory, practice, and research.

4. The theories presented in this chapter, although they view nursing from various perspectives, have brought to light these theorists' identification and development of the concepts of interest, thereby influencing the evolution of nursing as a discipline and framing nursing knowledge. How has the development of these and other nursing theories helped to frame knowledge and shape the role of the APN?

# References

American Nurses Association. (n.d.). Hall of fame: Virginia A. Henderson (1897–1996) 1996 inductee. Retrieved from http://www.nursingworld.org/FunctionalMenuCategories/AboutANA/Honoring-Nurses/HallofFame/19962000Inductees/hendva5545.aspx

Bandura, A. (1977). *Social learning theory.* Englewood Cliffs, NJ: Prentice Hall.

Bolton, K. (2006). Nightingale's philosophy in nursing practice. In M. R. Alligood & A. M. Tomey (Eds.), *Nursing theory: Utilization and application* (3rd ed., pp. 89–102). St. Louis, MO: Mosby.

Chinn, P. L., & Kramer, M. K. (2008). *Integrated knowledge development in nursing* (7th ed.). St. Louis, MO: Elsevier-Mosby.

Cook, E. (1913). *The life of Florence Nightingale* (Vols. 1 and 2). London, UK: Macmillan.

Dietz, D. D., & Lehozky, A. R. (1963). *History and modern nursing.* Philadelphia, PA: F. A. Davis.

Donahue, M. P. (1985). *Nursing: The finest art.* St. Louis, MO: Mosby.

Fawcett, J. (2005). *Contemporary nursing knowledge: Analysis and evaluation of nursing models and theories* (2nd ed.). Philadelphia, PA: F. A. Davis.

Fishbein, M. (1967). *Readings in attitude theory and measurement.* New York, NY: Wiley.

Furukawa, C. Y., & Howe, J. S. (2002). Definition and components of nursing: Virginia Henderson. In J. B. George (Ed.), *Nursing theories: The base for professional nursing practice* (5th ed., pp. 83–109). Upper Saddle River, NJ: Prentice Hall.

Gordon, S. C. (2001). Virginia Avenel Henderson: Definition of nursing. In M. Parker (Ed.), *Nursing theories and nursing practice* (pp. 143–149). Philadelphia, PA: F. A. Davis.

Harmer, B., & Henderson, V. (1939). *Textbook of the principles and practice of nursing* (4th ed.). New York, NY: Macmillan.

Harmer, B., & Henderson, V. (1955). *Textbook of the principles and practice of nursing* (5th ed.). New York, NY: Macmillan.

Henderson, V. (1964). The nature of nursing. *American Journal of Nursing, 64*, 62–68.

Henderson, V. (1966). *The nature of nursing: A definition and its implications for practice, research, and education.* New York, NY: Macmillan.

Henderson, V. (1991). *The nature of nursing: Reflections after 25 years.* New York, NY: National League for Nursing Press.

Henderson, V., & Nite, G. (1978). *Principles and practice of nursing* (6th ed.). New York, NY: Macmillan.

Holaday, B. (2006). Johnson's behavioral system model in nursing practice. In M. R. Alligood & A. M. Tomey (Eds.), *Nursing theory: Utilization and application* (3rd ed., pp. 157–180). St. Louis, MO: Mosby.

Holaday, B. (2010). Dorothy Johnson: Behavioral system model. In A. M. Tomey & M. R. Alligood (Eds.), *Nursing theorists and their work* (7th ed., pp. 366–390). St. Louis, MO: Mosby.

Johnson, D. E. (1959). The nature and science of nursing. *Nursing Outlook, 7*(5), 291–294.

Johnson, D. E. (1980). The behavioral system model for nursing. In J. Riehl & C. Roy (Eds.), *Conceptual models for nursing practice* (2nd ed., pp. 207–216). New York, NY: Appleton-Century-Crofts.

Johnson, D. E. (1990). The behavioral system model for nursing. In M. E. Parker (Ed.), *Nursing theories in practice* (pp. 23–32). New York, NY: National League for Nursing.

Johnson, B. M., & Webber, P. B. (2010). *An introduction to theory and reasoning in nursing* (3rd ed.). Philadelphia, PA: Lippincott Williams & Wilkins.

Lobo, M. L. (2002). Environmental model: Florence Nightingale. In J. B. George (Ed.), *Nursing theories: The base for professional nursing practice* (5th ed., pp. 155–188). Upper Saddle River, NJ: Prentice Hall.

Loveland-Cherry, C. J., & Wilkerson, S. A. (1989). Dorothy Johnson's behavioral system model. In J. J. Fitzpatrick & A. L. Whall (Eds.), *Conceptual models of nursing* (2nd ed., pp. 147–163). Englewood Cliffs, NJ: Prentice Hall.

McCullagh, M. C. (2009). Health promotion. In S. J. Peterson & T. S. Bredow, *Middle range theories: Application to nursing research* (2nd ed., pp. 290–303). Philadelphia, PA: Wolters Kluwer Health/Lippincott Williams & Wilkins.

Meleis, A. I. (2007). *Theoretical nursing: Development and progress* (4th ed.). Philadelphia, PA: Lippincott Williams & Wilkins.

Nightingale, F. (1858). *Subsidiary notes as to the introduction of female nursing into military hospitals in peace and war.* London, UK: Harrison and Sons.

Nightingale, F. (1860/1969). *Notes on nursing: What it is and what it is not.* New York, NY: Dover.

Pender, N. J. (1982). *Health promotion in nursing practice.* Norwalk, CT: Appleton-Century-Crofts.

Pender, N. J. (1996). *Health promotion in nursing practice* (3rd ed.). Stamford, CT: Appleton & Lange.

Pender, N. J., Murdaugh, C. L., & Parsons, M. A. (2002). *Health promotion in nursing practice* (4th ed.). Upper Saddle River, NJ: Prentice Hall.

Pender, N. J., Murdaugh, C. L., & Parsons, M. A. (2006). *Health promotion in nursing practice* (5th ed.). Upper Saddle River, NJ: Prentice Hall.

Pender, N. J., Murdaugh, C. L., & Parsons, M. A. (2011). *Health promotion in nursing practice* (6th ed.). Upper Saddle River, NJ: Pearson.

Pfettscher, S. A. (2010). Florence Nightingale: Modern nursing. In A. M. Tomey & M. R. Alligood (Eds.), *Nursing theorists and their work* (7th ed., pp. 71–90). St. Louis, MO: Mosby.

Pokorny, M. E. (2010). Nursing theorists of historical significance. In A. M. Tomey & M. R. Alligood (Eds.), *Nursing theorists and their work* (7th ed., pp. 54–68). St. Louis, MO: Mosby.

Reed, P. G., & Zurakowski, T. L. (1989). Nightingale revisited: A visionary model for nursing. In J. J. Fitzpatrick & A. L. Whall (Eds.), *Conceptual models of nursing: Analysis and application* (2nd ed., pp. 33–47). Norwalk, CT: Appleton & Lange.

Runk, J. A., & Muth Quillin, S. I. (1989). Henderson's comprehensive definition of nursing. In J. J. Fitzpatrick & A. L. Whall (Eds.), *Conceptual models of nursing: Analysis and application* (2nd ed., pp. 109–121). Norwalk, CT: Appleton & Lange.

Sakraida, T. J. (2010). The health promotion model. In A. M. Tomey & M. R. Alligood (Eds.), *Nursing theorists and their work* (7th ed., pp. 434–453). St. Louis, MO: Mosby.

Selanders, L. C. (1995). Life and times of Florence Nightingale. In C. M. McQuiston & A. A. Webb (Eds.), *Foundations of nursing theory: Contributions of 12 key theorists* (pp. 421–431). Thousand Oaks, CA: Sage.

Shelly, J. A., & Miller, A. B. (2006). *Called to care: A Christian worldview for nursing* (2nd ed.). Downers Grove, IL: InterVarsity Press.

Tomey, A. M. (2002). Virginia Henderson: Definition of nursing. In A. M. Tomey & M. R. Alligood (Eds.), *Nursing theorists and their work* (5th ed., pp. 98–111). St. Louis, MO: Mosby.

Tomey, A. M. (2006). Nursing theorists of historical significance. In A. M. Tomey & M. R. Alligood (Eds.), *Nursing theorists and their work* (6th ed., pp. 54–67). St. Louis, MO: Mosby.

Tooley, S. A. (1910). *The life of Florence Nightingale*. London, UK: Cassell.

Woodham-Smith, C. (1951). *Florence Nightingale*. New York, NY: McGraw-Hill.

# Models and Theories Focused on a Systems Approach

*Martha V. Whetsell*
*Yolanda M. Gonzalez*
*María Elisa Moreno-Fergusson*

## Introduction

Nursing professionals use theories in their practice to describe, explain, predict, and prescribe. The development and use of theories also is a way to generate and disseminate new knowledge in nursing. The application of nursing theory in practice depends on nurses' knowledge of theories, as well as their understanding of how philosophies, models, and theories relate to one another (Alligood, 2002). Using conceptual models as an overarching model for practice, research, education, and administration keeps nursing theory at the forefront of the profession and, ideally, leads advanced practice nurses (APNs) to become proficient in testing and generating theory. With the use of conceptual models and theory in clinical practice, nurses create new ways of thinking and introduce new and expanded ways of delivering health care.

This chapter focuses on three conceptual nursing models that are all based on the systems perspective—the Roy adaptation model, King's conceptual system, and the Neuman systems model. Systems science is an interdisciplinary field of physical, chemical, and psychological structures for nature and society. A system can be a single organism, an object, an organization, or a society.

## General Systems Theory

General systems theory grew from thermodynamics—a branch of physics, chemistry, and engineering. This theory is grounded in the premise that the world is composed of systems that are interconnected and influenced by one another. The two main assumptions of this theory are as follows: (1) energy is needed to maintain an organizational state and (2) a dysfunction in one system has an effect on other systems (Boulding, 1956). The origin of systems theory dates back at least to the 1920s, when theorists sought to explain the interrelatedness of organisms in ecosystems. In 1928, the biologist Ludwig von Bertalanffy became the first person to propose that a system is characterized by the interactions of its components and that the interactions are nonlinear. It was not until 1951, however, that von Bertalanffy extended the theory to include biological systems (McNeill & Freiberger, 1994). In 1968, he published the influential book *General System Theory*.

It might be said that Florence Nightingale introduced systems theory in nursing when she stated that nursing laws would be defined (Riehl & Roy, 1974). King (1964) presented the foundation for the general systems framework in her article titled "Nursing Theory: Problems and Prospect." It was not until 1970, however, that Roy implemented her systems model—known as the Roy adaptation model—as the basis of a nursing curriculum at Mount St. Mary's College in Los Angeles, California (Roy, 2009). Neuman introduced the Neuman systems model in 1970 at the University of California, Los Angeles, and in 1972 Neuman and Young published an article about the model.

The nursing systems models are based on a framework of organized complexity and an interaction among all of the models' components. Such models are dynamic in that they can be used to investigate the client's continuous relationship with the environment. According to Fawcett (2005), the use of systems thinking demands flexibility, which in turn demands the use of creativity to meet the challenges associated with the complex societal changes occurring in this century. This consideration is particularly significant given Fawcett's (2009) assertion that only a strong link between theory and research will advance nursing knowledge—this link supports the building of conceptual–theoretical–empirical (C-T-E) structures for research. Fawcett described two methods of C-T-E: one for theory-generating research and the other for theory-testing research (2009, p. 21).

# The Roy Adaptation Model

## The History

Sister Callista Roy recalled that the origins of her adaptation model date back to 1964, when she was a master's-level student at Mount St. Mary's College in Los Angeles. In 1970, she published the basic ideas of her conceptual model in an article titled "Adaptation: A Conceptual Framework for Nursing" in *Nursing Outlook*. In 1971 and 1973, the model was further explained in a chapter of Riehl and Roy's (1974) book, *Conceptual Models for Nursing Practice*. A more comprehensive explanation of the model can be found in Roy's (1976) book, *Introduction to Nursing: An Adaptation Model*. Further refinements of the model were published in the second edition of that book (Roy, 1984). Roy's clinical experiences in pediatric nursing and neurological nursing were important influences in the development of her model (Roy, 2009).

The primary influencers for defining the key aspects of Roy's adaptation model included the systems theory described by von Bertalanffy (1968) and the work of physiological psychologist Harry Helson (1964), who developed adaptation-level theory. Helson proposed that adaptation involves both psychological and physical processes when an individual faces environmental stimuli. He described three kinds of stimuli—focal, contextual, and residual—that come together and result in a pooled effect. Based on those principles, Roy described how adaptation could help people conserve the energy needed to heal and to cope with new life experiences (Roy & Whetsell, personal communication, 2005).

## The Philosophy and Assumptions

Roy's (2009) model was based on two underlying philosophical assumptions—humanism and veritivity. *Humanism* is the "broad movement in philosophy and psychology that recognizes the individual and subjective dimensions of human experiences as central to knowing and valuing" (p. 28). In 1988, Roy introduced the concept of *veritivity*—"a principle of human nature that affirms a common purposefulness of human existence" (Roy, 1988, as cited in Roy, 2009, p. 27). She described living systems as totalities made of parts that are unified by a purpose, not simply by cause–effect relationships. The veritivity principle is related to four aspects of human society: (1) human existence's purpose, (2) humankind's shared purpose, (3) activity and creativity for the common good, and (4) life sense value (Roy & Andrews, 1999).

Roy acknowledged that her spiritual orientation was a meaningful philosophical influence for development of her model. She also became interested in Teilhard de Chardin's work in 1955, largely because of its characteristic reconciliation of science and spirituality. According to Roy, nurses assume the responsibility of believing in each person's life purpose (Roy, 2009). People remain together in a common destiny and find sense in mutual relationships established with other persons, the world, and God. Roy emphasized the commonality that underlies people's unity and diversity (Roy, 2006). Activity and creativity for the common good are involved in veritivity, and each single human being is different from each other human being—that is, each individual has a unique identity (Roy, 2009). The principle of veritivity allows the nurse to meet the social mandate to help change the system by contributing to the common good through the application of knowledge in practice (Roy & Whetsell, personal conversation, 2005). Roy's last assumption about veritivity is life sense of value; thus the person is the main domain of interest (Roy, 1996). Similarly, Maritain (1966) viewed a person's life as having a higher value than mere social utility.

## The Model

Roy's first three books—published in 1976, 1984, and 1991—highlighted the many colleagues and students who were involved in her work. In 1987, nursing scholars calculated that more than 100,000 nurses were taught by nursing faculty or had graduated from schools that used Roy's model as a curricular framework (Roy, 1996).

Roy developed the Roy adaptation model while maintaining a unique focus on the changes that occur in the human adaptive system and in the environment. The model's central feature is adaptation. According to this model, problems in adaptation materialize when the adaptive systems of a person are unable to respond to stimuli from internal or external environments (Roy & Andrews, 1999).

### Major Elements

Roy did not define the metaparadigm concepts as human beings (person), health, environment, and nursing. Instead, Roy labeled the major elements as adaptation, person, environment, health, and goal of nursing.

***Adaptation.*** *Adaptation* is the process and outcome in which individuals and groups become integrated with their environment through conscious choices (Roy, 2009). Adaptive responses promote integrity in terms of human beings' goals, which are survival, growth, reproduction, mastery, and personal and environmental transformation. All responses that do not contribute to the integrity of the goals of the human system are recognized as ineffective responses.

***Person.*** Early in the development of her model, Roy defined the *person* as "a bio-psycho-social being, in constant interaction with a changing environment" (Roy & Andrews, 1999, p. 19). An expansion of the concept of person along with the addition of *groups* was incorporated in the 1980s as part of the model, in the adaptation systems. Described as totality made of parts behaving purposefully, the person uses innate and acquired mechanisms for biological, psychological, and social adaptation. These mechanisms serve as the regulator and cognator subsystems for individuals and the stabilizer and innovator subsystems for people in groups (Roy, 2009).

***Environment.*** *Environment* is defined as "every condition, circumstance and influence surrounding and affecting, particularly mutual, individual and group development and behavior" (Roy, 1984, as cited in Roy & Andrews, 1999, p. 31). The environment includes all focal, contextual, and residual stimuli (see the definitions in the subsection "Stimulus").

***Health.*** Over time, the concepts of Roy's model were expanded, with health being one of the main foci. In 1964, Roy described *health* as an inherent dimension of a person's life and noted how the health–sickness continuum may vary from severe illness to maximum well-being. More recently, Roy has described health as a "state and a process of being and becoming an integrated and whole person"

(Roy, 2009, p. 48). The concept of health is unidimensional, whereas the concept of nursing is represented by science and art. In Roy's systems theory, the scientific assumptions of the model link the adaptation-level theory described by Helson (1964) with the main concepts of her model. Individuals are regarded as holistic, adaptive systems that are more than the sum of their parts and that function as a whole in constant interaction with the environment (Roy & Andrews, 1999). Similar to how a system has inputs, processes, and outputs, people have stimulus inputs and an adaptation level.

**Goal of nursing.**    According to Roy and Andrews (1999), nursing is "the protection, promotion, and optimization of health and abilities, prevention and injury, alleviation of suffering through the diagnosis and treatment of human response, and advocacy in the care of individuals, families, communities, and populations" (p. 6). The *goal of nursing* is "to promote the health of individuals and societies" (Roy, 2009, p. 54). In pursuing this goal, nurses integrate specialized knowledge from the applied sciences to formulate health promotion and illness management strategies for people. Nursing knowledge is focused on how people—sick or well—interact with their environments to enhance well-being and flourishing.

## Adaptive Systems

*Adaptive systems* include stimuli, adaptation level, and behavior. They are holistic systems that are defined in terms of human beings.

**Stimulus.**    A *stimulus* is the trigger that provokes a response; it can be viewed as the point of interaction between the human system and the environment (Roy, 2009). The constructs of stimuli in Roy's model are based on Harry Helson's work relating to focal, contextual, and residual concepts. The focal stimulus evokes a primary internal or external awareness by the individual or the group, contextual stimuli are additional environmental factors that operate from within or outside the individual, and residual stimuli are other environmental factors that generate effects that may not be readily apparent in a given situation (Roy, 2009). Stimuli can change rapidly and often do so constantly because of the interactions between people and their environment.

**Adaptation level.**    *Adaptation level* includes three conditions of the human adaptive system: (1) integrated, (2) compensatory, and (3) compromised. As Roy stated, "The level of adaptation conveys that the human adaptive system is not passive in relation to the environment and that the person and the environment are in constant interaction with each other" (Roy, 2009, p. 37). The integrated level means that the structures and functions of the life processes work as one whole to meet the needs of humans. The compensatory level is where the cognator and regulator subsystems for individuals have been activated; or for groups, it is where the stabilizer and innovator subsystems have been activated. The compromised level is initiated in response to the system's diminishing adaptation, because the integrated and the compensatory levels are no longer working.

**Behavior.**    *Behavior* is defined as internal or external actions and reactions that occur under specific circumstances (Roy, 2009). Behavior is sometimes objectively observed and measured or subjectively reported by individuals or people in groups. Output behavior indicates how well a system can adapt while interacting with the environment—this relationship is the target of nursing interventions.

The behavioral response is evident in the coping process, but it remains independent of this process. The processes involving the human being as an adaptive system underscore the various ways in which people deal with the demands of their environment. These processes specifically focus on those behaviors that meet the goals for adaptation; they relate to responses that promote the integrity of the human system in terms of adaptation goals (Roy & Andrews, 1999). Put simply, the behavioral response can be either adaptive or ineffective, as described in the previous section on model elements.

## Coping Processes

*Coping processes* are "innate or acquired ways of interacting with—that is, responding to and influencing—the change environment" (Roy & Andrews, 1999, p. 41). The coping processes include the coping capacity, cognator and regulator subsystems for coping processes, and stabilizer and innovator subsystems for control processes.

**Coping capacity.**    *Coping capacity* is viewed as an important stimulus to enhance adaptation. One's coping ability as an adaptive system serves as a significant internal input for the person; output, in contrast, relates to the actual behavior. Coping involves the four dimensions already mentioned: regulator and cognator coping subsystems for individuals, and stabilizer and innovator control subsystems for groups.

**Cognator and regulator coping processes.**    The *cognator subsystem* for individuals is a coping process that interacts primarily with the other three modes. This system includes four cognitive–emotive channels: (1) perceptual and information processing, (2) learning, (3) judgment, and (4) emotion.

The *regulator subsystem* for individuals constitutes a major coping process that includes an extremely linked physiological mode. The neurochemical and endocrine systems respond unconsciously to stimuli through neural, chemical, and endocrine coping channels; thus, they affect the fluid, electrolyte, and acid–base balance, as well as the endocrine system. These responses are interrelated and act in concert with one another, rather than in isolation, to maintain the equilibrium of the systems.

**Stabilizer and innovator control processes.**    The *stabilizer subsystem* for groups is a control process associated with systems maintenance involving structures, values, and daily activities to fulfill the purpose of the social system. The *innovator subsystem* is a control process related to individuals in groups; it encompasses structures and processes associated with personal change and growth within social systems.

## Adaptive Modes

The coping process responses constitute the outputs of the human adaptive system. These responses are reflected in behaviors, which are interrelated *adaptive modes*. As such, adaptation is evident in four adaptive modes for individuals: (1) physiological, (2) self-concept, (3) role function, and (4) interdependence. For groups, the four adaptive modes are (1) physical, (2) identity, (3) role function, and (4) interdependence. Thus "behavior in one mode may have an effect on or act as stimulus for one or all the other modes" (Roy & Andrews, 1999, p. 51).

***Physiological/physical mode.*** The *physiological mode* reflects the way that individuals as physical beings interact with the environment. This mode consists of two components: the physiological mode and the physical mode. The physiological mode pertains to the individual. In this mode, persons manifest the physical processes and activities of living organisms (Roy, 2009). The behavior in this mode represents the physiological manifestations of a person's cells, organs, and systems. This mode has nine components: five basic needs (oxygenation, nutrition, elimination, activity and rest, and protection) and four processes (senses, fluid and electrolyte balance, neurological function, and endocrine function). The basic need of the physiological mode is physiologic integrity.

By comparison, the *physical mode* relates to "the way the human adaptive system of the group manifests adaptation relative to basic operating resources, that is, participants, physical facilities and fiscal resources" (Roy, 2009, p. 43). The fundamental need of the physical mode is resource adequacy.

***The self-concept/group identity mode.*** The *self-concept mode* reflects personal aspects of individuals related to behavior. A self-concept is "the composite of beliefs and feelings that an individual holds about him or herself at a given time" (Roy, 2009, p. 44). The basic need for the self is psychic and spiritual integrity—that is, the need to know who one is so that the person can live with a sense of unity and purposefulness in the universe (Roy, 2009). Self-concept includes three components: (1) physical self (body image and body sensations), (2) personal self (self-consistency, self-ideal), and (3) the moral–ethical–spiritual self.

The *group identity mode* reflects group aspects of behavior. It comprises four subdimensions: (1) interpersonal relationships, (2) group self-image, (3) social milieu, and (4) group culture. The basic need underlying this mode is identity integrity of the group.

***The role function mode.*** Focusing on the roles that the person has in society, the basic needs underlying the *role function mode* have been identified as social integrity, role clarity, and the need to know who one is in relation to others so that one can act. This mode relates to the function or responsibility that an individual or group has in society.

The individual has three types of roles:

1. *A primary role*, which is unchangeable because it is based on age, gender, and developmental stage.
2. *A secondary role*, which is related to the expectations of the individual and the primary role. This role is an important one because it relates to the life project of each individual.
3. *A tertiary role*, which is temporary, is linked to the first two roles. In general, the tertiary role can change and is derived from the secondary and primary roles. Tertiary roles are freely chosen and often relate to small tasks undertaken in the course of a person's life.

In relation to groups, Roy (2009) established that the role's functions are "the vehicle through which the goals of the social system are actually accomplished" (p. 44)—relating to their mission or the tasks associated with the functions of the group. The role function includes the function of administrators and staff, the management of information, and systems for decision making and maintaining order.

**The interdependence mode.**    The *interdependence mode* is the category of behavior related to relationships that individuals and groups establish with others. For individuals, this mode focuses on those interactions through which the individual receives and gives love, respect, and valuation. The basic need of this mode is nurturing relationships. For groups, this category reflects the group's social context.

The adaptive modes reflect the responses of the coping processes of the individual or group to the focal, contextual, and residual stimuli. These modes are interrelated, such that a response in one mode affects the responses in the other three modes and is expressed in an individual's behavior. Roy's adaptation model is a *systems* model, meaning that it has elements of an "interactional" model. It was developed specifically to be used in caring for individual clients, but it can also be adapted for use with families and communities.

## The Nursing Process

When implementing the nursing process according to the Roy adaptation model, human experiences and responses are approached in a nontraditional way. An individual or a group of individuals is viewed as a holistic adaptive system. Stimuli from the internal and external environments trigger the coping processes maintained by the four adaptive modes. The nurse assesses the behavior of the person or group and the influence of the stimuli on behavior; based on this assessment, the nurse then formulates nursing diagnoses.

Roy (2009) viewed the nursing process as relating to human beings as adaptive systems. This process includes six steps:

1. Assessment of behavior
2. Assessment of stimuli

3. Nursing diagnosis
4. Goal setting
5. Intervention
6. Evaluation

***Assessment of behavior.***     The first step involves gathering behavioral data. During the assessment, the nurse systematically examines responses in each adaptive mode, uses observational skills, and compares current measurements to preestablished measurements. Effective communication and caring take precedence—an approach that contributes to the effectiveness of nurse–patient interactions.

***Assessment of stimuli.***     The second step of the nursing process is an extension of the first and encompasses the identification of internal and external stimuli affecting particular behaviors. In completing this assessment, the nurse utilizes skills similar to those applied in the first step. Identifying the behavior that threatens the integrity of the system is the primary concern. During the identification process, the nurse pinpoints the focal, contextual, and residual stimuli that influence the response, as well as the adaptation level that contributes to adaptive or ineffective behavior.

***Nursing diagnosis.***     Nursing diagnosis, according to Roy, is a judgment process that confirms the adaptation status of the person or the group. In formulating a diagnosis, the nurse primarily uses critical thinking. The nursing diagnosis must include behaviors with the most relevant influencing stimuli (Roy, 2009, p. 68).

***Goal setting.***     Goal setting entails the establishment of clear statements vis-à-vis the outcomes of nursing care, as well as the time frame for the expected attainment of the goal. Goal setting is established following the nurse's assessment. The statement of a goal helps it to materialize and ensures that the behavior of the person or the group becomes the focus.

***Nursing intervention.***     The nursing intervention step requires that the nurse choose nursing interventions that promote the adaptation process. After the selection of nursing-appropriate interventions, nurses develop an approach to initiate the steps needed to change the focal stimuli and enhance coping abilities.

***Evaluation.***     Evaluation is the last step of the nursing process; it involves an assessment of the effectiveness of the nursing intervention based on the previously established goals. This step could be the last one in the process, but it might also serve as a change agent to begin a new intervention if the previous goal was not achieved.

The most valuable feature of this process is the collaboration between the person or group and the nurse in every step of the nursing process. Under the auspices of the Roy adaptation model, the effectiveness of the intervention depends on the nurse's knowledge of the situation and the way in which the nurse obtains collaboration from the person or persons involved.

## Application of the Model to Education, Research, and Practice

The use of the Roy adaptation model for nursing education is well documented. This model is used not only in the United States, but also in Asia, Europe, South America, Central America, and Mexico. One of the benefits of using the Roy adaptation model in education is that it provides students with a solid structure for thinking in a holistic manner and developing critical thinking skills. Indeed, the benefit of using this model as a framework for nursing practice has been demonstrated throughout the world, although the level of integration of the model into practice varies among hospitals and countries. Roy's model generally is found to be useful in focusing, organizing, and directing nurses' thoughts and actions regarding client care, resulting in a perception that the quality of nursing and client outcomes are improved. An example is easing the patient into a state of adaptability to care. The nursing role in this adaptation process is pivotal in maintaining adaptive responses and converting ineffective responses to adaptive ones to achieve health.

Research indicates that the Roy adaptation model is a conceptual model of nursing being used in nursing practice in the United States, Japan, Brazil, Colombia, Mexico, Panama, and Peru. Collectively, the studies in these countries demonstrate that using the model leads to better adaptability to care by patients and improved healthcare outcomes (Moreno & Alvarado, 2009).

Literature has shown that the Roy adaptation model is most useful as a tool when used in nursing research. Numerous quantitative and qualitative research studies have been conducted using Roy's model as a conceptual framework, and several research instruments have been derived from it (Fawcett, 2005). Many middle-range theories can be created and derived from Roy's conceptual system. A review of the literature revealed that the model has been used in descriptive studies of personal responses to environmental stimuli and correlations between the modes, manifestations of the stimuli, and effects of nursing interventions that are linked to propositions of the model.

# The King Conceptual System and Theory of Goal Attainment

## The History

Imogene King was the first nurse theorist to develop a nursing framework and a middle-range theory related to it (Sieloff & Frey, 2007). Born in 1923, King graduated with a diploma in nursing from St. John's Hospital in St. Louis, Missouri, in 1945, a bachelor's degree in nursing education from St. Louis University in 1948, a master's degree in nursing from St. Louis University in 1957, and a doctorate of education from Teachers College, Columbia University in New York City in 1961. Two decades later, in 1980, she was conferred an honorary doctorate from Southern Illinois University. King began her academic career at St. Louis University, then taught at Loyola University in Chicago, and ultimately moved to the University of South Florida, where, after a distinguished career, she became professor emeritus. In 1964, King was one of the pioneers who urged nursing professionals to focus on the organization of nursing knowledge, arguing that a theoretical body of knowledge was necessary for the advancement of nursing.

In her 1968 article titled "A Conceptual Frame of Reference for Nursing," King presented the concepts of social systems, health, interpersonal relationships, and perceptions as being universal to the discipline of nursing (King, 1968, 1995). In 1971, in her book *Toward a Theory for Nursing*, she began to refine the *conceptual system*. She further refined the conceptual system when she introduced the theory of goal attainment as part of her model in *A Theory for Nursing: Systems, Concepts, Process* (1981a). It is in this book that she presented the concepts of environment and person, suggested that fewer dichotomies exist between health and illness, changed the terminology in her theory from "adaptation" to "adjustment," and distinguished a person as a human being or individual rather than as "man."

## The Philosophy

King's philosophical worldview is a systems and interactional approach, as evidenced by her admonition that her framework should be read "from the perspective of General System Theory and a science of wholeness" (King, 1990, p. 74). King validated her philosophy as driven by Greek philosophy and grounded in the Aristotelian–Thomistic perspective, which includes that of individuals striving for the end goal of happiness and flourishing. Persons must be motivated and guided to understand the necessity of using new and consistent behaviors to facilitate the process of goal attainment.

## The Models
### The Conceptual System

The core of King's conceptual system is the notion that human beings are open systems interacting constantly with the environment (King, 1989). King's conceptual model incorporates three interacting systems: *personal, interpersonal,* and *social*. She discovered these three systems when she began categorizing health issues by way of a systems approach, which was shaped by von Bertalanffy's (1968) general systems theory and interaction theory.

King's (1989) model reflects the metaparadigm concepts of person, environment, health, and nursing as systems. The concept of person is represented by the three systems (personal system, interpersonal system, and social system); a set of concepts for each system provides a method for nurses to organize their knowledge, skills, and values. Client goals are met through the transaction between the nurse and client. This interaction, which occurs over time, constitutes a transaction, such that eventually the person's goal is met (King, 1997, 2001).

## Personal System

The hub of the personal system is the individual (person)—whether healthy or ill, who gathers and uses information to assist him or her in understanding another individual or group (King, 1975, 1995). The composition of the seven concepts—perception, self, growth and development, body image, time, personal space, and learning—form the whole, complex personal system. Human beings are open systems responding to and coping with stimuli based on their expectations, other people, events, and objects. The personal system is influenced by variables—namely, age, habits, situations, place in the family, and roles—that lead to the performance of the function.

## Interpersonal System

In King's (1981a) framework, interpersonal systems are groups (small or large) of people. Interpersonal systems enclose six concepts—communication, interaction, roles, stress, coping, and transaction, all of which transpire at some point during the nursing process. Perceptions shape the person-to-person and person-to-environment interactions, but communication is the mode through which individuals make transactions, such as setting goals, choosing the strategies for attaining the goals, and attempting to maintain their health.

## Social System

The social system is an "organized boundary system of social roles, behaviors and practices developed to maintain values and the mechanisms to regulate the practices and rules" (King, 1981a, p. 115). The social system addresses the needs of individuals and of the subgroups that are formed by certain commonalities, such as age, patterns of behavior, roles, and status. The concepts that make up the social system include authority, decision making, organization, power, and status.

## Other Concepts

Other concepts that King included in the conceptual system are authority, body image, communication, decision making, growth and development, interaction, organization, perception, power, role, self, space, status, time, and transaction. These complex concepts are interrelated in the interactions of human beings with their environment. The metaparadigm concepts used by King are environment, health, nursing, and person. (Refer to the personal system for an explanation of person.)

According to King (1981a), the environment is holistic and transformative because individuals continually adjust their internal environment to transform energy in order to adjust to the continuous changes of the external environment. Although King did not explicitly define *internal environment* and *external environment*, she recognized the environment as functioning to bring harmony to the internal and external interactions.

King's view of health is "a process of human growth and development and relates to the way individuals deal with stress of growth and development while functioning within the cultural pattern in which they were born and to which they attempt to conform" (1981a, p. 4). With this thought in mind, individuals undergo constant dynamic change in their state of health; they require continuous adjustment to stress to achieve physiological stability. King (1981a) did not identify health and illness on a linear continuum because she chose not to address certain abstract, and required, concepts, particularly wellness; rather, King saw illness as an imbalance in the person's physiological or psychological makeup, constituting a disturbance in the dynamic state of the person in her view.

The focus of nursing is the human being and human acts. Nursing is an observable behavior found in a society's many healthcare systems. It is a process of action, reaction, and interaction, whereby a nurse and client share information about their perceptions in the nursing situation (King, 1995). King (1971, 1991) based her framework on the assumption that nursing's focus is on interactions between individuals and their environment to promote, maintain, and restore their health. The nurse–client transactions, which are different in each situation, comprise a sequence of behaviors that establish expectations, mutual goals, and interdependent roles. Each nursing action and its effectiveness varies with each transaction, depending on the extent to which goals are realistic and nursing judgments are valid.

According to Sieloff and Frey (2007), the following propositions were included in early publications by King:

- The nursing process is conducted within a social system that includes five dimensions: (1) the nursing process, (2) the individuals involved in the nursing process, (3) the individuals involved in the environment within which the nursing process is activated, (4) the social organization within which the nursing process is activated, and (5) the community within which the social organization functions.
- The nursing process will differ, depending on the individual nurse and each recipient of nursing services.
- The nursing process will differ relative to all individuals in the environment.
- The nursing process will differ relative to the social organization in which the nursing process takes place.
- The relationship among the dimensions affects the nursing process.
- Nursing includes specific components: (1) nursing judgment, (2) nursing action, (3) communication, (4) evaluation, and (5) coordination.
- The nursing judgment will vary relative to each nursing action.
- The effectiveness of nursing action will vary in the extent to which it is communicated to those responsible for its implementation.
- Nursing action is more effective if the goals are communicated and standards of nursing performance have been established.
- Nursing action is based on facts, which may change; thus nursing judgments and actions are evaluated and revised as the situation changes.

- Nursing is a component of health care; thus, health care is affected by the coordination of nursing with health services. (1981a, pp. 401–402)

## Theory of Goal Attainment

King's theory of goal attainment, which was derived from her conceptual framework, focuses on holism and includes nursing as a process that is interactional in nature. These interactions lead to the critical transactions that result in goal attainment (King, 1992; Sieloff Evans, 1991). Emphasis is placed on interpersonal systems and the phenomena of process and outcomes (goals). These goals become criteria for measuring the effectiveness of nursing care.

**Assumptions.**    King's theory of goal attainment is based on the following assumptions:

- Individuals are social beings.
- Individuals are sentient beings.
- Individuals are rational beings.
- Individuals are reacting beings.
- Individuals are perceiving beings.
- Individuals are controlling beings.
- Individuals are purposeful beings.
- Individuals are action-oriented beings.
- Individuals are time-oriented beings.
- Perceptions of nurse and of client influence the interaction process.
- Goals, needs, and values of nurse and client influence the interaction process.
- Individuals have a right to knowledge about themselves.
- Individuals have a right to participate in decisions that influence their life, their health, and community services.
- Health professionals have a responsibility to share information that helps individuals make informed decisions about their health care.
- Individuals have a right to accept or reject health care.
- Goals of health professionals and goals of recipients of health care may be incongruent. (King, 1981b, pp. 143–144)

The major concepts of goal attainment include communication, growth and development, interaction, perception, role, space, stress, time, and transaction (King, 1981b). Decision making is a shared collaborative process where the nurse and client share information for the purpose of setting and attaining goals.

**Propositions.**    According to King (1981b), the major concepts mentioned in the last section are embedded in the following propositions of the theory of goal attainment:

1. If perceptual accuracy is present in the nurse–client interaction, transaction will occur.
2. If the nurse and the client make transactions, goals will be attained.

3. If goals are attained, satisfaction will occur.

4. If goals are attained, effective nursing care will occur.

5. If transactions are made in the nurse–client interaction, growth and development will be enhanced.

6. If role expectations and role performance as perceived by the nurse and the client are congruent, transaction will occur.

7. If role conflict is experienced by the nurse, the client, or both, stress in nurse–client interactions will occur.

8. If nurses with special knowledge and skills communicate appropriate information to clients, mutual goal setting and goal attainment will occur.

***Hypothesis.***    King (1981b, p. 156) developed the following hypothesis from the theory of goal attainment:

1. Perceptual accuracy in nurse–client interactions increases mutual goal setting.

2. Communication increases mutual goal setting between nurses and clients and leads to satisfaction.

3. Satisfaction in nurses and clients increases the likelihood of goal attainment.

4. Goal attainment decreases stress and anxiety in nursing situations.

5. Goal attainment increases client learning and coping ability in nursing situations.

6. Role conflict experienced by clients, nurses, or both decreases transactions in nurse–client interactions.

7. Congruence in role expectations and role performance increases transactions in nurse–client interactions.

## Nursing Application of King's Conceptual System and Theory of Goal Attainment

King's conceptual framework, both the conceptual system and the theory of goal attainment, are applicable to nursing practice, education, research, and administration. The discipline of nursing and nursing knowledge continue to be advanced by King's work on the nursing process, systems, and goal attainment. Many researchers and theorists have accelerated the progress made on King's work.

Fawcett (2005) emphasized that conceptual models, such as King's conceptual system, or grand theories, can serve as an overarching frame of reference for nursing and the phenomena of interest in nursing practice, but they cannot be applied directly to practice. Instead, middle-range theories must serve as theories for direct practice applicability, and the concepts within the middle-range theories must be consistent with the nurse's (or institution's) adopted conceptual model. Many nurses have aligned their frame of reference with King's systems framework in their practice, education, or administration.

King formulated her middle-range theory of goal attainment from her conceptual system. The theory of goal attainment provides a meaningful application for nurses. Nurses have long been interacting with clients and making goal-setting transactions with patients. Although the social systems concept was not a definite system in her theory of goal attainment, as it was in her conceptual system, the other two systems—personal and interpersonal—were clearly linked.

# The Neuman Systems Model

Betty Neuman described the Neuman systems model as "a unique systems-based perspective that provides a unifying focus for approaching a wide range of nursing concerns" (Neuman, 2002a, p. 3). This model is a comprehensive guide for nursing practice, research, education, and administration and has the potential for unifying health-related theories through the examination of the relationships between nursing intervention and patient response to stressors. The wellness, multidimensionality, and wholistic systemic perspective of the Neuman systems model has demonstrated its relevance and reliability in various clinical and educational settings in the United States and abroad (Neuman, 2002a).

## The Evolution of the Neuman Systems Model

Neuman was born in 1924 in Lowell, Ohio. In 1947, she received a registered nurse diploma from People's Hospital School of Nursing in Akron, Ohio. She later moved to California, where she gained experience as a hospital staff nurse, school nurse, industrial nurse, and clinical instructor in medical–surgical, critical care, and communicable disease nursing. In 1957, Neuman received a bachelor's degree from the University of California at Los Angeles (UCLA) with a double major in psychology and public health. In 1966, she received a master's degree in nursing from UCLA; she received a doctor of philosophy degree in clinical psychology from Pacific Western University in 1985.

Neuman was a pioneer in the community mental health movement in the late 1960s. In mid-1970, she introduced the Neuman systems model for nursing education and practice. A refinement of the model was published in the first edition of Riehl and Roy's 1974 book, *Conceptual Models for Nursing Practice*. Further refinements were presented in 1982 in the first edition of Neuman's own book, titled *The Neuman Systems Model: Application to Nursing Education and Practice* (Neuman, 1982).

Neuman's conceptual model has undergone many changes since its inception in 1970. Today the Neuman systems model provides nursing with a comprehensive, flexible, wholistic, and systems-based guide that focuses (1) on the response of the client systems to actual or potential environmental stressors and (2) on the use of primary, secondary, and tertiary nursing prevention interventions for retention, attainment, and maintenance of optimal client wellness (Neuman, 1996).

## The Philosophy

Neuman's philosophy is based on wholism, reality, and wellness, along with her assumptions about interactions of four metaparadigm concepts—person, environment, health, and nursing. She derived the term *wholism* from the holistic systems concept introduced by de Chardin (1955), a Catholic priest, scientist, and philosopher who believed in the wholeness of life as being the interconnectedness of the human spirit and mind. Neuman (1996) recognized her systems model as a wholistic conceptual framework for guiding nursing interactions with clients. A focal point in the Neuman model is nurses' insight and involvement in the response of the client system to actual or potential environmental stressors.

Neuman's notion about *reality* mirrors gestalt theory in three ways:

1. Emphasis on the perceived
2. Awareness of *what is* and not *what should be*
3. Completely understanding the patterns and structures in unity, or the whole situation in a perceptual field

Encasing the client system is a perceptual field in dynamic equilibrium, where all parts or variables work together as a whole. Reality is based on the client's perspective. Neuman (2002a) described the wholeness of the perceptual field as "the total organization of the field" (p. 12), or nurses "taking into consideration the simultaneous effects of the interacting variables—physiological, psychological, sociocultural, developmental, and spiritual" (p. 13).

Neuman classified her systems model as a wellness model—that is, as a model of retaining wellness and ensuring optimal wellness attainment (Neuman, 1995). *Wellness* is generally described by degrees. From Neuman's perspective, optimal wellness "represents the greatest possible degree of system stability at a given point in time" (1995, p. 25). Clients perceive their own degree of wellness and health, but the definition of health encompasses a broader perspective than just each client's perception of health. According to Neuman (1995), wellness needs to be defined and negotiated between the client and the nurse because of the interrelationship between the systems energy, the environment, and the nurse's perception of the client's health.

## The Model

The metaparadigm concepts within the Neuman systems model are human beings, environment, health, and nursing. This systems-based model includes two major components: stress and systematic feedback loops (Neuman, 1995). The client is considered an open system in which continual cycles of input, process, output, and feedback make up an active organizational pattern. The client is simultaneously an individual as well as part of a group, a family, or a community. Neuman considered all variables affecting a client's response to environmental stressors and explains that knowing something about one part of a system enables us to know something about another part. As systems become more complex, the internal conditions of regulation become more intricate. Even so, the nursing goal is to obtain wellness through retention and attainment of client system stability. Neuman (2002a) also stated that the interaction with the environment is mutual—meaning that both the client and environment could each have a positive or negative effect on the other.

The Neuman systems model reflects a wholistic orientation to wellness (Neuman, 1995). It is similar to gestalt theory in stating that each system is surrounded by a perceptual field that is in dynamic equilibrium (Edelson, 1970). The Neuman model also reflects Lazarus's (1999) and Selye's (1946) theories of stress, and Caplan's (1964) conceptual model of levels of prevention (Harris, Hermiz, Meininger, & Steinkeler, 1994). Moreover, Neuman suggested that in understanding the systems model from a wholistic point of view, we must consider five variables of the person: (1) physiological, (2) psychological, (3) sociocultural, (4) developmental, and (5) spiritual. Particular awareness of these variables must be exercised, though they are only connected with reference to the whole (Neuman, 2002a). In effect, the system has a core structure comprising basic survival factors that are common to species (George, 1996)—namely, system variables, genetic features, and the strengths and weaknesses of the system parts. Examples in the healthcare setting include hair, body temperature regulation ability, the homeostatic functioning of body systems, cognitive ability, physical strength, and factors that are encircled by concentric rings of barriers (the flexible line of defense, the normal line of defense, and the lines of resistance), which act as boundaries to provide protection to the system (Fawcett, 2005; Neuman, 2002a).

### Structure of the Model

The Neuman systems model is an open systems model that provides nursing with a unifying focus (Neuman, 2002a). The client system expands the perspective of nursing by taking into account all variables that will affect a client's response to stressors. In doing so, it explains how stability is obtained in relation to the stressors imposed on the client by the environment (Fawcett, 2005).

The basic structure is related to system variables, as well as to unique person variables. The model adopts a wholistic approach that views the client as an open system, the environment as both internal and external, and the interplay of human and environment as a process of interaction of matter and energy (Harris et al., 1994).

In Neuman's model, the total system interacts with the environment. The system relating to the client is affected by five variables—that is, five characteristics of the person (Harris et al., 1994). The basic structure is a combination of all the variables applicable to human survival and those variables unique to each individual. Homeostasis occurs when available energy exceeds the amount being used by the system. In this interaction process, matter, energy, and information are exchanged by a system and its environment through feedback from the process of intake and output. The goal is an equalization of energy gain and loss at a desired level to produce homeostasis. The variables reside within the basic structure, because they are part of the flexible line of defense (Neuman, 2002a).

***The flexible line of defense.***    The *flexible line of defense* forms the outer barrier to (or, put another way, cushions) the normal line of defense of the client system. This mechanism serves as a protective buffer system for the client's normal or stable state. The flexible line of defense is dynamic and can be altered in a relatively short period of time. If all possible defenses prevent the invasion of the stressors and keep the system free of symptomatology, then this line of defense acts like an accordion—expanding away from the normal line of defense and providing protection as it draws closer. When flexible lines of defense fail, the normal line of defense is activated (Neuman, 2002b).

***The normal line of defense.***    The *normal line of defense* denotes what the client has overcome, because it acts as a protective buffer system for the client's stable state. The normal line of defense is used also as a baseline from which to measure health deviation (Neuman, 2002b). Each line of defense is made up of similar protective elements related to the five variables; in other words, it keeps the system free from stressor reactions. The function of the normal line of defense is dynamic, rather than stable, and can be changed over a short period of time (Neuman, 2002b). Its expansion reflects an enhanced wellness state (Fawcett, 2005). When the flexible line of defense is no longer capable of protecting the client or fails to provide protection to the normal line of defense, however, the lines of resistance become activated.

The normal line of defense represents system stability over time; it is the solid boundary line that encircles the broken internal lines of resistance. Because it represents what each client has become over time, this line of defense can be used as a standard against which to measure wellness level or health deviation. The interrelationships of the five client systems variables with environmental stressors help to determine the extent to which a client is stable (Neuman, 2002a).

***Lines of resistance.***    The *lines of resistance* serve as a protective mechanism whose function is to stabilize the client system and return it to the normal wellness level (Neuman, 2002b). Graphically, these lines of resistance may be depicted as a series of concentric broken circles surrounding and protecting the basic structure. They become activated when environmental stressors invade the normal line of defense—for example, as in the activation of the platelets in response to a laceration. If the lines of resistance are effective, the system can reconstitute its defenses; if the lines of resistance are not effective, the resulting energy depletion can result in death.

***Stressors.***    *Stressors* are forces that disrupt and can operate within the system (Neuman, 2002b). They comprise environmental tension forces that cause system instability; these forces can each have a positive or negative effect on the system. The outcome of the effect depends on the system perception and ability to negotiate its effect. According to gestalt theory, stressors influence the reaction to all other stressors (Lazarus, 1999).

Stressors include three dimensions:

1. *Intrapersonal:* occur within the person or family relationships (e.g., emotions)
2. *Interpersonal:* occur between individuals or between the individual and the community (e.g., role expectations or family relationships)
3. *Extrapersonal:* occur outside the individual, such as community groups (e.g., healthcare policies)

The reaction of the client to any stressor will influence the treatment of the symptoms. The nurse can predict the client's adjustment based on past coping behavior, which in turn depends on the strength of the lines of resistance and defense. The nurse may also attempt to restore stability to the system by means of primary, secondary, and tertiary interventions. According to Lazarus (1999), cognitive appraisal determines the degree of stress felt, whereas coping functions mediate the reaction.

### Prevention as Intervention

According to Neuman, the point of entry to the healthcare system is the *primary prevention level*. Before a reaction occurs, it strengthens the clients and helps them to deal with stressors; at the same time, it influences the environment to reduce the stressors. It strengthens the flexible lines of defense through health promotion and maintenance of wellness (Neuman, 2002b). For example, doing exercise every day for 30 to 40 minutes benefits all body systems; teaching people to wash their hands before eating helps to prevent *E. coli* infection. In a community setting such as a daycare center for elderly people, the primary prevention could be a vaccination journey against pneumococcal and influenza infection.

*Secondary prevention* occurs after the client has reacted to a stressor. The goal of secondary prevention is not only to identify the stress point of entry, but also to protect the basic core structures. This level of prevention focuses on the types of interventions that could be used alone or simultaneously to prevent damage to the central core by strengthening the internal lines of resistance and/or removing the stressor. The notion of secondary prevention as intervention is related to the treatment of symptoms that follows the reaction of the stressors (Neuman, 2002a). Examples of secondary interventions include the treatment of pressure ulcers in a bedridden patient and the nursing care that a community needs after an earthquake.

*Tertiary prevention* follows after the system has been treated through secondary prevention. This level supports the client by adding or reducing energy so that the system can be reconstituted (Neuman, 2002a). An example of a tertiary prevention is the nursing care provided for a person who recently had a car accident and had a leg amputated. In this situation, the nurse is prompted to focus on the patient's actual symptoms, and later, to plan for the patient's achievement of long-term goals aimed at prevention of secondary complications.

## Neuman's Perception of Nursing

The Neuman systems model nursing process was designed specifically for the implementation of the model and has been developed to address three issues in this regard:

1. *Nursing diagnosis:* obtained through assessment and consideration of the five variables in three stressor areas
2. *Nursing goals:* negotiated with the client and taking into account both the client's and the nurse's perceptions
3. *Nursing outcomes:* considered in relation to five variables and achieved through primary, secondary, and tertiary interventions

According to Neuman, the major concern of nursing is to obtain significant and comprehensive client data in order to make a comprehensive objective diagnosis (Fawcett, 2005). The data synthesized in this way provide a rationale for future nursing action. A unique feature of the Neuman systems model nursing process is the determination of the perceptions held by the client and the nurse.

Neuman (1995) perceived health as energy that produces the finest system stability at any point in time. Thus health is a continuum with a wellness condition, marked by the highest available energy, at one extreme and death, which signifies total energy absence, at the other extreme. In using this model, the nurse focuses his or her practice on promoting system stability through attainment, retention, and maintenance of optimal wellness and wholeness. The concept of prevention as intervention facilitates the use of the nursing process in persons as individuals or groups with the goal of achieving client system stability and maintaining protective barriers. With primary prevention as intervention, nursing knowledge is applied to assessment and nursing intervention for the purposes of identification and reduction of risk factors associated with environmental stressors to prevent reaction. Primary prevention encompasses the goal of health. Secondary prevention involves treatment actions based on client symptomatology after system reaction. The goal in this circumstance is to provide correct treatment to obtain optimal client system stability. Secondary prevention is provided when primary prevention was not effective. Tertiary prevention involves actions that promote wellness after treatment. According to Neuman (2002b), if nurses are to keep a system stable, they must create a connection between the client, the environment, health, and nursing.

In the first step of the nursing process, the nurse acquires significant and comprehensive data related to the impact of the environmental stressors. Analysis of these data provides the rationale for nursing action (Neuman, 2002c). The nursing diagnostic statement should reflect the entire client condition.

### Outcome Identification and Planning

Outcome identification and planning involve negotiation between the caregiver and the client or recipient of care. The overall goal of the caregiver is to guide the client to conserve energy and to use energy as a force to move beyond the present (Neuman, 2002c).

### Nursing Goals

Neuman's goals for nursing are based on the synthesis of a comprehensive database about the client and the theory appropriate to the client's and the caregiver's perceptions and possibilities for functional competence in the environment. A unique feature of Neuman's systems model is the mutual determination of any interventions in order to formulate goals. During this step, the evaluation confirms that the anticipated or prescribed change has (or has not) occurred. Immediate- and long-range goals are structured in relation to the short-term goals (Neuman, 2002c).

### Evaluation

Neuman's evaluation component in the nursing process involves evaluating outcomes. Nurses evaluate the effectiveness of their interventions based on the degree to which clients met their goals. With evaluation, nurses determine the client's status in the health–illness continuum so that changes can be made as needed in the planning and implementation of care (Neuman, 2002c).

## Education

Neuman compels students to use logic, deduction, and induction in developing their nursing care plans. Most importantly, the model reveals to students that client perceptions are an integral part of the nursing process and should be included in the data collection and client outcome development steps (Neuman, 1995).

Newman, Neuman, and Fawcett (2002) offered some valuable guidelines for education:

- The curriculum focuses on the client system's reaction to environmental stressors.
- The curriculum content encompasses all of the concepts in the model.
- Education can occur in educational and technical programs.
- Students must critically think.
- Teaching–learning strategies must foster critical thinking and independent learning.

## Practice

The Neuman systems model provides APNs and other nurses with a different frame of reference for addressing health conditions within distinctive settings. In the literature describing the use of the Neuman systems model in practice, the reader can appreciate how the model guides wholistic approaches to client care. International research, for example, has revealed broad use of this model (Engberg, 1995; Vaughan & Gough, 1995). The Neuman systems model also supports the use of clinical tools that are practical and that guide wholistic assessment and prevention for individuals, families, communities, and organizations; these tools help to guide the practitioner's clinical practice.

The model has been used in several areas of practice. In the United States, the model has made a significant contribution in a neglected area of health care: postpartum mood disorders (PPMD). Kendall-Tackett (1993) contributed significantly to the prevention of health problems in young childbearing families by describing primary, secondary, and tertiary interventions for PPMD.

The following guidelines are delineated for practice (Freese, Neuman, & Fawcett, 2002):

- The purpose is to assist clients to retain, attain, or maintain optimal system stability.
- Practice problems include actual or potential reactions to stressors.
- Practice takes place in any healthcare setting.
- The participants are persons, families, and communities who are faced with stressors.
- The practice process of the model consists of three components: diagnosis, goals, and outcomes.

Along with these guidelines, other precepts exist for administration of healthcare systems (Shambaugh, Neuman, & Fawcett, 2002):

- The focus is the client system.
- The purpose is to facilitate the delivery of the primary, secondary, and tertiary prevention interventions directed toward maintaining optimal stability.
- Administrators and healthcare personnel must have knowledge of the content of the Neuman systems model to facilitate its implementation.
- Healthcare services are located in appropriate settings where primary, secondary, and tertiary prevention can be delivered.
- The management strategies focus on achieving optimal client stability.

## Research

The Neuman systems model has been the basis for a wide range of studies, from descriptions of the Neuman phenomena to experiments testing the effects of prevention intervention on multiple system outcomes (Fawcett, 2002). The following guidelines for research, which were based on the Neuman systems model, were extrapolated by Louis, Neuman, and Fawcett (2002) from several studies.

- The purpose of the model is to predict the effects of primary, secondary, and tertiary prevention interventions on retention, attainment, and maintenance of client stability, and to determine the cost–benefit trade-off and utility of prevention interventions.
- The phenomena of interest include physiological, psychological, sociocultural, developmental, and spiritual variables.

- The problems to be studied deal with the impact of stressors on the client's stability.
- The research methods include inductive and deductive research using quantitative and qualitative research.
- Study participants may include clients, families, groups, and communities.
- The model-based research contributes to the understanding of the influence of prevention on the relationship between stressors and client stability.

### Contributions to Nursing

According to Fawcett, the primary contribution of the Neuman systems model has been pragmatic, in that the model can be used as guide for nursing education and practice, it can be translated to other cultures, and it has the potential to facilitate resolution of universal nursing concerns (Fawcett, 2005). The Neuman systems model portrays the interest of the profession in seeing people as a wholistic system; this comprehensive system guides nursing practice, research, education, and administration; it helps nurses to organize their practice within a broad perspective. Neuman places a substantial degree of emphasis on wellness and the central role that clients play in setting goals and identifying prevention interventions. Her model also has the potential to unify other health professions through the clarification of the commonalities that exist in different disciplines.

A nursing process format and an assessment intervention tool are available that were designed to facilitate implementation of the Neuman systems model. The Neuman systems model is a good fit for approaches that emphasize the inter-relationships among the body, mind, and spirit of the client in a constantly changing environment and society.

# Analysis of the Models

In their models, Roy, King, and Neuman depicted nursing logically as a science, yet in their explanation of the connections between mind and intuition, they described nursing as an art. According to Fawcett (2005), these theorists and their models brought to light the diverse factors that constitute professional nursing. Nurses and nursing scholars began to see the profession's complexities that arose from the quick expansion of nursing knowledge development during this time period.

In 1964, King published discussions of nursing as a science rather than an occupation—she initiated the discourse about theory development related to nursing. During the early 1970s, Neuman's systems model was introduced for nursing education and practice; at approximately the same time, Roy developed her adaptation model for nursing education, nursing administration, and nursing research.

Conceptual models (or grand theories), according to Fawcett (2005), provide an overarching model for clinical practice, education, administration, methodology, and discipline inquiry, but they cannot be applied directly to practice.

Instead, middle-range theories must serve as theories for direct practice applicability, and the concepts within the middle-range theories must be consistent with the nurse's (or institution's) adopted conceptual model.

These three theorists—Roy, King, and Neuman—all integrated their systems' concepts with nursing phenomena, thereby clarifying and defining nursing knowledge in relation to the science. Organized in a unique manner, the models focus on a solution for the complex needs of the client. Adopting a conceptual model brings a certain reality and arrangement of the concepts to advanced practice. In this reality, APNs then process, integrate, and synthesize information through the cognitive, psychomotor, and affective domains to shape their clinical practice. Characteristics of the three models are summarized here:

1. The models represent the evolution of nursing as a profession (Silva & Rothbart, 1983), starting from the development of nursing knowledge based on the observation of human experience as it relates to the maintenance of health, to using the nursing process, which remains congruent with social expectations regarding nursing practice. The value of the models is not just that they promote the exploration of the effectiveness of new nursing interventions, theory testing, and development, but that they provoke deeper questions about how nurses can contribute to the well-being of humanity as a whole (Roy, 2009).

2. The models provide structure, process, function, resources, and goals for nursing as a discipline and a profession, leading to creative approaches for human care by defining the person, the environment, and health (Fawcett, 2005). These nursing models provide nurses with a framework for describing human phenomena and the tools needed to predict and control clinical outcomes in order to achieve better health outcomes for clients.

3. The models were derived from research, serve as the basis for researching phenomena that affect client stability, and serve as a basis for the development of new nursing strategies that will influence client recuperation and well-being (Fawcett, 2005).

4. These models provide a certain reality or conceptual arrangement to the phenomena of interest and the concepts involved. As APNs begin to understand and explain concepts and potential relationships within their chosen conceptual model, they can create and refine nursing interventions designed to diminish stress and enhance life patterns.

## Summary

This chapter was a review of three conceptual models and one middle-range theory based on a systems approach—the Roy adaptation model, King's conceptual system, King's theory of goal attainment, and the Neuman systems model. The models are useful for viewing nursing from different perspectives, such as health promotion, primary prevention, secondary prevention, and tertiary prevention. Roy's model is focused on adaptation and coping. King provided a conceptual system of interactions and transactions between nurses and clients within three systems—personal, interpersonal, and group. King's theory of goal attainment—namely an emphasis on mutual goal setting between the nurse and the client—was derived from her conceptual system. Neuman's model is focused on the wellness of the client in terms of environmental stressors and the client's reactions to those stressors. The three models are conceptual models, as defined by Fawcett (2005), and they provide nurses with a purposive reality and conceptual arrangement for nursing.

## Discussion Questions

1. Explore one research instrument or questionnaire that you could use to measure King's concept of goal setting from her theory of goal attainment.

2. What are the common propositions of each of the three conceptual models? How do they differ from one another?

3. Choose one of the three conceptual models described in this chapter. Search the databases to find at least one middle-range theory (except King's theory of goal attainment) that was derived from the chosen model. Explain how the concepts of the conceptual model and the middle-range theory are consistent and are linked.

## References

Alligood, M. (2002). Practice made perfect: Higher level aspirations for practice nurses. *Journal of Advanced Nursing, 40*(1), 122.

Boulding, K. E. (1956). General systems theory: The skeleton of science. *Management Science, 2*(3), 197–208.

Caplan, G. (1964). *Principles of prevention psychiatry.* Oxford, England: Basic Books.

de Chardin, P. T. (1955). *The phenomenon of man.* London, UK: Collins.

Edelson, M. (1970). *Sociotherapy and psychotherapy.* Chicago, IL: University of Chicago Press.

Engberg, I. B. (1995). Brief abstracts: Use of the Neuman systems model in Sweden. In B. Neuman (Ed.), *The Neuman systems model* (3rd ed., pp. 653–656). Norwalk, CT: Appleton & Lange.

Fawcett, J. (2002). *Analysis and evaluation of contemporary nursing knowledge, nursing models and theories.* Philadelphia, PA: F. A. Davis.

Fawcett, J. (2005). *Contemporary nursing knowledge: Analysis and evaluation of nursing models and theories* (2nd ed.). Philadelphia, PA: F. A. Davis.

Fawcett, J. (2009). *Analysis and evaluation of conceptual models of nursing.* Philadelphia, PA: F. A. Davis.

Freese, B. T., Neuman, B., & Fawcett, J. (2002). Guidelines for Neuman systems model-based clinical practice. In B. Neuman & J. Fawcett (Eds.), *The Neuman systems model* (4th ed., pp. 37–42). Upper Saddle River, NJ: Prentice Hall.

George, G. B. (1996). Betty Neuman. In J. B. George (Ed.), *Nursing theories: The base for professional nursing practice* (4th ed., pp. 252–279). Norwalk, CT: Appleton & Lange.

Harris, S. M., Hermiz, M. E., Meininger, M., & Steinkeler, S. E. (1994). Betty Neuman: Systems model. In A. Marriner-Tomey (Ed.). *Nursing theorists and their work* (3rd ed.). St. Louis, MO: Mosby.

Helson, H. (1964). *Adaptation level theory.* New York, NY: Harper & Row.

Kendall-Tackett, K. (1993). *Post-partum depression: A comprehensive approach for nurses.* Newbury Park, CA: Sage.

King, I. M. (1964). Nursing theory: Problems and prospect. *Nursing Science, 2,* 394–403.

King, I. M. (1968). A conceptual frame of reference for nursing. *Nursing Research, 17,* 27–31.

King, I. M. (1971). *Toward a theory for nursing: General concepts of human behavior.* New York, NY: Wiley.

King, I. M. (1975). A conceptual frame of reference for nursing. *Nursing Research, 17,* 27–31.

King, I. M. (1981a). *A theory for nursing: Systems, concepts, process.* New York, NY: Wiley.

King, I. M. (1981b). *A theory of goal attainment: General concepts of human behavior.* New York, NY: Wiley.

King, I. M. (1989). King's general systems framework and theory. In J. P. Riehl-Sisca (Ed.), *Conceptual models for nursing practice* (3rd ed., pp. 149–158). Norwalk, CT: Appleton & Lange.

King, I. M. (1990). Health as the goal for nursing. *Nursing Science Quarterly, 3,* 123–128.

King, I. M. (1991). Nursing theory 25 years later. *Nursing Science Quarterly, 4,* 94–95.

King, I. M. (1992). King's theory of goal attainment. *Nursing Science Quarterly, 5,* 19–26.

King, I. M. (1995). A systems framework for nursing. In M. A. Frey & C. L. Sieloff (Eds.), *Advancing King's systems framework and theory of nursing* (pp. 14–22). Thousand Oaks, CA: Sage.

King, I. M. (1997). King's theory of goal attainment. *Nursing Science Quarterly, 10,* 180–185.

King, I. M. (2001). Theory of goal attainment. In M. Parker (Ed.), *Nursing theories and nursing practice* (pp. 275–286). Philadelphia, PA: F. A. Davis.

Lazarus, R. (1999*). Stress and emotion: A new synthesis.* New York, NY: Springer.

Louis, M., Neuman, B., & Fawcett, J. (2002). Guidelines for Neuman systems model-based nursing research. In B. Neuman and J. Fawcett (Eds.), *The Neuman systems model* (4th ed., pp. 113–149). Upper Saddle River, NJ: Prentice Hall.

Maritain, J. (1966). *The person and the common good* (J. J. Fitzgerald, Trans.). Notre Dame, IN: University of Notre Dame Press.

McNeill, D., & Freiberger, P. (1994). *Fuzzy logic: The revolutionary computer technology that is changing our world.* New York, NY: Simon & Schuster.

Moreno, M. E., & Alvarado, A. (2009). Aplicación del modelo de adaptación de Callista Roy en Latinoamérica. *Aquichan, 9,* 62–72.

Neuman, B. (1982). *The Neuman systems model: Application to nursing education and practice.* Norwalk, CT: Appleton-Century-Crofts.

Neuman, B. (1995). *The Neuman systems model* (3rd ed.). Norwalk, CT: Appleton & Lange.

Neuman, B. (1996). The Neuman systems model in research and practice. *Nursing Science Quarterly, 9,* 67–70.

Neuman, B. (2002a). The Neuman systems model. In B. Neuman & J. Fawcett (Eds.), *The Neuman systems model* (4th ed., pp. 3–33). Upper Saddle River, NJ: Prentice Hall.

Neuman, B. (2002b). The future and the Neuman systems model. In B. Neuman & J. Fawcett (Eds.), *The Neuman systems model* (4th ed., pp. 319–321). Upper Saddle River, NJ: Prentice Hall.

Neuman, B. (2002c). Assessment and intervention based on the Neuman systems model. In B. Neuman & J. Fawcett (Eds.), *The Neuman systems model* (4th ed., pp. 347–359). Upper Saddle River, NJ: Prentice Hall.

Newman, M., Neuman, B., & Fawcett, J. (2002). Guidelines for Neuman systems model-based education for the health professions. In *The Neuman systems model* (4th ed., pp. 191–215). Upper Saddle River, NJ: Prentice Hall.

Riehl, J. P., & Roy, C. (1974). *Conceptual models for nursing practice*, New York, NY: Appleton-Century-Crofts.

Roy, C. (1970). Adaptation: A conceptual framework for nursing. *Nursing Outlook, 18*(3), 18–23.

Roy, C. (1976). *Introduction to nursing: An adaptation model.* Englewood Cliffs, NJ: Prentice Hall.

Roy, C. (1984). *Introduction to nursing: An introduction model* (2nd ed.). Englewood Cliffs, NJ: Prentice Hall.

Roy, C. (1988). An explication of the philosophical assumptions of the adaptation model. *Nursing Science Quarterly, 1*(1), 26–34.

Roy, C. (1991). *An adaptation model.* Thousand Oaks, CA: Sage.

Roy, C. (1996). Domain primacy: Use of a theoretical framework to guide the selection of subject matter for theory development and methods of inquiry. In the University of Rhode Island College of Nursing Conference Proceedings, *Building a cumulative knowledge base from fragmentation to congruence of philosophy, theory, method of inquiry and practice* (pp. 69–75). Proceedings of the 4th and 5th Symposia of the Knowledge Development Series. Kingston, RI: University of Rhode Island College of Nursing.

Roy, C. (2006). *The Roy adaptation model: Relevance to theory-based education, practice, and research.* Conference presentation. Roy Adaptation Association. Los Angeles, CA.

Roy, C. (2009). *The Roy adaptation model* (3rd ed., pp. 2–54). Upper Saddle River, NJ: Pearson Education.

Roy, C., & Andrews, H. A. (1999). *The adaptation model* (2nd ed.). Norwalk, CT: Appleton & Lange.

Selye, H. (1946). The general adaptation syndrome. *Journal of Clinical Endocrinology, 6*(2), 117–230.

Shambaugh, B. F., Neuman, B., & Fawcett, J. (2002). Guidelines for Neuman systems model-based administration of health care services. In *The Neuman systems model* (4th ed., pp. 265–270). Upper Saddle River, NJ: Prentice Hall.

Sieloff, C., & Frey, M. A. (2007). *King's structure, process, and outcome in the twenty-first century.* New York, NY: Springer.

Sieloff Evans, C. (1991). *Imogene King: A conceptual framework for nursing.* Newbury Park, CA: Sage.

Silva, M., & Rothbart, D. (1983). *An analysis of changing trends in philosophies of science.* New York, NY: Wiley.

Vaughan, B., & Gough, P. (1995). Use of the Neuman systems model in England: Abstracts. In B. Neuman, *The Neuman systems model* (3rd ed., pp. 599–605). Norwalk, CT: Appleton & Lange.

von Bertalanffy, L. (1968). *General system theory.* New York, NY: George Braziller.

# Models and Theories Focused on Human Existence and Universal Energy

*Violet M. Malinski*

---

## Introduction

---

Undoubtedly the nursing figure most associated with the focus on energy in nursing is Martha E. Rogers (1914–1994), who posited a radically different view of both the human being and the environment. Rogers is best remembered for having introduced a new world view in nursing with her revolutionary, future-oriented, basic nursing science, known as the science of unitary human beings. Although Rogers made descriptions of this worldview available throughout the 1970s on class handouts, the first formal publications of this perspective did not appear until 1986 (Madrid & Winstead-Fry, 1986; Malinski, 1986). Rogers (1992) included the final version in her seminal article in *Nursing Science Quarterly*. Briefly, she described shifts from an older to a newer worldview in a variety of areas—for example, from cell theory to field theory, from homeostasis to homeodynamics, from three-dimensionality to pandimensionality, from an entropic to a negentropic universe, from causation and adaptation to mutual process, and from person and environment as separate to unitary.

Initially, Rogers was the only theorist whose work fit this new worldview in nursing, but she was soon joined by Margaret Newman, with her theory of health as expanding consciousness (HEC), and by Rosemarie Rizzo Parse, with her theory of humanbecoming. Both of the later theorists offer a view of human transformation and emphasize the centrality of the nurse–person relationship via true presence (for Parse) and transforming presence (for Newman). Elizabeth Barrett, following the Rogerian assumption that change is ongoing, diverse, creative, and unpredictable, derived her theory of power as knowing participation in change from Rogerian nursing science. All of these perspectives describe nursing as having roots outside of the biomedical model, offering an alternative vision of nursing knowledge, practice, and research.

## Rogers' Science of Unitary Human Beings

Rogers (1970, 1990, 1992) was an early advocate for nursing as both science and art, as well as a learned profession in need of an organized body of nursing-specific knowledge. Her view of humans as irreducible wholes integrated with their environments in "a pandimensional universe of open systems, points to a new paradigm, and initiates the identity of nursing as a science. The purpose of nurses is to promote health and well-being for all persons wherever they are. The art of nursing, then, is the creative use of the science of nursing for human betterment" (Rogers, 1992, p. 28). Rogers' science of unitary human beings encompasses four postulates, three principles, and a range of theories derived initially by Rogers herself and later by other Rogerian theorists.

The four postulates—energy fields, openness, pattern, and pandimensionality—together express reality as described in this nursing science. Change that is predictable, resulting from a cause–effect sequence, yields to change that is unpredictable, diverse, and innovative. Starting with the idea that the infinite, continuously flowing energy field is fundamental to all life means that humans and environments are irreducible, pandimensional energy fields, distinct but not separate, engaging in a continuous mutual process where change occurs simultaneously for both. In an open universe of energy fields, there are no divisions or boundaries; thus, energy flows continuously through human and environmental fields in an unbroken wave, characterized by patterning.

Todaro-Franceschi's (1999) philosophical study of energy from multiple perspectives, including Rogerian nursing science, highlighted the communal, transformative nature of energy, an ongoing process of becoming that is, by nature, unpredictable. We cannot bring about change; "We can only participate in the inherent, communal process of energy transformation. . . ." (p. 111).

*Pattern* refers to the ever flowing motion of the energy field; it is described by Rogers (1992) as continuously changing while revealing itself through manifestations of the unitary human–environmental field mutual process. Pattern manifestations reveal increasing diversity of field patterning in characteristics such as lesser and greater diversity; longer, shorter, and seemingly continuous rhythms; slower, faster, and seemingly continuous motion; time experienced as slower, faster, and timelessness; pragmatic, imaginative, and visionary awareness; and longer sleeping, longer waking, and beyond waking experiences (Rogers, 1992).

*Pandimensionality* refers to "a nonlinear domain without spatial or temporal attributes" (Rogers, 1992, p. 29), thus transcending traditional ideas about space and time, with perceived boundaries not necessarily matching tangible ones. Pandimensional awareness, for example, encompasses phenomena commonly labeled paranormal, which in Rogerian nursing science are manifestations of a changing diversity of field patterning.

As part of her new worldview shift away from older ideas such as homeostasis, equilibrium, and adaptation, Rogers chose *homeodynamics* as the concept that her principles exemplified, in acknowledgment of the ever-changing nature of life and the world. The principles underlying homeodynamics are resonancy, helicy, and integrality (Rogers, 1992). Together they describe the nature and process of continuous change within the human–environmental field.

*Resonancy* is the "continuous change from lower to higher frequency wave patterns in human and environmental fields" (Rogers, 1992, p. 31). The principle of resonancy describes the way change occurs, fluctuating throughout lower- and higher-frequency wave patterns—sometimes one, sometimes the other. Rogers (1990) clarified that persons can "experience lesser diversity and greater diversity . . . time as slower, faster, or unmoving. Individuals are sometimes pragmatic, sometimes imaginative, and sometimes visionary" (p. 10). One manifestation is not valued more highly than the other; rather, both lower- and higher-frequency awareness are integral to the wholeness of the rhythmical pattern. As Phillips (1994, p. 15) noted, "When the rhythmicities of lower–higher frequencies work together, they yield innovative diverse patterns."

*Helicy* is the "continuous, innovative, unpredictable, increasing diversity of human and environmental field patterns" (Rogers, 1992, p. 31). The principle of helicy describes the nature of change in field patterning as ongoing, creative, and diverse. According to Phillips (2010a), this is a "becoming diversity of pattern that is innovative, creative, and unpredictable" (p. 57). *Integrality* is the "continuous mutual human and environmental field process" (Rogers, 1992, p. 31). It specifies that change occurs simultaneously for human and environment, because they constitute a unitary whole that cannot be divided into two separate fields.

Taken together, the three principles of homeodynamics describe the mutual patterning process of human and environmental fields as one that changes continuously, innovatively, and unpredictably, fluctuating throughout lower and higher frequencies. Rogers (1990) believed these principles would serve as a guide for practice and research flowing from her nursing science.

Rogers identified three theories, but she encouraged others to identify additional theories in the belief that multiple theories could be derived from her nursing science. First, the theory of accelerating change (originally accelerating evolution) suggests that change is accelerating in human–environment field patterning, offering the possibility of "new norms with a wider range of distribution of differences among individuals" (Rogers, 1992, p. 32). Indeed, perhaps the only norm is accelerating change. Aging provides an example, with Rogers suggesting that rather than a process of inevitable decline, aging of the human field is a creative process with increasing diversity in field manifestations such as sleeping, waking, dreaming, and perception of time passing.

Second, the theory of the emergence of paranormal phenomena suggests that experiences commonly labeled paranormal are actually manifestations of innovative field patterning and pandimensional awareness. For example, health patterning modalities such as imagery, meditation, and Therapeutic Touch transcend traditionally perceived limitations of time, space, and physical boundaries, opening the door to new, creative opportunities for healing and well-being.

There is an expanding view of living and dying. McEvoy (1990) hypothesized that the process of dying is one of expanding awareness encompassing so-called paranormal events such as out-of-body and apparitional experiences. Todaro-Franceschi (2006) identified the occurrence of synchronicities in the experiences of bereaved persons grieving the loss of a spouse, finding that such experiences helped them relate to their deceased loved ones in new, meaningful ways and showing that dying is a transition rather than an end. Malinski (2012) synthesized the unitary rhythm of dying–grieving, also illustrative of Rogers' (1970) belief that dying is a process at once creative and transforming, with no real beginning or ending.

Rogers' third theory, manifestations of field patterning in unitary human beings (formerly the correlates of pattern), was discussed earlier as the nonlinear, creative, unpredictable process of change in human–environmental field patterning. Rogers offered some manifestations of this relative diversity as examples, including rhythmical fluctuations of motion, time experience, and sleeping–waking, but she encouraged others to identify additional ones.

Rogers (1992) believed that her science "identifies nursing's uniqueness and signifies the potential of nurses to fulfill their social responsibility in human service" (p. 33). She adamantly maintained that "autonomous nursing practice directed by nurses holding valid baccalaureate and higher degrees with an upper division major in nursing science is central to the future" (p. 33). Her vision encompassed individualized, community-based services, including development of nursing centers and practice incorporating noninvasive therapeutic modalities such as Therapeutic Touch, imagery, meditation, humor, laughter, music, and movement. Although she believed that unconditional love and hope can facilitate healing and well-being, Rogers did not view caring as unique to nursing. Rather, she saw caring as a way of using knowledge—specifically, in terms of how nurses might use Rogerian nursing science for the betterment of humankind (Rogers, 1992).

Rogers called for an emphasis on human rights, client decision making, and noncompliance in the belief that clients know themselves best and have the right to make informed choices about health care. This belief, joined with her great sense of humor, was in evidence some years ago when Rogers had pencils printed up with the statement, "Be noncompliant, you'll live longer." She noted that her basic assumption of increasing diversity calls for the provision of healthcare services that are individualized to a greater degree than ever before—a feat that cannot be achieved with standardized tools or a normative approach to patient care.

Theory derivation from the science of unitary human beings continues today. Rogers noted that her science calls for nurses to envision creative new ways to describe and understand unitary phenomena within a pandimensional view of people and their world (Malinski, 2006). Selected examples of this ongoing work include Reed's (1991, 2003) theory of self-transcendence, Hills and Hanchett's (2001) theory of enlightenment, Butcher's (1993) theory of kaleidoscoping in life's turbulence, Bultemeier's (1997) theory of perceived dissonance, Alligood and McGuire's (2000) theory of aging, and Butcher's (2003) theory of aging as emerging brilliance, among others.

Although Rogers died in 1994, the science of unitary human beings lives on in the community of Rogerians who continue to use and refine it in their own conceptualizations, practice, and research. For example, Phillips (2010b) recently proposed and elaborated on the ideas of "energyspirit" and "Homo pandimensionalis" in an exploration of expanding "pandimensional relative present awareness" (p. 8). *Energyspirit* is the key to all life, all that is, and *Homo pandimensionalis* represents the unanticipated, creative, transformational changes taking place in the human–environment mutual process, in keeping with the basic ideas of Rogerian nursing science.

For a fuller explication of the historical evolution of this science, readers are referred to *Martha E. Rogers: Her Life and Her Work* (Malinski & Barrett, 1994).

## Barrett's Power as Knowing Participation in Change

A prime example of early and continuing theory development is Barrett's (1986, 1990, 1998, 2010) theory of power as knowing participation in change, which she first described in her 1983 dissertation, the culmination of her study with Rogers at New York University. Picking up on Rogers' (1970) assumption that change is continuous and humans can participate knowingly in change, Barrett identified this knowing participation in change as power. She developed a theory, power tool, and practice method, which Rogerians have been using for more than 25 years. In fact, in June 2008, a conference titled "A Celebration of Barrett's Theory of Power" was held in New York City to honor her work. Papers presented at this conference were included in the January 2010 issue of *Nursing Science Quarterly*.

The discussion in this section is based on the content of Barrett's interactive website, www.drelizabethbarrett.com (redesigned in late 2009), which carries the latest explication of her work. Barrett now differentiates between *power-as-freedom*, represented by her theory, and the traditional view of *power-as-control*, both of which manifest in the world in multiple forms. Power-as-freedom represents a spiritual worldview, whereas power-as-control represents a material worldview. Four inseparable dimensions characterize power, encapsulated in the following statement: "Power is being **aware** of what one is **choosing** to do, **feeling free** to do it and **doing it intentionally**" (emphasis in the original) (Barrett, 2009a). Power enhancement is represented by the acronym POWER, where P = possibilities, O = openness, W = will, E = energy, and R = reversing. "Power is openness to possibilities using the energy of the will to change through the principle of reversing" (Barrett, 2009b).

Barrett described the four observable dimensions of power as inseparable and continuously fluctuating. They are measured with the Power as Knowing Participation in Change Tool (PKPCT), also known as the Power Meter. This instrument consists of 52 items in a semantic differential format that assess the four dimensions of power. Taken together, they yield a person's or group's power profile, which identifies areas of greater and lesser power. Because change is a given in Rogerian science, this profile changes as the human–environmental mutual process changes, whether with individuals, families, or groups. The PKPCT is widely used in both research and practice.

Numerous studies have been conducted in several countries using the PKPCT. This tool has been translated into Finnish, Swedish, Japanese, Korean, and Portuguese. Caroselli and Barrett (1998) published a review of 39 studies conducted as of 1993. Kim (2009) conducted a review of 46 studies carried out since 1983, including 27 studies reviewed by Caroselli and Barrett and another 18 completed since their 1998 publication. Significant positive correlations have been noted between power or a power subscale and such variables as human field motion, life satisfaction, feminism, well-being, purpose, transformational leadership style, imagination, empathy, hope, spirituality, and perceived health. Significant negative correlations have been noted with such variables as chronic pain, distress, anxiety, hopelessness, alcohol dependence, and transactional leadership style.

Practice is conducted via Barrett's health patterning methodology, which takes into account both pattern manifestation knowing and voluntary mutual patterning. The first process consists of discovering what is going on and what the person wants. In the second process, the nurse assists the person to "freely choose with awareness ways to participate to make happen the changes they want to happen and to enhance their well-being by focusing on intention, aim, and direction with no attachment to outcome" (Barrett, 2009c). The two processes go on simultaneously, and both nurse and client jointly participate in them. Health patterning modalities, such as Therapeutic Touch, imagery, music, and movement, provide ways to facilitate a client's knowing participation in creating change and can serve as a framework for individualized power prescriptions.

The power profile, which identifies areas of greater and lesser power, assists the nurse in designing the power prescription—that is, the plan the client can follow to enhance awareness, choices, freedom, and involvement. The power profile varies as human–environmental field patterning changes. The changes tell us something about the nature of awareness, the type of choice being made, the degree to which a person feels free to act intentionally, and the manner in which a person is involved in creating change (Barrett, 1986, 2010). In living power-as-freedom, Barrett (2010) notes that people make and act on choices that promote health, consistent with what health means to them. We "can participate knowingly in changing any situation in our lives" (2010, p. 52). Barrett suggests that people ask themselves questions such as, "What am I aware of?" and "What choices am I making" followed by questions such as, "Do the changes I intend to create interfere with anyone else's freedom?" and "Do the changes I intend to create attempt to control, dominate, manipulate or bring harm to anyone?" (p. 52). Readers are referred to the website for an example of health patterning therapy.

## Other Rogerian-Based Practice Examples

Other Rogerians have met Rogers' challenge to develop innovative practice methods consistent with Rogerian nursing science. Cowling (1993, 1997), for example, offered a pattern appreciation method, consistent with Barrett's health patterning therapy, suggesting 10 constituents characteristic of Rogerian practice:

1. Field pattern manifestations are the focus.
2. The client's experiences, perceptions, and expressions are taken as manifestations of pattern and a focus for pattern appreciation.
3. Information about pattern in all forms, from sensory to lab data to feelings, is sought.
4. The nurse uses all forms of awareness—from sensory to intuition to tacit knowing—to cultivate pandimensional awareness in appreciating pattern information.
5. The nurse then engages in both synthesis and synopsis to view the information as manifestations of a unitary whole interpreted within a unitary perspective.
6. The nurse constructs a pattern profile that unites the client's experiences, perceptions, and expressions in a meaningful narrative or art form such as a picture, metaphor, or photograph.
7. This pattern profile is shared with and verified by the client, and the nurse and the client engage in mutual discussion of options, goals, and patterning strategies.
8. Health patterning is based on knowing participation in change.
9. The health patterning approaches are determined by the client.
10. Knowledge derived from pattern appreciation reflects the unique human–environmental field pattern of the client.

Butcher (Butcher, 2006; Butcher & Malinski, 2010; Butcher & Malinski, in press) synthesized the work of Barrett and Cowling in a comprehensive practice model, the unitary pattern-based practice (praxis) method. He identified the focus of nursing care as "recognizing manifestations of patterning through pattern manifestation knowing and appreciation and by facilitating the client's ability to participate knowingly in change, harmonizing person/environmental integrality, and promoting healing potentialities and well-being through voluntary mutual patterning" (Butcher, 2006, p. 170).

## Rogerian Research

Research in the science of unitary human beings "enables one to understand better the nature of human evolution and its multiple, unpredictable potentialities. Description, explanation, and vision strengthen a nurse's ability to practice according to the level and scope of preparation and knowledge in the science of nursing" (Rogers, 1992, p. 33). Vision replaces prediction given the focus on diverse, unpredictable potentialities in this nursing science. Rogers maintained that quantitative and qualitative methodologies might potentially be appropriate for conducting such research, depending on the nature of the research question, but she also called for the development of new methods and tools (Malinski, 2008).

Not surprisingly, early research in Rogerian nursing science focused on tool development, primarily tied to the proposed manifestations of change. Ference (1986) explored motion (slower/faster/seems continuous) as the focus for her Human Field Motion Test, in which the concepts "my motor is running" and "my field expansion" are rated using a semantic differential format. Time (slower/faster/timelessness) provided the focus for Paletta's (1990) Temporal Experience Scale, which consists of three subscales rating the three experiences of time passing using metaphors. Hastings-Tolsma (Watson, Barrett, Hastings-Tolsma, Johnston, & Gueldner, 1997) explored lesser diversity/ greater diversity in creating the Diversity of Human Field Pattern Scale, which assesses change occurring in the human–environmental field process using a 16-item Likert scale. Watson (Watson et al., 1997) identified dreaming as a beyond-waking manifestation in the manifestation of longer sleeping/longer waking/beyond waking, creating a 20-item Likert scale to assess diversity of dream experience. Gueldner (Gueldner, 1996; Watson et al., 1997) developed a picture tool composed of 18 pairs of black and white drawings designed to represent low- and high-frequency descriptors of concepts in her Index of Human Field Energy. This tool was later modified to become the Well-Being Picture Scale (Gueldner et al., 2005). Applications of this tool include validating it as a measure of mood (Johnston, Guadron, Verchot, & Gueldner, 2011) and to appraise well-being in pregnancy (Reis & Alligood, 2008). Anderson and Ashman (2011) found that the tool correlated with presenting symptom distress, as measured by the Brief Symptom Inventory-18 (BSI-18), in a group of patients with cancer undergoing radiation therapy. The Well-Being Picture Scale was also easier for nurses and patients to use than the BSI-18. Terwillinger, Gueldner, and Bronstein (2012) are evaluating a children's version of the Well-Being Scale.

Recognizing that concepts such as self-esteem and body image are not appropriate in Rogerian nursing science, Johnston (Johnston, 1994; Watson et al., 1997) used Phillips' (1990) idea of human field image and designed the Human Field Image Metaphor Test. Composed of 25 metaphors, this Likert-type tool is designed to measure the two domains of human field image, perceived potential and integrality, with human field image defined as "individual awareness of the infinite wholeness of the human field" (Watson et al., 1997, p. 94).

Carboni (Barrett, Cowling, Carboni, & Butcher, 1997; Carboni, 1992) argued that in the unitary view nurses could not intervene and, therefore, could not conduct research designed to quantitatively test hypotheses without violating basic assumptions of Rogerian nursing science. She developed a qualitative measure, the Mutual Exploration of the Healing Human Field–Environmental Field Relationship, "designed to capture changing configurations of energy field patterns" (Carboni, 1992, p. 137). Nurse and client complete this instrument together to understand their mutual healing process. Carboni's tool taps into descriptions of experiences and expressions of those experiences—for example, via metaphor and picture.

As indicated earlier, Rogers identified the need for new research methods as key to conducting research related to her proposed worldview. It is interesting to note that the three developed to date—the Rogerian process of inquiry, the unitary field pattern portrait research method, and unitary case inquiry—employ qualitative rather than quantitative methods, reflecting the debate in Rogerian circles over the appropriate methodology for research in Rogerian nursing science (Barrett et al., 1997).

Carboni (1995) developed a Rogerian process of inquiry designed "to investigate the enfolding–unfolding change of human field–environmental field energy field patterns in order to understand the nature of human evolution and its multiple, unpredictable potentialities" (p. 36). She identified 16 characteristics of this process of inquiry, starting with *a priori* nursing theory, grounded in the science of unitary human beings and theories derived from it, that guide the flow of Rogerian inquiry, which proceeds in the following way. First, the Rogerian researcher envisions multiple potentialities for change as field patterning flows in lower- or higher-frequency wave patterns, revealing configurations of lesser or greater diversity. This, in turn, yields visionary insights into such potentialities. Next, the Rogerian researcher maintains an explicit focus on energy fields, because field patterns reflect the whole, which "is the only valid concern of Rogerian research" (p. 25), and the only source of unitary meaning. Manifestations of field patterning are identified and explored, even as the researcher remains open to the possibility that new manifestations might emerge and be identified.

The Rogerian researcher conducts the process of inquiry in the pandimensional field enfolding researcher, participants, and the natural setting; observer and observed are integral to this investigation. Observations and shared descriptions are processed by the researcher and participants through mutual exploration and discovery, and the researcher uses unitary instruments such as the healing human field–environmental field relationship qualitative measure to generate shared descriptions of field patterns. All data are synthesized inductively and deductively to identify unitary constructs, which are then interpreted within Rogerian nursing science and explored for their potential to generate new insights and perhaps the synthesis of new theories. Carboni also developed a pandimensional unitary process report to present the study, its processes, and conclusions, along with special criteria for trustworthiness of the research in the form of credibility, unitary integrity, and auditability.

Butcher (1994, 1998, 2005) developed the unitary field pattern portrait method to create a unitary understanding of pattern manifestations with a focus on well-being and human betterment. Butcher identified eight aspects to be addressed:

1. Initial engagement
2. *A priori* nursing science
3. Immersion
4. Manifestation of knowing and appreciation
5. The unitary field pattern profile
6. The mutually constructed unitary field pattern profile
7. The unitary field pattern portrait
8. Theoretical unitary field pattern portrait

In addition, Butcher identified three processes: (1) creative pattern synthesis, (2) immersion and crystallization, and (3) evolutionary interpretation (Butcher & Malinski, 2010; Butcher & Malinski, in press). The criteria of trustworthiness and authenticity are used to ensure rigor (Butcher, 1998, 2005). Butcher (2006) used his method to study dispiritedness in later life, synthesizing a description of the experiences, perceptions, and expressions of dispiritedness that can be used to enhance nurses' understanding and appreciation of this phenomenon. He noted that sharing the pattern profile with clients can potentially enhance their knowing participation in change, perhaps inspiring clients as they work with nurses to enhance active involvement, intensify connectedness with persons and nature, and facilitate hope.

Cowling (1998) developed unitary case inquiry and identified unitary appreciative inquiry for use with individuals, groups, or communities to explore a phenomenon, concern, or situation from a unitary perspective (Cowling, 2001). With this approach, researcher and participants engage in a shared, mutual process where all experiences, perceptions, and expressions are viewed together as reflections of wholeness and field pattern and used to construct a pattern profile. This profile can be constructed jointly or by either researcher or participant. It may then be shared in the form of story, poetry, or art—whatever is most meaningful for the persons involved. Cowling's major focus in research and practice has been the experience of despair.

## Applications in Advanced Practice Nursing: Science of Unitary Human Beings

Healthcare consumer Mandl (1997) issued a plea to educate the public about Rogerian nursing science following her experience with Rogerian nursing at a major medical center. Unexpectedly hospitalized following a pancreatitis attack, she found herself no longer in the role of a competent businessperson, but rather she became a patient who was frightened and confused, emotionally distraught, and feeling like a victim. Healthcare providers came and went, all talking to one another but rarely to her. At 11:00 P.M., a nurse practitioner entered her room and sat with her. They talked and shared stories of their experiences:

> I didn't realize just how angry and scared I was until we started talking. She massaged my body, held my hand, stroked my head, adjusted the

pillows and the tubes, all the while soothing me with words and touch
. . . I felt calmed, I felt understood, I received compassion and healing.
(p. 237)

Once discharged, Mandl began reading Rogers' work and sought out health patterning with Barrett. She offered ways to bring Rogers into the mainstream, noting that people could find different ways to approach health issues once they
discover their power to change their expectations.

Madrid (1990), the advanced practice nurse mentioned in Mandl's vignette, described her Rogerian practice with Roger, a patient who was hospitalized with AIDS
and a gastrointestinal bleed. When he told her that nothing seemed to help him, including his medications, and that his skin felt on fire, Madrid began Therapeutic
Touch, which she continued for 30 minutes. Roger relaxed and told her he felt great.
She then taught him relaxation techniques and helped him focus on relaxing his muscles, after which he was able to sleep. When he awoke, he shared the story of his life.

When his body next contracted in pain, Madrid learned that the only way
Roger could urinate was to strain and force out short bursts of urine, an extremely painful process for him in which all his muscles contracted, increasing
his pain. She led him through deep breathing and relaxation by first having him
synchronize his breathing with hers, after which he was able gently to release a
stream of urine. After she washed his hair, Roger took interest in his appearance
and had the energy to shave and trim his mustache.

Next, Madrid enlisted Roger's participation in a more aesthetic arrangement
of the flowers in his room. He listened to music, noticing that it was like he was
hearing favorite pieces for the first time, feeling "boundless in nature . . . as if he
had lost all physical, spatial attributes and was infinite with the universe" (p. 98).
When he mentioned sadly that he would probably never have the chance to spend
another evening on the beach, Madrid led Roger through an imagery exercise so
that, once again, he could sit on the beach and enjoy the sunset, which moved
him deeply. He died the next day.

> It was not sophisticated technology that made such a difference that
> evening. It was the art of nursing . . . the caring and application of
> knowledge to human betterment . . . generated from the principles of
> resonancy, helicy, and integrality. (p. 99)

Several years after this experience, Madrid (1994) described her use of Barrett's
health patterning methodology with another hospitalized dying patient. She noted
the need for continuing pattern appraisal to guide practice strategies, because pattern manifestations were continuously changing. Storytelling, massage, Therapeutic Touch, and affirmations were among the uniquely nursing practices that
Madrid brought to her patient's care, along with the standard care provided to a
person with leukemia experiencing a blast crisis.

Gold (1997), an advanced practice certified holistic nurse, called for nurses to
understand and identify what is unique to nursing; this knowledge, she suggested,

should guide their vision in the practice of nursing and support nurses in finding meaning, value, and satisfaction in their practice. She provided examples of her work with patients, including her experiences with an 82-year-old man hospitalized with sepsis, atrial fibrillation, and pemphigus who spoke no English. Rather than concentrating on his medical diagnoses, she focused on behavioral manifestations of his energy field, which she described as a pattern of independence and passion. Using silence, active listening, caring facial expressions, and Therapeutic Touch, Gold and her patient accessed a place beyond words where each touched the other's heart: ". . . I continue to feel his pandimensional presence in my life" (p. 253).

## Newman's Theory of Health as Expanding Consciousness

Two pivotal experiences in the development of Newman's theory were her experiences as primary caregiver for her mother, who had amyotrophic lateral sclerosis (Lou Gehrig's disease), and her doctoral work at New York University with Martha Rogers (Newman, 2008). Through her interactions with her mother, Newman came to know her mother as a whole person, rather than as a patient defined by her disease, and she recognized how the restrictions her mother experienced in time, space, and movement became her restrictions as well. Movement, time, and space remained foundational concepts for Newman as she studied rehabilitation nursing and embarked on her doctoral dissertation exploring the relationship between time and movement. *Consciousness* emerged as another important concept once she realized how study subjects were compensating for imposed alterations of natural movement.

Newman was challenged to come up with her own view of health by Rogers' view of health and illness as aspects of the life process, rather than as a unique focus for nursing. In 1978, she began to develop this perspective in earnest when she was asked to make a presentation on her theory of health at the Nurse Educator Conference in New York City. Although she had presented her ideas in earlier publications, Newman's book, *Health as Expanding Consciousness*, did not appear until 1986; the second edition was published in 1994. As its title suggests, her major premise is that health is expanding consciousness: "Health encompasses disease and non-disease and is a manifestation of the underlying pattern of person–environment" (Newman, 1994, p. 11).

Newman (2008) credits Rogers' (1970) emphasis on mutual process as introducing a new focus—albeit one not immediately recognized or appreciated—on relational process, or the mutuality of the nurse–client relationship in research and practice rather than the traditional observer–observed focus prevalent at the time. As she transitioned from quantitative methods to an appreciation for qualitative methods as more appropriate for use with her theory, Newman realized that research is practice. As a consequence, she suggested that one cannot study a person, family, group, or community. Rather, the Newman nurse engages with the client in a unitary process that simultaneously contains the theory. This praxis is presented as theory–research–practice (Newman, 2008), a unitary whole. Once again, as in the more recently developed Rogerian research methods, the researcher is the instrument of data collection.

Another early influence on Newman was Bentov's (1977) idea that life is a process of expanding consciousness, which he defined as the informational capacity of the system as it interacts with the environment. Newman also found support for her theory in physicist David Bohm's (1980) formulation of the implicate and explicate orders of reality. The *implicate* is the underlying pattern of all that is, unbounded by space and time. In contrast, all that is observed and accepted as "real" serves as *explication* of this unseen reality, unfolding in perceived time and space. All observable manifestations, then, including disease, are manifestations of the underlying pattern of the whole.

Chemist Ilya Prigogine's theory of dissipative structures (Prigogine & Stengers, 1984) pointed to disorder as a path to higher consciousness. When disorder occurs in a previously ordered system, he suggested, the system moves in self-organizing but seemingly random ways toward a higher level of organization. Finally, Arthur Young (1976) described stages in expanding consciousness, using the downward–upward motion of a "V" or rhythmic wave format to indicate the descending and ascending shift from potential to absolute freedom. It is at the downward point that a choice point exists. The old ways are no longer working, there is a loss of freedom, and, for the system to evolve, a shift must occur with a choice that allows increasing freedom and higher consciousness.

For Newman (2008), all this translated into consciousness as the information of the system, a dynamic pattern. She suggested that the appropriate focus for nursing is the person, who serves as the pattern of the evolving whole, continually transforming throughout unpredictable and often seemingly chaotic processes.

Like Rogers, who described the older and newer worldviews in nursing, with the latter laying the groundwork for her nursing science, Newman (2008) recognized that her theoretical ideas, along with those of scientists whose work supported her ideas, necessitated a paradigm shift, one characterized by dynamic order and unity, where "order is revealed in the relationships that emerge" (p. 13). The focus, then, becomes the nurse–client relationship, whether the client is an individual, family, group, or community. This relationship, Newman suggested, must be allowed to unfold naturally.

Earlier, Newman, Sime, and Corcoran-Perry (1991) had described three philosophical perspectives that could help nurses understand differences in research and knowledge development in nursing. The first word in each pair of terms represents how phenomena are viewed, the second the nature of change that occurs (Newman, 2008). In the *particulate–deterministic* view, phenomena are seen as isolated and can be manipulated in experimental designs, with causal inferences being made and tested. In the *interactive–integrative* view, phenomena interact and cannot be isolated; multiple variables need to be considered, and change is probabilistic rather than predictable. In the *unitary–transformative* view, the focus is on the evolving pattern of the whole, and change represents a transformation in this patterning. This last pair describes a participatory view that necessitates a move to what Newman (2008) identified as *compassionate consciousness*, following through on the definition of nursing as caring in the human health experience identified earlier by Newman et al. (1991). Inherent values reflect "wholeness (health), caring, evolving pattern, mutual process, and transformation. The phenomenon of nursing is a dynamic nurse–client relationship viewed within a unitary perspective of health" (Newman, 2008, p. 19). Health is the pattern of the whole and reflects the chaos of transformation, which takes the participant to another phase of becoming and connectedness. "The thing that makes a difference in practice is the caring, creative presence of the nurse in recognizing the pattern of the whole" (Newman, 2005, p. 9).

The paradigm shift initiated by Rogers and continued by Newman (1994, 2008) encompasses a move from treating symptoms to searching for pattern, from viewing pain and disease as negative to seeing them as important sources of pattern information, from disease as entity to disease as process, and from the body as a machine to be repaired to the human as a dynamic energy field continuous with the larger environmental field (see **Box 19–1**).

Newman (2008) synthesized three basic assumptions of her theory of HEC:

1. Health is an evolving *unitary pattern* of the whole, including patterns of disease.
2. Consciousness is the *informational capacity* of the whole and is revealed in the evolving pattern.
3. Pattern identifies the human–environmental process and is characterized by *meaning*. (Emphasis in the original) (p. 6)

The manifestations of expanding consciousness are found in Newman's (1994) concepts of time and timing, integration via movement, expansion of space-time, choice point and beyond, and beyond space-time. Patterning of space, time, and movement is rhythmical and individualized. Preferred patterns of the individual, group, family, or community may be in or out of synchrony with the patterns of other people, healthcare settings, and events occurring around them, with such experiences of disorganization presenting opportunities for growth. In nurse–client relationships, as in all healthcare settings, it is important to sense readiness for connecting and relating so that timing is mutual and comfortable for all participants. In a classic article, Newman, Lamb, and Michaels (1991) highlighted the value of nurses being free to connect with clients in the community when the latter were ready, rather than by setting arbitrary appointments. Describing the practice at Carondelet St. Mary's Hospital and Health Center

## Box 19–1  Pattern Formation: Human as Dynamic Energy Field

Newman (2008) cites the example of a friend with medically uncontrolled hyperthyroidism treated by Dora Kunz, who, along with Dolores Krieger, developed Therapeutic Touch. Kunz described a pattern of diffused energy. On reflection, Newman realized that her friend did, indeed, expend energy in many ways, through commitments to family, friends, and work and that she neither ate regularly nor got enough sleep to refresh and energize her. Although her friend's thyroid was working hard to keep up with her fast-paced life, telling her to cut back on activities was working against her pattern, not with it. The friend followed Kunz's advice and made sure to increase sources of energy, thereby gaining pattern insight. Ultimately, this knowledge enabled her to decrease her intake of medication and avoid surgery. "Her disease was a manifestation of the whole, not a separate entity to be attacked as though it were alien to the person" (p. xvi).

Pharris (cited in Newman, 2008) offered the example of a man who made repeated visits to the emergency department (ED) for chest pain, resulting in multiple tests and admissions to rule out heart attack, but nothing helped him. On yet another visit to the ED, after provision of the initial care, Pharris sat and talked with him. During the conversation, she noted, "Your heart seems to be hurting" (p. 97). The patient told her that his wife had left him, and that he had a disability, which contributed to his feeling stuck emotionally and physically. They talked through what this experience meant to him and how he could get on with his life, including referral to a public health nurse. The man did not return to the ED. In this case, the focus on a meaningful life event revealed pattern and ways for transformative change.

A friend was experiencing severe shoulder and upper back pain. As we talked, we both came to the same realization: My friend felt as if she was carrying the weight of the world on her shoulders. She immediately began making changes in her life, including giving herself permission to say no.

Providing a relational, caring presence while focusing on pattern recognition enables the Newman nurse and client to learn about experiences, meaning, and transformative change together. Both health and illness become important sources of pattern information.

in Tucson, Arizona, where nurses were freed from the usual bureaucratic time constraints, these authors noted that nurses recognized the importance of timing in their relationships with clients and the rhythm of when to connect and when to separate, describing it as "a crucial dimension of authenticity in the nurse–client relationship" (p. 406) (see **Box 19–2**).

## Box 19–2  Application of Newman's Theory

From 1989 to 1990, Newman spent 3 months at Carondelet St. Mary's Hospital and Health Center in Tucson, Arizona. Her goals were twofold:

1. Describe the nature of nurse case management and its interrelationship with the broader nursing and healthcare community
2. Evaluate the relevance of her theory to the way nurses practiced in the setting

The nurse case managers at this hospital thought that Newman's theory could provide a new perspective on their existing practice based on the following components:

- Looking at the whole
- Caring and commitment to service
- Respecting clients' decisions and agendas
- Facilitating informed choices
- Providing cost-effective, quality care
- Working in ongoing partnerships with clients that crossed service settings
- Engaging in a nonhierarchical model of group practice

Dimensions of the nurse–client relationship were described as follows:

1. *Pattern recognition*
   - Seeing the client in hospital and home/community settings, in the context of family and friends
   - Seeing illness as a way of life and helping to expand awareness of choices

2. *Rhythm and timing*
   - Learning when to connect and when to separate within the nurse–client relationship
   - Opening to self and others, to alternate choices
   - Knowing when enough is enough
   - Moving in and out of the client's environment according to the readiness and needs of the client and the nurse case manager's comfort and knowledge

3. *Opening of self to client*
   - Using oneself therapeutically while being open to the client's needs, both expressed and unexpressed

4. *Mutual growth*
   - Sharing, learning, and growing together as an unfolding process

*(Continues)*

5. *Choices*
  - Respecting and facilitating clients' choices, supporting them non-judgmentally, and meeting them where they are

6. *Beginning and ending*
  - Selecting clients and frequency of visits
  - Deciding when it is time to let go, at least for one phase of care

All parties agreed that a parallel existed between nursing practice at St. Mary's Carondelet and Newman's HEC: Nurse and client came together at critical choice points, with rhythmicity and timing. There was a letting go of the need to control or direct the relationship. Pattern identification was seen as essential, and transformation occurred for both client and nurse.

*Source:* Newman, M., Lamb, G. S., & Michaels, C. (1991). Nurse case management: The coming together of theory and practice. *Nursing & Health Care, 12,* 404–408. *Nursing & Health care:* official publication of the National League for Nursing by National League for Nursing. Reproduced with permission of Technomic Publishing Co., Inc. in the format Republish in a book via Copyright Clearance Center.

HEC can be diagrammed along a "V" parallel to Young's (1976; cited in Newman, 1994) depiction of the evolution toward freedom and choice. For Young, the top left point of the V represented potential freedom, with steps moving down the left arm representing binding and centering, the move from loss of individuality to sense of self; coming to the choice point at the bottom of the V, a new awareness as one seeks to learn the laws governing life; initiating a move up the right arm of the V into decentering and unbinding, involving transcendence and awareness of greater purpose and meaning; and culminating in real freedom at the top of the right arm of the V. Newman (1994) used the V to represent potential consciousness at the top left point, moving down through space and time to the choice point and beyond at the base, and then up through infinite space and timelessness to absolute consciousness. All persons experience this rhythmic up-and-down flowing of evolving consciousness throughout our lives.

Movement is a basic expression of life and reflects, via rhythmical patterning of tempo, personal organization and environmental integration. Consciousness is expressed in movement, persons interact with the environment via movement, and communication reflects this rhythmic tempo (Newman, 1994). Restricted movement—such as is often experienced in situations involving illness, trauma, bed rest, and so forth—involves changing perceptions of time and space. This dynamic situation offers opportunities for reflection and evolving new patterns of relating, as the old ones no longer work, propelling one "into a realm beyond space-time" (Newman, 1994, p. 60). For example, Jonsdottir (1998) explored the life patterns of 10 people with chronic obstructive pulmonary disease, finding a common theme of isolation and being closed in as they experienced activity restrictions and difficulties in expressing themselves and relating to others. This theme was manifested in different life pattern configurations. Notably, Jonsdottir found indications that some of these patients were beginning to glimpse the choice point—that is, the turning point of pattern recognition.

When persons encounter a disorganized, disruptive pattern characterized by fluctuation, the opportunity for creative change emerges, with the potential for transformation. Through this evolution, the individual transcends the usual experiences of space and time, entering experiences beyond space and time that are potentially transforming not only for the person but for all their relationships.

It is at the choice point and beyond that a turning point in evolving consciousness can occur, as people reflect on the pattern of their lives and relationships in their lives, seeking new rules for themselves as consciousness evolves beyond space-time. Here lie opportunities for experiencing and appreciating a new reality or consciousness, one that lifts people out of themselves and incorporates others in a more loving, compassionate way.

Neill (2005) explored life patterns of seven women living with either multiple sclerosis (MS) or rheumatoid arthritis (RA). She distinguished choice points from turning points at the stage of movement, the downward point of the "V" discussed earlier, and identified four new ways of living that could help nurses recognize where clients are in stages of expanding consciousness. The four ways of living occurred during transcendent stages of expanding consciousness, representing both change and transformation (ascending arm of the V), and were drawn by Neill from narratives reflecting boundarylessness and timelessness. After reaching a choice point, the women found meaning that restored harmony in their lives, despite the failure to cure either MS or RA. For example, all seven women spoke of finding simple pleasures, unique to each. All focused on being positive, and most developed optimistic philosophies that enabled them to preserve their quality of life. The women with MS described gaining self-control and a sense of wholeness, captured by Neill as self-differentiation. Neill suggested that nurses can "harmonize their caring with individual person–environment interaction patterns" (p. 341). For example, when an individual is in early stages of time or space (the descending arm of the V), it is too soon to focus on self-transcendent activities. For someone who is progressing beyond the choice point and beginning to focus on strategies for finding simple pleasures, being positive, gaining self-control, and experiencing self-differentiation can assist in finding new ways of living.

Patterns connect; they identify relationships with people and the environment. As nurse and client come together in an interference pattern of resonating waves, a new pattern is formed. Resonance is the way nurses gain patterning information. As Pharris (2010) noted, nurses must be open, able to free the self of any preconceived ideas, expectations, judgments, or cultural beliefs and values, in order to resonate with patients. As they come together and then move apart, there is the potential for recognition of patterning, insight, choice, and transformation for both parties if the nurse is fully present with the client in a shared experience of the present. Then their meeting "forms a new rhythmic pattern of the combined fields" (Newman, 2008, p. 55). The process of pattern recognition focuses on meaning—that is, what is meaningful in the life of the person—and is elicited through story or narrative and reflected back by the nurse. Although relationships unfold unpredictably, the potential always exists for greater freedom, connectedness, and caring within relationships. Thus, Newman (1994, 2008) sees pattern recognition as a form of knowing from within, sensing into the pattern, and a form of caring.

## Newman Praxis

*Praxis* involves establishing the mutuality of an encounter, eliciting the story or narrative of meaningful events and people in a person's life, developing the narrative as segments over time to depict the emerging pattern, diagramming that pattern, sharing and verifying this understanding with the client, and applying the theory of HEC. Nurses provide a presence that is transforming, integrating, and healing. As they engage in praxis, they are also developing meaningful nursing knowledge.

When engaging in research, the Newman nurse expands on the previously described activities by seeking institutional review board approval as appropriate and obtaining informed consent from participants. The process of informed consent takes on new meaning within the theory of HEC. According to Hayes (2005), it is unethical to approach everyone in the same way; rather, patterning configurations must be taken into account when engaging with others. For example, restrictions in movement affect a person's sense of time and timing, so the nurse must be aware of and sensitive to these differences, striving for synchrony with the person in the sharing of information and asking the person to make a choice about whether to participate in research.

The dialog between nurse and client is usually audiotaped when used for research purposes. The phases described here, which were first outlined by Newman (2008), fit both research and practice. Specifically, the nurse practitioner/researcher (PR) begins with an *a priori* theory, being grounded in HEC. The first phase is engaging with the client/participant (CP), where the PR's intention is to be fully present with the CP. The PR asks for a description of the most meaningful persons and events in the CP's life. This phase 1 interview comprises a nondirective process, guided by the CP, with the nurse PR engaging in active listening, general prompting if necessary, clarifying, and using intuitive hunches to guide his or her participation in the dialog. Because this is a mutual process, the PR is free to share a personal story, if appropriate. It is meaning—rather than data or information—that is key in this phase, which ends with a natural pause or a feeling of closure.

In phase 2, development of the narrative, the PR identifies the statements considered most important by the CP and arranges them in a chronology depicting a narrative of the most significant relationships. This information can then be depicted pictorially using a flowing up and down trajectory in lines and rhythmic swirls with descriptions and/or metaphors representing person–environment patterns of relatedness.

In one or more follow-up meetings (phase 3), the PR and the CP review the data and the pictorial pattern together, with the CP adding or modifying data as appropriate and the PR asking for clarification as needed. Insight may occur as both parties reflect together, indicating signs of pattern recognition. According to Newman (2008), most researchers state at least three such follow-up meetings are necessary. If no pattern recognition occurs, this finding is considered equally meaningful: It may reflect the absence of an observable pattern.

The fourth phase reflects HEC theory application. Although the PR began with theory and reflected on it throughout the process, more intense examination of the theory occurs during phase 4, including possible comparisons to other theories that are compatible with HEC theory. The PR notes any transformational changes that took place, both for the CP and the nurse. Again, this is a mutual process.

During the course of this four-phase process, reciprocal patterns of family and community may become evident, which the PR can subsequently turn into dialog with family and/or community. An excellent example of this evolution is provided by Pharris (2005), who identified a community troubled by a rising rate of youth homicide and then used the HEC praxis, first with 12 young men incarcerated for murder, to explore this issue. She noted that her purpose was to find out what was meaningful for the youths, rather than which factors led them to murder someone. Her purpose was not to discover how the community should change; instead, Pharris trusted that meaningful insights would emerge through dialog. Her intention was not to empower the community, because she recognized that power was already embedded within the community; as a consequence, she believed, answers would emerge along with actions to be taken as the praxis unfolded.

What emerged from Pharris's series of dialogs with the young men were themes such as never being asked or asking themselves similar questions before and now finding an intensified quest for personal meaning and new conceptualizations of how they might get on with their lives while in prison. Pharris (2005) identified "not a common pattern of pathologically disturbed youth, but rather a common pattern of interaction with the community that surrounded them" (p. 88) that had failed to protect and engage them, characterized by abuse and/or separation, stigmatizing events between ages 9 to 12 with no adult to help them, truancy, casual sex, use of drugs and alcohol, feeling alienated, and easy access to guns. She then took the patterns and stories to 16 community agencies and groups, where all concerned experienced "ah-ha" moments as they discerned ways to "reweave their presence in young people's lives and in the lives of their families" (p. 89).

MacNeil (2012) described Newman's research praxis as an "interactive unity," as researcher and participant come together for the wholeness of the pattern to emerge in dialog (p. 262). In her study of the complexity of living with Hepatitis C in a group of adults, MacNeil identified the main theme of "the experience of struggling to overcome" (p. 263). Several participants discussed how difficult it was to find healthcare professionals who understood Hepatitis C, what it meant to the person, and who was willing to work with them, highlighting the potential value of understanding the experience from the person's perspective in order to provide effective nursing care. For an integrative review of research based in Newman's theory, see Smith (2011).

## Applications in Advanced Practice Nursing: Health as Expanding Consciousness

The advanced practice nurse following Newman's theory of HEC can make a difference in people's lives through transforming presence, or being fully present in the relationship (Newman, 2008). As an example, Newman cites Falkenstern's doctoral research exploring the nursing relationship with families of children having special care needs: "One does not practice nursing using this theory . . . One embodies the theory; the theory becomes a 'way of being' in presencing with the client" (Falkenstern, 2003, p. 213; Falkenstern, Gueldner, & Newman, 2009).

Jones (Clarke & Jones, 2011) emphasized the difference between the medical model, with its focus on fixing, removing, and curing quickly, and Newman's assertion that symptoms are an expression of the whole, not the diseased/malfunctioning part. Symptoms may be cured, but the underlying pattern persists and may manifest again. This is a process that occurs over time, not at some fixed point in time. "The nurse's goal is to be with persons, to be aware and intentionally present so the patients can look at their own patterns" (p. 224).

Noveletsky-Rosenthal and Solomon (2005) used a model of structured reflection with advanced practice nursing students to foster a nursing identity and help them develop a way to sense pattern. Although this experience was in an entry-level program, presenting unique challenges in the socialization process as professional nurses, these authors' points apply to other graduate programs where the educational focus is heavily biomedical. In Newman's theory, pattern evolves over time; pattern discovery is accomplished through examinations of multiple interactions over time to identify recurring themes. In Noveletsky-Rosenthal and Solomon's work, students from primary and ambulatory care settings used advanced practice clinical seminars as a forum for engaging in individual and collective reflection on practice and theory. The students came to understand that it was their connectedness with patients that separated their practice from that of other healthcare providers and that what was left unspoken was as meaningful as what was spoken. Students gained insight into their own patterns, as well as the patterns of clients, re-evaluating personal beliefs and ways of interacting and recognizing self-imposed barriers to connecting with clients (Noveletsky-Rosenthal & Solomon, 2005). Ongoing reflection is necessary if the nurse is to continue growing and changing, using insights that emerge to make informed choices.

Imagine the vistas opening for creative change if advanced practice nurses embodied the theory of HEC in every encounter with an individual, family, group, or community. Opportunities to enhance healing and well-being would expand exponentially, transcending specific roles, settings, and patient populations. On the Exemplars page of Newman's website (healthasexpandingconsciousness.org), Margaret Pharris provided a clinical example from the ED of a trauma center involving a woman who presented with severe dehydration related to nausea and vomiting secondary to AIDS. Recognizing that every encounter embodies the potential for transformation, the nurse was mindfully present and attentive to the wholeness of this woman as she performed the necessary medically oriented tasks. The essence of her nursing encounter, however, was the nurse's connectedness with the patient and the way she encouraged her to share her experiences. Pharris pointed out that if all she did were the tasks and her only focus was the patient's physical condition, then the nurse would be reinforcing that it is the physical condition that matters most. Although the interaction was brief, embodying the theory meant that both nurse and patient recognized that this was a point not only of physical deterioration but a time of potential spiritual growth, one at which health took on new meaning (Pharris, n.d.).

Newman's praxis process has helped nurses and clients understand patterning and achieve insights into the potential for transformative change among people living with such diverse conditions as cancer, cardiac disease, diabetes, MS, RA, dementia, chronic obstructive pulmonary disease, and chronic skin wounds. For example, Rosa (2006) used the praxis methodology to gain understanding of 18 men and women, ages 49 to 98, who were living with chronic skin wounds. She discovered a new way to look at the experience of physical threat and to consider how that state is integrated into patterning over time. Rosa's findings informed practice through the model of wholistic healing that she developed, which focuses on healing the whole person: "The *closing the gap: process model of wholistic healing and personal transformation* describes participants' healing journey when guided by the nurse through phases of self-awareness, deepening awareness, appreciating meaning, and transformation" (emphasis in the original) (p. 357). Rosa noted that this mutual partnership supports recognition of problems and facilitates both lifestyle choices and personal healing. Specific clinical outcomes included increases in self-awareness, body image, openness to support, commitment to change, well-being, and satisfaction with nursing care, along with improved wound healing. "In conclusion, the findings in this research study offer evidence that an advanced practice nurse–patient relationship focused on understanding a person's pattern encouraged personal lifestyle changes to improve chronic wound healing" (p. 357).

Pierre-Louis, Akoh, White, and Pharris (2011) engaged in Newman-theory guided community-based collaborative action research to understand the experience of African American women living with type 2 diabetes. This process provided a holistic view of health problems and disparities while facilitating insights leading to action. "Through dialogue, women come to understand the patterns of their lives and realize their own potential for action using their own wisdom to guide meaningful transformations" (p. 235).

MacLeod (2011) explored the experiences of spousal caregivers whose spouses had been discharged home following coronary artery bypass graft surgery.

Recommendations included re-evaluating the current discharge education provided, recognizing the importance of early interaction with the caregiving dyad, and improving strategies to understand the experience and better facilitate the "caregiver's ability to deal with the ensuing chaos and uncertainty found in the assumption of this role" (p. 255).

## Rosemarie Rizzo Parse's Humanbecoming School of Thought

Parse first introduced her theory of man–living–health in 1981; she has made significant changes to the theory over the ensuing years. One difference is the evolution from the original theory into a school of thought, a knowledge tradition shared by a community of scholars with a specific ontology represented by the assumptions and principles, an epistemology identifying the focus of inquiry, and appropriate methodology for practice and research (Parse, 1998).

Parse introduced a new paradigm of nursing grounded in the human sciences with her theory, which originally drew on ideas from Rogers (principles and postulates) along with existential phenomenology (i.e., the tenets of intentionality and human subjectivity along with the concepts of coconstitution, coexistence, and situated freedom). Her original synthesis of these ideas produced nine assumptions that have now been synthesized into three assumptions reflecting her major themes of meaning, rhythmicity, and transcendence (Parse, 1998). Briefly, they portray *humanbecoming* as (1) "freely choosing personal meanings situated in the intersubjective process of living value priorities," (2) "cocreating rhythmical patterns of relating in mutual process with the universe," and (3) "cotranscending multidimensionally with emerging possibles" (p. 29). Each assumption leads to a principle, and it is the three principles taken together that form the theory within the school of humanbecoming.

Humanbecoming is a unitary construct that portrays the "human's cocreation of rhythmical patterns of relating in mutual process with the universe" (Parse, 1998, p. 31). This mutual participation is reflected in quality of life and health. Health is becoming, a way of living, and a synthesis of personal values. Disease is also a pattern of this human–universe mutual process.

Parse's (1998) first principle states that "structuring meaning multidimensionally is cocreating reality through the languaging of valuing and imaging" (p. 35). Rather than confronting an independent, external reality, humans construct reality through the significance they give situations throughout the "was," "is," and "will be," all of which are experienced simultaneously. *Imaging* is a prereflective–reflective coming to know process of shaping personal knowledge explicitly–tacitly. Imaging or picturing our world involves comparing the new within the whole of one's personal framework or worldview. *Valuing* involves the rhythm of confirming–not confirming one's cherished personal beliefs reflected in the choosing–not choosing among imaged options. In this way new beliefs are examined and compared, with some being integrated into the construct of reality and others being abandoned. *Languaging* is the process of symbolizing one's chosen values through speaking–being silent and moving–being still. It is the content and context of the message using qualities or characteristics such as tonality, volume, gesture, and posture. Meaning changes continuously along with the individual.

Parse's (1998) second principle states that "cocreating rhythmical patterns of relating is living the paradoxical unity of revealing–concealing and enabling–limiting while connecting–separating" (p. 42). Patterns of relating exhibit timing (cadence) and flow (alternating rising and falling). Ways of becoming present this rhythmical flow of apparent opposites as foreground and background—that is, as two dimensions present simultaneously within paradoxical rhythms. As Rosen (1994) wrote, wholeness is embodied in paradox, with wholeness as "utterly fluid and dynamic, an unobstructed boundless flow" (p. 269) that "confounds the dichotomies built into ordinary thinking" (p. 120).

*Revealing–concealing* is the first paradoxical rhythm, with the human choosing to reveal (disclose) and conceal (not disclose) simultaneously in mutual process with others. The essence of humankind is mystery; there is always something that cannot be known. *Enabling–limiting* is the simultaneous living of opportunities and restrictions as we make choices among innumerable options, not all of which can be chosen at once or even in the course of a lifetime. *Connecting–separating* is simultaneously being with and apart from other people, situations, ideas, and the like that we encounter as we live our lives. To be present with one is to be distant from another. There is a cadence, an all at once moving with while moving away. All three of these rhythms are present as we cocreate rhythmical patterns of relating in the process of humanbecoming.

Parse's (1998) third principle states that "cotranscending with the possibles is powering unique ways of originating in the process of transforming" (p. 46). Humanbecoming is moving beyond what is to what might be (i.e., hopes and dreams) while pushing–resisting new ways of viewing both the familiar and the new. *Powering*, according to Parse (1998), is the "pushing–resisting process of affirming–not affirming being in light of nonbeing" (p. 47). *Nonbeing* involves the potential risk of loss as people deal with the not yet known; powering is the essential force behind a person's very existence. Pushing–resisting patterns exist in all human encounters, creating tension and sometimes conflict as people struggle between what is and what might be, but it is through this struggle that cotranscendence evolves. *Originating* helps people identify personal uniqueness as they create ways of conforming–not conforming in the certainty–uncertainty of living (Parse, 1998). Each human shares commonalities with others, yet also remains distinct. Choices are unpredictable, so there is no certainty of outcomes—only creative imaginings of what might be. *Change* is continuous, presenting both the familiar and the unfamiliar together. *Transforming* is struggling to integrate the unfamiliar with the familiar as creative new possibilities emerge.

Collectively, these three principles described humanbecoming, which Parse (1998) described as follows:

> [S]tructuring meaning multidimensionally in cocreating rhythmical patterns of relating while cotranscending with the possibles . . . The human participates with the universe in creating health and quality of life by choosing imaged values in multidimensional experiences that are the human's paradoxical ways of relating. (p. 55)

Humanbecoming continues to evolve as Parse creatively contemplates possible futures. Moving forward in 2007, as she envisioned the humanbecoming school of thought in the year 2050, Parse clarified important features of her theory. She highlighted the meaning of indivisible cocreation by merging terms to make both humanbecoming and humanuniverse become one word. She explicitly identified four postulates that had been embedded in the ontology of her theory and that permeate the three principles: (1) illimitability, (2) paradox, (3) freedom, and (4) mystery. She refined the wording of the principles while keeping the original intent:

> *Structuring meaning is the imaging and valuing of languaging . . . Configuring rhythmical patterns of relating is the revealing–concealing and enabling–limiting of connecting–separating . . . Cotranscending with possibles is the powering and originating of transforming.* (Emphasis in the original) (Parse, 2007, p. 309)

Humans structure personal meanings, configure rhythmical patterns of relating, and cotranscend with the possibles in "cocreating reality illimitably with paradoxical rhythms" and with "inherent freedom in the impenetrable mystery of being human" (p. 309).

Parse's vision for 2050 identifies nurses as living their art in all settings imaginable. In these environments, they focus on enhancing quality of life as defined by persons, families, and communities rather than carrying out orders or actions determined by members of other healthcare disciplines. Humanbecoming sciencing, according to Parse, will focus on relevant lived experiences changing over time as people and communities change. The values of human freedom and dignity will be a consistent focus for humanbecoming nurses, who will be "the preeminent *professional* healthcare presence" (emphasis in the original) (p. 309).

Current developments in the humanbecoming school of thought include delineation of the humanbecoming leading–following model (Parse, 2008a), the application of humanbecoming to practice situations (Doucet & Maillard-Struby, 2009), and the humanbecoming mentoring model (Parse, 2008b). In addition, Parse (2009) described her humanbecoming family model as an alternative to traditional views of family. Community has been conceptualized from the humanbecoming perspective, with specific community change concepts and processes identified (Parse, 2003, 2012) and creative sciencing within the community perspective described.

Parse (2010) recently identified human dignity as a humanbecoming ethical phenomenon, identifying the fundamental tenets of reverence, awe, betrayal, and shame. She suggested ways of sciencing (researching) these tenets while simultaneously living them.

## Humanbecoming Research

The ongoing process of inquiry in the humanbecoming school of thought is termed *sciencing* (White, 1938). It involves qualitative approaches used in "coming to know and understand the meaning of phenomena of concern to a discipline"—in this case, the meaning of lived experiences as described by the people experiencing them (Parse, 2001, p. 1). Two types of basic research appropriate to humanbecoming theory have been identified—the phenomenological–hermeneutic research method introduced by Parse and the humanbecoming hermeneutic method pioneered by Cody to study the meaning of lived experiences through print and art forms. The applied research method is the qualitative descriptive preproject–process–postproject method, which is used to evaluate what happens in settings that use humanbecoming theory to guide practice (Parse, 1998, 2001, 2010).

Parse (2001) identified four distinct characteristics of her method. First, universal lived experiences reflecting health and quality of life, such as joy and suffering, are described by participants in a variety of ways, including words, metaphors, poetry, photography, and music. Second, data are gathered in dialog, different from an interview, where the researcher engages in true presence with participants. Third, the researcher moves from essences extracted from the data provided by participants to higher levels of abstraction as the researcher first synthesizes essences in his or her theory language and then identifies propositions, core concepts, and finally the structure of the lived experience that provided the focus for the study. Fourth, this heuristic interpretation links findings back to the principles of humanbecoming theory. The three processes of this method are dialogical engagement, extraction–synthesis, and heuristic interpretation. In *dialogical engagement*, the researcher is in true presence with the participant (Parse, 2005). In *extraction–synthesis*, the researcher synthesizes a story and extracts essential essences in the participant's language, and then in the researcher's language, synthesizes core concepts and uses them to formulate a structure of the lived experience explored (Parse, 2005). In *heuristic interpretation*, the researcher weaves in the principles of humanbecoming theory and offers an artistic representation that symbolizes the lived experience (Parse, 2005).

Recent examples of method studies based on Parse's theory include the lived experiences of feeling disappointed (participants from a community health center's foot care clinic; Bunkers, 2012), feeling stronger (community-dwelling adults; Doucet, 2012), feeling unsure (community-dwelling adults; Maillard-Struby, 2012), doing the right thing (community-dwelling adults; Smith, 2012), and feeling bored (elders either residing in a long-term care facility or affiliated with a church outreach program; Baumann, 2013).

One example of international use of the Parse method is provided in a book edited by Parse (1999) that describes 13 studies conducted in nine countries (United States, Australia, Canada, Finland, Italy, Japan, Sweden, Taiwan, and the United Kingdom), whose participants ranged from individuals living in a leprosarium to families living with coronary disease to children and elders. All researchers explored the question, "What is the structure of the lived experience of hope?" (Parse, 1999, p. 6). Examples of core concepts that emerged included "expectancy among the arduous," "enduring with vitality," "benevolent affiliations," "creating anew with cherished priorities," "transfiguring enlightenment," "liberation and arduous restriction," "contentment of desired accomplishments," "resolute perseverance," "formidable ambiguity," and "trusting in potentiality" (pp. 291–292). In Bunkers and Daly's (1999) Australian study of hope in families living with coronary disease, the structure of hope was defined as "anticipating possibilities amid anguish, while enduring with vitality in intimate affiliations" (p. 57). Taken together, the findings from the 13 studies deepen understanding of the lived experience of hope as reflected in health and quality of life.

In the humanbecoming hermeneutic method, the researcher selects a published text or art form to ponder. He or she notes any insights and ideas that emerge from this source, records them, contemplates them, and remains open to new insights. Emergent meanings are then synthesized and written in a narrative, which conceptualizes facets of humanbecoming into a new understanding of the human experience under study (Parse, 2001). Cody (2001), for example, applied this method to multiple readings of Tennessee Williams' play *Cat on a Hot Tin Roof* and multiple viewings of the film version of this work. He identified the meaning of mendacity as the refusal to bear witness—a "turning-away-from" and an "unloving, judgmental way of being/becoming . . . that serves to alienate others and engender mistrust" (pp. 215–216). He noted how the importance of bearing witness has emerged in both nursing and non-nursing literature as a critical factor in affirming personhood and common humanity. Therefore, the refusal to bear witness "clearly contributes dangerously to experiences of devastation, horror, and misery in individuals, families, and communities" (p. 219).

The final research method employed in conjunction with Parse's humanbecoming school of thought is the qualitative descriptive preproject–process–postproject method, which is used in settings that have chosen humanbecoming theory as a framework for practice. Information is gathered before initiation of the project, midway through the project, and at the end. Once the initial information has been gathered, teaching–learning sessions on humanbecoming theory are provided for nurses and other healthcare providers. Once the midway information has been gathered, the teaching–learning sessions continue. Once the postproject information has been gathered, the researcher applies the process of analysis–synthesis to identify and synthesize themes from all information sources, ending in theory-based thematic conceptualizations.

Bournes (2002) looked at six such studies across a variety of settings and synthesized three themes reflecting changes in nurses' beliefs and practices. Transforming intent represented a shift in purpose, with nurses "becoming available, honoring the person's knowing, and shifting patterns of practice" (p. 191). Unburdening joy represented more meaningful, rewarding practice. Struggling with change captured the difficulties of living the theory in practice. Patients and families appreciated the attention and caring; many said that nurses made a difference in their lives and as a result they found care more meaningful and open. From these studies, Bournes synthesized a set of universal values for knowledge development in nursing—namely, being accountable to the people served, listening to what people say is important for health and honoring their opinions, and respecting the right to self-determination. "The human becoming [sic] nurse's goal is to be truly present with people as they enhance their quality of life" (Parse, 1998, p. 69). Quality of life can be described only by the person(s). The nurse lives the dimensions and processes (identified by italics in the following list) of the practice methodology consistent with the three principles:

1. Illuminating meaning is explicating what was, is, and will be. *Explicating* is making clear what is appearing now through languaging.
2. Synchronizing rhythms is dwelling with the pitch, yaw, and roll of the human–universe [sic] process. *Dwelling with* is immersing with the flow of connecting–separating.
3. Mobilizing transcendence is moving beyond the meaning moment with what is not-yet. *Moving beyond* is propelling with envisioned possibles of transforming. (Emphasis in the original) (pp. 69–70)

These dimensions and processes are not intended to be followed in a linear manner, but rather are lived all at once as the nurse engages in true presence with the individual, family, group, or community across a range of settings, wherever people are.

As part of his or her humanbecoming practice, the nurse invites the person, group, family, or community to discuss the meaning of a situation, moving with the flow in a dialog reflecting ups and downs, joys and struggles, reaching toward hopes and dreams, and moving beyond what is to what might be. In doing so, the nurse lives true presence with others, a special way of being with others in which the nurse bears witness to their living of personal values. The nurse is fully present, focused in the moment, entering the others' world as a not-knowing stranger, joining their reality without labeling or judging (Parse, 1998, p. 72). True presence is possible in face-to-face dialogs, silent immersions, and lingering presence. Dialogs may involve discussion or other forms of expression such as interpretations of stories, movies, art, music, and photography. Silent immersion is being without words, a silent bearing witness that is still fully present with the other. Lingering presence is the remembered presence, whether explicitly or tacitly recalled.

Individuals have the choice to change health patterns as they change value priorities in true presence with the nurse. Parse notes that this kind of decision making may occur during the course of such processes as creative imagining, affirming personal becoming, and glimpsing the paradoxical. Imagining what life or a situation might be like if lived in a different way and uncovering personal patterns of preferences and deciding which to change help create the opportunity to do so. Looking at incongruence sheds light on conflict and can help change one's view.

Parse (1998, 2001) identified guidelines for documentation of practice for the humanbecoming nurse. First is the personal health description: In dialog with the nurse, the person shares his or her perspective as meanings, hopes, and dreams surface, along with patterns of relating with others who are close to the person. Second is the description of the person's intent and priorities relating to patterns of becoming, which is written from the person's perspective and includes what the person wants from health care. Third is the person's description of experiences in the nurse–person process; recording of this description may be done by either the person or the nurse.

## Applications in Advanced Practice Nursing: Humanbecoming Theory

Cody (2003) described how the Charlotte Rainbow PRISM Model of community health nursing services delivery, affiliated with the Family and Community Nursing Department at the University of North Carolina at Charlotte, was derived from humanbecoming theory along with community-based and community health nursing. The term Rainbow in the model's name was chosen to express commitment to respect for diversity; PRISM is an acronym for *p*resence, *r*espect, *i*nformation, *s*ervices, and *m*ovement:

- *Presence* is being with, face-to-face, attending to, and staying with the community over time.
- *Respect* is honoring dignity and persons' rights and responsibilities to make choices, with nursing activities guided by the community's values, hopes, and dreams.
- *Information* is about and for clients. The nurse listens, is mindful that clients make their own choices, and makes information available that clients say they want to support decision making. Thus the teaching–learning process consists of client-directed education.
- *Services* are helpful acts that clients see as desirable and meaningful. They are provided by registered nurses (including undergraduate nursing students), advanced practice registered nurses (faculty, family nurse practitioners, graduate students), and advanced practice community health nurses (faculty and graduate students).
- *Movement* is change in desired directions, with nurses following the lead of people served. "Nurses encourage, support, and coparticipate in movement as determined by the community" (p. 52).

For nurse practitioners and nurse practitioner students, the usual care expectations are met, such as physical assessments, but all care is provided in a manner consistent with the PRISM model. For example, given the focus on constituents' desires and values, no smoking cessation programs were offered as part of this program, because cigarette smoking provided comfort to the women, who voiced no desire to stop. What one group of women did desire was an evening discussion and support group, so one was established. Although not all the nurses accepted bearing witness in true presence as the essence of practice, all learned about it and other elements of Parse's theory via orientation and periodic seminars (Cody, 2003).

Bunkers (2003) has described the Health Action Model for Partnership in Community (HAMPIC), developed in Sioux Falls, South Dakota, in 1997; formation of this model was guided by Parse's theory as well. In HAMPIC, community is defined as a process of living in relationships and advanced practice community nurses focus on the connections–disconnections within the community: "In creating health action plans the nurses work with the community in exploring hopes and fears for changing patterns of health, thus changing the community's quality of life" (p. 74). The three integral components of this model are advanced practice nurses, the steering committee, and site communities. "The intent of advanced community nursing in the HAMPIC 'is to connect in true presence with persons and communities and to understand their health experiences with connections–disconnections and their hopes for changing patterns of health'" (Bunkers, Nelson, Leuning, Crane, & Josephson, 1999, p. 96 as cited in Bunkers, 2003, p. 78). The nurses participate in an ongoing study of Parse's humanbecoming theory. The steering committee is composed of community agency personnel and persons served by the HAMPIC program who meet regularly to make sure the voices of those served are heard. Site communities are partners in the model and vary widely, from soup kitchens to residential housing for the homeless to community health centers.

Two advanced practice nurses also have described their work with HAMPIC. First, Josephson (2000) described her work with a group that included Native American women at a drop-in center for women and families needing a safe place. More than 100 women met over the years to focus on quality of life issues and serve as family for one another. They began with a women's club to discuss issues of common interest and then chose to develop a group health description and health action plan. The group named itself Women of Hope-Tiospaye, a Native American Dakota word meaning "kinship within an extended family." Second, Letcher (2000) described living the humanbecoming theory at one of the HAMPIC community health centers, sharing the evolving story of John, a Sudanese immigrant, through paradoxical rhythms that emerged and his living the person–community relationship and experiencing community interconnectedness within the HAMPIC program. (See Box 19–3.)

---

### Box 19–3  Living the Humanbecoming Theory

John was a refugee from Sudan. In broken English, he told Letcher the story of his life in a country where killing another human being was the way young men proved their manhood. John had lost five brothers to this killing ritual, and he spent his adolescence running from hunters in the bush on his way to school. For marginalized and disenfranchised individuals like John,

*(Continues)*

HAMPIC offered the collaborative relationship of family in community. Letcher used his story to show how advanced practice nurses can learn from this perspective of family in community through the lens of humanbecoming and the major HAMPIC concepts.

## Quality of Life

John chose to emigrate so that he could start a new life. Letcher engaged in true presence with him as he strove to define quality of life as an immigrant in a new country where he thought that people needed the means to buy their life.

## Health as Humanbecoming

John's personal health issues and goals determined the course of Letcher's work with him. Together they explored how John made choices in his new life based on his values. As he told his story, new choices emerged as he began to see ways out of "the very dark jungle" he saw as the metaphor for his life (p. 303).

## Synchronizing Rhythms

As Letcher offered connections and resources within the community, John became more energized.

- *Revealing–concealing* was seen as John discussed his despair and struggles with Letcher, but felt unable to do so with other Sudanese immigrants in the community.
- *Enabling–limiting* was seen as John found a full-time job with benefits that helped him pay his bills yet meant he had less time available to respond to requests for assistance from family and friends left behind.
- *Connecting–separating* was seen as John spoke of helping other Sudanese immigrants in the community, while simultaneously finding the need, at times, to take his phone off the hook to decrease the demands made of him.
- *Mobilizing transcendence*, for John, was seen when he was able to speak of hopes and dreams, despite feeling suicidal.

Together in true presence, nurse and client were able to see emerging ways of being for John. He became a coordinator for the local Sudanese community, finding a place of worship and organizing a celebration to recognize the liberation of New Sudan.

*Source:* Letcher, D. C. (2000). Buying your life. *Nursing Science Quarterly, 13,* 303–305. Copyright © 2000 by SAGE Publications. Reprinted by permission of SAGE Publications.

Williamson (2000), a client, movingly recounted her personal relationship with an advanced practice nurse living the humanbecoming theory and the changes she experienced through that relationship. Feeling worthless; being depressed; enduring antipsychotic drugs, shock treatments, and hospitalization at a state institution; ending up homeless and living in her car, Williamson encountered Diane, the humanbecoming nurse, as she did her laundry at the local HAMPIC drop-in center. Diane invited her to attend the on-site women's group. Food was served, so Williamson went. "The curious thing about the situation was that the group decided what health issues they wanted to learn about . . . Although it was hard to believe, Diane's attentions were always focused on each individual as each person spoke" (p. 126). Williamson discussed the gradual evolution of her relationship with Diane and its effects on her life: "Because of the true presence that Dr. Parse's theory teaches, and the way Diane lives it, I have become more of who I really am" (p. 126).

Over time, Williamson became part of the steering committee for the drop-in center. She attended and met Parse at a theory conference. Eventually, Williamson became a participant in and a recruiter for a Parse research study. She participated in cocreating her Personal Health Descriptions and Health Action Plan. In addition, she expressed herself in poetry. Notably, she rephrased a personally meaningful sentence from Ecclesiastes 3:2–8 as follows: "The possibles of the not-yet will become explicit" (p. 128).

Williamson's journey from feeling devalued and unimportant throughout her life to feeling important and being honored as a person is a powerful illustration of the value of true presence. Regardless of the specific advanced practice role and specialty focus, a hallmark of nursing practice is engaging in relationships with clients. That nursing self can be nurtured and honored through cultivation of true presence in living humanbecoming theory, whether the task at hand is physical assessment, pharmacological management, or teaching.

Karnick (2005) acknowledged that living humanbecoming can be a challenge for a nurse practitioner, especially in the current healthcare system. She gave a beautiful illustration of living humanbecoming with children, noting that colleagues who find this approach too time consuming still notice the qualitative difference in her practice and are intrigued by her way of relating with children and the closeness of the relationships she forms.

Kim, Lee, and Baumann (2011) illuminated the experiences of three North Korean refugee families living in South Korea from the perspective of the humanbecoming family model, noting the importance of working with families who have lived through extreme hardships without judging or being critical of the painful decisions they had to make. "The humanbecoming family model provides a framework for nursing that focuses on honoring the dignity and creative potential of persons and families without needing to label them or pathologize their behaviors" (p. 277). For examples of other practice applications, see Parse (2010).

# Summary

It is nursing theory-based practice that differentiates nurses from other healthcare providers and that resonates so meaningfully with the persons, groups, families, and communities served by nurses. Examples abound in the literature to assist advanced practice nurses who are interested in pursuing nursing theory-based practice. One cannot practice or live what one does not know. The first step, therefore, is immersing oneself in a chosen theory and finding like-minded colleagues to continue knowingly participating in personal and professional change. It is a journey worth making!

# Discussion Questions

1. What is meant by the concept of pattern for each theorist discussed in this chapter? What is the importance of pattern for advanced practice nurses?
2. How can advanced practice nurses live HEC, humanbecoming, or Rogerian theory in fast-paced settings where much of the work to be done is medically based?

# References

Alligood, M. R., & McGuire, S. L. (2000). Perception of time, sleep patterns and activity in senior citizens: A test of a Rogerian theory of aging. *Visions: The Journal of Rogerian Nursing Science, 8*, 6–14.

Anderson, F. R., & Ashman, J. (2011). Establishing the correlation between well-being and presenting symptomatology in persons who are seriously ill. *Visions: The Journal of Rogerian Nursing Science, 18*, 41–46.

Barrett, E. A. M. (1986). Investigation of the principle of helicy: The relationship of human field motion and power. In V. M. Malinski (Ed.), *Explorations on Martha Rogers' science of unitary human beings* (pp. 173–184). Norwalk, CT: Appleton-Century-Crofts.

Barrett, E. A. M. (1990). Rogers' science-based nursing practice. In E. A. M. Barrett (Ed.), *Visions of Rogers' science-based nursing* (pp. 31–44). New York, NY: National League for Nursing.

Barrett, E. A. M. (1998). A Rogerian practice methodology for health patterning. *Nursing Science Quarterly, 11*, 136–138.

Barrett, E. A. M. (2009a). Become your own powerhouse. Retrieved from http://www.drelizabethbarrett.com

Barrett, E. A. M. (2009b). The power as knowing participation in change theory. Retrieved from http://www.drelizabethbarrett.com/background/power-knowing-participation-change-theory

Barrett, E. A. M. (2009c). Health patterning modalities. Retrieved from http://www.drelizabethbarrett.com/what-i-do/health-patterning-modalities

Barrett, E. A. M. (2010). Power as knowing participation in change: What's new and what's next. *Nursing Science Quarterly, 23*, 47–54.

Barrett, E. A. M., Cowling, W. R., Carboni, J. T., & Butcher, H. K. (1997). Unitary perspectives on methodological practices. In M. Madrid (Ed.), *Patterns of Rogerian knowing* (pp. 47–62). New York, NY: National League for Nursing.

Baumann, S. L. (2013). Feeling bored: A Parse research method study with older adults. *Nursing Science Quarterly, 26,* 42–52.

Bentov, I. (1977). *Stalking the wild pendulum.* New York, NY: Dutton.

Bohm, D. (1980). *Wholeness and the implicate order.* London, UK: Routledge & Kegan Paul.

Bournes, D. A. (2002). Research evaluating human becoming in practice. *Nursing Science Quarterly, 15,* 190–195.

Bultemeier, K. (1997). Rogers' science of unitary human beings in nursing practice. In M. R. Alligood & A. Marriner-Tomey (Eds.), *Nursing theory: Utilization and practice* (pp. 153–174). St. Louis, MO: Mosby.

Bunkers, S. S. (2003). Community: An emerging mosaic of human becoming. In R. R. Parse (Ed.), *Community: A human becoming perspective* (pp. 73–95). Sudbury, MA: Jones and Bartlett.

Bunkers, S. S. (2012). The lived experience of feeling disappointed: A Parse research method study. *Nursing Science Quarterly, 25,* 53–61.

Bunkers, S. S., & Daly, J. (1999). The lived experience of hope for Australian families living with coronary disease. In R. R. Parse (Ed.), *Hope: An international human becoming perspective* (pp. 45–61). New York, NY: National League for Nursing.

Bunkers, S. S., Nelson, M., Leuning, C., Crane, J., & Josephson, D. (1999). The health action model: Academia's partnership with the community. In E. Cohen & V. DeBack (Eds.), *The outcomes mandate: Case management in health care today* (pp. 92–100). St. Louis, MO: Mosby.

Butcher, H. K. (1993). Kaleidoscoping in life's turbulence: From Seurat's art to Rogers' nursing science. In M. E. Parker (Ed.), *Patterns of nursing theories in practice* (pp. 183–198). New York, NY: National League for Nursing.

Butcher, H. K. (1994). The unitary field pattern portrait method: Development of a research method within Rogers' science of unitary human beings. In M. Madrid & E. A. M. Barrett (Eds.), *Rogers' scientific art of nursing practice* (pp. 397–429). New York, NY: National League for Nursing.

Butcher, H. K. (1998). Crystallizing the processes of the unitary field pattern portrait research method. *Visions: The Journal of Rogerian Nursing Science, 6,* 13–26.

Butcher, H. K. (2003). Aging as emerging brilliance: Advancing Rogers' unitary theory of aging. *Visions: The Journal of Rogerian Nursing Science, 11,* 55–66.

Butcher, H. K. (2005). The unitary field pattern portrait research method: Facets, processes, and findings. *Nursing Science Quarterly, 18,* 293–297.

Butcher, H. K. (2006). Unitary pattern-based praxis: A nexus of Rogerian cosmology, philosophy, and science. *Visions: The Journal of Rogerian Nursing Science, 14*(2), 8–33.

Butcher, H. K., & Malinski, V. M. (2010). Martha E. Rogers' science of unitary human beings. In M. E. Parker & M. Smith (Eds.), *Nursing theories and nursing practice* (3rd ed.). Philadelphia, PA: F. A. Davis.

Butcher, H. K., & Malinski, V. M. (in press). Martha E. Rogers' science of unitary human beings. In M. E. Parker & M. C. Smith (Eds.), *Nursing theories and nursing practice* (4th ed.). Philadelphia, PA: F. A. Davis.

Carboni, J. T. (1992). Instrument development and the measurement of unitary constructs. *Nursing Science Quarterly, 5,* 134–142.

Carboni, J. T. (1995). A Rogerian process of inquiry. *Nursing Science Quarterly, 8,* 22–37.

Caroselli, C., & Barrett, E. A. M. (1998). A review of the power as knowing participation in change literature. *Nursing Science Quarterly, 11,* 9–16.

Clarke, P. N., & Jones, D. A. (2011). Expanding consciousness in nursing education and practice. *Nursing Science Quarterly, 24*, 223–226.

Cody, W. K. (2001). "Mendacity" as the refusal to bear witness: A human becoming hermeneutic study of a theme from Tennessee Williams' "Cat on a Hot Tin Roof." In R. R. Parse (Ed.), *Qualitative inquiry: The path of sciencing* (pp. 205–220). Sudbury, MA: Jones and Bartlett.

Cody, W. K. (2003). Human becoming: Community change concepts in an academic nursing practice setting. In R. R. Parse (Ed.), *Community: A human becoming perspective* (pp. 49–71). Sudbury, MA: Jones and Bartlett.

Cowling, W. R. (1993). Unitary practice: Revisionary assumptions. In M. E. Parker (Ed.), *Patterns of nursing theories in practice* (pp. 199–212). New York, NY: National League for Nursing.

Cowling, W. R. (1997). Pattern appreciation: The unitary science/practice of reaching essence. In M. Madrid (Ed.), *Patterns of Rogerian knowing* (pp. 129–142). New York, NY: National League for Nursing.

Cowling, W. R. (1998). Unitary case inquiry. *Nursing Science Quarterly, 11*, 139–141.

Cowling, W. R. (2001). Unitary appreciative inquiry. *Advances in Nursing Science, 23*(4), 32–48.

Doucet, T. J. (2012). Feeling strong: A Parse research method study. *Nursing Science Quarterly, 25*, 62–71.

Doucet, T. J., & Maillard-Struby, F. (2009). The humanbecoming leading–following model in practice. *Nursing Science Quarterly, 22*, 333–338.

Falkenstern, S. (2003). *Nursing facilitation of health as expanding consciousness in families who have a child with special health care needs.* Unpublished PhD dissertation, Pennsylvania State University, University Park, PA.

Falkenstern, S. K., Gueldner, S. H., & Newman, S. H. (2009). Health as expanding consciousness with families with a child with special healthcare needs. *Nursing Science Quarterly, 22*, 267–279.

Ference, H. M. (1986). The relationship of time experience, creativity traits, differentiation, and human field motion. In V. M. Malinski (Ed.), *Explorations on Martha Rogers' science of unitary human beings* (pp. 95–105). Norwalk, CT: Appleton-Century-Crofts.

Gold, J. (1997). The practice of nursing from a unitary perspective. In M. Madrid (Ed.), *Patterns of Rogerian knowing* (pp. 249–256). New York, NY: National League for Nursing.

Gueldner, S. H. (1996). Index of field energy. *Rogerian Nursing Science News, 8*(4), 6.

Gueldner, S. H., Michel, Y., Bramlett, M. H., Liu, C. F., Johnston, L. W., Endo, E., . . . Carlyle, M. S. (2005). The well-being picture scale: A revision of the index of field energy. *Nursing Science Quarterly, 18*, 42–50.

Hayes, C. (2005). Linking Newman's theory of health as expanding consciousness to ethics and caring. In C. Picard & D. Jones (Eds.), *Giving voice to what we know: Margaret Newman's theory of health as expanding consciousness in nursing practice, research, and education* (pp. 27–39). Sudbury, MA: Jones and Bartlett.

Hills, R. G., & Hanchett, E. (2001). Human change and individuation in pivotal life situations: Developing and testing the theory of enlightenment. *Visions: The Journal of Rogerian Nursing Science, 9*, 6–19.

Johnston, L. W. (1994). Psychometric analysis of Johnston's human field image metaphor scale. *Visions: The Journal of Rogerian Nursing Science, 2*, 7–11.

Johnston, N., Guadron, M., Verchot, C., & Gueldner, S. (2011). Validation of the well-being picture scale (WPS) as a measure of mood. *Visions: The Journal of Rogerian Nursing Science, 18*, 8–21.

Jonsdottir, H. (1998). Life patterns of people with chronic obstructive pulmonary disease: Isolation and being closed in. *Nursing Science Quarterly, 11*, 160–166.

Josephson, D. K. (2000). Women of Hope-Tiospaye. *Nursing Science Quarterly, 13,* 300–302.

Karnick, P. M. (2005). Human becoming theory with children. *Nursing Science Quarterly, 18,* 221–226.

Kim, H. K., Lee, O. J., & Baumann, S. L. (2011). Nursing practice with families without a country. *Nursing Science Quarterly, 24,* 273–278.

Kim, T. S. (2009). The theory of power as knowing participation in change: A literature review update. *Visions: The Journal of Rogerian Nursing Science, 16*(1), 19–39.

Letcher, D. C. (2000). Buying your life. *Nursing Science Quarterly, 13,* 303–305.

MacLeod, C. E. (2011). Understanding experiences of spousal caregivers with health as expanding consciousness. *Nursing Science Quarterly, 24,* 245–255.

MacNeil, J. M. (2012). The complexity of living with Hepatitis C: A Newman perspective. *Nursing Science Quarterly, 25,* 261–266.

Madrid, M. (1990). The participating process of human field patterning in an acute-care environment. In E. A. M. Barrett (Ed.), *Visions of Rogers' science-based nursing* (pp. 93–104). New York, NY: National League for Nursing.

Madrid, M. (1994). Participating in the process of dying. In M. Madrid & E. A. M. Barrett (Eds.), *Rogers' scientific art of nursing practice* (pp. 91–100). New York, NY: National League for Nursing.

Madrid, M., & Winstead-Fry, P. (1986). Rogers' conceptual model. In P. Winstead-Fry (Ed.), *Case studies in nursing theory* (pp. 73–102). New York, NY: National League for Nursing.

Maillard-Struby, F. (2012). Feeling unsure: A lived experience of humanbecoming. *Nursing Science Quarterly, 25,* 72–81.

Malinski, V. M. (1986). Further ideas from Martha Rogers. In V. M. Malinski (Ed.), *Explorations on Martha Rogers' science of unitary human beings* (pp. 9–14). Norwalk, CT: Appleton-Century-Crofts.

Malinski, V. M. (2006). Rogerian science-based nursing theories. *Nursing Science Quarterly, 19,* 7–12.

Malinski, V. M. (2008). Research diversity from the perspective of the science of unitary human beings. *Nursing Science Quarterly, 21,* 291–293.

Malinski, V. M. (2012). Meditations on the unitary rhythm of dying-grieving. *Nursing Science Quarterly, 25,* 239–244.

Malinski, V. M., & Barrett, E. A. M. (Eds.). (1994). *Martha E. Rogers: Her life and her work.* Philadelphia, PA: F. A. Davis.

Mandl, A. (1997). A plea to educate the public about Martha Rogers' science of unitary human beings. In M. Madrid (Ed.), *Patterns of Rogerian nursing* (pp. 236–238). New York, NY: National League for Nursing.

McEvoy, M. D. (1990). The relationships among the experience of dying, the experience of paranormal events, and creativity in adults. In E. A. M. Barrett (Ed.), *Visions of Rogers' science-based nursing* (pp. 209–228). New York, NY: National League for Nursing.

Neill, J. (2005). Health as expanding consciousness: Seven women living with multiple sclerosis or rheumatoid arthritis. *Nursing Science Quarterly, 18,* 334–343.

Newman, M. A. (1994). *Health as expanding consciousness* (2nd ed.). New York, NY: National League for Nursing.

Newman, M. A. (2005). Caring in the human health experience. In C. Picard & D. Jones (Eds.), *Giving voice to what we know: Margaret Newman's theory of health as expanding consciousness in nursing practice, research, and education* (pp. 3–10). Sudbury, MA: Jones and Bartlett. Reprinted from the *International Journal of Human Caring, 6*(2), 2002.

Newman, M. A. (2008). *Transforming presence: The difference that nursing makes*. Philadelphia, PA: F. A. Davis.

Newman, M., Lamb, G. S., & Michaels, C. (1991). Nurse case management: The coming together of theory and practice. *Nursing and Health Care, 12*(8), 404–408.

Newman, M. A., Sime, A. M., & Corcoran-Perry, S. A. (1991). The focus of the discipline of nursing. *Advances in Nursing Science, 14*(1), 1–6.

Noveletsky-Rosenthal, H., & Solomon, K. (2005). Cultivating a way to sense pattern with advanced practice nursing students. In C. Picard & D. Jones (Eds.), *Giving voice to what we know: Margaret Newman's theory of health as expanding consciousness in nursing practice, research, and education* (pp. 179–186). Sudbury, MA: Jones and Bartlett.

Paletta, J. L. (1990). The relationship of temporal experience to human time. In E. A. M. Barrett (Ed.), *Visions of Rogers' science-based nursing* (pp. 239–253). New York, NY: National League for Nursing.

Parse, R. R. (1998). *The human becoming school of thought: A perspective for nurses and other health professionals*. Thousand Oaks, CA: Sage.

Parse, R. R. (Ed.). (1999). *Hope: An international human becoming perspective*. New York, NY: National League for Nursing.

Parse, R. R. (Ed.). (2001). *Qualitative inquiry: The path of sciencing*. Sudbury, MA: Jones and Bartlett.

Parse, R. R. (Ed.). (2003). *Community: A human becoming perspective*. Sudbury, MA: Jones and Bartlett.

Parse, R. R. (2005). The human becoming modes of inquiry: Emerging science. *Nursing Science Quarterly, 18,* 297–300.

Parse, R. R. (2007). The humanbecoming school of thought in 2050. *Nursing Science Quarterly, 20,* 308–310.

Parse, R. R. (2008a). The humanbecoming leading–following model. *Nursing Science Quarterly, 21,* 369–375.

Parse, R. R. (2008b). A humanbecoming mentoring model. *Nursing Science Quarterly, 21,* 195–198.

Parse, R. R. (2009). The humanbecoming family model. *Nursing Science Quarterly, 22,* 305–309.

Parse, R. R. (2010). Rosemarie Rizzo Parse's humanbecoming school of thought. In M. E. Parker & M. C. Smith (Eds.). *Nursing theories & nursing practice* (3rd ed., pp. 277–289). Philadelphia, PA: F. A. Davis.

Parse, R. R. (2012). New humanbecoming conceptualizations and the humanbecoming community model: Expansions with sciencing and living the art. *Nursing Science Quarterly, 25,* 44–52.

Pharris, M. D. (2005). Engaging with communities in a pattern recognition process. In C. Picard & D. Jones (Eds.), *Giving voice to what we know: Margaret Newman's theory of health as expanding consciousness in nursing practice, research, and education* (pp. 83–94). Sudbury, MA: Jones and Bartlett.

Pharris, M. D. (n.d.). Exemplars of HEC nursing practice. Retrieved from http://healthasexpandingconsciousness.org/home/index.php?option=com_content&task=view&id=18&Itemid=34

Pharris, M. D. (2010). Margaret Newman's theory of health as expanding consciousness. In M. E. Parker & M. C. Smith (Eds.). *Nursing theories & nursing practice* (3rd ed., 290–313). Philadelphia, PA: F. A. Davis.

Phillips, J. R. (1990). Research and the riddle of change. *Nursing Science Quarterly, 3,* 55–56.

Phillips, J. R. (1994). The open-ended nature of the science of unitary human beings. In M. Madrid & E. A. M. Barrett (Eds.), *Rogers' scientific art of nursing practice* (pp. 11–25). New York, NY: National League for Nursing.

Phillips, J. R. (2010a). The universality of Rogers' science of unitary human beings. *Nursing Science Quarterly, 23*, 55–59.

Phillips, J. R. (2010b). Perspectives of Rogers' relative present. *Visions: The Journal of Rogerian Nursing Science, 17*, 8–18.

Pierre-Louis, B., Akoh, V., White, P., & Pharris, M. D. (2011). Patterns in the lives of African American women with diabetes. *Nursing Science Quarterly, 24*, 227–236.

Prigogine, I., & Stengers, I. (1984). *Order out of chaos: Man's new dialogue with nature.* Boulder, CO: Shambhala.

Reed, P. G. (1991). Toward a theory of self-transcendence: Deductive reformulation using developmental theory. *Advances in Nursing Science, 13*(4), 64–77.

Reed, P. G. (2003). The theory of self-transcendence. In M. J. Smith & P. R. Liehr (Eds.), *Middle range theory for nursing* (pp. 145–166). New York, NY: Springer.

Reis, P. J., & Alligood, M. R. (2008). Well-being in pregnancy: A pilot study using the well-being picture scale. *Visions: The Journal of Rogerian Nursing Science, 15*, 8–17.

Rogers, M. E. (1970). *An introduction to the theoretical basis of nursing.* Philadelphia, PA: F. A. Davis.

Rogers, M. E. (1990). Nursing: Science of unitary, irreducible human beings: Update 1990. In E. A. M. Barrett (Ed.), *Visions of Rogers' science-based nursing* (pp. 5–11). New York, NY: National League for Nursing.

Rogers, M. E. (1992). Nursing and the space age. *Nursing Science Quarterly, 5*, 27–34.

Rosa, K. C. (2006). A process model of healing and personal transformation in persons with chronic skin wounds. *Nursing Science Quarterly, 19*, 349–358.

Rosen, S. M. (1994). *Science, paradox, and the Moebius principle: The evolution of a "transcultural" approach to wholeness.* Albany, NY: State University of New York.

Smith, M. C. (2011). Integrative review of research related to Margaret Newman's theory of health as expanding consciousness. *Nursing Science Quarterly, 24*, 256–272.

Smith, S. M. (2012). The lived experience of doing the right thing: A Parse method study. *Nursing Science Quarterly, 25*, 82–89.

Terwilliger, S. H., Gueldner, S. H., & Bronstein, L. (2012). A preliminary evaluation of the well-being picture scale-children's version (WPS-CV) in a sample of fourth and fifth graders. *Nursing Science Quarterly, 25*, 155–159.

Todaro-Franceschi, V. (1999). *The enigma of energy: Where science and religion converge.* New York, NY: Crossroad.

Todaro-Franceschi, V. (2006). Synchronicity related to dead loved ones: A natural healing modality. *Spirituality and Health International, 7*, 151–161.

Watson, J., Barrett, E. A. M., Hastings-Tolsma, M., Johnston, L., & Gueldner, S. (1997). Measurement in Rogerian science: A review of selected instruments. In M. Madrid (Ed.), *Patterns of Rogerian knowing* (pp. 87–99). New York, NY: National League for Nursing.

White, L. (1938). Science is sciencing. *Philosophy of Science, 5*(4), 369–389.

Williamson, G. J. (2000). The test of a nursing theory: A personal view. *Nursing Science Quarterly, 13*, 124–128.

Young, A. (1976). *The reflexive universe: Evolution of consciousness.* San Francisco, CA: Briggs.

# CHAPTER 20

# Models and Theories Focused on Competencies and Skills

*Mary W. Stewart*

## Introduction

Each of us can remember our early days in nursing school. Regardless of our entry level into practice, our educational journeys started in a common way: learning the competencies and skills to be a nurse. At that point, we were primarily focused on concrete skills, looking forward to our first opportunity to stick someone with a needle with much anticipation! Competencies, by comparison, were vague aspirations to which our instructors referred. Nevertheless, the educational process moved us beyond our initial triumphs to a greater understanding of the expertise of professional nursing. We began to see—often retrospectively—that our toolbox was becoming filled with more and more resources. Our ability to care for patients was multidimensional and grounded in theory, knowledge, experience, and intuition. The focus of this chapter is on three theoretical approaches that underpin competency and skills approaches to nursing care, with specific attention to theoretical contributions at the advanced practice level.

Nursing science is grounded in philosophies and theories that define the discipline. A dynamic construct, nursing knowledge is gleaned from diverse approaches. Today's nurses no longer depend solely on traditional positivist methods. Quite the contrary, nursing is accepting the value of contexts (personal, historical, linguistic) for both the researcher and the researched in discovering knowledge structures (Chinn & Kramer, 2004). As we look at these theories of competencies and skills, we are challenged to identify their potential contributions to the emerging global view of science and knowledge.

When discussing theoretical pillars of nursing, we must recognize nursing's moral obligation as a discipline and science. Nursing is aimed at contributing to the health of individuals and the health of society (Grace, 2006). In a climate characterized by the vociferous "health care for all" debate, nursing has been unwavering in the principle of health as a human good. Advanced practice nurses (APNs) are responsible for sounding nursing's voice. Evaluating theoretical support for the principle of individual and societal health plays a substantial role in determining the relevance and applicability of theoretical tenets of nursing practice.

## From Novice to Expert (Patricia Benner)

Based on Dreyfus and Dreyfus's model of skill acquisition and skill development, Benner distinguished five levels of nursing practice: (1) novice, (2) advanced beginner, (3) competent, (4) proficient, and (5) expert (Benner, 1984; see **Table 20–1**). Additionally, Benner identified two aspects that discriminate among these levels:

1. Clinicians live in different worlds depending on their level of practice.
2. Clinicians develop *agency,* or a sense of responsibility toward their patients (Mitre, Alexander, & Keller, 1998). In their unique worlds, clinicians utilize different guides for taking action.

Benner's (1984) model of skill acquisition provides three general aspects of changes across these skilled competency levels:

1. Movement from reliance on abstract principles (novice) to experiences (expert) to view and guide practice
2. Movement from seeing all pieces of a situation as equally relevant (novice) to seeing the whole with varying degrees of relevant pieces (expert)
3. Movement from the detached observer (novice) to the engaged doer (expert)

Using Heideggerian principles of text interpretation, context, and holistic inquiry, Benner (1984) synthesized interviews to describe nursing knowledge as embedded in nursing practice. She referred to this approach as a "hybrid of theory and experience" (p. 41). Although the explication of interpretive phenomenology is beyond the scope of this chapter, it is important to note that Benner utilized this approach to find *meaning* in her research:

> The goal of studying persons, events, and practices in their own terms is to understand world, self, and other. The interpreter moves back and forth between the foreground and background, between situations, and between the practical worlds of the participants. (Benner, 1994, pp. 99–100)

This to-and-fro movement is central to understanding the participants' stories. At the same time, one assumption of this process is that the world can never be fully known (Benner, 1994).

**TABLE 20–1   Benner's Stages of Clinical Competence**

| | |
|---|---|
| Stage I: Novice | Beginners with no experience |
| | Rule-governed performance in all contexts |
| | Inflexible |
| | "Tell me what to do, and I'll do it." |
| Stage II: Advanced Beginner | Some experience (lived or mentored) |
| | Identifies meaningful components in situations |
| | Begins formation of guiding principles, based on experience |
| Stage III: Competent | Increased experience in practice (2–3 years) |
| | Sees long-term effects of actions |
| | Plans consciously and deliberately |
| | Improved efficiency and organization |
| | Sense of mastery and coping ability |
| | Moves slowly and without flexibility |
| | Lacks ability to prioritize |
| Stage IV: Proficient | Anticipates needs based on past experiences |
| | Perceives whole situation and long-term goals |
| | Identifies critical aspects and relevant nuances |
| | Maxims guide decision making |
| Stage V: Expert | No reliance on rules, guidelines, or maxims |
| | Extensive and varied experiences |
| | Highly developed intuitive sense |
| | Understands total situation in depth |
| | Prioritizes, acts quickly and fluidly |
| | Uses keen analytical skills and problem solving when situations do not go as anticipated |

*Source:* Benner, P. Commemorative edition, 1st edition (2001). *From novice to expert: Excellence and power in clinical nursing practice.* Adapted by permission of Pearson Education, Inc., Upper Saddle River, NJ.

The logical development of Benner's theory is appealing. She identified expert competencies, which were then classified into seven domains of nursing practice (1984):

1. The helping role
2. The teaching–coaching function
3. The diagnostic and patient-monitoring function

4. Effective management of rapidly changing situations
5. Administering and monitoring therapeutic interventions and regimens
6. Monitoring and ensuring the quality of healthcare practices
7. Organizational and work-role competencies

According to Benner (1984), her research aim was "to uncover meanings and knowledge embedded in skilled practice. By bringing these meanings, skills, and knowledge into public discourse, new knowledge and understanding are constituted" (p. 218).

Although depicted two-dimensionally, the domains and competencies have no specific beginning or ending. The nurse moves in and out of the relationship with the patient at whatever place best meets the patient's need. Unlike a linear model that lists tasks in sequential order, Benner's theory is both situation based and interpretive (Benner, 1984). The *embodiment* of nursing expertise (i.e., the nurse's body) takes over the clinical skill, allowing the nurse to know with feelings, senses, and thinking (Brykczynski, 2006). This knowing guides the nurse to undertake the right action. APNs have developed expertise through their interactions with patients in various settings over time; this investment is a resource that positions the APN in the expert role.

As a practice discipline, nursing extends beyond the science that guides it and includes the testing out—the questioning—of that research in the clinical setting. Practice is the setting for working out relationships. Nurses' narratives indicate understanding that a list of tasks and analytical supports to direct practice alone are insufficient in achieving best practices; ethical principles and aesthetic knowing are also essential.

The APN recognizes the value of past experiences, clinical guidelines, and procedural aids. At the same time, the APN gives careful attention to his or her intuition that supersedes these rudimentary practices. Because of this developed sense of knowing, APNs pay attention to detail, recognize potential outcomes, and take action to prevent deleterious events. In a crisis, the APN evolves as a leader, directing the actions needed and managing multiple interventions simultaneously. The expert nurse recognizes that science is vital, yet it is insufficient when applied alone.

Clinical forethought is another contribution of APNs. Even when the nurse is wrong about the outcome of a patient situation, forethought allows for pausing, questioning, and contemplating. APNs listen to patients and respond accordingly. They prioritize their interventions based on patient needs and recognize that "keeping up" is impossible. It is possible, however, to stay ahead of a situation through diligent observation, common sense, and quick action (Benner, Hooper-Kyriakidis, & Stannard, 1999).

At the core of the APN's competencies, domains, assumptions, and stages is *caring*—the primacy of nursing (Benner & Wrubel, 1989). Caring "means that persons, events, projects, and things matter to people" (p. 1). Care represents connection of thought, feeling, and action—of knowing and being.

Because caring makes involvement possible, caring is essential for coping. "Coping cannot cure or abolish loss and pain. Coping can help one manage those experiences, but coping based on caring also allows for the possibility of joy, the satisfactions of attachment" (Benner & Wrubel, 1989, p. 3).

Caring is specific and relational. The nurse's understanding of illness allows for joining of the patient's experience and the illness. When a nurse is able to be with a patient—that is, through the sharing of presence—recognition of their common humanity ensues. This awareness defines caring as the basis for nursing practice (Benner & Wrubel, 1989). The APN is in the best position to see and seize these moments, to lead others by example, and to enrich the stories of the patients and families who trust in the nurse's care.

Benner's work on caring as central to nursing practice emphasizes the key role of human morality in this interplay. The human situation—the context— was a critical component of her identification of nursing domains and competencies. One reason why her work has gained such wide acceptance is its research base and derivation from real-world practice experiences (Brykczynski, 2006).

As experts, APNs can be more sensitive and responsive to the insecurities of the novice or advanced beginner nurse. Likewise, the APN can deal with the tension between the educational setting and the clinical expectations. The beginner relies on abstract principles, models, and theories to perform safely. The expert, in contrast, deviates from this basis to engage in a deeper level of questioning in clinical situations. In addition to past experiences, the expert has a matured level of perception that goes beyond facts, concepts, and theories. "Thus, the theoretician must always depend on the practitioner for clinical knowledge development and for finding puzzles and questions that current theorizing does not predict or cover" (Benner, 1984, p. 187).

The relational aspect of Benner's work is paramount. "Nursing is relational and therefore cannot be adequately described by strategies that leave out content, context, and function" (Benner, 1984, p. 42). Nursing is holistic, nonprocedural, and relationship dependent. As a result of their extensive experiences, APNs inherently possess a knowing that cannot be explicated with words; they have a developed sense of intuition that moves them beyond knowing facts to knowing how to meet the patient in a relationship.

Relationships based on mutual respect and caring lead to healing. The envelopment of genuinely caring for patients provides nurses with a unique power that is both modest and wise. Benner (1984) identified six qualities of powers associated with nurses' caring: (1) transformative power, (2) integrative caring, (3) advocacy, (4) healing power, (5) participative/affirmative power, and (6) problem solving. Nurses' humility concerning this power may cause them to mute their voices, especially as novices and advanced beginners. In contrast, APNs have a matured sense of power, with accompanying opportunities to utilize that influence in ways that benefit the individual patient and society as a whole.

## Application of the Novice-to-Expert Model

Benner's work has found its place in a multitude of settings. In particular, the novice-to-expert model is frequently used in the development of mentorship programs (Dracup & Bryan-Brown, 2004; Nedd, Galindo-Ciocon, & Belgrave, 2006; Wolak, McCann, & Madigan, 2008). In addition, many agencies have adopted this model to develop career ladders and guide practice in field settings (Marble, 2009; Murphy, 2005). Even the information technology discipline has used Benner's framework to illuminate challenges and opportunities throughout the implementation of clinical decision support systems (CDSSs) in nursing practice (Courtney, Alexander, & Demiris, 2008). Courtney and colleagues defined the nurse's role and perspective at each level of implementation and noted subsequent implications for information technology to facilitate movement to full integration and enhancement of the CDSS in clinical practice.

Nursing education has weaved Benner's work into curriculum development, faculty evaluation, faculty mentorship, clinical decision making, and APN preparation (Carlson, Crawford, & Contrades, 1989; Field, 1987; Hawkins & Fontenot, 2009). Latham and Fahey (2006) used the model for APN role self-assessment. In their advanced practice study, through activities of reflection, APN students were guided to identify their point of view about where they were on the novice-to-expert continuum. Students recognized that some characteristics of the novice were dominant as they "began again" in preparation for their new APN role. Faculty used the students' baseline as a place of understanding and mapped their plan for growth. Further, faculty emphasized the emotional feelings and educational needs of the APN students at each level of competency.

Benner's contributions have been subjected to critiques and inspired debate. Altmann (2007) proposed that Benner's work best represents a philosophy, rather than a testable theory. She referred to it as "seminal qualitative research which lays the foundation for understanding nursing expertise and skill acquisition" (p. 122). Quick to acknowledge the value of Benner's work, Altmann aimed to put the model into its place as a support for nursing, education, practice, and research.

In a 4-year debate, English (1993), Darbyshire (1994), and Paley (1996) presented their perspectives on the value of Benner's model. First, English (1993) questioned Benner's definition of intuition and what he perceived as the ambiguity of the expert role. He proposed that intuition be redefined in cognitive terms—using cognitive psychology models of memory to give clearer explanations. English questioned the claim that not all nurses could be experts and called for ways to test Benner's claims.

In a response, Darbyshire (1994) criticized English for an apparent ignorance of the interpretive phenomenological method. Defending Benner vigorously, Darbyshire addressed several of English's comments, including the notion that Benner's work was "denigrating to nurses." Arguing the contrary position, Darbyshire cited evidence of empowerment and guidance for nurses in various fields.

In 1996, Paley replied to the previous opinions and focused on the rift between positivist science and interpretive phenomenology. He advised releasing both absolutist views and moving beyond the divisive rhetoric. According to Paley, attention should be given instead to the study and understanding of contemporary philosophy; we should learn about "recent philosophy of science and put that to work" (p. 671).

# The American Association of Critical-Care Nurses Synergy Model for Patient Care

A more recent model for understanding and guiding practice, specifically in the critical care area, is the American Association of Critical-Care Nurses (AACN, n.d.) synergy model for patient care. The AACN sought to develop a model of care that was driven by patient needs, aiming to articulate nursing competencies brought to meet those patient care needs. The hope was to link clinical practice with patient outcomes.

Hardin (2009) has described the timeline for this model's development (see **Table 20–2**). The process started with the AACN's assumptions that critical care

**TABLE 20–2   Evolution of the AACN Synergy Model for Patient Care**

| Time | Activity | Results |
|---|---|---|
| 1990s | AACN goal to identify model for critical care that moved beyond a list of tasks | Assumptions:<br>• Critical care nurses bring a unique skill set to the bedside.<br>• Care is holistic; it is greater than the sum of the tasks. |
| 1993 | Think tank to identify certified nursing practice concepts and quality outcomes | 6 outcomes<br>13 patient needs<br>9 nurse characteristics |
| 1995 | Committee of subject matter experts to refine model | Eliminated list of tasks for certification<br>8 nurse characteristics<br>8 patient characteristics |
| 2000 | Five assumptions of model | |
| 2003 | Addition of four assumptions<br>Delineation of nurse<br>  characteristics to<br>    descriptive behaviors:<br>novice, competent, and expert | |

*Source:* Hardin, S. R. (2009). The AACN synergy model. In S. J. Peterson & T. S. Bredow (Eds.), *Middle range theories: Application to nursing research* (2nd ed., pp. 100–114). Philadelphia, PA: Wolters Kluwer/ Lippincott Williams & Wilkins. Reprinted by permission of Wolters Kluwer Health and the author.

nurses bring a unique skill set to the bedside and that the whole of critical care nursing is greater than the sum of its parts (i.e., critical care tasks). At that time, certification required a certain number of hours in the critical care setting, completion of a list of critical care tasks, and a defined measure of professional development and continuing education credits. With this understanding, work groups convened over the next several years to develop and refine the AACN synergy model for patient care. As a result of this effort, the list of tasks is no longer required, and 20% of the examination itself is based on application of principles from the synergy model.

Early in the model's development, a think-tank group identified six quality outcomes related to nursing: (1) patient and family satisfaction, (2) rate of adverse incidents, (3) complication rate, (4) adherence to discharge plan, (5) mortality rate, and (6) length of stay (Hardin, 2009). Outcomes derived from the patients include functional changes, behavioral changes, trust, satisfaction, comfort, and quality of life. Those derived from nursing include physiological changes, complications, and the extent to which treatment objectives were met. Finally, outcomes from the healthcare system include readmission rate, length of stay, and cost utilization per case (Curley, 1998). The synergy model was found to be congruent with these patient, nursing, and system outcomes (Hardin & Kaplow, 2005).

In 1995, eight nurse characteristics and eight patient characteristics were identified (Hardin, 2009). In the years following, the nurse characteristics were delineated into levels of expertise ranging from novice (1) to expert (5). Likewise, the patient characteristics were found to range from the worst patient state (1) to the best patient state (5). Definitions for levels 2 and 4 remain undetermined (see **Table 20–3** and **Table 20–4**).

Synergy occurs when the needs of the patient and the competencies of the nurse are well matched. Optimal outcomes result from this synergistic relationship. For example, a patient with complex needs requires a highly competent nurse. When that pairing exists, the best patient outcomes become possible. Currently, nine assumptions underlie the synergy model (Becker, Kaplow, Muenzen, & Hartigan, 2006). The first five were identified in 2000; the latter four in 2003 (Hardin & Kaplow, 2005).

1. A patient is a holistic entity who is at a particular developmental stage and must be considered as a whole (body, mind, spirit) being.
2. The patient, family, and community provide a context for the nurse–patient relationship.
3. Patients can be described by a variety of characteristics, which are connected and contribute to one another; they cannot be looked at in isolation.
4. Nurses can be described on a number of dimensions. The interrelated dimensions paint a profile of the nurse.
5. A goal of nursing is to restore each patient to an optimal level of wellness as defined by the patient. Death can be an acceptable outcome, where the nurse helps move a patient toward a peaceful end-of-life experience.
6. Nurses create the care environment, and the environment affects what a nurse can do.

**TABLE 20–3    Characteristics of Patients in the AACN Synergy Model for Patient Care**

| Characteristic | Definition | Levels |
|---|---|---|
| *Resiliency* | Capacity to return to restorative level of functioning using compensatory or coping mechanisms | 1. *Minimal:* unable to mount a response, failure of compensatory/coping mechanisms, minimal reserves, brittle<br>3. *Moderate:* able to mount a moderate response, able to initiate some degree of compensation, moderate reserves<br>5. *High:* able to mount and maintain a response, intact compensatory/coping mechanisms, strong reserves, endurance |
| *Vulnerability* | Susceptibility to actual or potential stressors that may adversely affect patient outcomes | 1. *High:* susceptible; unprotected, fragile<br>3. *Moderate:* somewhat susceptible; somewhat protected<br>5. *Minimal:* safe; out of the woods; protect fragile others |
| *Stability* | Ability to maintain a steady-state equilibrium | 1. *Minimal:* labile; unstable; unresponsive to therapies; high risk of death<br>3. *Moderate:* able to maintain steady state for limited period of time; some responsiveness to therapies<br>5. *High:* constant; responsive to therapies; low risk of death |
| *Complexity* | Intricate entanglement of two or more systems | 1. *High:* intricate; complex patient/family dynamics; ambiguous/vague; atypical presentation<br>3. *Moderate:* moderately involved patient/family dynamics<br>5. *Minimal:* straightforward; routine patient/family dynamics; simple/clear cut; typical presentation |
| *Resource availability* | Extent of resource that the patient, family, and community bring to the situation | 1. *Few resources:* necessary knowledge, skills, financial support not available; minimal personal/psychological supportive resources; few social systems resources<br>3. *Moderate resources:* limited knowledge, skills, financial support available; limited personal/psychological supportive resources; limited social systems resources |

*(continues)*

**TABLE 20–3   Characteristics of Patients in the AACN Synergy Model for Patient Care (Continued)**

| Characteristic | Definition | Levels |
|---|---|---|
| | | 5. *Many resources:* extensive knowledge and skills available and accessible; financial resources readily available; strong personal/psychological supportive resources; strong social systems resources |
| *Participation in care* | Extent to which the patient and family engage in aspects of care | 1. *No participation:* patient and family unable or unwilling to participate in care<br>3. *Moderate level of participation:* patient and family need assistance in care<br>5. *Full participation:* patient and family fully able to participate in care |
| *Participation in decision making* | Extent to which the patient and family engage in decision making | 1. *No participation:* patient and family have no capacity for decision-making; requires surrogacy<br>3. *Moderate level of participation:* patient and family have limited capacity; seeks input/advice from others in decision-making<br>5. *Full participation:* patient and family have capacity, and makes decision for self |
| *Predictability* | Characteristic that allows one to expect a certain course of events or course of illness | 1. *Not predictable:* uncertain; uncommon patient population/illness; unusual or unexpected course; does not follow critical pathway, or no critical pathway developed<br>3. *Moderate:* wavering; occasionally noted patient population or illness<br>5. *High:* certain; common patient population/illness; usual and expected course; follows critical pathway |

*Source:* http://www.aacn.org/WD/Certifications/Content/synmodel.pcms. Reprinted by permission of American Association of Colleges of Nursing.

7. Impact areas are interrelated, and the nature of that interrelatedness may change as a function of experience, situation, or setting changes.
8. Nurses may work to optimize outcomes for patients, their families, healthcare providers, and the healthcare system.
9. Nurses bring their background to each situation, including their education/knowledge and skills/experience.

**TABLE 20-4  Characteristics of Nurses in the AACN Synergy Model for Patient Care**

| Characteristic | Definition | Level 1 (Novice) | Level 3 (Competent) | Level 5 (Expert) |
|---|---|---|---|---|
| Clinical Judgment | Clinical reasoning, which includes clinical decision making, critical thinking, and a global grasp of the situation, coupled with nursing skills acquired through a process of integrating formal and informal experiential knowledge and evidence-based guidelines | Collects basic-level data; follows algorithms, decision trees, and protocols with all populations and is uncomfortable deviating from them; matches formal knowledge with clinical event to make decisions; questions the limits of one's ability to make clinical decisions and delegates the decision making to other clinicians; includes extraneous detail | Collects and interprets complex patient data; makes clinical judgments based on an immediate grasp of the whole picture for common or routine patient populations; recognizes patterns and trends that may predict the direction of illness; recognizes limits and seeks appropriate help; focuses on key elements of case while sorting out extraneous details | Synthesizes and interprets multiple, sometimes conflicting, sources of data; makes judgment based on an immediate grasp of the whole picture, unless working with new patient populations; uses past experiences to anticipate problems; helps patient and family see the *big picture*; recognizes the limits of clinical judgment and seeks multidisciplinary collaboration and consultation with comfort; recognizes and responds to the dynamic situation |
| Advocacy and Moral Agency | Working on another's behalf and representing the concerns of the patient/family and nursing staff; serving as a moral agent in identifying and helping | Works on behalf of patient; self-assesses personal values; aware of ethical conflicts/ issues that may surface in clinical setting; makes ethical/moral | Works on behalf of patient and family; considers patient values and incorporates in care, even when differing from personal values; supports colleagues in | Works on behalf of patient, family, and community; advocates from patient/ family perspective, whether similar to or different from personal values; advocates ethical conflict and issues |

*(continues)*

**TABLE 20–4  Characteristics of Nurses in the AACN Synergy Model for Patient Care (*Continued*)**

| Characteristic | Definition | Level 1 (Novice) | Level 3 (Competent) | Level 5 (Expert) |
|---|---|---|---|---|
| Advocacy and Moral Agency (*continued*) | to resolve ethical and clinical concerns within and outside the clinical setting | decisions based on rules; represents patient when the patient cannot represent self; aware of patients' rights | ethical and clinical issues; moral decision making can deviate from rules; demonstrates give and take with patient's family, allowing them to speak/represent themselves when possible; aware of patient and family rights | from patient/family perspective; suspends rules—patient and family drive moral decision making; empowers the patient and family to speak for/represent themselves; achieves mutuality within patient/professional relationships |
| Caring Practices | Nursing activities that create a compassionate, supportive, and therapeutic environment for patients and staff, with the aim of promoting comfort and healing and preventing unnecessary suffering. Includes, but is not limited to, vigilance, engagement, and responsiveness of caregivers, including family and healthcare personnel | Focuses on the usual and customary needs of the patient; no anticipation of future needs; bases care on standards and protocols; maintains a safe physical environment; acknowledges death as a potential outcome | Responds to subtle patient and family changes; engages with the patient as a unique patient in a compassionate manner; recognizes and tailors caring practices to the individuality of patient and family; domesticates the patient's and family's environment; recognizes that death may be an acceptable outcome | Has astute awareness and anticipates patient and family changes and needs; fully engaged with and sensing how to stand alongside the patient, family, and community; caring practices follow the patient and family lead; anticipates hazards and avoids them, and promotes safety throughout patient's and family's transitions along the healthcare continuum; orchestrates the process that ensures patient's and family's comfort and concerns surrounding issues of death and dying are met |

| Characteristic | Definition | Level 1 (Novice) | Level 3 (Competent) | Level 5 (Expert) |
|---|---|---|---|---|
| Collaboration | Working with others in a way that promotes each person's contributions toward achieving optimal/realistic patient/family goals. Involves intra- and inter-disciplinary work with colleagues and community | Willing to be taught, coached, and/or mentored; participates in team meetings and discussions regarding patient care and/or practice issues; open to various team members' contributions | Seeks opportunities to be taught, coached, and/or mentored; elicits others' advice and perspectives; initiates and participates in team meetings and discussions regarding patient care and/or practice issues; recognizes and suggests various team members' participation | Seeks opportunities to teach, coach, and mentor and to be taught, coached, and mentored; facilitates active involvement and complementary contributions of others in team meetings and discussions regarding patient care and/or practice issues; involves/recruits diverse resources when appropriate to optimize patient outcomes |
| Systems Thinking | Body of knowledge and tools that allow the nurse to manage whatever environmental and system resources exist for the patient/ family and staff, within or across healthcare and non-healthcare systems | Uses a limited array of strategies; limited outlook—sees the pieces or components; does not recognize negotiation as an alternative; sees patient and family within the isolated environment of the unit; sees self as key resource | Develops strategies based on needs and strengths of patient/ family; able to make connections within components; sees opportunity to negotiate but may not have strategies; developing a view of the patient/family transition process; recognizes how to obtain resources beyond self | Develops, integrates, and applies a variety of strategies that are driven by the needs and strengths of the patient/ family; global or holistic outlook—sees the whole rather than the pieces; knows when and how to negotiate and navigate through the system on behalf of patients and families; anticipates needs of patients and families as they move through the healthcare system; utilizes untapped and alternative resources as necessary |

*(continues)*

**TABLE 20–4  Characteristics of Nurses in the AACN Synergy Model for Patient Care (*Continued*)**

| Characteristic | Definition | Level 1 (Novice) | Level 3 (Competent) | Level 5 (Expert) |
|---|---|---|---|---|
| Response to Diversity | Sensitivity to recognize, appreciate, and incorporate differences into the provision of care. Differences may include, but are not limited to, cultural differences, spiritual beliefs, gender, race, ethnicity, lifestyle, socioeconomic status, wage, and values | Assesses cultural diversity; provides care based on own belief system; learns the culture of the healthcare environment | Inquires about cultural differences and considers their impact on care; accommodates personal and professional differences in the plan of care; helps patient/family understand the culture of the healthcare system | Responds to, anticipates, and integrates cultural differences into patient/family care; appreciates and incorporates differences, including alternative therapies, into care; tailors healthcare culture, to the extent possible, to meet the diverse needs and strengths of the patient/family |
| Facilitation of Learning | Ability to facilitate learning for patients/families, nursing staff, other members of the healthcare team, and community. Includes both formal and informal facilitation of learning | Follows planned educational programs; sees patient/family education as a separate task from delivery of care; provides data without seeking to assess patient's readiness or understanding; has limited knowledge of the totality of the educational needs; focuses on a nurse's perspective; sees the patient as a passive recipient | Adapts planned educational programs; begins to recognize and integrate different ways of teaching into delivery of care; incorporates patient's understanding into practice; sees the overlapping of educational plans from different healthcare providers' perspectives; begins to see the patient as having input into goals; begins to see individualism | Creatively modifies or develops patient/family education programs; integrates patient/family education throughout delivery of care; evaluates patient's understanding by observing behavior changes related to learning; is able to collaborate and incorporate all healthcare providers' and educational plans into the patient/family educational program; sets patient-driven goals for education; sees patient/family as having choices and consequences that are negotiated in relation to education |

*Source:* http://www.aacn.org/WD/Certifications/Content/synmodel.pcms. Reprinted by permission of American Association of Colleges of Nursing.

The AACN synergy model for patient care is relationship focused. For example, nurses construct the patient and nurse relationship by identifying patient needs and matching them with nursing competencies. The relationships between nurses are also important. A healthy connection allows for improved teamwork and maximized use of personnel to enhance patient safety. Finally, the nurse–healthcare system relationship allows for analysis of the political, economic, and financial realities of health care. The synergy created from these relationships positions the patient, nurse, and healthcare system for optimal clinical outcomes.

## Application of the AACN Synergy Model for Patient Care

Since its inception, the AACN synergy model has been widely used in critical care areas. Becker and colleagues (2006), for example, surveyed acute care nurse practitioners (NPs) and clinical nurse specialists (CNSs) using an instrument based on the synergy model. The APNs described their work according to the eight nurse competencies and completed an experience inventory. Tasks performed by the APNs were similar; however, the two groups differed on their ratings of the most critical activities. CNS participants were more evenly engaged in clinical judgment, caring practices, facilitation of learning, and clinical inquiry. By comparison, the NP participants concentrated the majority of their activities on clinical judgment and advocacy actions. Authors concluded that the practice of NPs and CNSs in the acute care setting differed and the two specialties should be respected as making unique contributions to critical care nursing.

To assess patients' perceptions of nurses' skill, Wysong and Driver (2009) used the AACN synergy model to determine the extent to which nurses' attributes corresponded to nurses' characteristics. Patients' comments regarding nurses' skill fit well with seven of the eight nurse characteristics/competencies delineated in the AACN model. Clinical inquiry was not recognized by any of the 32 patients. In contrast, nurses' caring practices were identified as the most important trait of a skilled nurse; all patients identified this factor as important. Acting as a facilitator of learning and clinical judgment followed in importance, with approximately half of the participant patients identifying them as important characteristics of a skilled nurse. "Friendly nurses seem like they know everything" (p. 34).

Alspach (2009) reported on a three-part survey screening for incompetence among critical care nurses. Part 2 of the survey was based on the eight nurse competencies identified in the AACN synergy model. After converting definitions of the competencies into negative language, patients were asked to select either "witnessed" or "not witnessed" in reference to the characteristic. For example, clinical judgment was reworded as "used faulty/poor (erroneous, incomplete, inappropriate for situation) clinical judgment" (p. 12). Results indicated that the majority of the 80 respondents witnessed incompetence in all areas except "response to diversity." Most frequently, 93% witnessed incompetence in clinical judgment, followed by clinical inquiry (88%), caring practices (76%), systems thinking and facilitation of learning (72%), collaboration (69%), and advocacy (65%).

Although this study had many limitations—including problems related to sampling and generalizability—it was the first to use the AACN synergy model to identify nursing incompetency. More work is needed to see if these issues are related to poor patient outcomes.

Other uses of the model include development of critical care preceptor/orientation programs based on the competencies and measured by nursing satisfaction (Welch & Austin, 2008). Brewer and colleagues (2007) tested a case report form based on the model in a population of adult and pediatric patients. Results showed that the form was internally consistent, and nurses who were unskilled in use of the tool were able to use it to assess patients without difficulty. Kelleher (2006) applied the AACN synergy model to patient care assessment and the critical care nurse's personal reflection of the assessment.

In the critical care unit, Smith (2006) applied the AACN synergy model to address spirituality. One underlying assumption of this model is that the patient is a holistic being, including a spiritual dimension. Smith identified four areas of the model related to spiritual character: resiliency and resources (characteristics of patients) and caring practices and response to diversity (characteristics of nurses). Smith suggested the model could be used to organize and guide five nursing interventions:

1. Caring practices: accurately identify spiritual needs
2. Response to diversity: make congruent matches
3. Support resiliency: make appropriate referrals
4. Support resiliency: make space and time for group and individual religious rituals and spiritual practices
5. Support resource availability: make connections between patients and their spiritual support systems (Smith, 2006, p. 45)

Smith concluded that more research on spiritual care—particularly the frequency and monitoring of spiritual assessments—is needed. Further, the AACN synergy model provides a basis for that examination.

The AACN model has also been examined outside the critical care setting. For example, Cox and Galante (2003) incorporated the AACN synergy model in a master's-level curriculum preparing critical care nurse specialists. Cox (2003) described its use by CNSs to care for victims of intimate-partner violence. In an outpatient congestive heart failure (CHF) clinic, Hardin and Hussey (2003) reviewed the model's applicability to a CHF patient case study. These researchers looked at the patient characteristics as existing along a continuum, just as the nursing competencies can be placed on a continuum. Because the patient characteristics change with the patient's condition, the nurse recognizes that nursing competencies must change to maintain synergy and optimal patient outcomes. Hardin and Hussey commented that critical care patients are often cared for outside hospital walls, and the model's flexibility allows it to be appropriately applied with various patient populations in nontraditional settings.

Other applications of the AACN synergy model have drawn on the patient and nurse characteristics as a discussion guide in nursing rounds (Mullen, 2002). Annis (2002) demonstrated teamwork with a patient in acute respiratory distress syndrome, where the team used the model from condition onset to the patient's death, including family support.

Curley (1998) is credited with a classic report on the AACN synergy model for patient care and its use in optimizing patient outcomes. In Curley's foundational work, the characteristics and competencies are amply described. Case studies and questions for certification examination review are also included. Curley outlined the model's contribution of providing defined nurse characteristics/competencies and patient characteristics/needs and explained how the "best fit" of these characteristics can lead to the best possible patient outcomes. As the fundamental principle, the patient's needs drive the nurse's competencies. Thus the AACN synergy model holds the promise of opening new dialogue across many settings and disciplines (Curley, 1998; Pope, 2002).

# Relationship-Based Care:
# A Model for Transforming Practice

As in the two models previously discussed, Koloroutis (2004) posited that relationships are central to health care. The relationship-based care (RBC) model for transforming practice consists of six core components: (1) leadership, (2) teamwork, (3) professional nursing practice, (4) patient care delivery system, (5) resources, and (6) outcomes measurement. The patient and family are at the center of all of the components.

Three crucial elements make up the RBC model:

1. The care provider's relationship with patients/families
2. The care provider's relationship with self
3. The care provider's relationship with colleagues

> We experience the essence of care in the moment when one human being connects to another. When compassion and care are conveyed through touch, through a kind act, through competent clinical interventions, or through listening and seeking to understand the other's experience, a healing relationship is created. This is the heart of RBC. (Koloroutis, 2004, p. 5)

In the preface to Koloroutis's book, Jean Watson identified three requirements for transformation: (1) leaders committed to change, (2) an organization's adoption of a way to change, and (3) clear communication of goals (Koloroutis, 2004, p. vii). Watson went on to say that these three things combine with the 12 basic value assumptions of the model (see **Table 20–5**) and guide the transformative process. Together, they change what is current into something new.

**TABLE 20-5    Twelve Basic Value Assumptions of the Relationship-Based Care Model**

1. The meaning and essence of care are experienced in the moment when one human being connects with another.
2. Feeling connected to one another creates harmony and healing; feeling isolated destroys spirit.
3. Each and every member of an organization, in all disciplines and departments, has a valuable contribution to make.
4. The relationship between patients and their families and members of the clinical team belongs at the heart of care delivery.
5. Care providers' knowledge of self and self-care are fundamental requirements for quality care and healthy interpersonal relationships.
6. Healthy relationships among members of the healthcare team lead to the delivery of quality care and result in high levels of patient, physician, and staff satisfaction.
7. People are most satisfied when their roles and daily work practices are in alignment with their personal and professional values—when they know they are making a positive difference for patients, families, and their colleagues.
8. The value of relationships in patient care must be understood, valued, and agreed to by all members of the healthcare organization.
9. A therapeutic relationship between a patient/family and a professional nurse is essential to quality patient care.
10. Patient experiences improve measurably when staff members "own" their practice and know that they are valued for their contributions.
11. People willingly change when they are inspired and share a common vision, when an infrastructure is implemented to support the new ways of working, when relevant education is provided for personal and professional development, and when they see evidence of the success of the new plan.
12. Transformational change happens one relationship at a time.

*Source:* Koloroutis, M. (Ed.). (2004). *Relationship-based care: A model for transforming practice.* Minneapolis, MN: Creative Health Care Management. Used with permission. © Creative Health Care Management. www.chcm.com

The key relationship is between the nurse and the patient; this bond forms the core of the healing environment. The second relationship—the nurse to self—is often overlooked, but it is critical to the nurse's ability to form a relationship with the patient. Caring for oneself may be seen as selfish, and by strict definition, it is. However, selfishness—being focused on self—is a "health-full" endeavor that cannot be foregone. Restoring oneself is a precursor to aiding in the restoration of others. The third relationship is between the nurse and the healthcare system. This broader community operates best when the first two relationships are strong and vital. The interdependence of all three relationships propels us toward optimal healthcare outcomes.

A caring and healing environment is the context for these relationships and the way in which RBC thrives. Within that environment, the six key elements previously mentioned surround the relationship between the nurse and patient/family: (1) leadership, (2) outcomes measurement, (3) resources, (4) patient care delivery, (5) professional nursing, and (6) teamwork (see **Table 20–6**).

Koloroutis (2004) defined four elements for transforming the patient care delivery environment: $I_1$ = inspiration; $I_2$ = infrastructure; $E_1$ = education; and $E_2$ = evidence. When these elements work in sync, as evidenced by the formula $(I_2E_2)$, they simplify the process of engaging people to enjoy success while continuing to change the care environment.

- *Inspiration* promotes movement, a "drawing forth" within an organization. People are valued and consequently inspired. Patient-centered care inspires others.
- *Infrastructure* refers to the practices, systems, and processes through which vision is achieved. It is the foundation that allows change to occur.
- *Education* promotes competence, confidence, and personal commitment. An assumption is made that people want to do a good job. Personal growth and professional development are inseparable.
- *Evidence* indicates that change has happened and is viable within the organization. Evidence then links back to inspiration: Seeing results inspires further investment in the transformation process.

Leaders (often APNs) must know and follow the five conditions for $I_2E_2$ to work. Specifically, they need to meet the following criteria: (1) clarity—know where they are going; (2) competency—know expectations and have support to acquire the skills needed to meet those expectations; (3) confidence—believe that one possesses necessary knowledge and skills; (4) collaboration—work together toward a common goal; and (5) commitment—each person makes contributions, takes ownership, and collaborates with others. When leaders ensure the existence of these five conditions, goals are achieved. In this way, RBC provides the chance to clarify roles, responsibilities, authority, and accountability in APNs' work. This model includes individual and collective proficiency, clinical skills, critical/creative thinking, and interpersonal skills. It is the "essence of leadership at the point of care" (Dingman, 2005, p. 136).

A founder of the movement toward primary care nursing, Marie Manthey discussed her view of RBC in a 2006 interview (Manthey & Lewis-Hunstiger, 2006). Manthey viewed RBC as a return to nursing's roots in primary care. Using the start of the first Nightingale schools in 1873 as a beginning point, she noted that nurses did not work in hospitals for the first 60 years of nursing's existence. Instead, student nurses worked in hospitals with a registered nurse (RN) as director of both the nursing school and the nursing service. Citing the 1920 census, Manthey explained that during that time, 80% of RNs worked as independent

**TABLE 20-6  Key Elements of the Relationship-Based Care Model**

| Key Element | Description |
|---|---|
| Leadership | Leaders exist at all levels of an organization. |
| | Leaders create caring cultures that are healing. |
| | Leaders know the vision, model it, take action toward it, and support others to fulfill it. |
| | Leaders solve problems. |
| Outcomes measurement | RBC has a positive impact on patient outcomes. |
| | Data are meaningful and motivational. |
| | Achieving outcomes requires planning, periodic assessment of measured outcomes, and perseverance. |
| Resources | Nursing staff and managers share responsibility for resources—their acquisition, judicious use, and appropriate management. |
| | Effective use of resources requires critical and creative thinking. |
| | The resources needed for practice are determined by the nurse–patient relationship. |
| Patient care delivery | The system provides support for caregivers in collegial relationships. |
| | Professional development is encouraged and supported. |
| | Patient care delivery is organized and driven by the nurse–patient relationship. |
| Professional nursing | The nurse–patient relationship is sacred and the basis for professional nursing. |
| | The nurse has a social responsibility and is accountable for working within the scope of practice. |
| | The nurse has six practice roles—sentry, guide, healer, collaborator, teacher, and leader. |
| | Effective nursing practice requires an understanding of the human condition. |
| | Caring is the essence of professional nursing. |
| Teamwork | Teamwork is a predictor of quality patient care. |
| | Diverse interdisciplinary members share a common purpose and work toward that aim. |
| | All members contribute. |
| | Group energy and interdependence lead to excellent patient care delivery and outcomes. |

*Source:* Koloroutis, M. (Ed.). (2004). *Relationship-based care: A model for transforming practice.* Minneapolis, MN: Creative Health Care Management. Used with permission. © Creative Health Care Management. www.chcm.com

practitioners (fee-for-service caregivers in homes), 10% ran hospitals, and 10% were in public health. During the Great Depression, however, nurses needed work and exchanged their services for room and board in hospitals. That pattern continued until 1968, with the advent of professional primary care nursing based on the nurse–patient relationship.

In the 1990s, economic pressures replaced primary nursing with "team" nursing. Manthey and Lewis-Hunstiger referred to this approach as "FRED—Frantically Running Every Day" (2006, p. 7). In contrast, RBC is a hopeful response to FRED. RBC calls APNs back to the concepts of responsibility, accountability, and authority. These principles of decentralized nursing departments must also apply to APNs' personal lives. Being in the right relationship with ourselves includes the knowledge that we have the choice to think, feel, and act in certain ways.

Three kinds of thinking are inherent in RBC (Manthey & Koloroutis, 2004):

1. *Critical thinking:* systematic; multidimensional; sees what is there and what is not; includes critical feeling; involves humility in choosing what to do
2. *Creative thinking:* questions what the day will look like; encourages tolerance of ambiguity
3. *Reflective thinking:* time and space to pause; silence for reflection and to rejuvenate

To date, critical thinking has garnered the most significant attention and inspired the most debate. Creative thinking, by comparison, has remained largely out of the spotlight. Critics claim that creative thinking takes too much time, when in truth, sitting at the bedside with a patient to discuss how the patient envisions the day takes only a moment. Reflective thinking, although desirable and pursued, is difficult to do in most work environments. Places of calm, quiet, and solemnity do not exist for most nurses in the workplace. Traveling to and from work provides some opportunity for reflection but is often jumbled with thoughts of tasks—to do, done, and left undone (Manthey & Koloroutis, 2004).

RBC provides a systems framework where one cares for patients, self, and others. In this setting, positive outcomes (e.g., clinical safety, clinical quality, satisfaction, recruitment and retention, high morale, and achievement of goals) become possible. The potential for these outcomes has led to the adoption of RBC as a model of nursing care (Beaty, 2006).

## Application of the Relationship-Based Care Model

Maklebust and Suchy (2007) implemented the RBC model in a comprehensive cancer center and used it in practical ways. Job descriptions were rewritten to reflect caring behaviors. Nurses sat with patients to identify mutual goals. Staff names and goals were written on whiteboards in patient rooms. Shift report began to include communication of patient goals and preferences. Around the center, posters with pictures of staff demonstrating RBC actions were displayed. Weekly continuing education offerings were conducted to inform and inspire the staff. Authors reported wide acceptance of the model with improved patient and nurse satisfaction.

Nurses at the University of Mississippi Medical Center's Hospitals and Clinics recently surveyed various models to guide their journey toward Magnet status. Janet Harris, chief nursing executive officer, reported that nurses selected the RBC model as the framework to support this endeavor and transform practice at the Medical Center (presentation by J. Harris, November 30, 2009).

Although Koloroutis was not credited with the development of the model, Rivas-Vazquez and colleagues (2009) used the RBC terminology as the conceptual framework for their study involving psychiatric patients in the criminal justice system. Members of the homeless mentally ill population entered an RBC program to ensure them access to psychiatric and primary care. The number of post-program arrests was significantly reduced for patients in the RBC group. In another report, RBC principles were used to describe individually focused care that led to positive patient outcomes (Francavilla, 2008). Nurses had the authority and autonomy to manage an anticoagulation clinic and produced improved outcomes for patients under that program.

The question of how to integrate RBC in today's world poses a significant challenge. Notably, 12-hour shifts and reduced lengths of patient stays threaten the continuity of the nurse–patient relationship that is central to RBC. To overcome these obstacles, nurses are reminded that presence—being with the patient—is not necessarily a time-intensive activity. As we perform tasks, we can connect with the patient. We can exchange ideas. We can listen to the patient's perspective (Manthey & Lewis-Hunstiger, 2006).

Nurse educators are challenged to move beyond the mere teaching of time assessment and management. In the past, we have focused on thinking critically but have largely ignored the need to articulate that thinking to others. Now, however, we must recognize that we need to teach students to prioritize and to articulate their rationale for prioritizing and meeting needs.

The reality of practice is that the nurse's time must be parceled out—and balanced—between needs, priorities, and resources. The two factors that drive nursing's work are orders and patient acuity. There is not enough time to do it all. As with all important work, the nature of nursing is rooted in its perpetual responsibilities. Inexperienced nurses do not prioritize and they may let things fall off the list, whereas experienced nurses prioritize and manage detailed responsibilities (Benner, 1984; Manthey & Lewis-Hunstiger, 2006). Nurses need to find a way to reconcile not getting everything done. We have to release our tendency to see ourselves as victims and begin to adopt a long-term perspective. The RBC culture represents a step in that direction. In adopting its tenets, it would behoove APNs to remember that nursing is licensed by society to make prioritization judgments.

## Box 20–1 APN Skills and Competencies Undergirding Trust in the Nurse-Patient Relationship

- APNs have expertise owing to their numerous interactions with patients in various settings over time. The continuum of the expert (Benner, 1984) can serve as a guide for the roles and responsibilities of the APN.
- APNs have the opportunity and responsibility to guide neophyte nurses in clinical teaching.
- APNs need to read about and understand the debates related to models of practice. At the same time, they must avoid becoming so engaged in the weeds (rhetoric) that they lose the view from the trees (holistic perspective).
- APNs are leaders in the establishment and growth of nurse–patient relationships.
- APNs strengthen nurse–nurse relationships by responsible use of personnel.
- APNs are expected to engage in politics and the economics of the nurse–system relationship.
- Leading by example, APNs model friendliness and a sense of competence that reassures their patients, colleagues, and society.

## Conclusion

Each of the models described in this chapter, in its own way, guides us back to the basics of nursing—primarily, the relationship between the nurse and the patient. The rare trust embodied in that connection has existed since nursing's inception and continues to thrive today in all settings and populations. Our professional and personal responsibility is to invest in that relationship, using a variety of skills and competencies (see **Box 20–1**). When promoting house sales, realtors often say the most critical factors are "Location, location, location." In the sacred profession of nursing, our cornerstone is "Relationships, relationships, relationships." May we guard that prize with our whole being.

## Discussion Questions

1. Using the novice-to-expert model, explain what your approach as an APN would be if a nurse with 2 years of medical–surgical experience came to you for professional guidance.

2. As an APN, which practice areas do you see as favorable for adoption of the AACN synergy model for patient care? How would you lead in that effort?

3. Describe what RBC would look like in your area of advanced nursing practice. In that setting, how would you measure outcomes at the nurse–patient, nurse–nurse, and nurse–system levels?

# References

Alspach, G. (2009). Incompetence among critical care nurses: A survey report. *Critical Care Nurse, 29*(1), 12–17.

Altmann, T. K. (2007). An evaluation of the seminal work of Patricia Benner: Theory or philosophy? *Contemporary Nurse, 25*(1–2), 114–123.

American Association of Critical-Care Nurses. (n.d.). The AACN synergy model for patient care. Retrieved from http://www.aacn.org/WD/Certifications/Content/synmodel.pcms

Annis, T. D. (2002). The synergy model in practice: The interdisciplinary team across the continuum of care. *Critical Care Nurse, 22*(5), 76–79.

Beaty, B. (2006). Relationship-based care: A true evolution of primary nursing. *Creative Nursing, 12*(1), 3.

Becker, D., Kaplow, R., Muenzen, P. M., & Hartigan, C. (2006). Activities performed by acute and critical care advanced practice nurses: American Association of Critical-Care Nurses study of practice. *American Journal of Critical Care, 15*, 130–148.

Benner, P. (1984). *From novice to expert: Excellence and power in clinical nursing practice.* Menlo Park, CA: Addison-Wesley.

Benner, P. (1994). The tradition and skill of interpretive phenomenology in studying health, illness, and caring practices. In P. Benner (Ed.), *Interpretive phenomenology: Embodiment, caring, and ethics in health and illness* (pp. 99–127). Thousand Oaks, CA: Sage.

Benner, P., Hooper-Kyriakidis, P., & Stannard, D. (1999). *Clinical wisdom and interventions in critical care: A thinking-in-action approach.* Philadelphia, PA: Saunders.

Benner, P., & Wrubel, J. (1989). *The primacy of caring: Stress and coping in health and illness.* Menlo Park, CA: Addison-Wesley.

Brewer, B., Wojner-Alexandrov, A. W., Triola, N., Pacini, C., Cline, M., Rust, J. E., & Kerfoot, K. (2007). AACN synergy model's characteristics of patients: Psychometric analyses in a tertiary care health system. *American Journal of Critical Care, 16*, 158–167.

Brykczynski, K. A. (2006). Benner's philosophy in nursing practice. In M. R. Alligood & A. M. Tomey (Eds.), *Nursing theory: Utilization and application* (3rd ed., pp. 131–156). St. Louis, MO: Mosby-Elsevier.

Carlson, L., Crawford, N., & Contrades, S. (1989). Nursing student novice to expert: Benner's research applied to education. *Journal of Nursing Education, 28*, 188–190.

Chinn, P. L., & Kramer, M. K. (2004). *Integrated knowledge development in nursing* (6th ed.). St. Louis, MO: Mosby.

Courtney, K. L., Alexander, G. L., & Demiris, G. (2008). Information technology from novice to expert: Implementation implications. *Journal of Nursing Management, 16*, 692–699.

Cox, C. W., & Galante, C. M. (2003). An MSN curriculum in preparation of CCNSs: A model for consideration. *Critical Care Nurse, 23*(6), 74–80.

Cox, E. (2003). Synergy in practice: Caring for victims of intimate partner violence. *Critical Care Nursing Quarterly, 26*, 323–330.

Curley, M. (1998). Patient–nurse synergy: Optimizing patients' outcomes. *American Journal of Critical Care, 7*(1), 64–72.

Darbyshire, P. (1994). Skilled expert practice: Is it "all in the mind"? A response to English's critique of Benner's novice to expert model. *Journal of Advanced Nursing, 19,* 755–761.

Dingman, S. (2005). A dialogue on relationship-based care: Reflection on practice. *International Journal for Human Caring, 9,* 136.

Dracup, K., & Bryan-Brown, C. W. (2004). From novice to expert to mentor: Shaping the future. *American Journal of Critical Care, 13,* 448–450.

English, I. (1993). Intuition as a function of the expert nurse: A critique of Benner's novice to expert model. *Journal of Advanced Nursing, 18,* 387–393.

Field, P. A. (1987). The impact of nursing theory on the clinical decision making process. *Journal of Advanced Nursing, 12,* 563–571.

Francavilla, C. L. (2008). Registered nurse–managed anticoagulation clinic: Improving patient outcomes. *Nursing Economics, 26,* 130–132.

Grace, P. J. (2006). Philosophies, models, and theories: Moral obligations. In M. R. Alligood & A. M. Tomey (Eds.), *Nursing theory: Utilization and application* (3rd ed., pp. 67–85). St. Louis, MO: Mosby-Elsevier.

Hardin, S. R. (2009). The AACN synergy model. In S. J. Peterson & T. S. Bredow (Eds.), *Middle range theories: Application to nursing research* (2nd ed., pp. 100–114). Philadelphia, PA: Wolters Kluwer/Lippincott Williams & Wilkins.

Hardin, S. R., & Hussey, L. (2003). AACN synergy model for patient care: Case study of a CHF patient. *Critical Care Nurse, 23*(1), 73–76.

Hardin, S. R., & Kaplow, R. (2005). *Synergy for clinical excellence: The AACN synergy model for patient care.* Sudbury, MA: Jones and Bartlett.

Harris, J. (2009, November 30). *Nursing at University of Mississippi hospitals and clinics.* Oral presentation in the University of Mississippi Medical Center School of Nursing.

Hawkins, J. W., & Fontenot, H. (2009). What do you mean you want me to teach, do research, engage in service, and clinical practice? Views from the trenches: The novice and expert. *Journal of the American Academy of Nurse Practitioners, 21,* 358–361.

Kelleher, S. (2006). Providing patient-centered care in an intensive care unit. *Nursing Standard, 21*(13), 35–40.

Koloroutis, M. (Ed.). (2004). *Relationship-based care: A model for transforming practice.* Minneapolis, MN: Creative Health Care Management.

Latham, C. L., & Fahey, L. J. (2006). Novice to expert advanced practice nurse role transition: Guided student self-reflection. *Journal of Nursing Education, 45*(1), 46–48.

Maklebust, J., & Suchy, S. (2007). Implementing relationship-based care in a comprehensive cancer center [Abstract]. *Oncology Nursing Forum, 34,* 571.

Manthey, M., & Koloroutis, M. (2004). Resource driven practice. In M. Koloroutis (Ed.), *Relationship-based care: A model for transforming practice* (pp. 183–214). Minneapolis, MN: Creative Health Care Management.

Manthey, M., & Lewis-Hunstiger, M. (2006). Relationship-based care: Customized primary nursing. *Creative Nursing, 12*(1), 4–11.

Marble, S. G. (2009). Five-step model of professional excellence. *Clinical Journal of Oncology Nursing, 13,* 310–315.

Mitre, J. C., Alexander, J. E., & Keller, S. L. (1998). Patricia Benner: From novice to expert: Excellence and power in clinical nursing practice. In A. M. Tomey & M. R. Alligood (Eds.), *Nursing theorists and their work* (4th ed., pp. 157–172). St. Louis, MO: Mosby.

Mullen, J. E. (2002). The synergy model in practice: The synergy model as a framework for nursing rounds. *Critical Care Nurse, 22*(6), 66–68.

Murphy, F. (2005). Preparing for the field: Developing competence as an ethnographic field worker. *Nurse Researcher, 12*(3), 52–60.

Nedd, N., Galindo-Ciocon, D., & Belgrave, G. (2006). Guided growth intervention: From novice to expert through a mentoring program. *Journal of Nursing Care Quality, 21*(1), 20–23.

Paley, J. (1996). Intuition and expertise: Comments on the Benner debate. *Journal of Advanced Nursing, 23, 665–671.*

Pope, B. (2002). Working together to meet patient and family needs. *Nursing 2002, 32*(7), 6–7.

Rivas-Vazquez, R. A., Sarria, M., Rey, G., Rivas-Vazquez, A. A., Rodriguez, J., & Jardon, M. E. (2009). A relationship-based care model for jail diversion. *Psychiatric Services, 60, 766–771.*

Smith, A. R. (2006). Using the synergy model to provide spiritual nursing care in critical care settings. *Critical Care Nurse, 26*(4), 41–47.

Welch, S., & Austin, C. (2008). Development of an ICU preceptor program based on the AACN synergy model for patient care (abstract). *Critical Care Nurse, 28*(2), e6.

Wolak, E. S., McCann, M. F., & Madigan, C. K. (2008). Bridging the gap between the novice and expert nurse: The development of a mentoring program [Abstract]. *Critical Care Nurse, 28*(2), e23.

Wysong, P. R., & Driver, R. (2009). Patients' perceptions of nurses' skill. *Critical Care Nurse, 29*(4), 24–37.

# Theories Focused on Caring

*Joanne R. Duffy*

## Introduction

Caring is a belief or value (Watson, 1979, 1985, 1990), an intention (Duffy, 2009), a process (Swanson, 1991), and a way of being human (Roach, 1987) that enhances personhood (Boykin & Schoenhofer, 1993). When practiced authentically, it leads to feeling "cared for," a precursor to optimal health outcomes (Duffy, 2009; Duffy & Hoskins, 2003). It has been the subject of much focus in nursing for the last 30 years, having been described as the "moral ideal of nursing" (Watson, 1985, p. 29) and used to guide research, develop measurements, lead, educate, and practice professionally (Duffy, 2009; 2013). Some nurses have contended that caring is the essence of nursing (Leininger, 1984; Watson, 1979, 1985). When caring is present in the patient–nurse relationship, health outcomes are enhanced (Duffy, 2009).

Caring is a universal phenomenon that occurs in all societies and cultures (Leininger, 1978, 1991), but it is manifested most clearly in families. In the parent–child relationship, for example, parents can be observed providing both physical and emotional actions that enhance safety, promote physical growth, and encourage emotional and cognitive development in their children. According to Mayerhoff (1970), caring is essential for the attainment of human goals. Thus, caring relationships are transforming in that they facilitate human change, growth, and progress, adding meaning to life. In the parent–child relationship, parental caring actions are founded on a loving bond or connection between parent and child that assumes future advancement or expanded abilities in the children. In the patient–nurse relationship, caring actions are founded on disciplinary values and interaction strategies that provide the context for specific activities and ultimately future advancement (in terms of health outcomes).

In the context of health care, the vulnerability of persons of all ages and backgrounds creates an unusual dependency on healthcare providers (usually women) for behaviors, skills, and attitudes that engender safety, health, and general well-being. As patients try to negotiate the complex healthcare system and discover the meaning of their illness experience, expert nurses can enhance the care experience through caring relationships that advance healing and health. Caring in this instance is not just an attitude or a series of kind acts, but rather a collection of values, knowledge-based actions, and mannerisms guided by the human-to-human patient–provider relationship. It is in this relationship that the uniqueness of the patient becomes known to the nurse and the meaning of the illness experience can be fully appreciated. Caring relationships, therefore, are the medium for healthcare decisions, interventions, and, ultimately, healing and health.

According to Duffy (2013), caring relationships make patients and families feel cared for. It is this positive emotion that often stimulates patients and families to participate, learn, follow through, interact, and persist in meeting their health goals. Furthermore, nurses benefit from caring patient relationships in that they make nurses' work meaningful and satisfying, because such relationships are consistent with professional nursing values.

Caring, along with its explicit knowledge, specialized skills, and attitudes, provides the conduit for healthcare delivery. Consequently, health services grounded in caring are vital to establish the basis for ongoing interactions, accurately gather pertinent assessment data, establish relevant diagnoses, provide interventions, and ensure safe and high-quality outcomes, including satisfying experiences of care. Several theoretical frameworks and some empirical studies have linked caring relationships to improved patient care quality and work satisfaction for the provider. To better appreciate the phenomenon of caring, four theories are presented in this chapter: (1) the nurse as caring theory, (2) the theory of human caring, (3) the middle-range theory of caring, and (4) the Quality–Caring model.

## The Nursing as Caring Theory (Anne Boykin and Savina Schoenhofer)

The nursing as caring theory is considered a grand theory (Boykin & Schoenhofer, 1993) and was heavily influenced by Mayerhoff's (1970) and Gaut's (1984) philosophical and theoretical discussions of caring, Roach's (1987) five C's (compassion, competence, confidence, conscience, and commitment), and Paterson and Zderad's (1988) humanistic views of nursing. While considering the curricular infrastructure at Florida Atlantic University, Boykin and Schoenhofer (1990, 1993) carefully analyzed existing work on caring using an organizing framework that helped identify common themes and unique stances among several caring scholars. Their resulting theory was intended to be a practice theory that honors the special nature of all persons as caring. The central premise of the theory—that all persons are caring by virtue of their humanness—underlies its major concepts: personhood, the nursing situation, calls for nursing, and nursing as caring.

*Personhood* is "a process of living grounded in caring" (Schoenhofer & Boykin, 1993, p. 83) and is enhanced in "nurturing relationships with caring others" (p. 83). The *nursing situation* is the lived experience between a patient and a nurse that affects one's personhood. Each nursing situation is unique and dynamic. In this situation, the nurse brings his or her caring self and comes to know the other person as a caring human. In this nursing situation, *calls for nursing* that request specific forms of caring can be heard by the nurse. As the nurse responds to these calls, the other's unique experience and personal growth can be enhanced. In this theory, *nursing is caring*; that is, caring is the body of knowledge from which professional nursing uniquely responds to its social duty. Finally, intentionality of the nurse, defined as "consistently choosing personhood as a way of life and the aim of nursing" (Schoenhofer, 2002, p. 39), generates commitment and fuels resulting nursing actions.

The major assumptions of the nursing as care theory are summarized here:

- Persons are caring by virtue of their humanness.
- Persons are caring from moment to moment.
- Persons are whole or complete in the moment.
- Personhood is a process of living grounded in caring.
- Personhood is enhanced through participating in nurturing relationships with caring others.
- Nursing is both a discipline and a profession (Boykin & Schoenhofer, 1993).

Boykin, Schoenhofer, Smith, St. Jean's, and Aleman's (2003) view of all persons as whole or complete just as they are does not incorporate the nursing process, because it assumes some modification or change in persons is needed. Rather, these authors see nursing as "coming to know persons as caring" (p. 224) and creating caring responses that advance personhood. They view nursing as both a discipline and a profession, and the use of storytelling of the nursing situation as a form of evidence of nursing service. Other methodologies that advocate studying the phenomenon of caring in nursing include group interpretative phenomenology and research as praxis (Schoenhofer, 2002).

The nursing as caring theory has been used both in curricular design and in various implementation and research projects. For example, Boykin and Schoenhofer (2003), together with hospital-based investigators, reported the results of a project in which an 18-bed telemetry unit in a 350-bed for-profit hospital implemented the nursing as caring model. Through the use of dialog and specific practice strategies, patient and nurse satisfaction in this unit improved; lessons learned included returning to fundamental nursing values to create transformation.

Another innovative application of the theory is detailed by Bulfin (2005). A partnership between a university (Florida Atlantic University) and a community hospital (Boca Raton Community Hospital) used the nursing as caring theory to design and implement a professional practice model. Through four phases (education, understanding self, storytelling, and specific practice strategies), the model was evaluated using pre-intervention and post-intervention patient satisfaction measures. Post-satisfaction scores improved, although significance testing was not described. Qualitative approaches, such as patient letters, were also used in the evaluation of the project.

In a systems implementation of the model (Pross, Hilton, Boykin & Thomas, 2011), the process of transforming ways of relating is described as an important foundation for sustained change. Likewise, integrating caring theory into education and practice was explained through an academic service partnership where faculty members, staff, and students were exposed to and expected to practice caring together (Dyess, Boykin, & Riggs, 2010).

Although progress is being made in terms of gathering evidence related to the value of the nursing as caring theory, systematic evaluation of its benefits to both patients and nurses is warranted. Future research using qualitative methods such as focus groups, for example, could elicit the lived experience of this theory from both nurses' and patients' perspectives. Descriptive studies examining relationships between patients who receive nursing care based on the theory and nursing-sensitive outcomes are needed as well. Finally, testing specific nursing interventions grounded in the theory using quasi-experimental or experimental designs would provide evidence of its benefits.

## The Theory of Human Caring (Jean Watson)

From a strong foundation in educational counseling and psychology, Jean Watson developed the theory of human caring while designing an integrated baccalaureate curriculum in a large school of nursing (Watson, 1979). Watson's goal was to present nursing as a distinct entity, a profession, a discipline and science in its own right, separate from, but complementary to, medicine.

The theory of human caring was more formally articulated in 1985, when Watson authored the book *Nursing: Human Science and Human Care*. In this text, Watson elaborated on the caring occasion, the transpersonal nature of caring, the 10 carative factors, phenomenal fields, the influence of time (past, present, and future), and human growth—all of which are major concepts in the theory. In this theory, all persons are considered to be unique and to have a life history, including social norms and experiences, that generates a subjective reality or phenomenal field. A caring occasion occurs whenever the nurse and another person come together with their unique subjective realities, seeking to connect to each other in the present. During this moment, if the carative factors are authentically present, the relationship is considered to be transpersonal (unified body, mind, and spirit; collective consciousness; one with the universe). Through such relationships, humans grow, learn, and develop. Thus both the carer and the one being cared for benefit from the encounter (Watson, 1985).

The 10 carative factors originally considered foundational to the theory are as follows:

1. Formation of a humanistic–altruistic system of values
2. Instillation of faith and hope
3. Cultivation of sensitivity to oneself and to others
4. Development of a helping–trusting human caring relationship
5. Promotion and acceptance of the expression of both positive and negative feelings
6. Systematic use of a creative problem-solving caring process
7. Promotion of transpersonal teaching–learning
8. Provision for a supportive, protective, and/or corrective mental, physical, societal, and spiritual environment
9. Assistance with gratification of human needs
10. Allowance for existential–phenomenological–spiritual forces

Later, more spiritual and energy-related aspects of caring were articulated with heightened awareness of the nurse's intentionality and own personal evolution (Watson, 1999). Also, a sacred dimension of nursing's work with a philosophical–ethical–moral dimension was presented in Watson's (2006) book, *Caring Science as Sacred Science*. Moreover, Watson has showcased her evolving views on caring resulting from personal experiences, fresh perspectives on the convergence of transpersonal caring and unitary science theories (Watson & Smith, 2002), and metaphysical orientations. In doing so, Watson has suggested that caring is a foundational framework of all caring–healing professions and laid the groundwork for the more recent evolution to *caritas consciousness* or *clinical caritas*.

*Caritas* comes from the Greek word meaning "to cherish"; it connotes something that is very precious. Watson's wending path to this way of thinking highlights the connections between caring, spirituality, and human love. In other words, patient–nurse relationships are held in reverence and considered sacred and life enriching for both the patient and the nurse (Watson, 2002). The nurse thus embraces an expanded connectedness between the cosmic field of universal love, acknowledging the mysteries of birth, life, death, illness, and healing. Working this way allows the nurse to experience the deeper connections between the human condition and universal love. Related to this evolving theoretical stance on caring, Watson (2007) reflected, "I consider my work more a philosophical, ethical, intellectual blueprint for nursing's evolving disciplinary/professional matrix, rather than a specific theory per se" (para. 9).

A major concept in this evolved theory is the *caritas field*, which is described as a conscious healing presence founded on caring and love that profoundly changes the relational experience for nurses and patients alike (Watson, 2002). Thus, the carative factors have evolved to clinical caritas processes:

1. Embrace altruistic values and practice loving kindness with self and others.
2. Instill faith and hope and honor others.
3. Be sensitive to self and others by nurturing individual beliefs and practices.
4. Develop helping–trusting–caring relationships.
5. Promote and accept positive and negative feelings as you authentically listen to another's story.
6. Use creative scientific problem-solving methods for caring decision making.
7. Share teaching and learning that addresses individual needs and comprehension styles.
8. Create a healing environment for the physical and spiritual self that respects human dignity.
9. Assist with basic physical, emotional, and spiritual human needs.
10. Be open to mystery and allow miracles to enter (Watson, 2007).

The evolution of Watson's theory of human caring is a good example of the practical side of theory development. Changing worldviews, new insights and experiences, and evidence provided the background for new or revised concepts and relationships over the course of the theory's development. Many organizations have adopted the theory as a professional practice model, and it has been used as a foundation for measurement and research. For example, using Watson's model as the foundation, hospitals throughout the United States have integrated this theory into various patient care delivery systems (Watson & Foster, 2003). Furthermore, schools of nursing have used the model for curricular planning for teaching–learning strategies and course content (Beck, 2001; Cook & Cullen, 2003). Finally, tools to measure caring (Watson, 2009) and research studies (Erci, 2003; Smith, Kemp, Hemphill, & Vojir, 2002; Suliman, Welman, Thomas, & Omer, 2009) have used the theory as their foundation, albeit the theory of human caring as it was originally conceptualized. According to Watson (2006), research in caring embraces inquiries that are both reflective and subjective, as well as objective–empirical.

Watson's theory of caring has played a major role in helping professional nurses honor their unique and distinct values. Most recently, *Human Caring Science* (Watson, 2011) has provided a more evolved approach to guide the more mature nursing profession into the future. However, the theory does not conform to the biomedical, bureaucratic healthcare system and sometimes presents practical difficulties for nurses' work. The newly evolving theory of caritas consciousness or clinical caritas requires more evaluation in terms of its authentic application and its benefits to both patients and nurses.

## The Middle-Range Theory of Caring (Kristen Swanson)

Kristen Swanson's middle-range theory of caring was developed empirically through inductive methods while studying three groups of women. In this theory, caring is defined as "a nurturing way of relating to a valued other toward whom one feels a personal sense of commitment and responsibility" (Swanson, 1991). Using data from women who miscarried, neonatal intensive care unit caregivers (both parents and professionals), and at-risk mothers, five caring processes—maintaining belief, knowing, being with, doing for, and enabling—were described. Swanson maintained that while caring was not unique to nursing, it informed those relationships central to nursing: nurse to client, nurse to nurse, and nurse to self.

*Maintaining belief* demonstrates faith in the capacity of others and provides nurses with the foundation for the commitment to serve (both society in general and individual patients). *Knowing* refers to understanding how others' lives have meaning; it avoids assumptions and focuses on the one being cared for in order to better comprehend the client's lived reality. *Being with* incorporates emotional presence. It conveys to clients that they matter and assures them that their reality is appreciated. It includes physical presence as well as ongoing availability. *Doing for* involves nursing behaviors that preserve another's wholeness. It includes comforting, anticipating, protecting, maintaining confidentiality and dignity, interpersonal listening, teaching, coaching, referring, supporting and guiding, providing feedback, and validating the other's reality. *Enabling* implies facilitating another's capacity through providing information, being present, and sharing, and assisting behaviors.

In 1993, Swanson structured these processes such that they were ordered to influence the intended outcome—namely, client well-being. Later, Swanson (1999) completed a meta-analysis of the state of caring research. In this review of 130 empirical studies, she provided evidence of the consequences of caring and noncaring both for nurses and for patients. More importantly, she highlighted the clear significance of caring knowledge to current nursing practice and identified its implications for the nursing practice of the future.

Using knowledge of caring and the inductively developed theory of caring, Swanson set out on a program of research that focused on responses to miscarriage and interventions to promote healing subsequent to early pregnancy loss. She first tested an intervention based on her theory in a study of 242 women who had miscarried (Swanson, 1999). Using a caring-based counseling intervention, she used a randomized trial Solomon four-group design to test the intervention on several outcomes. Findings revealed that the caring intervention had a positive effect on disturbed mood, anger, and level of depression. In addition, a majority of the patients reported satisfaction with the caring intervention. Dr. Swanson followed up with a conceptual model of miscarriage (Wojner, Swanson, & Adolfsson, 2011).

Another intervention-focused study using 341 couples compared three types of couples-focused interventions to no treatment, with the goal being to identify strategies to help men and women resolve depression and grief during the first year after a miscarriage (Swanson, Chen, Graham, Wojnar, & Petras, 2009). Through this rigorous experimental design, findings revealed that overall, while participation in any of the three intervention arms accelerated women's grief resolution, their resolution of depression was best enhanced by the three nurse-led counseling sessions. Women who received three nurse counseling sessions were three to eight times more likely to see a faster decline in their symptoms of depression than women who received similar but limited help or no such help.

Swanson (2002) also developed the Caring Professional Scale to evaluate nurses' and consumers' perceptions of care received during miscarriage. Items on this instrument were derived from the five caring processes, and psychometric properties were evaluated. Despite the limitations imposed by her use of predominantly white and heterosexual samples, Swanson was able to demonstrate the benefits of caring interventions in terms of decreased depression, improved mood, less anger, and intervention satisfaction for persons who had experienced a pregnancy loss. Continued study with more diverse samples and efficiency measures would greatly advance this program of research.

The middle-range theory of caring is used to guide practice and curricula internationally, and Swanson continues to develop and refine the theory through ongoing research. For example, recently, the caring theory was implemented in a large health system and improvements were noted in patient and nurse satisfaction levels, patient pain, and response to call lights (Tonges & Ray, 2011). Dr. Swanson's persistence in testing, applying, and validating the theory provides an exemplary model for future researchers.

## The Quality–Caring Model (Joanne R. Duffy)

Developed in 2003 to fill a perceived practice and research void, the Quality–Caring Model was informed by earlier experiences with hospitalized patients who verbalized, "Nurses don't seem to care." In her experience with acutely ill hospitalized adults, Duffy observed that the foundational caring behaviors, skills, and attitudes of professional nursing had been marginalized as the emphasis in modern health care shifted to procedures and tasks, technology, and cost containment. This incongruity between professional values and behaviors was considered serious because it was linked to health outcomes, as well as to the work satisfaction and motivation of professional nurses. Going beyond the limitations of the patient–nurse relationship, Duffy also studied the influence of nurse–physician relationships on patient outcomes while participating in the national APACHE study of intensive care units (Zimmerman et al., 1993).

Corroborated by the literature on noncaring, Duffy set out to narrow the gap between professional values and professional practice and to improve patient outcomes by studying the linkage between nurse caring and quality care. After developing the Caring Assessment Tool (CAT) to measure patients' perceptions of caring, Duffy (1992) used this instrument to conduct a correlational study that linked nurse caring to patient satisfaction. The CAT was later adapted to assess staff nurses' perceptions of nurse managers' caring (CAT-adm), where findings demonstrated a positive relationship between nurse manager caring behaviors and staff nurse satisfaction (Duffy, 1993).

In the process of developing a caring-based nursing intervention for heart failure patients (Duffy, Hoskins, & Dudley-Brown, 2005), Duffy was struck by the lack of attention in the literature to the quality–caring link. Working with Dr. Lois Hoskins, she developed the Quality–Caring Model to guide their research. This model is considered middle range and deductive, drawing heavily on the works of Watson (1979, 1985); King (1981); Donabedian (1966); Mitchell, Ferketich, & Jennings (1988); and Irvine, Sidani, & Hall (1998). It was designed to "expose the hidden value of nursing" and support the connections between nurse caring and quality health outcomes. Participants, caring relationships, feeling cared for, and health represent the major concepts in this model. *Participants* include the individuals involved in the healthcare experience and can be identified as patients, providers, or the system (the organization) itself. Individuals are considered unique bio-psycho-socio-cultural-spiritual beings who possess characteristics (certain descriptive features), attitudes and behaviors, and life experiences. Individuals' subjective reality or phenomenal field is believed to influence the meaning of their experiences, including health and illness.

*Caring relationships* are human interactions grounded in caring factors—specific activities (doing), as well as specific attitudes (being with). Caring behaviors require specialized knowledge, attitudes, and behaviors that are directed toward health and healing. The model holds that caring relationships established with patients and families are independent functions that are implemented autonomously, and for which nurses are solely held accountable. Collaborative relationships, in contrast, are multidisciplinary in nature and include those activities and responsibilities that nurses share with other members of the healthcare team. Collaborative relationships are enhanced when mutual partnerships exist among the various professionals and are focused on the best interests of patients and their families. Such partnerships ensure that continuity is maintained and that patients and families, as well as team members, feel cared for. These three-way encounters are relationship centered when they are grounded in caring processes or factors.

Caring behaviors require specialized knowledge, attitudes, and behaviors that are directed toward an individual for the purposes of health and healing. A consequence of caring relationships, as espoused in the Quality–Caring Model, is feeling *cared for*. This emotion is important because it is associated with contentment, met needs, acceptance, and validation (Duffy & Hoskins, 2003). As individuals perceive being cared for by their healthcare providers, they experience ease, protection from harm, and maintenance of their human dignity. In this state,

"a sense of security develops that makes it easier to learn new things, change behaviors, take risks, and follow guidelines" (Duffy & Hoskins, 2003, p. 83). The
sense of feeling cared for is considered an antecedent to self-advancement, particularly to nursing-sensitive outcomes such as increased knowledge, safety, comfort, decreased anxiety, maintenance of human dignity, and positive experiences
of care. Self-advancing systems in this model are closely related to quality and are
multidimensional, dynamic, and holistic. Blending measurable health outcomes
with the unique caring relationships central to daily nursing practice represents
a practical, postmodern approach. Thus, this model emphasizes the centrality of
caring relationships and provides a practical way to generate evidence of its value.

In 2009, Duffy revised the Quality–Caring Model to reflect the more complex, interdependent nature of health systems. Drawing on complexity theory,
the model begins by illustrating the complex relationships that are continuously
evolving in health care through multiple, ongoing reciprocal interactions. In this
way of thinking, relationships are considered interdependent. When allowed to
develop, they naturally reveal how systems advance, even in changing conditions.
In this revised version of the model, four such relationships are considered necessary for quality caring (see **Figure 21–1**). The overarching concept, humans in
relationships, refers to the multidimensional nature of humans as they exist in
relation to themselves and their communities. The relationship with self includes

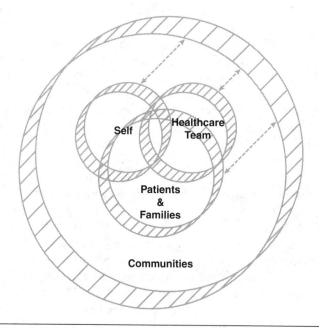

**FIGURE 21–1   Four relationships essential to quality caring.**
*Source: Quality caring in nursing and health systems: Implications for clinicians, educators, and leaders,*
(2nd ed.) Joanne R. Duffy, PhD, RN, FAAN. (2013). Reproduced with the permission of Springer Publishing
Company, LLC ISBN: 9780826110145. Adapted from Figure 4.2 – "Fundamental Relationships in the
Quality–Caring Model."

accessing the inner wisdom drawn from practice and using this guidance to know and value the self as a prerequisite for engaging in caring interactions. Caring relationships with communities build the capacity to address challenges and contribute to the welfare and development of community members, including nurses themselves. Furthermore, when nurses are involved professionally in their communities, they derive added meaning from their work.

During healthcare encounters, nurses' relationships with patients and families are considered to be the primary and uniquely discipline-specific relationship in the model. Using eight caring factors preliminarily validated through research (Duffy, Hoskins, & Seifert, 2007), nurses cultivate authentic mutually reciprocal interactions with patients and families that inform future interactions and contribute to health outcomes. It also is hypothesized that caring relationships with patients and families benefit nurses in terms of the latter's professional growth and work satisfaction.

> The caring factors, namely, mutual problem-solving, attentive reassurance, human respect, encouraging manner, healing environment, appreciation of unique meanings, affiliation needs, and basic human needs are fundamental and unique to the revised Quality–Caring Model because, although derived from theory, they have been preliminarily validated (Duffy, Hoskins, & Seifert, 2007). These factors, when applied expertly and over time, lead to "feeling cared for" in the recipient. (Duffy, 2009, p. 196)

Relationships with other members of the healthcare team are essential to the revised model, given that high-quality outcomes are enhanced when multiple healthcare providers work together as a team.

Other concepts in the revised model include relationship-centered professional encounters, feeling cared for, and self-advancing systems, expressed as dynamic positive progress that enhances a system's well-being (Duffy, 2009, p. 196). Self-advancing systems are considered quality systems because they enhance well-being and positive growth.

Assumptions of the revised Quality–Caring Model (see **Figure 21–2**) include the following:

- Humans are multidimensional beings capable of growth and change.
- Humans exist in relation to themselves, others, communities or groups, nature (or the environment), and the universe.
- Humans evolve over time and in space.
- Humans are inherently worthy.
- Caring is embedded in the daily work of nursing.
- Caring is a tangible concept that can be measured.
- Caring relationships benefit both the carer and the one being cared for.
- Caring relationships benefit society.
- Caring is done "in relationship."
- Feeling "cared for" is a positive emotion (Duffy, 2009, pp. 197–198).

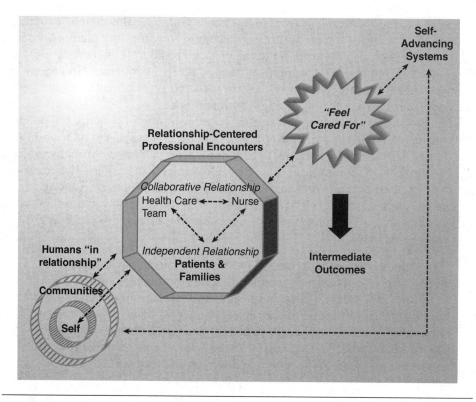

**FIGURE 21–2  Revised quality-caring model.**

*Source: Quality caring in nursing: Applying theory to clinical practice, education, and leadership* by Duffy, Joanne. Reproduced with permission of Springer Publishing Company Inc. in the format Republish in a book via Copyright Clearance Center.

Additionally, Duffy has advanced several propositions:

- Human caring capacity can be developed.
- Feeling "cared for" is an antecedent to self-advancing systems.
- Self-advancing systems are naturally self-caring or self-healing.
- Relationships characterized as caring contribute to individual, group, and system self-advancement (Duffy, 2009).

The revised Quality–Caring Model shifts the primary focus of professional nursing to a perspective characterized by relationships. Duffy offers specific responsibilities for the professional nurse (see **Table 21–1**) and suggests that "the clinical nurse of the future will be admired as an essential member of the health care workforce and will be included in important health care decisions" (Duffy, 2009, p. 203).

In 2013, the Quality-Caring Model was again revised (Duffy, 2013) in light of the larger health system. In this incarnation, nurses are urged to create value in health systems through caring relationships. Aspects of the model are presented more in depth and nurses are asked to work interprofessionally using caring relationships to lead the health system into the future.

**Table 21–1 Specific Responsibilities of the Professional Nurse**

- Attain and continuously advance knowledge and expertise in the caring factors
- Initiate, cultivate, and sustain caring relationships with patients and families
- Initiate, cultivate, and sustain caring relationships with other nurses and all members of the healthcare team
- Maintain an awareness of the patient's and family's points of view
- Carry on self-caring activities, including personal and professional development
- Integrate caring relationships with specific evidenced-based nursing interventions to positively influence health
- Advance quality health care through research and continuous improvement
- Using the expertise of caring relationships embedded in nursing, actively participate in community groups
- Recognize that feeling "cared for" influences the attainment of intermediate and terminal health outcomes
- Recognize that self-advancement is a nonlinear, complex process that emerges over time and in space
- Recognize that self-advancing systems are naturally self-caring or self-healing
- Acknowledge that relationships characterized as caring contribute to individual, group, and system self-advancement
- Contribute to the knowledge of caring and, ultimately, the profession of nursing using all forms of knowing
- Maintain an open, flexible approach

*Source*: Duffy, J. (2009). *Quality caring in nursing: Applying theory to clinical practice, education, and leadership*. New York, NY: Springer Publishing. Reproduced with permission of the Springer Publishing Company Inc. in the format Republish in a book via Copyright Clearance Center.

In the context of advanced nursing practice, the Quality–Caring Model accounts for the complexity of healthcare systems and honors the vital role that caring relationships play in advancing quality and reducing costs. This offers a strong basis for practice that can assist in the development of relevant organizational processes and procedures. The doctor of nursing practice graduate, for example, may be involved in translating model concepts into clinical practice, use the model to guide clinical decision making, generate and evaluate evidence of the model's value (in terms of patient outcomes), implement clinical innovations (derived from the model) that change practice, and work with others in caring ways (use the caring factors) to change individual and team behavior or impact organizational-level change. For example, advanced practice nurses may use team rounding as a forum to facilitate clinical decisions based on the model (perhaps including the patient in the decision) and present this as a learning tool to others. Another example is the creation of an innovative method for assessing discharge readiness (drawing on model concepts) that could be evaluated for its success in reducing 30-day readmission rates.

The Quality–Caring Model, based on its unique concepts and propositions, could also be used as the foundation for research or evaluation projects. For example, the CAT (Duffy, Brewer, & Weaver, 2010) is a valid and reliable 27-item instrument that measures patients' perceptions of caring relationships, providing a unique view of patient-centered care. Using the CAT, advanced practice nurses can correlate caring relationships with nursing-sensitive outcome indicators in their institutions, or measure longitudinal success of Quality–Caring implementation projects, evaluate health professionals' caring competence, and benchmark their organizations with others to improve quality. Recently, an electronic version of the CAT (the e-CAT) was used with hospitalized older adults to evaluate patient-centered care during hospitalization (Duffy, Kooken, Wolverton, & Weaver, 2012). In this pilot study, older adults expressed a preference for this way of evaluating their care; they were able to use the technology with little assistance. The e-CAT may now provide the opportunity to assess patient–provider relationships in real time and result in actionable practice changes. In fact, this measure could easily be incorporated into user-friendly information systems to transform quality improvement activities.

In the direct care role, a nurse with advanced education may use the Quality–Caring Model to role-model self-caring; complete systematic and holistic assessments of individuals, communities, or systems; cultivate and sustain caring relationships with patients and families; educate patients and families; make clinical decisions; and advance collaborative relationships with other health professionals. The model provides a guide for self-caring that includes remaining more aware (or mindful) as a particularly healthy way to work that deepen a nurse's ability to be present for patients and families. In fact, health professionals need to acknowledge and allow themselves to experience the feelings associated with their work, including suffering. Duffy asserts that this form of self-caring may be a necessary antecedent to caring for others. When role-modeled by advanced practice nurses, others may begin to incorporate such practices of their own.

Currently, more than 40 U.S. hospitals are using the Quality–Caring Model as the basis for practice, and several have developed unique patient care delivery systems based on this model. Duffy continues her research on caring relationships, most recently designing an intervention to improve the delivery of patient-centered care in hospitalized older adults. In this intervention, Duffy designed a unit-level intervention in which education, a technology-enhanced quality improvement program, and regular group reflection is integrated into clinical workflow (nursing work). In addition, she has developed a model of interprofessional collaboration for vulnerable populations. Duffy offered a series of suggestions for education, ongoing research, and leadership to support clinical practice in her latest text (Duffy, 2013). More evaluation of the Quality–Caring Model is needed in diverse populations using specific nursing-sensitive and cost-efficiency outcomes measures.

# Conclusion

No one universal theoretical approach to caring in nursing exists. In fact, two of the theories presented in this chapter use a philosophical/ethical approach (Boykin and Schoenhofer; Watson), one was developed inductively (Swanson), and one was developed deductively (Duffy). Each of these theories incorporates unique concepts, yet all share commonalities to some extent. Specifically, the relationship nature of caring, patient well-being, and some benefit to nurses are features found in all of the theories reviewed in this chapter.

Professional practice models founded on these theories are now being used on a widespread basis, and nursing students at all levels are being exposed to the theories. Advanced practice nurses are now in positions where they can make real contributions to evaluating the evidence for these theoretical perspectives (in terms of improved quality and reduced costs). Included in this evaluation are assessments of barriers and facilitators to their implementation, as well as specific interventions that can accelerate, change, improve, and sustain the use of caring theories in practice. Practicing nurses, educators, other health professionals, and those in leadership and policy positions are beginning to appreciate the relational aspect of health care and are demanding approaches that incorporate caring relationships to advance high-value health outcomes.

## Discussion Questions

1. Reflect on the vital nature of caring in health care. What are your thoughts?

2. Which sorts of knowledge, skills, and attitudes are required for caring professional practice?

3. How does the concept of personhood as used in the nursing as caring model (Boykin) relate to nurses?

4. Describe the evolution of the carative factors to clinical caritas processes (Watson).

5. Describe the systematic process used in the development and validation of the middle-range theory of caring (Swanson).

6. Which theoretical contributions were used in the development of the Quality–Caring Model?

7. What are the assumptions and major propositions of the Quality–Caring Model?

8. Reflect on the many interdependent relationships that exist in complex health systems. How do they shape these systems?

9. Describe a situation in which you cultivated a caring interprofessional relationship. What happened? What was your role? What did you learn from this experience?

10. As a nurse, how do you come to know the patient and his or her unique experience of illness?

11. As an advanced practice nurse, how do you role model self-caring?

12. How would you advise professional nurses to better incorporate caring relationships in their practice? Which strengths can you bring to help address the importance of caring relationships? How would you evaluate this effort?

13. How does a new graduate experience caring relationships at your institution? How does this affect caring professional practice?

14. Which continuing education activities at your institution promote quality caring?

15. Develop three evaluation questions based on one of the models presented in this chapter. What will you do with these questions?

# References

Beck, C. T. (2001). Caring within nursing education: A metasynthesis. *Journal of Nursing Education, 40,* 101–109.

Boykin, A., & Schoenhofer, S. O. (1990). Caring in nursing: Analysis of extant theory. *Nursing Science Quarterly, 4,* 149–155.

Boykin, A., & Schoenhofer, S. O. (1993). *Nursing as caring: A model for transforming practice.* New York, NY: National League for Nursing.

Boykin, A., Schoenhofer, S. O., Smith, N., St. Jean, J., & Aleman, D. (2003). Transforming practice using a caring-based nursing model. *Nursing Administration Quarterly, 27*(3), 223–230.

Bulfin, S. (2005). Nursing as caring theory: Living caring in practice. *Nursing Science Quarterly, 18*(4), 313–319.

Cook, P. R., & Cullen, J. A. (2003). Caring as an imperative for nursing education. *Nursing Education Perspectives, 24*(4), 192–197.

Donabedian, A. (1966). Evaluating the quality of medical care. *Milbank Memorial Fund Quarterly, 44*(Part 2), 166–203.

Duffy, J. (1992). The impact of nurse caring on patient outcomes. In D. Gaut (Ed.), *The presence of caring in nursing* (pp. 113–136). New York, NY: National League for Nursing Press.

Duffy, J. (1993). Caring behaviors of nurse managers: Relationships to staff nurse satisfaction and retention. In D. Gaut (Ed.), *Caring: A global agenda* (pp. 365–377). New York, NY: National League for Nursing Press.

Duffy, J. (2009). *Quality caring in nursing: Applying theory to clinical practice, education, and leadership.* New York, NY: Springer.

Duffy, J. (2013). *Quality caring in nursing and health systems: Applying theory to clinical practice, education, and leadership* (2nd ed.). New York, NY: Springer.

Duffy, J., Brewer, B., & Weaver, M. (2010). Revision and psychometric properties of the Caring Assessment Tool. *Clinical Nursing Research.* doi:10.1177/1054773810369827

Duffy, J., & Hoskins, L. (2003). The Quality–Caring Model: Blending dual paradigms. *Advances in Nursing Science, 26*(1), 77–88.

Duffy, J., Hoskins, L., & Dudley-Brown, S. (2005). Development and testing of a caring-based intervention for older adults with heart failure. *Journal of Cardiovascular Nursing, 20*(3), 1–9.

Duffy, J., Hoskins, L. M., & Seifert, R. F. (2007). Dimensions of caring: Psychometric properties of the Caring Assessment Tool. *Advances in Nursing Science, 30*(3), 235–245.

Duffy, J., Kooken, W., Wolverton, C., & Weaver, M. T. (2012). Evaluating patient-centered care: Feasibility of electronic data collection in hospitalized older adults. *Journal of Nursing Care Quality, 27*(4), 307–315.

Dyess, S., Boykin, A., & Riggs, C. (2010). Integrating caring theory with nursing practice and education: Connecting with what matters. *Journal of Nursing Administration, 40*(11), 498–503.

Erci, B. (2003). The effectiveness of Watson's caring model on the quality of life and blood pressure of patients with hypertension. *Journal of Advanced Nursing, 41*(2), 1–10.

Gaut, D. (1984). A theoretic description of caring as action. In M. Leininger (Ed.), *Care: The essence of nursing and health* (pp. 27–44). Thorofare, NJ: Charles B. Slack.

King, I. M. (1981). *A theory of nursing: Systems, concepts, process.* New York, NY: Wiley.

Irvine, D. M., Sidani, S., & Hall, L. M. (1998). Linking outcomes to nurses' roles in health care. *Nursing Economics, 16*(2), 58–64.

Leininger, M. (1978). *Transcultural nursing: Concepts, theories, practices.* New York, NY: Wiley.

Leininger, M. M. (1984). Caring is nursing: Understanding the meaning, importance, and issues. In M. M. Leininger (Ed.), *Care: The essence of nursing and health* (pp. 83–93). Thorofare, NJ: Charles B. Slack.

Leininger, M. M. (1991). *Culture care diversity and universality: A theory of nursing.* New York, NY: National League for Nursing Press.

Mayerhoff, M. (1970). *On caring.* New York, NY: Harper & Row.

Mitchell, P., Ferketich, S., & Jennings, B. M. (1998). American Academy of Nursing Expert Panel on Quality Health Care: Quality health outcomes model. *Journal of Nursing Scholarship, 30*(1), 43–46.

Paterson, J., & Zderad, L. (1988). *Humanistic nursing* (2nd ed.). New York, NY: National League for Nursing.

Pross, E., Hilton, N., Boykin, A., & Thomas, C. (2011). The dance of caring persons. *Nursing Management, 42*(10), 25–30.

Roach, S. (1987). *The human act of caring.* Ottawa, Canada: Canadian Hospital Association.

Schoenhofer, S. O. (2002). Choosing personhood: Intentionality and choosing nursing as caring. *Holistic Nursing Practice, 14*(4), 36–40.

Schoenhofer, S., & Boykin, A. (1993). Nursing as caring: An emerging general theory of nursing. In M. E. Parker, *Patterns of nursing theories in practice* (pp. 83–102). New York, NY: National League for Nursing.

Smith, M. C., Kemp, J., Hemphill, L., & Vojir, C. (2002). Outcomes of massage therapy for cancer patients. *Journal of Nursing Scholarship, 34*(3), 257–262.

Suliman, W., Welman, E., Thomas, L., & Omer T. (2009). Applying Watson's nursing theory to assess patient perception of being cared for in a multicultural environment *Journal of Nursing Research, 17*(4), 293–300.

Swanson, K. (1991). Empirical development of a middle range theory of caring. *Nursing Research, 40*(3), 161–166.

Swanson, K. (1993). Nursing as informed caring for the well-being of others. *Image: The Journal of Nursing Scholarship, 25*(4), 352–357.

Swanson, K. (1999). Effects of caring, measurement, and time on miscarriage impact and women's well-being. *Nursing Research, 48*(6), 288–298.

Swanson, K. M. (2002). Caring Professional Scale. In J. Watson (Ed.), *Assessing and measuring caring in nursing and health science* (pp. 203–206). New York, NY: Springer.

Swanson, K. M., Chen, H. T., Graham, J. C., Wojnar, D. M., & Petras, A. (2009). Resolution of depression and grief during the first year after miscarriage: A randomized controlled clinical trial of couples-focused interventions. *Journal of Women's Health, 18*(8), 1245–1257.

Tonges, M., & Ray, J. (2011). Translating caring theory into practice: The Carolina Care Model. *Journal of Nursing Administration, 41*(9), 374–381.

Watson, J. (1979). *Nursing: The philosophy and science of caring.* Boston, MA: Little, Brown.

Watson, J. (1985). *Nursing: Human science and human care.* Norwalk, CT: Appleton-Century.

Watson, J. (1990). Caring knowledge and informed moral passion. *Advances in Nursing Science, 13*(1), 15–24.

Watson, J. (1999). *Postmodern nursing and beyond.* Toronto, Canada: Churchill Livingstone.

Watson, J. (2002). *Instruments for assessing and measuring caring in nursing and health sciences.* New York, NY: Springer.

Watson, J. (2006). *Caring science as sacred science.* Philadelphia, PA: F. A. Davis.

Watson, J. (2007). Ten Caritas Processes. Retrieved from http://watsoncaringscience.org/about-us/caring-science-definitions-processes-theory/

Watson, J. (2009). *Assessing and measuring caring in nursing and health science* (2nd ed.). New York, NY: Springer.

Watson, J. (2011). *Human caring science: A theory of nursing.* Sudbury, MA: Jones & Bartlett Learning.

Watson, J., & Foster, R. (2003). The attending nurse caring model: Integrating theory, evidence and advanced caring–healing therapeutics for transforming professional practice. *Journal of Clinical Nursing, 12,* 360–365.

Watson, J., & Smith, M. (2002). Transpersonal caring science and the science of unitary human beings: A transtheoretical discourse for nursing knowledge development. *International Journal of Advanced Nursing, 37*(5), 452–461.

Wojnar, D. M., Swanson, K. M., & Adolfsson, A. S. (2011). Confronting the inevitable: A conceptual model of miscarriage for use in clinical practice and research. *Death Studies, 35*(6), 536–558.

Zimmerman, J., Shortell, S., Rousseau, D., Duffy, J., Gillies, R., Knaus, W., . . . Draper, E. A. (1993). Improving intensive care: Observations based on organizational case studies in nine intensive units: A prospective, multicenter study. *Critical Care Medicine, 21*(10), 1443–1451.

# Models and Theories Focused on Culture

*Larry Purnell*

## Introduction

This chapter provides an overview of selected cultural models and theories commonly used in nursing practice, education, administration, and research. Although the main focus of this chapter is the Purnell model for cultural competence, other models and theories are also described. Some of these cultural models are not intended for research, but they have value when used in education, practice, and administration. Advanced practice nurses (APNs) have preparation in all of these areas and use cultural models, theories, and approaches accordingly. Exemplars are given for cultural models and theories that have been used in nursing and healthcare research.

## Overview of Cultural Models and Theories

Many differing definitions and meanings of theory exist both within and outside of the nursing profession. Theory is not reality; it is abstract and complex and must be so that research can be generated to guide practice. According to Fawcett and DeSanto-Madeya (2012), theory is one or more relatively concrete and abstract concepts that are derived from a conceptual model, the propositions that describe those concepts, and the propositions that state specific relationships between two or more of the concepts. A theory can be grand or middle range, depending on its level and scope. Moreover, a theory must have (1) a purpose; (2) concepts that are systematically linked, defined, and interconnect the ideas of the theory; and (3) explicit and implicit assumptions. Nursing theory, of which there are four levels—metatheory, grand theory, middle-range theory, and practice theory—comprises either one or a combination of the following four types:

1. *Descriptive theory* identifies properties and components of a discipline, identifies meaning and observations, and describes which elements exist.
2. *Explanatory theory* identifies how the properties and components relate to one another and accounts for the functions of the discipline.
3. *Predictive theory* conjectures the relationships between the components of a phenomenon and predicts under which conditions the phenomena will occur.
4. *Prescriptive theory* addresses therapeutics and consequences of interventions (Fawcett & DeSanto-Madeya, 2012).

Because there is no agreement in the scientific community regarding the definitions of a conceptual model, conceptual framework, theoretical model, and theoretical framework, these terms are used interchangeably in this chapter. A *conceptual model* can be represented by words, diagrams, or pictures. Each theoretical/ conceptual model or theory is evaluated based on its clarity, simplicity, generality, empirical precision, and derivable consequences. Clarity is concerned with the logical and adequate arrangements of constructs and concepts. Simplicity is concerned with the number and complexity of concepts in the model. Generality is concerned with how the model or theory can be useful to APNs. Empirical precision is concerned with the ability of the model or theory to hold up over time. Derivable consequences refer to how practical and useful the theory or model is in relation to achieving important health outcomes (Purnell, 2000a).

Given the increasing complexity of culture, faculty in continuing education and schools of nursing are frequently looking for resources for teaching culture along with evidence-based materials. A few resources are the textbook by Jeffreys (2010), the American Association of Colleges of Nursing's (AACN's) Toolkit for Cultural Competent Education (2008), the AACN's doctor of nursing practice essentials (2009), and the Purnell textbook website. In addition, the American Academy of Nursing, along with members of the Transcultural Nursing Society, established a task force to develop standards of practice for culturally competent nursing care (Douglas et al., 2011).

The content of this chapter is not focused on the numerous simplistic approaches that use acronyms as a guide for cultural assessment. Although some of these simplistic techniques can be used for collecting initial interview data, they do not work well with all ethnic and cultural groups, nor are they comprehensive. Two examples of acronymic approaches are BATHE and LEARN. The LEARN approach includes the following guidelines: **L**isten to your patients from their perspectives; **E**xplain your concerns and your reasons for asking for personal information; **A**cknowledge your patients' concerns; **R**ecommend a course of action; and **N**egotiate a plan of care that considers cultural norms and personal lifestyles

(Berlin & Fowkes, 1983). The BATHE acronym stands for Background information, Affect [sic] the problem has on the patient, Trouble the problem causes for the patient, Handling of the problem by the patient, and Empathy conveyed by the healthcare provider (McCullough, Ramesar, & Peterson, 1998).

## Essential Terminology Related to Culture

Many different definitions exist for culturally related terms. Most of the definitions used in this chapter were created by the Expert Panel on Cultural Competence of the American Academy of Nursing (Giger, Davidhizar, Purnell, Harden, Phillips, & Strickland, 2007). These definitions were developed in an attempt to reach a standard worldwide consensus and thereby decrease confusion related to the inconsistent definitions of culture-related terms. The confusion arises because a variety of terms and definitions that describe cultural awareness, cultural sensitivity, and cultural competence are used interchangeably in the literature. They have been presented in several international conferences. A few of these definitions are listed here:

- *Cultural awareness* is being knowledgeable about one's own thoughts, feelings, and sensations and having an appreciation of diversity in terms of the objective (material) culture, such as arts, clothing, foods, and other external signs of diversity.
- *Cultural sensitivity* is experienced when neutral language, both verbal and nonverbal, is used in a way that reflects sensitivity and appreciation for the diversity of another. Cultural sensitivity is conveyed through words, phrases, and categorizations that are intentionally avoided, especially when referring to an individual who may interpret them as impolite or offensive.
- *Cultural imposition* intrusively applies the majority cultural view to individuals and families. An example of this is prescribing a special diet without regard to a person's culture and limiting visitors to immediate family border on cultural imposition. In this context, healthcare providers must be careful in expressing their cultural values too strongly until cultural issues are more fully understood.
- *Cultural imperialism* is the practice of extending the policies and procedure of one organization—usually the dominant one—to disenfranchised and minority groups. Proponents of cultural imperialism appeal to universal human rights values and standards. Opponents posit that universal standards are a guise under which the dominant culture seeks to destroy or eradicate traditional cultures by setting worldwide public policy.
- *Cultural relativism* is the belief that behaviors and practices of people should be judged only in the context of their cultural system. Proponents argue that issues such as abortion, euthanasia, female circumcision, and physical punishment in childrearing should be accepted as cultural values without judgment from the outside world. Opponents argue that cultural

relativism may undermine condemnation of human rights violations and that family violence cannot be justified or excused on a cultural basis.

- *Ethnocentrism* is a universal tendency to believe that one's own worldview is superior to another's worldview. It is often experienced in the healthcare arena, in particular when the healthcare provider's own culture or ethnic group is considered superior to another.
- *Stereotype* encompasses a simplified and standardized conception, opinion, or belief about a person or group. A healthcare provider who fails to recognize individuality within a group is jumping to conclusions about the individual or family.
- *Generalization* begins with assumptions about the individual or family within an ethnocultural group but leads to further information seeking about the individual or family.
- *Race* is a viable term that relates to biology but also has sociological implications. Members of a particular race share distinguishing physical features such as skin color, bone structure, or blood group. Race as a social construct can limit or increase opportunities, depending on the setting.
- *Racism* refers to feelings of prejudice against persons of another race or group of people. Racist practices lead to interpersonal tension, isolation, discrimination, and overt anger.
- An *ethnic group* is a group of people whose members have different experiences and backgrounds from the dominant culture in terms of status, background, residence, religion, education, or other factors that functionally unify the group and act collectively in their effects.
- *Stigma* is a characteristic or trait that puts a strain on or reproaches a group or individual's reputation or being.
- *Culture* is a learned, patterned behavioral response acquired over time that includes implicit versus explicit beliefs, attitudes, values, customs, norms, taboos, arts, and life ways accepted by a community of individuals. Culture is primarily learned and transmitted through the family and other social organizations, is shared by the majority of the group, includes an individualized worldview, guides decision making, and influences self-worth and self-esteem.

## Cultural Self-Awareness

Culture has a powerful unconscious impact on both patients and health professionals (Purnell, 2013). Each clinical encounter with an APN adds a unique dimension to the complexity of providing culturally competent care. The way APNs perceive themselves as competent is often reflected in the way they communicate with clients. Thus, it is essential for APNs to take time to think about themselves, their behaviors, and their communication styles in relation to their perceptions of different cultures.

Before addressing the multicultural backgrounds and unique individual perspectives of their patients, APNs must first address their own personal and professional knowledge, values, beliefs, ethics, and life experiences in a manner that optimizes assessment of and interactions with clients who come from cultures different from those of the APN. Self-awareness in cultural competence is a deliberate and conscious cognitive and emotional process of getting to know oneself; one's own personality, values, beliefs, professional knowledge, standards, and ethics; and the effects of these factors on the various roles one plays when interacting with individuals who are different from oneself. The ability to understand oneself sets the stage for integrating new knowledge related to cultural differences into the APN's knowledge base and perceptions of health interventions (Purnell, 2013).

# Selected Cultural Models and Theories

The limited space available here does not permit an exhaustive description of the numerous models and theories centered on culture. A brief description of the models most commonly used in practice, education, administration, and research follows. A more thorough description of the Purnell model for cultural competence is described in detail in the next section.

## The Campinha-Bacote Model

The Campinha-Bacote model is a practice model that was originally developed in 1991. It has been revised several times since then. It focuses on the process of cultural competence in the delivery of healthcare services. This model, which is currently referred to as a *volcano model* (Campinha-Bacote, 2011), is used primarily in practice and education; it does not have an accompanying organizational framework. In fact, a literature review did not reveal any research using the Campinha-Bacote model.

According to Campinha-Bacote (2011), individuals, as well as organizations and institutions, begin the journey to cultural competence by first demonstrating an intrinsic motivation to engage in the process of cultural competence. The five concepts in this model are described as follows:

1. *Cultural awareness.* The nurse becomes sensitive to the values, beliefs, lifestyle, and practices of the patient, and explores his or her own values, biases, and prejudices. Unless nurses go through this process in a conscious, deliberate, and reflective manner, there is always the risk of nurses imposing their own cultural values during the encounter.
2. *Cultural knowledge.* Cultural knowledge is the process through which nurses find out more about other cultures and the different worldviews held by people from other cultures. Understanding the values, beliefs, practices, and problem-solving strategies of culturally/ethnically diverse groups enables nurses to gain confidence in their cultural encounters.

3. *Cultural skill.* Cultural skill as a process is concerned with carrying out a cultural assessment. Based on cultural knowledge, nurses are able to conduct an assessment in partnership with patients.
4. *Cultural encounter.* Cultural encounter is the process that provides the primary and experiential exposure to cross-cultural interactions with people who are culturally/ethnically diverse from oneself.
5. *Cultural desire.* Cultural desire is a self-motivational aspect of individuals and organizations that encourages them to want to engage in the process of cultural competence.

Campinha-Bacote has emphasized that a cultural assessment is needed for every client, because every person has values, beliefs, and practices that must be considered when the nurse is delivering healthcare services. Therefore, cultural assessments should not be limited to specific ethnic groups, but rather conducted with each patient (Campinha-Bacote, 2011). Although this model does not have an assessment guide, it does meet the criteria for simplicity, clarity, generality, and empirical precision. A graphical display and additional information about the Campinha-Bacote model can be found at the Transcultural C.A.R.E. Associates website (http://www.transculturalcare.net).

## The Giger and Davidhizar Model

The transcultural assessment model developed by Giger & Davidhizar (2002; Geiger, 2012) focuses on assessment and intervention from a transcultural nursing perspective. In this model, each person is seen as a unique cultural being influenced by culture, ethnicity, and religion. The model has been used in education, practice, administration, and research. The six areas of human diversity and variation in the model are described as follows:

1. *Communication.* The factors that influence communication are universal, but they vary among culture-specific groups in terms of language spoken, voice quality, pronunciation, and use of nonverbal communication, including silence.
2. *Space.* People perceive physical and personal space through their biological senses. The cultural aspect of space reflects the degree of comfort one feels in proximity to others, in body movement, and in perception of personal, intimate, and public space.
3. *Social orientation.* Components of social organization vary by culture, with differences observed in what constitutes one's understanding of culture, race, ethnicity, family role and function, work, leisure, church, and friends in day-to-day life.
4. *Time.* Time is perceived, measured, and valued differently across cultures. Time is conceptualized in reference to the life span in terms of growth and development, perception of time in relation to duration of events, and time as an external entity outside of an individual's control.

5. *Environmental control.* Environment is more than just the place where one lives; it involves systems and processes that influence, and are influenced by, individuals and groups. Culture influences the understanding of how individuals and groups shape their environments and how environments constrain or enable individual health behaviors.
6. *Biological variations.* Biological variations include dimensions such as body structure, body weight, skin color, and internal biological mechanisms such as genetic and enzymatic predisposition to certain diseases, drug interactions, and metabolism.

The Giger and Davidhizar model proposes a framework that facilitates assessment of the individual. A set of questions is constructed under each of the six areas to generate information useful in planning care that is congruent with an individual's cultural orientation and needs. The model also represents a learning tool that can be used to explore issues about any of the six broad areas in practice. For nurses, flexibility and the involvement of the patient as an equal partner in the cultural assessment of needs are encouraged. The Giger and Davidhizar model can be used to elicit general explanatory models of health and illness. It meets the criteria for clarity, simplicity, generality, empirical precision, and derivable consequences (Giger & Davidhizar, 2002).

## The Papadopoulos, Tilki, and Taylor Model

The Papadopoulos, Tilki, and Taylor model—which focuses on the process of cultural competence in the delivery of healthcare services—was first published in 1998 and is used in education, practice, and administration. This model does not have an assessment guide or organizing framework. The four main components of this model are described as follows (Leonardo da Vinci Partnership Project, 2012):

1. *Cultural awareness.* Cultural awareness represents the first step toward cultural competence. It incorporates self-awareness, cultural identity, cultural adherence, ethnocentricity, stereotyping, and ethnohistory.
2. *Cultural knowledge.* Cultural knowledge is the second step toward cultural competence. It includes health beliefs and behaviors; anthropological, sociopolitical, and biological understanding; similarities and differences among cultures; and health inequities.
3. *Cultural competence.* Cultural competence includes assessment skills, diagnostic skills, and challenging and addressing prejudice, discrimination, and inequalities.
4. *Cultural sensitivity.* Cultural sensitivity includes empathy, interpersonal communication skills, trust and respect, acceptance, appropriateness, and barriers to cultural sensitivity.

This model meets the criteria for clarity, simplicity, generality, and empirical precision. A graphical display of this model can be found through the Leonardo da

Vinci Partnership Project website (http://www.ieneproject.eu/download/Outputs/intercultural%20model.pdf).

## Leininger's Cultural Care Diversity and Universality Theory and Model

Leininger's cultural care diversity and universality theory and the sunrise model that depicts her theory are perhaps the most well known in nursing literature on culture and health (Leininger & McFarland, 2006). The theory draws from anthropological observations and studies of culture and cultural values, beliefs, and practices. The theory of transcultural nursing promotes understanding of both the universally held and common understandings of care among humans and the culture-specific caring beliefs and behaviors that define any particular caring context or interaction. According to Leininger, this theory is intended to be holistic: Culture is the specific pattern of behavior that distinguishes any society from others and gives meaning to human expressions of care (Leininger, 2002).

The theory of cultural care diversity and universality is heavily used in education and research. It incorporates the following assumptions about care and caring as they relate to cultural competency (Leininger, 2002):

- Care (caring) is essential to curing and healing, for there can be no curing without caring.
- Every human culture has generic, folk, or indigenous care knowledge and practices and usually some professional care knowledge and practices that vary transculturally.
- Culture care values, beliefs, and practices are influenced by and tend to be embedded in the worldview, language, philosophy, religion and spirituality, kinship, social, political, legal, educational, economic, technological, ethnohistorical, and environmental contexts of cultures.
- A client who experiences nursing care that fails to be reasonably congruent with his or her beliefs, values, and caring life ways will show signs of cultural conflict, noncompliance, stress, and ethical or moral concern.
- Within a cultural care diversity and universality framework, nurses may take any or all of three culturally congruent action modes: (1) cultural preservation/maintenance, (2) cultural care accommodation/negotiation, and (3) cultural care repatterning/restructuring.

According to Leininger, *cultural care preservation/maintenance* refers to assistive, supportive, facilitative, or enabling professional actions and decisions that help individuals, families, and communities of a particular culture retain and preserve care values so that they can maintain well-being, recover from illness, or face possible handicap or death. *Cultural care accommodation/negotiation* refers to assistive, supportive, facilitative, or enabling professional actions and potential decisions that help individuals, families, and communities of a particular culture adapt to or negotiate with others for satisfying healthcare outcomes with professional caregivers. *Cultural care repatterning/restructuring* refers to the assistive, supportive, facilitative, and enabling roles filled by nurses and other healthcare providers to promote actions and decisions that may help the person, family, or community change or modify behaviors affecting their life ways, thereby achieving a new and different health pattern (Leininger & McFarland, 2006). These three action modes are sometimes used with other cultural theories and models.

Leininger recognized the comparative aspects of caring within and between cultures—hence the theory's acknowledgment of similarities as much as differences in caring in diverse cultures. Her transcultural model has implications for how nurses assess, plan, implement, and evaluate care of people from diverse cultural backgrounds. The sunrise model and theory have clarity, but they are complex. The model has generality for nursing, empirical precision, and derivable consequences. The sunrise model can be found on the Transcultural Nursing Society's website (http://tcns.org/Theories).

## Spector's HEALTH Traditions Model

Spector's health traditions model incorporates three main theories: Estes and Zitzow's heritage consistency theory, the HEALTH traditions model, and Giger and Davidhizar's theory about the cultural phenomena affecting health. *Heritage consistency* originally described the extent to which a person's lifestyle reflected his or her tribal culture but has since been expanded to study a person's traditional cultural background, such as European, Asian, African, or Hispanic. The values indicating heritage consistency exist on a continuum.

The HEALTH traditions model is based on the concept of holistic health and explores what people do to maintain, protect, or restore health. This model emphasizes the interrelationship between physical, mental, and spiritual health with personal methods of maintaining, protecting, and restoring health. To maintain physical health, for example, an individual may use traditional foods and clothing that have proven effective within the culture in the past. Protection of one's mental health may be achieved by receiving emotional and social support from family members and the community. Religious rituals may be performed, with the belief that they will assist in restoring health (Spector, 2009).

Spector also provides a Heritage Assessment Tool to determine the degree to which people or families adhere to their traditions. A traditional person observes his or her cultural traditions more closely. A more acculturated individual's practice is less observant of traditional practices (Spector, 2009). The model has clarity, simplicity, generality, and empirical precision.

# The Purnell Model for Cultural Competence

The Purnell model for cultural competence originated from education and practice. In 1989, I took third-year nursing students to a community hospital that was not accustomed to having students. Soon after the clinical experience began, it became obvious that the students and staff needed additional knowledge concerning culture. The students primarily came from middle-class and upper-middle-class white families, but most of the patients and staff came from lower-socioeconomic backgrounds or had a heritage rooted in Appalachia. As part of postconferences, I began having sessions with students and staff that centered on patients' cultures.

The next semester, I had senior nursing students in five different emergency departments. Again, it became obvious that both students and staff could benefit from a cultural assessment guide, as well as from greater knowledge about the specific cultural groups to whom they were providing care.

The first step in formalizing the cultural educational experience was to develop a comprehensive organizing framework that was usable by both staff and students. I continue to attest that the more APNs know about a specific ethnic or cultural group, the better their assessment of patients from these groups will be.

For example, if APNs are not aware of the various traditional healthcare practitioners used by many Hispanic or Latino people (e.g., *curanderos, sobadores, masajistas, y(j)erberos, espiritistas, sacerdotes*), they will not know to ask about them (Purnell, 2013).

Over the next few years, I further developed the organizing framework and expanded the model to include holographic and complexity theory. *Holographic* simply means that the theory is not confined to one discipline, but rather has applicability across health-related disciplines. In *complexity theory*, there is usually an accompanying organizing framework to simplify the theory. Complexity theory, similar to chaos theory, is characterized by large numbers of similar but independent domains; continuous change in the phenomena of interest, leading to adaptation to the environment to ensure survival; and self-organization over time. The system never reaches equilibrium because societal events necessitate ongoing change in beliefs and values (Rickles, Hawe, & Shiell, 2007).

This model has been used (1) in practice (Purnell, 2009); (2) in education as a guide to incorporate culture into baccalaureate, master's, and doctoral programs (Calvillo et al., 2009; Krainovich-Miller et al., 2008); (3) in research (Braithwaite, 2003; Crandall, George, Marion, & Davis, 2003; Purnell, 1999, 2000b, 2005, 2007; Purnell & Foster, 2003a, 2003b; Voyer, Rail, Laberge, & Purnell, 2005); and (4) in administration (Keynote Recap, 2004). It also has been used by non-nursing disciplines, such as physical therapy (Black-Lattanzi & Purnell, 2006), medicine (Braithwaite, 2003; Crandall et al., 2003; Purnell, 2003a, 2003b), and occupational therapy (Nayar & Tse, 2006). In addition, the model has been translated into Arabic, Flemish, German, Italian, Korean, Portuguese, Spanish, Swedish, and Turkish, testifying to its use on a worldwide basis. I have also consulted and made presentations about cultural competence in nursing and health care at more than 50 universities and healthcare organizations in Australia, Belize, Belgium, China, Colombia, Costa Rica, Denmark, England, Hungary, Italy, Korea, Panama, Portugal, Scotland, Spain, Sweden, Turkey, and the United States, testifying to its utility on an international scale.

## Assumptions of the Purnell Model

The explicit assumptions upon which the model is based include the following:

1. All healthcare professions need similar information about cultural diversity.
2. All healthcare professions share the metaparadigm concepts of global society, family, person, and health.
3. One culture is not better than another culture; they are just different.
4. There are core similarities shared by all cultures.
5. There are differences within, between, and among cultures.
6. Cultures change slowly over time.
7. The variant cultural characteristics determine the degree to which one varies from the dominant culture.
8. If clients are coparticipants in their care and have a choice in health-related goals, plans, and interventions, their compliance and health outcomes will be improved.
9. Culture has a powerful influence on an individual's interpretation of and responses to health care.
10. Individuals and families belong to several subcultures.
11. Each individual has the right to be respected for his or her uniqueness and cultural heritage.
12. APNs need both cultural-general and cultural-specific information to provide culturally sensitive and culturally competent care.
13. Caregivers who can assess, plan, intervene, and evaluate in a culturally competent manner will improve the care of clients for whom they care.
14. Learning culture is an ongoing process that develops in a variety of ways, but primarily through cultural encounters (Campinha-Bacote, 2011).
15. Prejudices and biases can be minimized with cultural understanding.
16. To be effective, health care must reflect the unique understanding of the values, beliefs, attitudes, life ways, and worldview of diverse populations and individual acculturation patterns.
17. Differences in race and culture often require adaptations to standard interventions.
18. Cultural awareness improves the caregiver's self-awareness.
19. Professions, organizations, and associations have their own cultures, which can be analyzed using a grand theory of culture.
20. Every client encounter is a cultural encounter.

## Variant Cultural Characteristics

Major influences that shape individuals' worldview and the extent to which people identify with their cultural group of origin are called variant cultural characteristics and include the following: nationality, race, color, gender, age, religious affiliation, educational status, socioeconomic status, occupation, military experience, political beliefs, urban versus rural residence, enclave identity, marital status, parental status, physical characteristics, sexual orientation, gender issues, reason for migration (e.g., sojourner, immigrant, or undocumented status), and length of time away from the country of origin. Moreover, immigration status also influences a person's worldview. For example, people who voluntarily immigrate generally acculturate and assimilate into a new society more easily. Conversely, sojourners who immigrate with the intention of remaining in their new homeland for only a short time or refugees who think they may return to their home country may not have the need or desire to acculturate or assimilate. Additionally, undocumented individuals (illegal immigrants) may have a different worldview from those who have arrived legally (Purnell, 2013). Some of these variant cultural characteristics change over time, while others do not. In addition, a stigma may occur for some, either the individual or the family, if they do change (e.g., changing religious affiliation from Judaism to Pentecostal).

## Cultural Competence According to the Purnell Model

Cultural competence is multifactorial in nature. To be comprehensive, this term is defined as developing an awareness of one's own existence, sensations, thoughts, and environment, without letting those factors have an undue influence on persons from other backgrounds. It incorporates the following aspects of care:

1. Demonstrating knowledge and understanding of the client's culture, health-related needs, and culturally specific meanings of health and illness.
2. Continuing to learn about the cultures of clients to whom one provides care.
3. Recognizing that the primary and secondary characteristics of culture determine the degree to which clients adhere to the beliefs, values, and practices of their dominant culture.
4. Accepting and respecting cultural differences in a manner that facilitates clients' and families' abilities to make decisions to meet their needs and beliefs.
5. Not assuming that the healthcare provider's beliefs and values are the same as the client's.
6. Resisting judgmental attitudes such as "different is not as good."
7. Being open to cultural encounters.
8. Being comfortable with cultural encounters.
9. Adapting care to be congruent with the client's culture.
10. Engaging in cultural competence as a conscious process and not necessarily a linear one.
11. Accepting responsibility for one's own education in cultural competence by attending conferences, reading professional literature, and observing cultural practices.

## Description of the Purnell Model

The Purnell model for cultural competence and its organizing framework can be used in all kinds of practice settings and by all kinds of healthcare providers. The model is depicted graphically as a series of circles, where the outlying rim represents global society, the second rim represents community, the third rim represents family, and the inner rim represents the person (see **Figure 22–1**).

The Purnell Model for Cultural Competence

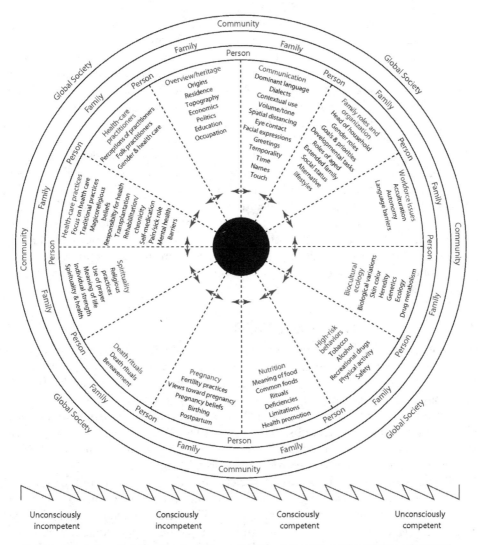

Variant cultural characteristics: age, generation, nationality, race, color, gender, religion, educational status, socioeconomic status, occupation, military status, political beliefs, urban versus rural residence, enclave identity, marital status, parental status, physical characteristics, sexual orientation, gender issues, and reason for migration (sojourner, immigrant, undocumented status)

Unconsciously incompetent: not being aware that one is lacking knowledge about another culture
Consciously incompetent: being aware that one is lacking knowledge about another culture
Consciously competent: learning about the client's culture, verifying generalizations about the client's culture, and providing culturally specific interventions
Unconsciously competent: automatically providing culturally congruent care to clients of diverse cultures

**FIGURE 22–1    The Purnell model for cultural competence.**
*Source:* Purnell Model for Cultural Competence reprinted with permission of Larry D. Purnell, PhD, RN, FAAN.

The interior of the circle is divided into 12 pie-shaped wedges depicting cultural domains (constructs) and their associated concepts. The dark center of the circle represents unknown phenomena. Along the bottom of the model is a jagged line representing the nonlinear concept of cultural consciousness.

The 12 cultural domains and their concepts provide the organizing framework. Each domain includes concepts that need to be addressed when assessing patients in various settings. Moreover, APNs can use these same concepts to better understand their own cultural beliefs, attitudes, values, practices, and behaviors. An especially important concept is the notion that no single domain stands alone; rather, all of the domains are inextricably interconnected. The 12 domains are (1) overview/heritage, (2) communications, (3) family roles and organization, (4) workforce issues, (5) biocultural ecology, (6) high-risk health behaviors, (7) nutrition, (8) pregnancy and the childbearing family, (9) death rituals, (10) spirituality, (11) healthcare practices, and (12) healthcare practitioners (see Figure 22–1).

The Purnell model has clarity, generality, empirical precision, and derivable consequences. The model in its entirety is complex. The practitioner would rarely complete a full assessment using all of the concepts in the 12 domains, especially in any one setting. This cultural model is one of the most thoroughly developed to date (Catalano, 2011).

## Macro Aspects of the Purnell Model

The macro aspects of this interactional model include the metaparadigm concepts of global society, community, family, person, and conscious competence. The theory and model are conceptualized from foundations in biology, anthropology, sociology, economics, geography, history, ecology, physiology, psychology, political science, pharmacology, and nutrition, as well as theories from communication, family development, and social support. The model can be used in clinical practice, education, research, and the administration and management of healthcare services; it also can be used to analyze organizational culture.

Phenomena related to a global society include world communication and politics; conflicts and warfare; natural disasters and famines; international exchanges in education, business, commerce, and information technology; advances in health science; space exploration; and the expanded opportunities for people to travel around the world and interact with diverse societies. Information about global events that is widely disseminated by television, radio, satellite transmission, newsprint, and information technology affects all societies, either directly or indirectly. Such events create chaos while consciously and unconsciously forcing people to alter their life ways and worldviews.

In its broadest definition, *community* is a group of people having a common interest or identity; it goes beyond the physical environment. Community includes the physical, social, and symbolic characteristics that cause people to connect. Bodies of water, mountains, rural versus urban living, and even railroad tracks help people define their physical concept of community. Of course, technology and the Internet now allow people to readily expand their community beyond the physical boundaries that defined communities in the past. Economics, religion, politics, age, generation, and marital status delineate the social concepts of community. Moreover, sharing a specific language or dialect, lifestyle, history, dress, art, or musical interest are symbolic characteristics of a community. People actively and passively interact with the community, necessitating adaptation and assimilation for equilibrium and homeostasis in their worldview. Individuals may willingly change their physical, social, and symbolic community when it no longer meets their needs.

A *family* is two or more people who are emotionally connected. They may—but do not necessarily—live in close proximity to one another. Family may include physically and emotionally close and distant consanguineous relatives, as well as physically and emotionally connected and distant non-blood-related significant others. Family structure and roles change according to age, generation, marital status, relocation or immigration, and socioeconomic status, requiring each person to rethink his or her individual beliefs and life ways.

A *person* is a bio-psycho-sociocultural being who is constantly adapting to his or her community. Human beings adapt biologically and physiologically with the aging process; psychologically in the context of social relationships, stress, and relaxation; socially as they interact with the changing community; and ethnoculturally within the broad global society. In Western cultures, a person is considered a separate physical and unique psychological being and a singular member of society; that is, the self remains separate from others. In contrast, in Asian and some other primarily collectivistic cultures, the individual is defined in relation to the family or other group, rather than as a basic unit of nature.

*Health* is a state of wellness as defined by the individual within his or her ethnocultural group. Health generally includes physical, mental, and spiritual states because group members interact with the family, community, and global society. The concept of health, which permeates all metaparadigm concepts of culture, is defined globally, nationally, regionally, locally, and individually. Thus, people can speak about their personal health status or the health status of the nation or community. Health also can be subjective or objective in nature (Purnell, 2013).

## Domains of the Purnell Model and the Organizing Framework

The 12 domains in the Purnell model are listed in this section, along with the major concepts, key questions, and observations to make for each domain.

### *Overview and Heritage*

The overview and heritage domain includes concepts related to the country of origin and current residence, such as the effects of the topography of the country of origin and the current residence on health, economics, politics, reasons for migration, educational status, and occupations. **Box 22–1** lists specific questions and a sample rationale that the APN should consider for this domain.

### Box 22–1 Overview, Inhabited Localities, and Topography

The following are suggested questions, each accompanied by a sample rationale, that the APN can ask in a cultural assessment.

1. Where do you currently live? *Sample rationale:* Someone living in the inner city may be at increased risk for illnesses such as emphysema and asthma because of increased air pollution.
2. What is your ancestry? *Sample rationale:* Members of the Amish community have high rates of glutaric acidemia, dwarfism, cartilage-hair hypoplasia, and hemophilia B.
3. Where were you born? *Sample rationale:* Some studies of the Chernobyl (Russia) nuclear incident show an increase in genetic mutations and hereditary defects related to radioactive contamination.
4. How many years have you lived in the United States (or other country, as appropriate)? *Sample rationale:* May show degree of assimilation and acculturation.
5. Were your parents born in the United States (or other country, as appropriate)? *Sample rationale:* May show degree of assimilation and acculturation.
6. What brought you (your parents/ancestors) to the United States (or other country, as appropriate)? *Sample rationale:* Refugees may have post-traumatic stress disorders related to their stay in refugee camps.
7. Describe the land or countryside where you live. Is it mountainous, swampy, and so on? *Sample rationale:* People living in or around wooded areas and who have vague symptoms of fever, fatigue, and headache with or without skin rash may have Lyme disease.
8. Have you lived other places in the United States/world? *Sample rationale:* People immigrating from, or who have recently visited parts of, Central America or Africa and who present with fever, chills, headache, and fatigue may need to be assessed for malaria or dengue fever.
9. What was the land or countryside like when you lived there? *Sample rationale:* People who have lived near a contaminated (Superfund) site may be at risk for increased incidence of cancer.
10. What is your income level? *Sample rationale:* May provide information about the ability to afford prescription medication and other treatment aids such as dressings and prescriptive devices.
11. Does your income allow you to afford the essentials of life? *Sample rationale:* May have implications for the ability to purchase "fresh fruits and vegetables."
12. Are you able to afford health insurance on your salary? *Sample rationale:* An individual may have the financial wherewithal to afford

*(Continues)*

insurance, but some persons who have a present orientation may not see the value in obtaining health insurance.

13. Do you have health insurance? *Sample rationale:* If the patient does not have health insurance, he or she may be referred to social services for financial support.

14. What is your educational level (formal/informal/self-taught)? *Sample rationale:* May have implications for health literacy and teaching.

15. What is your current occupation? If the individual is retired, ask about previous occupations. *Sample rationale:* A person may currently work in the construction industry but previously have worked in coal mines, which increases the risk for radiation poisoning and black lung.

16. Have you worked in other occupations? What were they? *Sample rationale:* An individual may currently work in carpentry but previously have worked in welding and therefore have an increased risk for cataracts.

17. Are there (were there) any particular health hazards associated with your job(s)? *Sample rationale:* People who work in the ornamental nursery industry and farming are at high risk for health problems related to the use of pesticides.

Questions and observations related to the primary and secondary characteristics of culture not covered in the previous questions include the following:

1. Have you been in the military? If so, in which foreign countries were you stationed? *Sample rationale:* People who have served in Afghanistan are at high risk for water- and foodborne diseases.

2. Are you married? *Sample rationale:* Part of a standard assessment and may provide information about support.

3. How many children do you have? *Sample rationale:* Part of a standard assessment and may provide information about support.

## Communication

The communication domain includes concepts related to the dominant language, dialects, and the contextual use of the language; paralanguage variations such as voice volume, tone, intonations, inflections, and willingness to share thoughts and feelings; nonverbal communications such as eye contact, gesturing, facial expressions, use of touch, body language, spatial distancing practices, and acceptable greetings; temporality in terms of past, present, and future orientation of worldview; clock versus social time; and the amount of formality in use of names. **Box 22–2** lists specific questions and a sample rationale that the APN should consider for this domain.

### Box 22–2  Communication

The following are suggested questions, each accompanied by a sample rationale, that the APN can ask in a cultural assessment.

1. What is your full name? *Sample rationale:* Part of a standard assessment. Complex naming can create difficulties for medical record keeping.

2. What is your legal name? *Sample rationale:* Hispanic/Latino individuals have an extended name format that includes a first name, middle name, father's last name, and mother's last name, with an additional last name of the husband if a woman is married. In these cases, a person selects any combination of last names for his or her legal name.

3. By which name do you wish to be called? *Sample rationale:* Helps establish trust and increases comfort level of the patient.

4. What is your primary language? *Sample rationale:* The primary language is usually best for patient education, but the APN should ask about the preferred language.

5. Do you speak a specific dialect? *Sample rationale:* A dialect-specific interpreter is preferred. For example, people from northern China speak a different dialect than people from southern China.

6. Which other languages do you speak? *Sample rationale:* May be helpful for interpretation if the preferred language interpreter is not available. For example, many Vietnamese persons speak French as a secondary language.

7. Do you find it difficult to share your thoughts, feelings, and ideas with family? Friends? Healthcare providers? *Sample rationale:* For people who find it difficult to share their feelings, additional time may be needed to establish trust and get full disclosure, especially with sensitive topics.

8. Do you mind being touched by friends? Strangers? Healthcare workers? *Sample rationale:* Reinforces the necessity to ask permission before touching. Always explain the rationale for touching.

9. How do you wish to be greeted? Handshake? Nod of the head? Something else? *Sample rationale:* Preferred greetings help establish trust.

10. Are you usually on time for appointments? *Sample rationale:* A clear rationale can be given for intolerance of lateness; for example, some healthcare organizations will not see the patient if he or she is more than 15 minutes late and some still may charge for the visit.

11. Are you usually on time for social engagements? *Sample rationale:* Ask only if the question is pertinent.

*(Continues)*

12. Observe the client's speech pattern. Does the speech pattern demonstrate a high or low context? *Sample rationale:* Clients from highly contexted cultures place greater value on silence and may take more time to give a response.

13. Observe the client when physical contact is made. Does he or she withdraw from the touch or become tense? *Sample rationale:* Helps establish trust and reinforces the necessity of explaining the reason for touch.

14. How close does the client stand when talking with family members? With healthcare providers? *Sample rationale:* The APN should not take offense if a patient stands closer to or farther away than the distance to which the APN is accustomed. Spatial distancing is culture bound.

15. Does the client maintain eye contact when talking with the APN? *Sample rationale:* Some cultures avoid eye contact with people in hierarchal positions (the APN is in a hierarchal position in the healthcare setting) as a sign of respect.

## Family Roles and Organization

The family roles and organization domain includes concepts related to the head of the household, gender roles (a product of biology and culture), family goals and priorities, developmental tasks of children and adolescents, roles of the aged and extended family, individual and family social status in the community, and acceptance of alternative lifestyles such as single parenting, nontraditional sexual orientations, childless marriages, and divorce. **Box 22–3** lists specific questions and a sample rationale that the APN should consider for this domain.

## Workforce Issues

The workforce issues domain includes concepts related to autonomy, acculturation, assimilation, gender roles, ethnic communication styles, and healthcare practices of the country of origin. **Box 22–4** lists specific questions and a sample rationale that the APN should consider for this domain.

## Biocultural Ecology

The biocultural ecology domain includes physical, biological, and physiological variations among ethnic and racial groups such as skin color (the most evident) and physical differences in body habitus; genetic, hereditary, endemic, and topographical diseases; psychological makeup of individuals; and the physiological differences that affect the way drugs are metabolized by the body. In general,

## Box 22–3 Family Roles and Organization

The following are suggested questions, each accompanied by a sample rationale, that the APN can ask in a cultural assessment.

1. Who makes most of the decisions in your family? *Sample rationale:* If the decision maker is not accessed, no decision will be made and time will be wasted.
2. Which types of decisions do(es) the female(s) in your family make? *Sample rationale:* In many traditional families, the female makes decisions about the household and child care, but not always.
3. Which types of decisions do(es) the male(s) in your family make? *Sample rationale:* In many traditional families, the male is the primary decision maker regarding affairs outside the household, but not always.
4. What are the duties of the women in the family? *Sample rationale:* Looking for division of labor, which can become important when illness occurs.
5. What are the duties of the men in the family? *Sample rationale:* Looking for division of labor, which can become important when illness occurs.
6. What should children do to make a good impression for themselves and for the family? *Sample rationale:* Important to note in school health and family counseling. A child's behavior can bring shame upon or honor to the family.
7. What would children do that would *not* make a good impression for themselves and for the family? *Sample rationale:* Among traditional Chinese, children are to do well in school or shame may come to the family.
8. What are children forbidden to do? *Sample rationale:* Among traditional Germans, taboo behaviors include talking back to elders and touching another person's possessions.
9. What should young adults do to make a good impression for themselves and for the family? *Sample rationale:* Among most Koreans, one of the most important things young adults can do to bring pride to themselves and their families is to do well in school. Otherwise, shame can occur to the extent that many students have committed suicide.
10. What would young adults do that would *not* make a good impression for themselves and for the family? *Sample rationale:* Among traditional Mexican families, young adults should not dress in a provocative manner. Otherwise, shame can come to them or their family.
11. What are adolescents forbidden to do? *Sample rationale:* Taboo behaviors for young adults in Iran include using illicit drugs or engaging in sexual activity before marriage. This behavior can bring shame upon the family.

*(Continues)*

12. What are the priorities for your family? *Sample rationale:* For a lower-socioeconomic family, the priority may be having adequate food and shelter with stress on the present. Health care and education may not be priorities if the basic needs are not met.

13. What are the roles of older adults in your family? Are they sought for their advice? *Sample rationale:* Among traditional Koreans, no decision is made until the advice of older adults has been sought.

14. Are there extended family members in your household? Who else lives in your household? *Sample rationale:* Being aware of the household membership is important for health teaching and adequacy of care for sick family members. Most members of traditional Asian cultures live in extended family arrangements.

15. What are the roles of extended family members in this household? *Sample rationale:* In many Filipino families, extended family members provide significant financial and social support and are important resources for child care.

16. What gives you and your family status? *Sample rationale:* Among the Navajo, status is obtained by sharing what you have with others.

17. Is it acceptable to you for people to have children out of wedlock? *Sample rationale:* Among traditional Arab families, shame may occur if a pregnancy occurs outside of marriage.

18. Is it acceptable to you for people to live together and not be married? *Sample rationale:* Among many Asian cultures, if a man and a woman live together without being married, that relationship may cause them to be rejected by their families.

19. Are you accepting of gay, lesbian, or transgendered people? *Sample rationale:* Not all cultures and individuals are accepting of gay, lesbian, or transgendered populations. Do not disclose these relationships to family members.

20. What is your sexual preference/orientation? (if appropriate, and then later in the assessment after a modicum of trust has been established). *Sample rationale:* Important for health counseling if sexually active.

most diseases and illnesses may be classified into one of three categories based on their causes:

1. *Lifestyle causes* include cultural practices and behaviors that can generally be controlled—for example, smoking, diet, and stress.

2. *Environmental causes* refer to the external environment (e.g., air and water pollution) and situations over which the individual has little or no control (e.g., presence of malarial mosquitoes, exposure to chemicals and pesticides, access to care, and associated diseases).

3. *Genetic conditions* are caused by genes.

## Box 22–4  Workforce Issues

The following are suggested questions, each accompanied by a sample rationale, that the APN can ask in a cultural assessment.

1. Do you usually report to work on time? *Sample rationale:* For present-oriented people who are accustomed to a lack of timeliness in the workforce, the supervisor needs to be very clear about the importance of timeliness and any repercussions if timeliness becomes a concern.
2. Do you usually report to meetings on time? *Sample rationale:* In some cultures, such as among Panamanians, a meeting starts when most people have arrived.
3. Which concerns do you have about working with someone of the opposite gender? *Sample rationale:* Strict Muslim separation of the sexes means that there may be family disharmony if men and women are expected to work in close proximity.
4. Do you consider yourself a "loyal" employee? *Sample rationale:* In Japanese culture, an employer may expect absolute loyalty, and employees often remain with the same company for their entire lives.
5. How long do you expect to remain in your position? *Sample rationale:* May have implications for health insurance and seeking health care in the United States.
6. What do you do when you do not know how to do something related to your job? *Sample rationale:* Among many traditional Koreans, when an employee does not know how to do something, rather than going to a supervisor, a coworker of the same nationality (if available) is sought out.
7. Do you consider yourself to be assertive in your job? *Sample rationale:* Traditional Filipinos are frequently not seen as assertive as some U.S. employers would like.
8. What difficulty does English (or another language) give you in the workforce? *Sample rationale:* May have implications for accuracy in fulfilling job requirements, both verbally and in writing.

**Box 22–5** lists specific questions and a sample rationale that the APN should consider for this domain.

### High-Risk Health Behaviors

The high-risk health behaviors domain includes substance use and misuse of tobacco, alcohol, and recreational drugs; lack of physical activity; increased calorie consumption; nonuse of safety measures such as seat belts, helmets, and safe driving practices; and not taking safety measures to prevent oneself from contracting

## Box 22–5  Biocultural Ecology

The following are suggested questions, each accompanied by a sample rationale, that the APN can ask in a cultural assessment.

1. Are you allergic to any medications? *Sample rationale:* Standard for any assessment.

2. Which problems did you have when you took over-the-counter medications? *Sample rationale:* Looking for possible allergies and side effects; standard for any assessment. The APN should ask about medicines purchased in countries outside the United States. In Mexico and other countries, a wide variety of medicines can be purchased over the counter that would require a prescription in the United States.

3. Which problems did you have when you took prescription medications? *Sample rationale:* Looking for possible allergies and side effects; standard for any assessment.

4. What are the major illnesses and diseases in your family? *Sample rationale:* Part of standard assessment; looking for opportunities for health promotion and teaching. In addition, many Asians and Pacific Islanders have high incidences of glucose-6-phosphate dehydrogenase deficiency and alpha-thalassemia.

5. Are you aware of any genetic diseases in your family? *Sample rationale:* Members of Amish and Jewish populations have many hereditary and genetic illnesses, and heritage can be important for counseling.

6. What are the major health problems in the country from which you come (if appropriate)? *Sample rationale:* Vietnamese immigrants and people who have spent time in refugee camps have a high incidence of hepatitis A.

7. With which race do you identify? *Sample rationale:* May be important for organizational demographics for grants.

8. Observe skin coloration and physical characteristics. *Sample rationale:* To assess for rashes on people with dark skin, the APN may need to palpate the area rather than relying on visual cues.

9. Observe for physical handicaps and disabilities. *Sample rationale:* Part of standard assessment. Many people do not disclose handicaps or disabilities upon initial encounter unless specifically asked, especially learning disabilities.

HIV and sexually transmitted infections. **Box 22–6** lists specific questions and a sample rationale that the APN should consider for this domain.

## Nutrition

The nutrition domain includes the meaning of food, common foods and rituals, nutritional deficiencies and food limitations, and the use of food for health promotion, restoration, illness, and disease prevention. **Box 22–7** lists specific questions and a sample rationale that the APN should consider for this domain.

---

### Box 22–6 High-Risk Health Behaviors

The following are suggested questions, each accompanied by a sample rationale, that the APN can ask in a cultural assessment.

1. How many cigarettes per day do you smoke? *Sample rationale:* Standard for any assessment. Because smoking carries a stigma in some cultures, the APN should assess smoking with a nonjudgmental attitude.

2. Do you smoke a pipe (or cigars)? *Sample rationale:* Standard for any assessment. Because smoking carries a stigma in some cultures, the APN should assess smoking with a nonjudgmental attitude.

3. Do you chew tobacco? *Sample rationale:* In parts of rural Appalachia and other areas of the world, chewing tobacco is common; this increases the risk for oropharyngeal cancer.

4. For how many years have you smoked/chewed tobacco? *Sample rationale:* Part of a standard assessment if there is a history of tobacco use.

5. How much do you drink each day? Ask about wine, beer, spirits, coffee, and energy drinks. *Sample rationale:* Part of a standard assessment; important for follow-up with laboratory tests.

6. Which recreational drugs do you use? *Sample rationale:* Part of a standard assessment. The APN should ask this question in a nonjudgmental manner to encourage the patient to disclose this sensitive information.

7. How often do you use recreational drugs? *Sample rationale:* Part of a standard assessment for determining the degree of risk.

8. Do you exercise each day? What type of exercise? For how long? *Sample rationale:* Part of a standard assessment for health promotion and wellness.

9. Do you use seat belts/helmets? *Sample rationale:* Part of a standard assessment for injury prevention.

10. Which precautions do you take to prevent getting a sexually transmitted infection/HIV? *Sample rationale:* Part of a standard assessment for health promotion and wellness and illness and disease prevention.

## Box 22-7 Nutrition

The following are suggested questions, each accompanied by a sample rationale, that the APN can ask in a cultural assessment.

1. Are you satisfied with your weight? *Sample rationale:* In many cultures, being overweight is seen as positive; members of these cultures do not adhere to the U.S. weight recommendations.
2. Which foods do you eat to maintain your health? *Sample rationale:* Food choices are seen as a means for promoting health. In the dominant U.S. culture, fresh fruits and vegetables are encouraged for health promotion.
3. Do you avoid certain foods to maintain your health? *Sample rationale:* Most Mexicans, as well as members of other cultures, try to avoid foods with high fat content.
4. Why do you avoid these foods? *Sample rationale:* People may avoid specific foods because they were not part of their diet when growing up, because they do not like the taste of the food, or because they do not like the appearance of the food. Recommending foods that the patient does not find pleasing diminishes the chance that the recommendations will be followed.
5. Which foods do you eat when you are ill? *Sample rationale:* In many cultures, common foods eaten when ill include toast and tea or ginger ale.
6. Which foods do you avoid when you are ill? *Sample rationale:* Recommending a food that the person culturally or personally avoids diminishes the chance that the recommendations will be followed.
7. Why do you avoid these foods (if appropriate)? *Sample rationale:* Foods may be avoided for a number of reasons.
8. For which illnesses do you eat certain foods? *Sample rationale:* In many cultures, people drink a "hot toddy" for a cold or minor illness. The ingredients for a hot toddy vary but generally include tea, lemon or lime, sugar or honey, and some type of liquor such as whiskey or rum.
9. Which foods do you eat to balance your diet? *Sample rationale:* Not all cultures adhere to the U.S. government's food pyramid because the food choices are not part of their cultural diet. Many Asians, Hispanics, and African Americans have lactose intolerance and, therefore, cannot follow the recommendations in this food pyramid.
10. Which foods do you eat every day? *Sample rationale:* Most people have specific foods that they eat on almost a daily basis. Incorporating these foods into dietary prescriptions will increase compliance with dietary instructions.

*(Continues)*

### Box 22–7 Nutrition (*Continued*)

11. Which foods do you eat every week? *Sample rationale:* Most people have specific foods that they eat on almost a weekly basis. Incorporating these foods into dietary prescriptions will increase compliance with dietary instructions.

12. Which foods do you eat that are part of your cultural heritage? *Sample rationale:* Including culturally preferred foods into nutritional recommendations increases compliance.

13. Which foods are high-status foods in your family/culture? *Sample rationale:* High-status foods vary according to cost and availability. Among Panamanians, canned sausages are high-status foods; the same items are low-status foods in the United States. Lobster is low status in the Philippines because of its ready availability but is high status in the United States because of its cost.

14. Which foods are eaten only by men? Women? Children? Teenagers? Older people? *Sample rationale:* Among some Guatemalan highland indigenous populations, primarily men eat eggs for the added protein value. The belief is that because men do heavy labor, they need more protein. However, they are supposed to share the protein foods on their plates with children.

15. How many meals do you eat each day? *Sample rationale:* Not all cultures eat the standard U.S. three meals per day. Among many Turks, people eat four to six times per day, but they consume smaller amounts at these meals than most European Americans do.

16. What time do you eat each meal? *Sample rationale:* May have implications for medication administration.

17. Do you snack between meals? *Sample rationale:* Studies have demonstrated that young adults in Appalachia snack frequently without eating a regular meal.

18. Which foods do you eat when you snack? *Sample rationale:* Many snacks are not considered healthy food choices. The APN can recommend healthy snacks to replace less healthy food choices.

19. Which holidays do you celebrate? *Sample rationale:* Holidays are a time for special meals and a time when many people consume excessive amounts of calories. Many Hispanic/Latino cultures celebrate all of the Catholic religious holidays, as well as the patron saint of their state or their province, their village, their school, and other celebrations.

20. Which foods do you eat on particular holidays? *Sample rationale:* Foods are an important part of maintaining one's culture and diet is one measure of acculturation.

(*Continues*)

21. Who usually buys the food in your household? *Sample rationale:* Many times it is just as important for the APN to talk with the person who purchases the food as with the person who prepares the meals. In migrant worker camps, the person who purchases the meals is not the person who cooks for the group. If one member of the group needs a special diet (e.g., a diabetic individual), the purchaser of the food needs to be included in nutritional education.

22. Who does the cooking in your household? *Sample rationale:* The person who does the cooking should be included in dietary counseling and education for special diets.

23. Do you have a refrigerator? *Sample rationale:* For homeless persons, proper food storage must be taken into consideration.

24. How do you cook your food? *Sample rationale:* Preparation practices can add significant calories to meals.

25. How do you prepare meat? *Sample rationale:* Preparation practices can add significant calories to meals.

26. How do you prepare vegetables? *Sample rationale:* Preparation practices can add significant calories to meals.

27. What do you drink with your meals? *Sample rationale:* Beverages can add significant calories to meals.

28. Do you drink special teas? *Sample rationale:* Teas are used by many people for health promotion and wellness and in times of illness.

29. Do you have any food allergies/intolerances? *Sample rationale:* Many African Americans and Asians have lactose intolerance. Encouraging milk and milk products in the diet would not be beneficial for these persons.

30. Are there certain foods that cause problems when you eat them? *Sample rationale:* Looking for allergies or food to avoid in dietary counseling.

31. How does your diet change with each season? *Sample rationale:* Most people's diet changes with the seasons. For those individuals who live in colder climates, fresh fruits and vegetables may be too expensive in the winter.

32. Are your food habits different on days you work from when you are not working? *Sample rationale:* A common occurrence is for some people to eat less healthy foods during the busy workweek, especially those who are single.

### Pregnancy and Childbearing Practices

The pregnancy and childbearing practices domain includes culturally sanctioned and unsanctioned fertility practices, views on pregnancy, and prescriptive, restrictive, and taboo practices related to pregnancy, birthing, and the postpartum period. **Box 22–8** lists specific questions and a sample rationale that the APN should consider for this domain.

---

### Box 22–8 Pregnancy and Childbearing Practices

The following are suggested questions, each accompanied by a sample rationale, that the APN can ask in a cultural assessment.

1. How many children do you have? *Sample rationale:* Part of a standard assessment.
2. Have you ever had an abortion? Stillborn? Miscarriage? *Sample rationale:* Part of a standard obstetrical/gynecological assessment.
3. What do you use for birth control? *Sample rationale:* Each cultural and religious group has acceptable and unacceptable methods of birth control. Islamic jurists have ruled that the use of "reversible" forms of birth control is "undesirable but not forbidden."
4. What does it mean to you and your family when you are pregnant? *Sample rationale:* In some cultures, a woman is not a true woman and has not reached her potential until she becomes pregnant.
5. Which special foods do you eat when you are pregnant? *Sample rationale:* Although there are no specifically prescribed foods for a pregnant Polish woman, she is expected to eat for two.
6. Which foods do you avoid when you are pregnant? *Sample rationale:* Korean women who are pregnant avoid coffee, spicy foods, chicken, and crab.
7. Which activities do you avoid when you are pregnant? *Sample rationale:* A belief among traditional Mexicans is that a pregnant woman should not walk in the moonlight for fear that the baby will be born with a cleft lip or palate.
8. Do you do anything special when you are pregnant? *Sample rationale:* A belief in many cultures is that a pregnant woman should not reach over her head for fear the cord will wrap around the baby's neck.
9. Do you eat nonfood substances when you are pregnant? *Sample rationale:* Eating nonfood substances is common among many cultural groups. Many African Americans eat clay in the belief that it has important minerals that the fetus needs.

*(Continues)*

10. Who do you want with you when you deliver your baby? *Sample rationale:* Most Filipino women prefer their mothers or another female family member to be present during the delivery, rather than husbands.

11. In which position do you want to be when you deliver your baby? *Sample rationale:* Traditional Indian women in Guatemala prefer to deliver in a squatting position rather than in the supine position.

12. Which special foods do you eat after delivery? *Sample rationale:* Haitian women are encouraged to eat rice, porridge, plantains, and red beans after delivery to build up the blood.

13. Which foods do you avoid after delivery? *Sample rationale:* Chinese women avoid cold fruits and vegetables after delivery; instead, they eat cooked foods.

14. Which activities do you avoid after you deliver? *Sample rationale:* Russian women do no strenuous activity after delivery to prevent any complications.

15. Do you do anything special after delivery? *Sample rationale:* Traditional Haitian women have a series of three special baths that are given to them by family members.

16. Who will help you with the baby after delivery? *Sample rationale:* Looking for home support for the mother and rest of the family.

17. Which bathing restrictions do you have after you deliver? *Sample rationale:* Many Arab women may be reluctant to bathe postpartum because they believe air may get into the mother and cause illness.

18. Do you want to keep the placenta? *Sample rationale:* Traditional Guatemalan women burn the placenta to keep away evil spirits.

19. What do you do to care for the baby's umbilical cord? *Sample rationale:* A common practice among Central American Indians is to place a coin or metal object, held on with an abdominal binder, to prevent the umbilicus from protruding.

## Death Rituals

The death rituals domain includes how an individual and society view death and euthanasia, rituals to prepare for death, burial practices, and bereavement behaviors. In most cultures, death rituals are slow to change. **Box 22–9** lists specific questions and a sample rationale that the APN should consider for this domain.

## Spirituality

The spirituality domain includes formal religious beliefs related to faith and affiliation and the use of prayer, behavior practices that give meaning to life, and

## Box 22–9  Death Rituals

The following are suggested questions, each accompanied by a sample rationale, that the APN can ask in a cultural assessment.

1. Which special activities need to be performed to prepare for death? *Sample rationale:* When death is impending, Muslims want the bed to face toward Mecca.
2. Would you want to know about your impending death? *Sample rationale:* A belief among traditional Hindus is that people might give up hope if impending death is made known to them.
3. What is your preferred burial practice? Burial? Cremation? *Sample rationale:* The patient's wishes should be granted and the family should be encouraged to honor them.
4. How soon after death does burial occur? *Sample rationale:* For traditional Jews, burial should occur before sundown the next day.
5. How do men grieve in your culture? *Sample rationale:* A wide range of grieving practices exists, and all practices should be unconditionally accepted.
6. How do women grieve in your culture? *Sample rationale:* A wide range of grieving practices exists and all practices should be unconditionally accepted.
7. What does death mean to you? *Sample rationale:* According to Muslim beliefs, death is foreordained and worldly life is but a preparation for eternal life.
8. Do you believe in an afterlife? *Sample rationale:* Most Germans and German Americans believe that there is a better life after death.
9. Are children included in death rituals? *Sample rationale:* Members of Amish groups include children in all aspects of dying and burial.

individual sources of strength. **Box 22–10** lists specific questions and a sample rationale that the APN should consider for this domain.

## Healthcare Practices

The healthcare practices domain includes the focus of health care (acute versus preventive); traditional, magicoreligious, and biomedical beliefs and practices; individual responsibility for health; self-medicating practices; and views on mental illness, chronicity, rehabilitation, acceptance of blood and blood products, and organ donation and transplantation. **Box 22–11** lists specific questions and a sample rationale that the APN should consider for this domain.

## Box 22–10  Spirituality

The following are suggested questions, each accompanied by a sample rationale, that the APN can ask in a cultural assessment.

1. What is your religion? *Sample rationale:* Traditional Judaism is more than a religion and prescribes male and female relationships as well as nutritional practices.
2. Do you consider yourself deeply religious? *Sample rationale:* Some people are religious but do not attend church on a regular basis.
3. How many times per day do you pray? *Sample rationale:* Islam requires prayer five times per day.
4. What items do you need to pray? *Sample rationale:* If possible, Muslims need a prayer rug.
5. Do you meditate? *Sample rationale:* Meditation may or may not be part of religious practice.
6. What gives strength and meaning to your life? *Sample rationale:* For some persons, religion is the most important thing in life; for others, the priority might be family or even work.
7. In which spiritual practices do you engage for your physical and emotional health? *Sample rationale:* For some people this is prayer, for others meditation, and for others just having quiet time.

## Box 22–11  Healthcare Practices

The following are suggested questions, each accompanied by a sample rationale, that the APN can ask in a cultural assessment.

1. In which prevention activities do you engage to maintain your health? *Sample rationale:* A strong value in the dominant European American culture is to have regularly scheduled health checkups, including breast self-examinations and mammograms.
2. Who in your family takes responsibility for your health? *Sample rationale:* In many Hispanic/Latino cultures, the female in the family assumes the primary responsibility for the health of the family.
3. Which over-the-counter medicines do you use? *Sample rationale:* Most cultural groups and individuals use over-the-counter medication, but some use them to the exclusion of prescription medicines. For many persons who have relatives in other countries, a large variety of prescription medications may be purchased and sent to family members in the United States.

*(Continues)*

## Box 22–11 Healthcare Practices (*Continued*)

4. Which herbal teas and folk medicines do you use? *Sample rationale:* Guatemalans, like members of many Hispanic/Latino populations, use a wide variety of herbal teas for many health conditions.

5. For which conditions do you use herbal medicines? *Sample rationale:* Many Panamanian men use "cat's claw" tea for prostate problems and delay going to a Western health professional.

6. What do you usually do when you are in pain? *Sample rationale:* Traditional Chinese individuals cope with pain by using externally applied treatments such as oils and massage.

7. How do you express your pain? *Sample rationale:* Many Filipinos view pain as part of living an honorable life and, therefore, may appear stoic and tolerate a high degree of pain.

8. How are people in your culture viewed or treated when they have a mental illness? *Sample rationale:* In many rural areas of Appalachia, rather than agreeing that a person has a mental health illness, they are likely to say the person is "odd" or "quite turned."

9. How are people with physical disabilities treated in your culture? *Sample rationale:* In Haitian culture, people with a disability are seen as being as important as anyone else and are incorporated into all family and social activities.

10. What do you do when you are sick? Stay in bed, continue your normal activities, or something else? *Sample rationale:* For many people from an Eastern European heritage, a belief is "If you are not dead, take something for relief and continue with your daily routines."

11. What are your beliefs about rehabilitation? *Sample rationale:* Studies demonstrate that Germans are more accepting of rehabilitation than other groups who have been studied. If rehabilitation is needed to function at maximum capacity, then all rehabilitation exercises are done.

12. How are people with chronic illnesses viewed or treated in your culture? *Sample rationale:* In cases of chronic illness among African Americans, close family and spiritual ties ensure that one's responsibilities are taken care of (by the family and even church members).

13. Are you averse to blood transfusions? *Sample rationale:* There is a religious prohibition against a Jehovah Witness receiving blood. In addition, many people do not want a blood transfusion for fear of contracting HIV/AIDS.

14. Is organ donation acceptable to you? *Sample rationale:* Jewish law views organ transplants from four perspectives: the recipient, the living donor, the cadaver donor, and the dying donor. Because life is sacred, if the recipient's life can be prolonged without considerable risk, then the transplant is favorably viewed.

*(Continues)*

15. Are you an organ donor? *Sample rationale:* Part of a standard health assessment. Many misconceptions exist about organ donations, and the APN can play a significant role in clarifying these misconceptions.

16. Would you consider having an organ transplant if needed? *Sample rationale:* Organ donation and transplantation among Koreans are rare, reflecting traditional attitudes toward integrity and purity. The APN can have a significant influence on Koreans' decisions about organ donation and transplantation by providing factual information.

17. Are healthcare services readily available to you? *Sample rationale:* APNs need to be aware of access problems for health care.

18. Do you have transportation problems in trying to access needed healthcare services? *Sample rationale:* Many organizations provide vouchers for public transportation if necessary.

19. Can you afford health care? *Sample rationale:* If the patient does not have adequate resources for health care, a social worker should be contacted for assistance.

20. Do you feel welcome when you see a healthcare professional? *Sample rationale:* If the answer is no, determine the reason. Just greeting the patient in a preferred manner, such as being formal with older African Americans, can make them feel welcome.

21. Which traditional healthcare practices do you use? Acupuncture, acupressure, *cai gao*, moxibustion, aromatherapy, coining/cupping, or something else? *Sample rationale:* If the APN is familiar with traditional practices in the culture, more specific information can be obtained.

22. Which home difficulties do you have that might prevent you from receiving health care? *Sample rationale:* Lack of support at home for child care may mean that a mother might not obtain regularly scheduled preventive care such as mammograms or Pap smears.

### Healthcare Practitioners

The healthcare practitioners domain includes the status, use, and perceptions of traditional, magicoreligious, and biomedical healthcare providers and the gender of the healthcare provider. **Box 22–12** lists specific questions and a sample rationale that the APN should consider for this domain.

# Individual Professional Cultural Competence

Much debate, especially in the last decade, has focused on the process of objectively measuring individual competence. Most tools for measuring cultural competence are self-reported and subjective in nature. A number of tools have

## Box 22–12 Healthcare Practitioners

The following are suggested questions, each accompanied by a sample rationale, that the APN can ask in a cultural assessment.

1. Which healthcare providers do you see when you are ill? Physicians? Nurses? *Sample rationale:* Not all patients see Western allopathic practitioners for illnesses, at least not as the first contact. The APN should also determine which treatments have been recommended by complementary alternative practitioners.
2. Do you prefer a same-sex healthcare provider for routine health problems? For intimate care? *Sample rationale:* Among traditional Islamic patients, a male healthcare provider should not tend to a female patient unless it is an emergency.
3. Which healers do you use in addition to physicians and nurses? *Sample rationale:* If the APN is familiar with the specific culture, he or she can ask more informed questions. Among many Hispanic/Latino groups, traditional healers include *curanderos, yerberos, masajistas, sacerdotes, sobadores,* and *espiritistas.*
4. For which conditions do you use healers? *Sample rationale:* Many Hispanics/Latinos use a variety of traditional healers. APNs who are caring for these populations should familiarize themselves with the specific groups' traditional healers and be able to ask the question in a nonjudgmental manner. Being able to integrate traditional healers with allopathic professionals will increase compliance with recommendations.

been developed to assess individual and organizational cultural competence. Some of these tools have been validated and are specific to a discipline or area of practice, whereas others are more general in nature. Most of these tools are available online. To view and select a specific plan, go to Google Scholar (www.scholar.google.com) and type "cultural competence measurement" or "cultural competence assessment tools" in the search field. The Office of Minority Health also has published a document on cultural competence standards (http://minorityhealth.hhs.gov/).

Cultural competence is a journey, rather than a skill mastered once and then used in an unchanging manner for the remainder of one's career. Its success relies on the willingness and ability of an individual to deliver culturally congruent and acceptable health and nursing care to clients. Individual cultural competence can be arbitrarily divided among cultural-general approaches, the clinical encounter, and language.

## Cultural-General Competence

APNs need a cultural general framework for assessment, as well as culturally specific knowledge about the clients to whom care is provided. Some cultural-general concepts follow:

1. Developing an awareness of one's own existence, sensations, thoughts, and environment without letting this have an undue influence on those from other backgrounds.
2. Continuing to learn about the cultures of clients to whom one provides care.
3. Demonstrating knowledge and understanding of the client's culture, health-related needs, and meanings of health and illness.
4. Accepting and respecting cultural differences in a manner that facilitates the client's and family's ability to make decisions to meet their needs and beliefs.
5. Recognizing that the APN's beliefs and values may not be the same as the client's.
6. Resisting judgmental attitudes such as "different is not as good."
7. Being open to new cultural encounters.
8. Recognizing that the primary and secondary characteristics of culture determine the degree to which clients adhere to the beliefs, values, and practices of their dominant culture.
9. Having contact and experience with the communities from which clients come.
10. Being willing to work with clients of diverse cultures and subcultures.
11. Accepting responsibility for one's own education in cultural competence by attending conferences, reading the literature, and observing cultural practices.
12. Promoting respect for individuals by discouraging racial and ethnic slurs among coworkers.
13. Intervening with staff behavior that is insensitive, lacks cultural understanding, or reflects prejudice.

## The Clinical Encounter

Some principles and guidelines for APNs in the clinical encounter follow:

1. Adapting care to be congruent with the client's culture.
2. Responding respectively to all clients and their families (including addressing clients and family members in the manner that they prefer, either formally or informally).
3. Collecting cultural data on assessments.
4. Forming generalizations as a method for formulating questions rather than stereotyping.
5. Recognizing culturally based healthcare beliefs and practices.

6. Knowing the most common diseases and illnesses affecting the unique population to whom care is provided.
7. Individualizing care plans to be consistent with the client's cultural beliefs.
8. Having knowledge of the communication styles of clients to whom you provide care.
9. Accepting varied gender roles and childrearing practices from clients to whom you provide care.
10. Having a working knowledge of the religious and spiritual practices of clients to whom you provide care.
11. Having an understanding of the family dynamics of clients to whom you provide care.
12. Using faces and language pain scales in the ethnicity and preferred languages of the clients.
13. Recognizing and accepting traditional, complementary, and alternative practices of clients to whom you provide care.
14. Incorporating clients' cultural food choices and dietary practices into care plans.
15. Incorporating clients' health literacy into care plans and health education initiatives.

## Language

Language ability has been determined to be one of the most important aspects in APNs' ability to obtain an adequate assessment for many culturally diverse patients. Some guidelines for language follow:

1. Developing skills and using interpreters (includes sign language) with clients and families who have limited English proficiency.
2. Providing clients with educational documents that are translated into their preferred language.
3. Providing discharge instructions at a level that the client and family understand and in the language that the client and family prefer.
4. Providing medication and treatment instruction in the language that the client prefers.
5. Using pain scales in the language of the client.

# Organizational Cultural Competence

Individual cultural competence is not sufficient to ensure the delivery of culturally competent care—the organization delivering the care must also demonstrate a commitment to cultural competence. Several things must be in place for an organization to demonstrate cultural competence. A list of attributes of culturally competent organizations, organized arbitrarily by governance and administration, education and orientation, and language, follows (Purnell et al., 2011; Purnell, 2013).

## Governance and Administration

1. The organization has a mission statement and policies that address diversity.
2. The board of governance includes members of the ethnicity of the community that the organization serves.
3. A committee for cultural competence exists and includes staff, managers, administrators, chaplains, and members who are representative of the community.
4. The organization engages in community diversity fairs.
5. The organization seeks resources from federal, state, and private agencies to continually upgrade and integrate cultural competence into its care.
6. The organization partners with diverse community agencies.
7. The organization networks with diverse community leaders.
8. Administrators, managers, and staff are encouraged to be active in developing public policy for the client base to whom they deliver care.
9. Policy statements include efforts to eliminate bias and prejudice on the part of both clients and staff.
10. Programs reflect the needs of the diverse community.
11. The organization's programs are advertised in community newspapers and on the radio and television in the languages of the community.
12. There is a willingness to support a mentoring program to entice recruitment into the health professions.
13. Data collected include race, ethnicity, culture, and language preferences of the staff and client base.
14. Patient rights documents are available in the major languages of the community.
15. Cultural and linguistic standards are adhered to by all members of the organization.
16. Fiscal resources are available for interpretation.
17. Strategic planning reflects the needs of the community.
18. Input on research priorities is sought from consumers.
19. Researchers are reflective of the staff, clients, and community.
20. Human resources recruitment and hiring activities reflect the diversity of the community.
21. The job analysis procedure includes scoring for ethnocultural and language ability.
22. Position descriptions and evaluation practices reflect cultural competence.
23. Conflict and grievance procedures reflect the language of the staff.
24. The organization actively recruits bilingual staff.
25. Staff members are compensated for bilingual ability and certification.
26. The ethics committee includes members who are reflective of the staff and clients.
27. The hours of operation of clinics are adjusted to meet the needs of the community.

28. Pictures and posters are reflective of the client base.
29. Food choices are reflective of the client and staff preferences.
30. The holiday calendar represents the holidays recognized by the client population base.
31. Intake forms reflect cultural assessment.
32. Pain scales are available in the diverse languages used by the population served.
33. Culturally appropriate toys are available (e.g., Hispanic Santa, African American dolls).
34. If staff members are used as interpreters or if professional interpretation is available, a plan is in effect to address their job duties while interpreting for patients and staff (also a requirement established by The Joint Commission).
35. Education and orientation diversity are addressed as part of new employees' orientation, in-service, and continuing education programs.
36. Nursing care delivery systems, the U.S. system of insurance reimbursement, and issues related to culture and autonomy are discussed.
37. Mentoring programs exist for diverse student and staff populations.
38. Diversity of the health professions is included in orientation.
39. All employees are offered education on both general cultural topics and the culture-specific needs of populations for whom they provide care.
40. Cultural celebrations are reflective of the staff and clients.
41. Resources are available to staff both the clinical unit and the library.
42. Staff members are trained in language interpretation.
43. Health classes are offered to clients whom the community serves.
44. Certification in culture for staff is offered at various levels.
45. Pharmacists, nurses, and physicians are educated in ethnopharmacology.
46. Lunch-and-learn series support the ongoing development of cultural competence.

## Language

1. There are mechanisms in place for translation of written materials in the preferred language of the client.
2. Policies address interpretation services.
3. Resources are available for translation of educational materials and discharge instructions in the languages of the client population.
4. The organization engages in activities that address the health literacy of the population whom it serves.
5. Written documents undergo a cultural sensitivity review.
6. Consent and procedure forms are translated into the languages of the population served.
7. "English as a second language" classes exist for staff.
8. Language classes are offered to clients and family (in English and the language of the population served).

9. Waiting areas have literature in the language of the population served.
10. Directions to referral facilities are in the languages of the client base.
11. Videos are in the language of the client base and have pictures reflective of the client base.
12. Diverse language includes sign language.
13. The need for an interpreter is determined ahead of time.
14. The telephone system prompts are in the languages of the community.
15. Television programs are available in the languages of the community.
16. Satisfaction surveys are available in the languages of the community.
17. Staff surveys are available in the languages of the employees.
18. Audiovisual materials for staff and clients are available in their preferred languages.
19. Wellness and health promotion classes are offered in the languages of the client base.

# Conclusion

APNs—whether they work in clinical practice, education, research, policy, or administration and management—will inevitably work with multicultural patients and with diverse disciplines. When one considers the cultures of the patient, the APN, the profession, and the organization with a diverse workforce, culture competency becomes exceedingly complex. Even though the APN may have exceedingly excellent clinical practice skills, if he or she does not understand and include patients' culture into the nursing process, recommendations will not be followed.

APNs have a crucial role in helping eliminate health disparities, addressing social justice, collaborating with other health disciplines, advancing policy formulation, and participating in or conducting research. The Graduate Cultural Competencies developed by the AACN clearly outline APN core competencies:

- Prioritize the social and cultural factors that affect health in designing and delivering care across multiple contents
- Construct socially and empirically derived cultural knowledge of people and populations to guide practice and research
- Assume leadership in developing, implementing, and evaluating culturally competent nursing and other healthcare services
- Transform systems to address social justice and health disparities
- Provide leadership to educators and members of the healthcare or research team in learning, applying, and evaluating continuous cultural competence development
- Conduct culturally competent scholarship that can be utilized in practice (AACN, 2009)

To this end, culturally competent care is not a luxury for APNs—it is a necessity.

The Purnell model for cultural competence provides a comprehensive guide for developing culturally competent health and nursing care. To date, this model has been used in organizational cultural competence with administration and management (Purnell et al., 2011).

## References

American Association of Colleges of Nursing. (2008). Toolkit for cultural competent education. Retrieved from http://www.aacn.nche.edu/Education/cultural.htm

American Association of Colleges of Nursing. (2009). Graduate cultural competencies: Establishing a culturally competent master's and doctorally prepared nursing workforce. Retrieved from http://www.aacn.nche.edu/education-resources/CulturalComp.pdf

Berlin, E. A., & Fowkes, W. C. (1983). A teaching framework for cross-cultural health care: Application in family practice. *Western Journal of Medicine, 139*(12), 93–98.

Black-Lattanzi, J., & Purnell, L. (2006). *Developing cultural competence in physical therapy practice.* Philadelphia, PA: F. A. Davis.

Braithwaite, A. (2003). Selection of a conceptual model/framework for guiding research interventions. *Internet Journal of Advanced Nursing Practice, 6*(1), 73–93.

Calvillo, E., Clark, L., Purnell, L., Pacquiao, D., Ballantyne, J., & Villaruel, S. (2009). Cultural competencies in health care: Emerging changes in baccalaureate nursing education. *Journal of Transcultural Nursing, 20*(2), 137–145.

Campinha-Bacote, J. (2011). Transcultural C.A.R.E. Associates. Retrieved from http://www.transculturalcare.net/

Catalano, J. T. (2011). *Nursing now: Today's issues, tomorrow's trends* (3rd ed.). Philadelphia, PA: F. A. Davis.

Crandall, S. J., George, G., Marion, G. S., & Davis, S. (2003). Applying theory to the design of cultural competency training for medical students: A case study. *Academic Medicine, 78*(6), 588–594.

Douglas, M., Pierce, J., Rosenkoetter, M., Clark Callister, L., Hattar-Pollara, M., Lauderdale, J., . . . Purnell, L. (2011). Standards of practice for culturally competent nursing care. *Journal of Transcultural Nursing, 229*(4), 317–334.

Fawcett, J., & DeSanto-Madeya, S. (2012). *Contemporary nursing knowledge: Analysis and evaluation of nursing models and theories.* Philadelphia, PA: F. A. Davis.

Giger, J. (2012). *Transcultural nursing: Assessment and intervention* (6th ed.). Philadelphia, PA: Elsevier.

Giger, J., & Davidhizar, R. (2002). The Giger and Davidhizar transcultural assessment model. *Journal of Transcultural Nursing, 13*(3), 185–188.

Giger, J., Davidhizar, R., Purnell, L., Harden, J., Phillips, J., & Strickland, O. (2007). American Academy of Nursing Expert Panel report: Developing cultural competence to eliminate health disparities in ethnic minorities and other vulnerable populations. *Journal of Transcultural Nursing, 18*(2), 95–102.

Jeffreys, M. (2010). *Teaching cultural competence in nursing and health care: Inquiry, action, and innovation.* New York, NY: Springer.

Keynote Recap. (2004). Men in nursing: Meeting a world of health care needs: Cultural competence, diversity, and recruitment. *InterAction, 22*(4), 3–7.

Krainovich-Miller, B., Yost, J., Norman, R., Auerhahn, C., Rosedale, M., Lowry, M., & Moffa, C. (2008). Measuring cultural awareness of nursing students: A first step toward cultural competency. *Journal of Transcultural Nursing, 19*(30), 250–258.

Leininger, M. (2002). Culture care theory: A major contribution to advance transcultural nursing knowledge and practices. *Journal of Transcultural Nursing, 13*(3), 189–192.

Leininger, M., & McFarland, M. (2006). *Culture care diversity and universality: A worldwide nursing theory.* Sudbury, MA: Jones and Bartlett.

Leonardo da Vinci Partnership Project. (2012). The Papadopoulos, Tilki and Taylor model for developing cultural competence. Retrieved from http://www.ieneproject.eu/download/Outputs/intercultural%20model.pdf

McCullough, J., Ramesar, S., & Peterson, H. (1998). Psychotherapy in primary care: The BATHE technique. *American Family Physician, 57*(9). Retrieved from http://www.aafp.org/afp/980501ap/mcculloc.html

Nayar, S., & Tse, S. (2006). Cultural competence and models in mental health: Working with Asian service users. *International Journal of Psychosocial Rehabilitation, 10*(2), 79–87.

Purnell, L. (1999). Panamanians' practices for health promotion and the meaning of respect afforded them by healthcare providers. *Journal of Transcultural Nursing, 10*(4), 333–340.

Purnell, L. (2000a). A description of the Purnell Model for Cultural Competence. *Journal of Transcultural Nursing, 11*(1), 40–46.

Purnell, L. (2000b). Guatemalans' practices for health promotion and wellness and the meaning of respect afforded them by healthcare providers. *Journal of Transcultural Nursing, 11*(3), 40–46.

Purnell, L. (2003a, March–August). *Cultural diversity for older Americans: Cultural competence for the physical therapist working with clients with alternative lifestyles* [Monograph]. American Physical Therapy Association.

Purnell, L. (2003b). The Purnell model for cultural competence: A model for all healthcare providers. *Medical Network, 1*(1), 8–17.

Purnell, L. (2005). Keynote article, special edition: The Purnell model for cultural competence. *Journal of Multicultural Nursing and Health, 11*(2), 7–15.

Purnell, L. (2007). Commentary on "Current approaches to integrating elements of cultural competence in nursing education." *Journal of Transcultural Nursing, 18*(Suppl.), 23–24.

Purnell, L. (2009). Understanding cultural language. *OR Nurse, 3*(4), 49–52.

Purnell, L. (2013). *Transcultural health care: A culturally competent approach* (4th ed.). Philadelphia, PA: F. A. Davis.

Purnell, L., Davidhizar, R., Giger, J., Strickland, O., Fishman, D., & Allison, D. (2011). Guide to culturally competent organizations. *Journal of Transcultural Nursing, 22*(1), 5–14.

Purnell, L., & Foster, J. (2003a). Cultural aspects of alcohol use: Part I. *Drug and Alcohol Professional, 3*(2), 17–23.

Purnell, L., & Foster, J. (2003b). Cultural aspects of alcohol use: Part II. *Drug and Alcohol Professional, 3*(3), 3–8.

Rickles, D., Hawe, P., & Shiell, A. (2007). A simple guide to chaos and complexity. *Journal of Epidemiology and Community Health, 61*, 933–937.

Spector, R. (2009). *Cultural diversity in health and illness* (7th ed.). Upper Saddle River, NJ: Pearson Prentice Hall.

Voyer, P., Rail, G., Laberge, S., & Purnell, L. (2005). Cultural minority older women's attitudes toward medication and implications for adherence to a drug regimen. *Journal of Diversity in Health and Social Care, 2*(1), 47–61.

# The Praxis Theory of Suffering

*Janice M. Morse*

---

## Introduction

The praxis theory of suffering provides a way to conceptualize an individual's and family's emotional response to the losses that occur because of accidental injury or illness, or during dying and bereavement. What a patient and their family *feel* is evident in their behavior. Nurses, in turn, can "read" or interpret these cues or signals of distress—whether they be signs of pain or discomfort, or emotions such as feeling scared, frightened, or terrified—and quickly respond with comforting strategies. These nursing responses may take the form of an appropriate behavioral or verbal interaction, or a nursing intervention intended to reduce the physical or emotional distress. The nurse then immediately reevaluates the patient's signals of distress and either continues with the comforting strategy or changes to a different intervention.

Thus the *praxis* part of the praxis theory of suffering refers to pragmatic interventions—that is, the nursing strategies that ease and relieve the suffering (i.e., comfort patients and families). This theory is clinically useful: Nursing assessments and interventions often take place within an interaction. As such, nurses, by recognizing behavioral cues and instantly responding, serve as the "front line" of intervention.

People often ask how it is possible to "intervene" if the problem is not known. In fact, it is not necessary to know details of the "problem," at least initially, and rarely does a nurse have more than a brief account prior to taking action. What the nurse sees is the person's emotional behavior—in this case, the suffering behaviors—and then responds to it. To recognize the state of suffering, the nurse does not need to know the *reasons* or the details of the cause—just as when a person enters a room full of laughing people, the person does not need to know the reason for their happiness, or to have heard the joke, to recognize that they are happy. What is important, in the case of suffering, is that the person approaching the suffering person reads the person's behavioral cues and responds accordingly. The "intervener" (in this case, the nurse) must take his or her cues from the person who is suffering, must provide behavioral responses that match those cues, and must change those responses as the sufferer's behavioral cues change. In this way, the interaction is dynamic and, ideally, the suffering diminishes as the comforting continues.

## The Praxis Theory of Suffering

### The Development of the Praxis Theory of Suffering

The *praxis theory of suffering* is a qualitatively derived theory; it has been developed from a synthesis of three decades of qualitative studies (see **Table 23–1**). In the 1980s, master's-level students were conducting research on various illness experiences using grounded theory, and some of these studies were published in *The Illness Experience: Dimensions of Suffering* (Morse & Johnson, 1991). The final chapter of the Morse and Johnson book provides a synthesis of the commonalities in all of these chapters. Titled the *illness-constellation model,* it depicts the individual and his or her family's response to illness. The publication of this theory was one of the first qualitative metasyntheses. The illness-constellation model became a part of undergraduate curricula in Europe (e.g., in the Netherlands and Belgium) and is still used in the United States in some physical therapy programs.

About this time, Morse received a 3-year foreign award from the National Institute of Nursing Research (NINR) to delineate comfort and comfort concepts (1991–1994) and to develop the comfort interaction model. A 5-year continuation grant then enabled the identification of comforting strategies during trauma care:

- The Comfort Talk Register—a linguistic register used by nurses to assist patients in excruciating pain to endure and cooperate with trauma care, thereby expediting and increasing its safety (Morse & Proctor, 1998; Proctor, Morse, & Khonsari, 1996).
- A comparison of successful and unsuccessful attempts at nasogastric tube insertion, noting ways that nurses facilitated patient endurance and decreased distress during the procedure (Morse, Penrod, Kassab, & Dellasega, 2000; Penrod, Morse, & Wilson, 1999).
- Integration of the family into trauma resuscitation, classification of their suffering behaviors, and identification of helpful and unhelpful interactions with staff (Morse & Pooler, 2002).

**TABLE 23-1    Research Program for the Development of the Praxis Theory of Suffering: Components, Progress, and Funding Received**

### 1. Background (1985–1991)

**Goal:** To develop grounded theories of illness experience/trajectory of suffering: for example, trajectories of myocardial infarction, hysterectomy, discharge form psychiatric hospital adolescent abortion, impact of chemotherapy on the family

**Funding:** Small grants

**Publications:** See references 1–9 in Appendix 23–1

**Metasynthesis:** The illness experience: dimensions of suffering[10]

⬇

### 2. Delineation of comfort and comforting (1991–1994)

**Goal:** To delineate the concepts inherent in comforting

**Concepts:** Caring, empathy, trust, social support, reciprocity, compathy; patterns of touch (infants)

**Funding:** NRC NIH R01 (3-year foreign award)

**Publications:** See references 11–26 in Appendix 23–1

⬇

### 3. Identification of role of suffering in comforting (1994–1996)

**Goal:** Identification of role of suffering in comforting

**Strategies:** Comfort talk register, nasogastric tube insertion, family presence in trauma care, pain dialogues, normalization

**Funding:** NINR NIH R01 continuation grant (5 years)

**Publications:** See references 27–36 in Appendix 23–1

⬇

### 4. Explication of suffering behaviors (1997–2001)

**Goal:** Development of praxis theory of suffering

Model of "preserving self"; development of praxis theory of suffering; model of reformulated self

**Funding:** NINR NIH R01 (continuation)

**Publications:** See references 37–56 in Appendix 23–1

⬇

### 5. Identification of patterns of suffering (2001–2006)

**Goal:** Identification of patterns of suffering and further development of the praxis theory of suffering; facial coding system for expressions of suffering; synchrony of suffering; patterns of suffering during breast cancer diagnosis

**Funding:** CIHR, Canadian Breast CA FDN

**Publications:** See references 57–63 in Appendix 23–1

⬇

### 6. Anticipated outcomes of this application (2010–2015)

Verified theory

Compendium of enduring behaviors

Clinical implementation model

We also identified a model of "preserving self" with burn patients (Morse, 1997; Morse & O'Brien, 1995) and analyzed their disembodying language as they spoke about their bodies when in agonizing pain (Morse & Mitcham, 1998). We interviewed emergency department/trauma room nurses about suffering and identified *compathy*—the physical equivalent to empathy, referring to the contagion of pain. We delineated this concept and developed a model of compathetic caregiving (Morse & Mitcham, 1997; Morse, Mitcham, & van der Steen, 1998). By 1996, with Barbara Carter, we recognized that there were two primary behavioral states in suffering: enduring (in which the emotions were suppressed) and emotional suffering (in which the emotions were released) (Morse 2000a; Morse & Carter, 1996). Finally, Morse developed (2001) and refined (2005) the model known as the praxis theory of suffering. According to this model, a suffering individual exits the suffering state as the reformulated self, with a new perspective on life (Carter, 1994; Morse & Carter, 1996; see **Figure 23–1**).

In 2001, the investigation continued with a 3-year grant from the Canadian Institutes of Health to further delineate the behaviors of suffering. As part of this study, we videotaped interviews with patients who had been critically ill and relatives of patients who had died (Morse, Beres, Spiers, Mayan, & Olson, 2003). We conducted qualitative ethology of these videotaped interviews, exploring

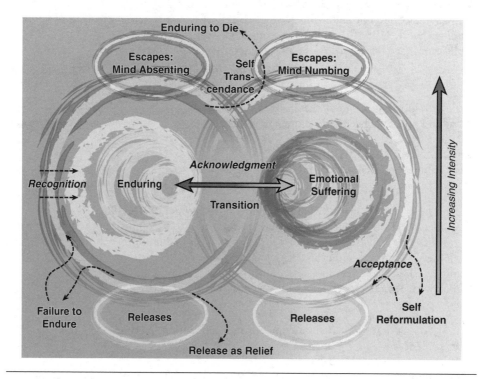

**FIGURE 23–1   Praxis theory of suffering.**

the transitions between the states of enduring and emotional suffering. We used Ekman's Emotional Facial Action Coding System (EMFACS), which is a modified version of the Facial Action Coding System (Ekman & Friesen, 1978; Ekman, Irwin, & Rosenberg, 1994). We described facial expressions of enduring and emotional suffering in the interviews, and we recorded patterned behavioral indices of transitions between enduring and emotional suffering, which lasted from 7.5 to 35 seconds.

More recently, we interviewed women who were awaiting a diagnosis (either positive or negative) of breast cancer and who had negative results to determine further patterns of suffering. Funding from the Alberta Cancer Foundation enabled us to determine whether women who were in the state of enduring must enter a state of emotional suffering to release the suppressed emotions (while enduring) to exit the suffering model, or whether they exited directly from enduring (see Figure 23–1). We found that some exited directly from enduring, releasing emotions as relief and laughter; others exited the model by transitioning through emotional suffering in a torrent of tears; and still others remained either in enduring or in emotional suffering, believing that the negative results were an error and that the physician simply had not found the cancer yet.

## The Components of the Praxis Theory of Suffering

The praxis theory of suffering is a *state* theory: Suffering is an emotional experience; emotion is reflected in, and evidenced in, the suffering person's behaviors. However, while these emotions are observable in distinctive behaviors, they may also be "covered" or concealed. Suffering is a patient-centered, patient-led, dynamic model, and the responses to suffering are individualized and may vary according to a given person's way of responding to loss, the context, cultural and social norms, and the amount of privacy afforded.

*Suffering* is defined as a basic human response to a threat to one's physical or psychosocial integrity (such as occurs in illness or disability, pain, or the death of a loved one), or in untenable life situations (such as abuse or accident). The suffering response may vary in intensity from slight to severe, according to the significance of the loss to the person. It is an emotional response that is manifested behaviorally, that occurs in response to a perceived, threatened (anticipated), or actual loss. The goal of the suffering response is to "shut down" the body or mind to protect the self.

Suffering consists of two major states: enduring and emotional suffering. *Enduring* is a state in which a person's emotions are suppressed and the person focuses on the present. In this situation, the past, which has resulted in the loss, is too painful to recall, and the altered future is too painful to contemplate. Suffering persons are aware that if they respond emotionally to the loss, they might "break down"—that is, they would be unable to function in daily activities and do whatever needs to be done. The emotional suppression is visible and evident in the person's posture, facial expression, interaction with others, and speech. The person who is enduring stands erect, has a mask-like expression, and moves "like a robot" with a lumbering gait that is devoid of spontaneous movement. These people stand apart from one another, tend to be silent, and respond to any attempt at conversation with a single word, nod, or gesture.

When a person is "ready to take it"—that is, to accept whatever is being suffered—he or she transitions into emotional suffering. This shift in state occurs when an individual acknowledges the actuality of their loss. The emotional resources can no longer be controlled and are manifested as states of despair, grief, and sorrow.

*Emotional suffering* is a state in which the emotions of distress are released and a person acknowledges the incomprehensible past, the altered present, and the anticipated future. Persons who are in a state of emotional suffering may cry or weep and have a sorrowful expression. They often want to talk incessantly about the loss to whoever will listen; they have a hunched posture that invites others to hold and comfort them.

These states—enduring and emotional suffering—do not occur simultaneously, nor is the praxis theory of suffering a stage model. Instead, a person may flip back and forth between enduring and emotional suffering. Eventually, when a person has "suffered enough," hope seeps in and the emotions change. He or she gains a new perspective about the experience of suffering—that is, *reformulates* (see self-reformulation in Figure 23–1; Carter, 1994; Morse & Carter, 1996). Individuals who have suffered reevaluate the experience and their altered lives. They are able to consider whatever has made them suffer in a new light, even valuing the experience. Suffering has given them a new appreciation for living, and they leave the states of suffering with a new perspective.

## Enduring

Enduring (see Figure 23–1) is defined as a response to the actual or threatened loss that causes feelings of chaos. When individuals speak of the antecedents to enduring, they describe feeling "blown away," of having "the wind knocked out of them," being "devastated," "crushed"—feelings of shock as they learn of, or experience, the loss. This antecedent event is something that is unavoidable, incomprehensible, and, if anticipated, dreaded. In the face of this loss, individuals respond by attempting to control the internal chaos by containing chaotic emotional responses. "Shutting down" emotionally allows a person to "hold on" or "last through" the threat to the self.

### Attributes of Enduring

As a concept, enduring consists of attributes, or characteristics, that are common to all instances of enduring: (1) maintaining control of self, (2) living in the present moment, (3) removing oneself from the situation, and (4) being aware of the danger or consequences of emotional disintegration.

***Maintaining Control of Self.***    How do those who are enduring hold on? Enduring is attained by *maintaining control of self,* primarily by deliberately suppressing the emotions of despair, grief, terror, or panic. Based on interview data, the initial response to an intrusive event appears to be one of shock, horror, terror, panic, or feeling very scared. When learning their diagnosis, fear may "grip at the heart." People in this state instinctively suppress their emotions so that they may remain in control, until the diagnosis is *real,* and they may think what to do and who to tell, when and where and how. Enduring requires deliberate effort and focus to keep going, to do what is required to get through each day, and to bear whatever must be endured.

How do individuals suppress these emotions? They refuse to let the sorrow show in their face for fear of upsetting others. They refuse to cry; if they do cry, they conceal their tears. Cognitively, they refuse to weep, moan, complain, and "break down." They suppress their feelings to the extent that they may feel calm, competent, and believe they are "managing" well, maintaining normality. Aware that a display of emotions would be distressing to others, they conceal any signals of distress.

This suppression of emotions may be so extreme that it inhibits motor movement in a form of forced self-composure. People in the enduring state feel it is important to maintain dignity: They stand erect but sometimes literally "hold themselves together" by standing with their arms crossed over their chest, clasping the opposite upper arm. They have a distinctive facial expression—one characterized by the lack of movement, a blank unfocused stare. Even if asked a question, they will respond with a monosyllable or a barely perceptible nod. These people do not initiate conversation. Their gait loses spontaneous movement, and they lumber from side to side as they walk. They stand apart from others, and family members may stand at each side flanking the suffering person. They walk in a line, or stand apart from each other, with spaces between. The implicit cue sent out from the enduring person is, "I am okay. Leave me alone." and "Do not touch me."

***Living in the Present Moment.***    Individuals in the enduring state are present focused, concentrating on what is happening now and unable to think about their past or contemplate their future. They feel overwhelmed and are unable to consider several tasks at once, focusing on one small thing at a time instead. They hope to get through the next hour—or sometimes only the next minute—and are unable to comprehend what must be done in a whole day.

For instance, trauma victims narrow their perception by focusing on breathing in and out in an attempt to maintain control; burn victims in the intensive care unit watch the hands of the clock move or count the tiles of the roof or the number of treatments. Those bereaving take "one step at a time." All state that they cannot see the big picture and instead focus on simply getting through the next minute, hour, or day.

***Removing Oneself from the Situation.*** Individuals may remove themselves physically from situations where whatever is being suffered would be publicly acknowledged—for instance, by not going to church or to the store, where others may offer condolences. Such acknowledgment brings whatever is being suffered to the fore and may result in a rush of emotions—the emotions that the individual has been trying to hold in check. For this reason, sympathy cards are valued by those who are enduring, because they may be read when the person is ready to handle the emotions.

Cognitively, individuals put whatever is being endured deliberately at the back of their mind. They may refuse to let thoughts that may cause suffering enter their consciousness. They work hard, focusing intensely and concentrating on work or on special tasks they have set themselves.

Those who are ill may focus on their therapies—for example, counting pills or tests, so that therapy itself becomes the distraction. Nurses' "small talk" becomes important, psychologically removing the person from the sick bed to the life "outside." Patients grab onto the smallest, most feeble joke they hear, repeating it endlessly. Finally, it is no accident that so many jigsaw puzzles can be found in rehabilitation facilities—they are there to distract disabled patients and to remove patients, albeit temporarily, from their present situation.

***Being Aware of the Danger and Consequences of Emotional Disintegration.*** Persons who are enduring resist crying and report they are afraid to cry—afraid they will not be able to stop, afraid they will not be there to do what needs to be done, and metaphorically afraid that they will break down and will not be there for others. They resist sympathetic or empathetic interactions, avoiding those who may offer condolences, because such responses "break through" the stoicism of enduring.

### Recognizing Facial Expressions of Enduring

When assessed using Ekman's EMFACS (Ekman & Friesen, 1978; Ekman et al., 1994), the suppressed emotion gives the face a blank appearance. Facial muscles lack tone and shape. The lips and mouths move only slightly during speech, the eyes are unfocused and rarely blink, and the gaze is centered in the distance, away from the interviewer (see **Figure 23–2**; Morse et al., 2003).

### Escaping from Enduring

When enduring, individuals use *escapes* to vent suppressed emotions. These escapes are *mind-absenting strategies,* or actions that occupy individuals so they do not have to think about whatever it is they are enduring. They include tactics such as keeping busy, concentrating on work, or doing puzzles. Occasionally the suppressed energy cannot be controlled or contained, however; it is then released as anger, fury, excessive exercise, or hysterical laughter. While releases remove the emotional pressure and help individuals remain in control, exhaustion and

**FIGURE 23–2    Faces of enduring.**
*Source:* Morse J. M., Beres M. A., Spiers J. A., Mayan, M., & Olson K. (2003). *Qualitative Health Research, 13*(8), p. 1071, Sage Publications. Reprinted by permission of Sage Publications.

the fatigue of illness without a release may also weaken an individual's ability to endure (i.e., contain the emotions) and cause him or her to lose control.

## Conceptual Boundaries of Enduring

A conceptual boundary separates what enduring is and what it is not. Enduring has not occurred (*fails to endure*) when an individual in the trauma room shifts to an out-of-control state. Out-of-control behavior is an event in which an individual resists care and fights caregivers. Persons in this state shout, swear, and may vocalize nonsensically instead of being able to articulate their emotions and thoughts (see "failure to endure" in Figure 23–1).

## Styles of Enduring

Styles of enduring differ according to (1) role expectations (with males more prone than females to endure), (2) culturally sanctioned behaviors, and (3) context. In Japan, for example, and with the American and Canadian native peoples, enduring is a "public" response and emotional suffering remains largely a private behavior. In other cultures, emotional suffering is likely to be sanctioned culturally but would be expected behavior at funerals, for instance.

## Releases from Enduring

A person cannot remain in a state of enduring indefinitely—the suppressed energy must go somewhere. The emotions emerge and break through explosively as anger or hysterical laughter. If anger emerges, it is usually targeted toward someone "safe" who will not jeopardize care. For example, if it occurs in the emergency department, relatives are more likely to kick the soda machine than to shout at the physician who is providing care.

**FIGURE 23–3    Faces of transition.**
*Source:* Morse J. M., Beres M. A., Spiers J. A., Mayan, M., & Olson K. (2003). *Qualitative Health Research, 13*(8), p. 1072, Sage Publications. Reprinted by permission of Sage Publications.

## Transition

The transition from a state of enduring into the state of emotional suffering is usually deliberate and can be resisted by "fighting" the rising emotions. Most often, a person moves into emotional suffering when he or she feels emotionally ready. Our research group (Morse et al., 2003) studied this transition by conducting videotaped interviews, asking people to tell us their story of the death of a loved one or their illness. As participants told their story, they relived the emotions experienced at that time ("emotional reenactment"; see Morse & Pooler, 2002). Thus, the states of enduring and emotional suffering, and the transitions between the two states, could be microanalyzed, and the dialog simultaneously analyzed as well (see **Figure 23–3**).

### *Facial Expression During Transition*

Transitioning from enduring to emotional suffering tended to take from 7.5 seconds to 35 seconds (mean, 18 seconds). The first indicator of transition from enduring to emotional suffering was the movement of participants' eyes, which made frequent and rapid undirected movements. Their eyes would dart around the room yet remained unseeing and unfocused. Then, as their emotions "broke through" their neutral facial expressions, participants frowned, with their inner forehead raised and their middlebrow lowered. As they lost control, their lips quivered, causing them to tighten and raise their chin to attempt to control the quivering and increasing expression of emotion. Often, at this point participants placed their hands over their mouths. If they continued talking, their upper lips and cheeks began to rise, and lips would begin to stretch as they tried to control their lower face and mouth to keep talking (see **Figure 23–4**; Morse et al., 2003).

| State | Enduring (suppressing emotions) | Transition | Releasing (Emotional suffering) |
|---|---|---|---|
| | nodding | tilts head left   head down (slightly) | |
| | eye movements | eyes blinking–(eyes down) | |
| AU's | | 14+24 → 10+14+24 → | 10+20+ → 10+14+24 → 10+20+24/10+14+24 → 20+24+25 → 10+14+24 → |
| | | 1+4 | 1+4+7 |
| | | breath in | hard swallow |
| Text | and, um, within hours Dr. X called and asked   if I   could have my Dad   at 3 o'clock (Pause | | ) And,   when Dr. X got up and hugged my dad |

Seconds: 0    5    10    15    20    24

**Key: EMFACS Codes (Ekman, Irwin & Rosenberg, 1994)**

| Action Unit (AU) | Corresponding Action | Action Unit (AU) | Corresponding Action | Action Unit (AU) | Corresponding Action |
|---|---|---|---|---|---|
| 1 | inner brow raise | 12 | lip corner pull | 17 | chin raise |
| 4 | brow lower | 14 | dimpler | 23 | lip tight |
| 10 | upper lip raise | 15 | lip corner depress | 24 | lip press |

**FIGURE 23–4   The transition from enduring (emotional suppression) to releasing (emotional suffering).**
*Source:* Morse J. M., Beres M. A., Spiers J. A., Mayan, M., & Olson K. (2003). *Qualitative Health Research, 13*(8), p. 1069, Sage Publications. Reprinted by permission of Sage Publications.

### *The Process of Transition*

In this study of transition, we videotaped 19 participants' stories of suffering. In these interviews were 28 transitions, ranging from 1 to 8 transitions per interview. Transitions from 9 participants were microanalyzed (Morse et al., 2003).

Facial expression and interview text were interdependent. In almost every case, the movement from enduring and reference to self and the future ramifications of the event being suffered was evident, with tearing or crying indicating the onset of emotional releasing. For example:

> 199 =    John (husband) said to me, "I-I think I am dying." (1.3 sec)
> So, um, (4.6 sec) =
> 200 =    he didn't <u>seem</u> any different than he had, (0.5 sec) you know? He was still =
> 201 =    John (0.7 sec) (husband) and still very much <u>alert</u>. (2.5 sec) I guess I didn't =
> 202 =    see the changes as much as every body else (1 sec), you know, because I, =
> 203 =    (0.9 sec) I went through the different stages with him. (2 sec) Part of me =
> 204 =    (.hhh) (5.1 sec) <u>part of me</u> (voice breaking) <u>was dying</u> (.h h .h h) (2.9 sec) =
> 205 =    as <u>John</u> (husband) <u>was dying</u>. (crying) (15.1 sec).

In the preceding text, notice how the language changes from "John" to "I" or "me" as the person transitions into emotional suffering.

## Emotional Suffering

Emotional suffering occurs when the individual acknowledges the actuality of the loss. The emotional resources can no longer be controlled and become manifested as states of despair, grief, and sorrow. During emotional suffering, individuals release emotions to mourn the lost past and altered future. They may cry, weep, or sob; they have a hunched posture and a sorrowful expression. Their posture and their tears touch others emotionally, who are moved to step forward and console the suffering person. Sufferers seek others to be there with them. They talk about the event and their loss incessantly to whoever will listen, psychologically working through and mourning their lost past and their altered future. They accept touch, sympathy, and empathy. When the pain of emotionally suffering is too much to bear, these individuals use escapes—mind-numbing strategies—such as watching television or sleeping incessantly (Morse, 2001)—to dull the emotional pain of suffering.

### *Recognizing Facial Expressions of Emotional Suffering*

When emotionally suffering, participants revealed a furrowed brow, the corners of their mouths dimpled, and they raised their chins as they pressed their lips

**FIGURE 23–5    Faces of emotional suffering.**
*Source:* Morse J. M., Beres M. A., Spiers J. A., Mayan, M., & Olson K. (2003). *Qualitative Health Research, 13*(8), p. 1073, Sage Publications. Reprinted by permission of Sage Publications.

together. Verbally, they moved the conversation to the self ("I" or "me"), and their speech was marked with swallowing, cracking of the voice, pausing, and uneven pacing (see **Figure 23–5**; Morse et al., 2003).

## The Synchrony of Suffering

Of importance to nursing is the synchrony of enduring and emotional suffering in family groups. Individuals within family groups move from enduring to suffering, and back to enduring, in a synchronized manner. Emotional suffering is often a private behavior that is concealed from others. We may watch family members endure as they walk down the corridor and into the cubical where their ill relative rests. Because they recognize that their own emotional suffering may cause distress in the sick person, family members endure while in the presence of the sick person, making jovial small talk and so forth. Then, after the visit, and as family members walk back to the family room, they may transition into emotional suffering, sobbing in the family room or the bathroom.

In family groups, family members take turns enduring and "holding the family together," acting as comforter and taking care of others. When family members are emotionally suffering, one may become the endurer, remaining strong enough to comfort and support those who are emotional suffering. Later, they may switch roles.

In our studies, we were able to explore the patterns of interactions between those who were enduring and those who were suffering by examining the videotapes of family groups as they entered the trauma room and visited their injured or ill family member (Morse & Pooler, 2002). In emergency situations, families are usually in shock, trying to grapple with what has happened. As such, the family members are usually in states of enduring, standing apart from one another and trying to hold themselves together. As the crisis passes, they move into suffering, with one member remaining in enduring to hold and comfort the others, talk to the staff, and make decisions.

## Coming Out of Suffering

Once a person has been able to accept what has happened and envision a new and altered future, hope seeps in. Using techniques of theoretical coalescence in our studies, we were able to "open" the concepts and examine processes of emotional suffering and hope and document the interaction of these two concepts. We were able to identify the linkage of these two concepts (the process of hope initially links to emotional suffering in the despair associated with emotional suffering) and to show how hoping enables an individual to make the effort to emerge from emotional suffering (Mayan, Morse, & Eldershaw, 2006; Morse & Penrod, 1999).

If the person who is suffering is dying, the outcome of emotional suffering is resolution of the suffering as *transcendence*; in such a case, the person does not have the energy to emotionally suffer and "fades away," dying in a state of enduring ("enduring to die"). If the person is in rehabilitation or is not ill, he or she exits emotional suffering as a *reformulated self*. Using techniques of concept analysis, we are able to show that transcendence is reached by using hope to find new meaning in a situation. *Reformulation* takes longer than transcendence, with the person living the renewed perspective by giving back to others—for instance, by volunteering for self-help groups or assisting in a cancer unit. In this state, people reevaluate their lives and change their values and goals accordingly.

### Enduring to Die

Facing one's own death when receiving palliative care, we reasoned, must be extraordinarily distressful. Therefore, we expected that extensive emotional suffering would be apparent in palliative care settings. "Not so," the nurses reported. Some patients did become distraught now and then (and this distress usually occurred in private). Very occasionally they had a patient who was "often" distressed, but by and large the patients manifested behaviors that could be described as enduring.

To investigate this matter further, we conducted a study interviewing patients and nurses (Olson, Morse, Smith, Mayan, & Hammond, 2000–2001) about emotions in palliative care. During this study, the patients' emotional states were, indeed, aptly described as enduring. As patients became increasingly sick and nearer to death, enduring behaviors continued, until the patients simply "faded away" as they became increasingly unaware, lost consciousness, and died. An important relationship was discovered between fatigue and emotional suffering—namely, "to emotionally suffer," energy is required. Palliative patients simply did not have the energy to emotionally suffer and, to conserve energy, maintained a state of enduring.

## Is It Possible to Exit the Model from Enduring?

By 2000, it was clear that assumptions of the praxis theory of suffering needed to be further explored. The original model was not linear, but rather dynamic. Persons could vary in intensity of enduring and emotional suffering and could move through the transition into suffering and then return to enduring; they could even move into a transitional state from enduring and then resist emotional suffering and return to enduring. What was uncertain was, except in the scenario of "enduring to die," whether a person must exit the model through emotional suffering to release the suppressed emotions of enduring. *Was it possible to exit the model directly from enduring in situations other then dying?*

We designed a study to explore this question, examining the release of enduring when the condition being endured was removed. We chose the instance of undergoing diagnostic tests for breast cancer—specifically, when the mammography was initially indicative of cancer, but later the result of the breast biopsy was found to be negative for cancer.

## Suffering Breast Cancer Diagnosis

We deliberately selected a situation that required maximal enduring to "get through," but then the conditions necessary to endure were removed. Women have described discovering a breast lump or having a suspicious mammogram, and subsequently waiting for the diagnosis, as "the worst experience of their lives." When a subsequent breast biopsy revealed that the lesion was benign, we conjectured that when the woman was informed that she did not have cancer, she would then enter emotional suffering to release the suppressed emotions of enduring, rather than moving directly from enduring without emotional release.

Our first assumption, that women would be *intensely* enduring, proved only partly correct. Some women did endure the threat of cancer; others were able to endure only partially and did emotionally suffer on occasions, switching back and forth between enduring and suffering as they contemplated their future cancer and death. A third group of women were not able to endure well and almost constantly displayed emotional suffering while waiting for their test results, already convinced that they had cancer.

Indeed, when told they did not have cancer, some women did enter emotional suffering and then displayed relief. The physician reported that it is these patients, "who do not have cancer, who cry at this time." Others exited enduring directly to a state of relief, laughing and celebrating. Surprisingly, despite the negative results, a third group continued enduring and emotionally suffering. They did *not* believe that they did not have cancer; they were certain that they did have cancer, but that the physician had simply not found it yet. Perhaps listening to the tentative nature of the physicians' request for long-term follow-up and mammograms at 6-month intervals supported their skepticism.

Nevertheless, the implications for the development of the praxis theory of suffering were that it was clear that the suppressed energy from enduring could be released directly from enduring as other emotions. The person did not have to enter emotional suffering, although this was certainly a path selected by some participants in the study.

### Learning to Recognize Behavioral States of Suffering

This model is titled the *praxis* theory because it has clear implications for nursing practice. By learning to read the behavioral cues of those who are suffering, nurses can determine if a person is enduring or emotionally suffering—a critical consideration because nurses' interactions with a person who is enduring are very different from the interventions that should be used with a person who is emotionally suffering.

When a person is enduring, the role of the nurse should be to support the enduring behaviors. People in this state are grappling and cognitively struggling to come to terms with whatever has happened to cause them to endure, or they may be enduring by moving the events to the back of their mind so they do not have to face or handle them at that particular moment. Because they are suppressing emotions, any empathetic expression or the use of comforting touch could bring the negative events to the fore and give them something else to endure. These people respond best to the caregiver *being with* them in silence, standing apart, and being available should they need anything. They may not converse. They will not respond well to questions about how they *feel*; they may withdraw if touched. Later, they may respond to distractions, grabbing onto any conversation that is about anything other than what is being endured, and struggle to maintain a normal appearance to the household routine.

In contrast, persons who are emotionally suffering send a message to caregivers that they need to be comforted. They respond to touch, being held, being stroked, and being listened to. They accept empathetic and comforting words, and need (and will accept) assistance.

Ideally, all nurses should learn to read bodily cues to discover individuals' states of mind (Morse, 2000a). The way a nurse interacts with a patient, for example, is determined by that individual's state. A nurse responds to a patient who is enduring by standing apart from that patient and providing concrete information in a factual manner. A nurse responds to a patient in emotional suffering quite differently: The nurse may express condolences, touch the person, or even place an arm around the individual.

This is a forgiving model: If a nurse makes a mistake—for instance, uses touch inappropriately with a person who is enduring—that person will instantly withdraw. Sensing this rejection, the nurse can immediately apologize and correct his or her approach. However, if the nurse does not attend to patients' cues of withdrawal and continues with the touch approach, he or she may cause persons to collapse, because empathetic statements and comforting touch *confirm* that the "worst has happened." Persons are then eligible for all of the social supports that are offered to individuals in crisis, hence forcing persons to accept what has happened before they are cognitively able to accept the event.

For nursing, the praxis theory of suffering is interlaced with comforting interventions. Comforting is the intervention to ease suffering: It enables enduring, and it relieves emotional suffering.

Using this perspective on suffering (i.e., that the suffering experience is observable) means that the nurse can assess a patient's state without using instruments, questionnaires, or interviews. The nurse can also determine a patient's state of suffering—and identify the patient's comfort needs—both quickly and accurately (Morse, 2000a). *Does the nurse need to know the details of what is being suffered?* Often nurses do not; they must move in to assist before they have that information, or perhaps to obtain that information. In fact, nurses must often move toward comforting a distressed person to find out "what the matter is" so that comfort begins before assessment is complete.

## Degrees of Enduring/Modes of Enduring

The preceding model incorporates two major states, enduring and emotional suffering. It would be naïve to suggest that there are only two behavioral states in patients. We can also identify degrees of the two states—for instance, emotional suffering ranging from sad to distraught.

While conducting research in the trauma care, we listened to nurses' descriptions of patients and then assessed these *emic* categorizations of behavioral states and characteristics displayed by patients and the modes of comforting interaction by nurses. Each of these states may be conceptualized in the praxis theory of suffering as evidence of a certain degree of either enduring or failure to endure.

*Scared.* Patients who are scared are relatively quiet and, if spoken to, may respond with a single word or a silent nod. Verbalizations are not offered spontaneously, but rather are given only in response to direct questions. For example, the patient responds with such words as "what," "yes," and "no," and uses vocalizations such as "mm" and "huh, huh":

| | |
|---|---|
| Physician: | Does your arm hurt anywhere? |
| Patient: | No. |
| Physician: | How about this arm (reaching across to patient's right arm)? |
| Patient: | No. |
| Physician: | Can you squeeze my fingers? Squeeze my finger over here real tight. Okay, now your left hand. Squeeze my fingers again, real tight. Squeeze my fingers. |
| Patient: | Um huh. |
| Physician: | Is that as hard as you can? |
| Patient: | Yeah, uh huh [don't know if this is right]. |

Volume, or loudness of the voice, can range from soft to normal. Voice modulation can range from normal to some quivering. These patients are generally quiet and are absorbing everything that is going on, so that the quiet, minimal behavior is pragmatically functional. They appear to listen intently to whatever is being said about them.

Scared patients do not have any spontaneous movements and lie very still ("scared stiff"). If a nurse moves their arm, they will keep that arm in that position until the nurse moves it again. If they cry, the tear will roll out of the corner of their eyes without being wiped away.

*Comforting interactions* with these patients are *being there,* with the nurse sometimes providing a "running commentary" of what he or she is doing: "I am here, just behind your head, changing your IV."

***Anxious.***   In contrast to scared patients, anxious patients are often hyperverbal and produce a continuous flow of words, perhaps in an attempt to control their anxiety. This hyperverbal behavior is manifested by constant talking; patients provide more information than is needed; caregivers tend to interrupt them to move the assessment along. Anxious patients' affects may vary; these patients may present with joking, flirting, frequent excessive praising of the staff, or comments to minimize their injury. At the same time, they may constantly verbalize their concern about their injury, the treatment, or general concern about others involved in the accident. The essential feature is that patients keep talking: "Oh I'm, I'm okay. I tell you, you girls are doing a great job with me. Great job."

Patients' volume is normal with efforts to control the levels of intensity; this attempted control may give the voice a restrained quality. When the restraint threatens to be lost, a tremulous quality is reflected in the voice. Some patients may exhibit whining behavior, particularly in children ("Mommmy" or "I, I, I, I'm, I'm, sooooo thirsty"). It seems that the children's alternative to hyperverbalization is this whining.

| | |
|---|---|
| Patient: | When are you going let me up? [sound dampened] |
| Nurse: | Listen, we put a little tube into your penis. So you can pee, okay? You don't have to stand up. It's already, go . . . you're already going. |
| Patient: | Where's it going to go? |
| Nurse: | It's going to go into a little bag here. We have a bag for it, so you can just go ahead and go. We have to make sure your back's okay. |
| Patient: | Owwww [whining]. |
| Nurse: | I know . . . we'll take it out once it's . . . once we're all done, okay? |
| Patient: | Owwww. |
| Nurse: | So don't pull it because it will hurt if you pull it out. |
| Patient: | Can I go to the bathroom? [Kind of tentative now] |

***Frightened.***   The critical and distinctive features of being frightened are complaining, moaning, groaning, whimpering, and begging interspersed with rapid questioning ("What are you doing?"), repeated requests, and demands for changes in care practices.

| | |
|---|---|
| Patient: | No! Can I bend my knee? [Struggles to free herself from another nurse who was holding her legs.] |
| Physician: | You can bend your knees. |
| Patient: | Jesusss. |
| Physician: | Don't move around there [sound dampened]. |
| Patient: | All rightttt! |
| Nurse: | You don't have to be so nasty. We're here to help you! |
| Patient: | I don't feel like you're helping very much right now! I feel like you're hurting me! |
| Physician: | Physically? |

Frightened patients are not reticent about letting the staff know when procedures are painful or when their level of discomfort is unbearable. Their speech is peppered with expressions such as "ouch," "ooohh," and "stoppp," vocalized in a commanding voice quality.

Patients who are frightened speak at moderate volume, which seems to be used as a mechanism to reduce their fear. When they are verbalizing, the content has an unsteady quality in that they produce longer chunks of language before the nurse hears a break in the voice. In all age groups, crying can be heard. This is the only behavioral state in which crying with vocalization occurs.

Frightened patients may withdraw from care and treatments, although if nurses and other staff hold their hands, they will not pull away from care and do not need to be restrained. They watch—monitor—all staff movements very carefully.

***Terrified.*** In the terrified state, patients vocalize in short phrases or short sentences, during which they loudly protest, swear, shout, and beg the staff. These short sentences or phrases are usually up to five words in length. These patients vacillate between loud intensity and a moderate volume, and they include vocalizations that take the form of loud protestations ("Noooooo," "Please, oh God please God!"). Vocal modulation has an emphatic and exclamatory nature, and a lot of anger and hostility is often evident. Note that these patients are irrationally refusing care despite the urgent nature of the care. Physically, they may struggle to get up from the gurney, are restless, may be combative and fight caregivers, and may have to be restrained. (The numbers in the following comments and in other places in this chapter represent the line numbers, the time, or the seconds from the interview transcriptions.)

| | |
|---|---|
| Patient: | Aw come on now! . . . I want to go home. (3.00) |
| Patient: | I want to go home. [Said in almost a normal voice] (3.03) |
| Patient: | Ow, no. [In response to procedures being applied] (3.09) |

|   |   |
|---|---|
| **Patient:** | I just want the fuck out! [Patient struggling] (3.11) |
| **Physician:** | Don't move. (3.14) |
| **Patient:** | Come on now! (3.21) |
| **Patient:** | Please, come on. (3.23) |
| **Patient:** | Look, I'm not your guinea pig. |
| **Nurse:** | You're not a guinea pig. We do this to everyone that comes in this way, okay? (3.30) |
| **Patient:** | Oh god, ow . . . |
| **Physician:** | Put your head down! |
| **Patient:** | Ouch, it hurts man! (3.33) |
| **Patient:** | Ouch, it hurts man. (3.34) |
| **Nurse:** | I know it does . . . |
| **Patient:** | I thought you'd be fucking nice to me! |

Both frightened and terrified patients respond to a nurse being there for them and *talking them through* the experience (Morse & Proctor, 1998; Proctor et al., 1996). More recently, this response has been proven effective with frightened patients in second-stage labor (Bergstrom, Richards, Morse, & Roberts, 2010; Bergstrom et al., 2009). Talking them through as a nursing intervention is discussed in more detail later in this chapter.

***Out of Control.***    Out-of-control patients exhibit hysterical, screaming, bellowing behavior. They are beyond coherent verbalizations, although occasionally a single word may be intelligible. Some attempts to verbalize are characterized by babbling, and short verbalizations will often be heard between screams.

The sound ranges from very loud to piercing and continuous. Voice modulation is erratic and inconsistent. This piercing and vacillating voice quality is accompanied by guttural sounds, such as "Aghuh gh gh gh gh" or "Aghuhuhhuh Owww Owwww Owwww." This kind of volatile patient often loses the ability to modulate his or her voice and produces maximum volume, yelling and screaming at the highest possible level. Staff interaction with these patients ceases, and it is difficult when a patient is out of control to communicate or to stop the vocalizations.

|   |   |
|---|---|
| **Patient:** | Aghuh aghuh. |
| **Physician:** | Don't move! |
| **Patient:** | Aghuh gh gh gh gh, |
| **Physician:** | Easy . . . |
| **Patient:** | Aghuh gh gh gh gh, |
| **Physician:** | Hold still . . . |

Out-of-control patients must be restrained so that emergency care can be administered, or they must be anesthetized as quickly as possible. They can be so distraught that they lose the ability to speak and vocalize shouts of rage. At this point, any discourse with the patient stops and caregivers go ahead, attending to the person's injuries.

Nurses can identify other behavioral states in the clinical areas and select the most appropriate modes of nursing interactions with those patients. There is much work to do in this area. Nurses see severe suffering on a daily basis, but they also see the suffering resulting from minor discomforts—for example, from a sore back from lying in bed, from nausea, from worries about how the family is managing at home while the mother is in the hospital. Nurses become adept at quickly and easily recognizing the cues that indicate something is not quite right. Sometimes comforting is providing an analgesic, giving a back rub, talking, listening, or just being there.

## Comfort and Comforting

What, then, is comfort? *Comfort* is a concept that incorporates the caring focus of nursing—which enables us to see the cues and signals of suffering and motivates us to comfort—and a comforting action or task (Morse, 2000b). Note that when comfort is the central concept for nursing, nursing care is focused on the patient—in contrast to caring, which is focused on the nurse. Within this framework, nurses' use of touch and talk are not indicators of caring per se; rather, they are comforting strategies that are responses to *signals of suffering*. They are *strategies for alleviating suffering* (Morse, 1992). Comfort, therefore, cannot be separated from suffering.

Comforting is not a "one-shot" intervention; it is a process that occurs in many iterative steps within the interaction and the developing relationship. During the *comforting interaction loop* in which a comforting action occurs, the patient is reevaluated and another comforting action is provided, and so forth. Examples of the comforting interaction loop follow:

- Observing that the patient appears to be in pain (noting the signal of suffering or cues of distress), verifying the pain with the patient (action), administering an analgesic action (comforting action), and observing signs that the pain was subsequently alleviated
- Observing that the patient appears cold and is shivering (noting the behavioral cue), fetching a warm blanket (comforting action), and observing the patient appears more relaxed and warmer

As nursing tasks increase in complexity, so do the comforting actions:

- During childbirth, the nurse observes that the patient is becoming distressed (signal of suffering) and uses his or her voice (comforting interaction, "talking through") to assist in synchronizing the second-stage labor until the woman regains control (Bergstrom et al., 2010).
- In the trauma room during resuscitation, a patient is scared but lying still (caring observation). The nurse provides a "running commentary" by talking constantly, describing everything that he or she and the trauma team are doing. Later, the patient reports that she "just listened to that nurse's voice and held on."

- During trauma resuscitation, the nurse observes that the patient is terrified (signal of suffering). He or she uses the *comfort talk register* to enable the patient to hold on, and hold still (comforting action) until the analgesics take effect (Morse & Proctor, 1998; Proctor et al., 1996).

Comforting continues until it is no longer needed or demanded by the patient. Thus, comfort is defined as a relative and optimal state of well-being that may occur during any stage of the illness–health continuum. Responding to signals of suffering by making the patient comfortable is the goal of nursing (Morse, 1992).

## The Comforting Interaction

The *comforting interaction* comprises the patient cue or a signal of distress from the patient, the cue or signal observed by the nurse, and the nurse's assessment of the patient and provision of a comfort strategy (Morse, Havens, DeLuca, & Wilson, 1997). The nurse then assesses the effectiveness of the strategy and, if the need has not been resolved, provides another strategy. This cycle may be slow and deliberate, or as quick and almost subconscious as an interaction. As the comforting interactions accrue, the trust in the nurse–patient relationship builds. The relationship itself changes from a clinical relationship to a therapeutic relationship; then, to a connected relationship (Morse, 1991); the patient feels safe and relinquishes himself or herself to the nurse's care (Morse, 1992).

The comforting interaction is patient led. In our observations of postoperative infants, for example, comforting always occurred in response to the infant's cues. If the infant did not, or could not, "demand" a comforting strategy, it was usually not provided. For instance, because the infants were intubated, they cried silently, unable to vocalize their distress. As a result, nurses rarely used their voices to comfort the infants (Morse, Solberg, & Edwards, 1993; Solberg & Morse, 1991).

The nurse needs to provide care that is appropriate to the patient's state, and each state is associated with a different compendium of comforting strategies. If the nurse provides the wrong strategy, then the patient's state escalates. Ideally, the nurse will immediately correct the error and change the comforting intervention (Morse et al., 1997).

*How important are these comforting interventions?* Did you know that the way a nurse talks to the patient while inserting a nasogastric tube affects the success of the procedure (Morse et al., 2000; Penrod et al., 1999)? If the nurse, either by using technical talk (talk that focuses solely on what the patient should do) or by using solely caring terms of endearment, is overly receptive to the patient's cues of distress and does not include instructions for the patient, then the nurse will require more trials to place the tube correctly. The optimal way to talk to patients is a blend of technical and caring talk. Our research has shown that when the nurse uses the optimal style of talking, the nasogastric tube is successfully inserted with the smallest number of trials.

*How important is comfort talk in trauma care?* Trauma patients may be highly anxious, terrified, or out of control. Out of control is a very dangerous state—these patients could be irrational and try to fight the caregivers, and such effort both slows the delivery of emergency care and exacerbates injuries.

Can you imagine how pushing off caregivers and fighting care increases intracranial pressure? If the patient has a head injury, such actions could produce a large amount of cerebral damage. In the window of time before the patient can be given analgesics, the nurse assists the patient in maintaining control. The nurse talks the patient through the experience, using the *comfort talk register* (Morse & Proctor, 1998; Proctor et al., 1996), positions himself or herself over the patient's head, and holds his or her gaze (see **Figure 23–6**). The nurse then talks to the patient using a high "sing-song" register with distinct verbal contours. The nurse immediately interrupts any patient utterances and cries, urges the patient to "hold on," constantly warns the patient of painful procedures, and informs the patient how much longer the procedures will last.

The practice of talking through also serves other important functions in trauma care. All communications to and from the patient go through the nurse. The nurse receives and communicates information about the patient's condition; he or she provides explanations, and the nurse's explanations then pace the trauma team. Procedures are performed one at a time, and only once the patient

**FIGURE 23–6   Posturing in "talking through" using the comfort talk register.**

has been told what will happen. For instance, the nurse might say, "You will feel a finger in your bum, okay? Okay? **Okay?**"; only then is the rectal examination conducted. Without this information and pacing, the patient is very likely to lose control.

In a trauma situation, comfort is clearly a combination of touching, talking, posturing, and being immediately available to the patient. This assists the patient in maintaining control and is essential for the provision of safe care. These states in which care is given are known as *relinquishment to care* (Morse, 2000b). Various types of relinquishment are as follows:

- *Complete relinquishment:* The patient is unconscious or the patient cedes control totally to the nurse, urging the nurse to do "whatever is necessary."
- *Relaxed relinquishment:* The patient passively lies or dozes and lets the nurse give care. The patient trusts the nurse and senses the degree of vigilance, "watching over," and monitoring of the patient's condition, as with scared states.
- *Guarded relinquishment:* The patient watches what the nurse does and follows the nurse's action with his or her eyes. The patient holds still and permits care but does not trust the nurse or has limited trust.
- *Conditional relinquishment:* Bargaining takes place between the patient and the caregiver: The patient demands information about the procedure, sometimes in great detail. This behavior is often seen in children or highly anxious patients.
- *Reluctant relinquishment:* After bargaining, the patient continues to protest throughout the procedure. The patient often must be persuaded with a bribe.
- *Forced relinquishment:* The patient protests, refuses care, and must be held down. Patients constantly try to pull away, shout, or beg the nurse to "Hurry!" These patients are often terrified.

In trauma care, for instance, patients who feel in control relinquish to care; that is, they are responsive, cooperative, and receptive. Despite the pain, they try to remain passive and hold still, to "take it," to "bear it," and not to cry out. They work with staff—the patient who has completely relinquished realizes that care is necessary and submits to "whatever needs to be done." The result is that care is given quickly and safely. Again, the comfort level is a dynamic continuum, and patients generally fall somewhere between complete relinquishment and forced relinquishment (Morse, 2000b, p. 36). Nevertheless, the nurse–patient relationship is complex, and the patient does not immediately move to complete relinquishment, unless the patient's needs are great and life threatening.

### The Patient's Comfort Level

Interestingly, nursing is just beginning to develop a solid theoretical base for providing comfort. When in the clinical areas, nurses would be well advised to listen for the ways that other nurses talk about patient states and communicate information about the patient's comfort states. Often, nurses will hear references to the patient's *comfort* level (Sasano & Morse, 2006). The comfort level is actually not a level of comfort, but rather the level of *distress* and the extent to which pain (or whatever is causing the distress) is being tolerated. For instance, a nurse may ask, "What is the patient's comfort level?" and be told, "He is tolerating it quite well"—which means that the patient is enduring the procedure, and it is not necessary to provide an analgesic immediately. Conversely, the nurse may reply, "He is really scared" or "He is out of control—we really need a hand in the trauma room!" Again, the comfort level is not the amount of pain that is being experienced, but rather how well it is being tolerated. Description of this level enables the rapid communication of the patient's behavioral state of suffering.

## Compendium of Comforting Strategies

Comforting strategies available to nurses are numerous, and only some have been mentioned thus far. It is beyond the scope of this chapter to list them all. A brief classification of comforting strategies—by no means complete—is provided here.

Some strategies are present in the everyday interaction, without premeditation, as we console, or commiserate. Other strategies are used thoughtfully, and with care, such as providing empathy or formal counseling strategies. Some comforting strategies are prescribed, such as administering an analgesic. Some are standardized as a part of excellent nursing care, such as a back rub, position change, or bed bath. Some are in the control of nursing but are not routine, such as placing a patient on an air mattress. Some are indirect, such as controlling the environment—noise level or temperature, for example. The point is that all of these strategies are intended to enhance enduring, to help the patient "get through," and to reduce or to minimize the patient's suffering.

# Summary

Developed first from a synthesis of many research projects, and later by systematic research to test conjectures or to fill gaps, the praxis theory of suffering links myriad patient emotional states with comforting strategies. The model is patient led. With the nurse being responsive to patients' needs and the effects of nursing interventions, the model is dynamic and provides a means by which the nurse can systematically provide comfort. It is a malleable model, so that if a nurse provides an inappropriate strategy and the patient withdraws or has a negative response, the nurse may immediately change the strategy and move again toward comforting.

*Is the model culturally bound? Can it be used cross-culturally?* Because the nurse follows a patient's cues and signals of distress, this theory may be used to provide interventions with any culture.

*Is the model limited to acute care or to trauma care?* While most of the observational work has been done in areas of extreme distress, this model could be used in any setting, in home care, in clinics, in nursing homes—indeed, in any caregiving situation. Because the nurse "reads" the patient's behavior, the praxis theory of suffering offers many benefits over other models in which assessment is much slower, is more complex, or requires psychometric instruments. This model is compatible with actual patient care, bereavement, and rehabilitation.

A significant amount of work remains to be done on this theory, such as identification of patient states, signals and cues of distress, and comforting strategies, as well as development of the model. For instance, much work remains to be done on the state of enduring, on styles of enduring, and on the ways in which people self-console. We need to be able to develop and apply the model clinically: Can nurses, for instance, teach strategies of enduring, and if so, will those strategies decrease the length of time spent in rehabilitation?

## Discussion Questions

1. Search the Web for groups of people who are suffering. If you use "suffering" as the search term, for example, you will retrieve great works of art, depicting emotional suffering. But if you search for current events that have caused suffering—earthquakes, floods, fires, accidents, and so forth—you will get very interesting pictures from which you can easily identify states of enduring or emotional suffering. Examine both the person whom the photographer has targeted and the states of the people in the background. Often the target person is emotionally suffering and those in the background are enduring. Why do photographers target those who are emotionally suffering rather than enduring? Examine the proximal relationships of groups of people. Who are the supporters and who is releasing emotions? Who are the comforters? Note the states (enduring or emotional suffering) of each person.

2. Examine photographs of formal ceremonies, such as funerals. Do you think conventions and ceremonies support enduring or emotional suffering behaviors in the bereaved? How? Why?

3. Both enduring and emotional suffering trigger emotions in observers. How do these emotions differ? Which kinds of responses in the observer do they elicit?

## References

Bergstrom, L., Richards, L., Morse, J., & Roberts, J. (2010). How caregivers manage pain and distress in second stage labor. *Midwifery, 55*(1), 38–45.

Bergstrom, L., Richards, L., Proctor, A., Bohrer-Avila, L., Morse, J., & Roberts, J. (2009). Birth talk in second stage labor. *Qualitative Health Research, 19,* 954–964.

Carter, B. J. (1994). Surviving breast cancer. *Cancer Practice, 2*(2), 135–140.

Ekman, P., & Friesen, W. V. (1978). *Facial action coding system: A technique for the measurement of facial movement.* Palo Alto, CA: Consulting Psychologists.

Ekman, P., Irwin, W., & Rosenberg, E. (1994). *EMFACS: Coders instructions (EMFACS-8).* San Francisco, CA: University of California, San Francisco.

Mayan, M., Morse, J. M., & Eldershaw, L. P. (2006). Developing the concept of self reformulation. *QHW: International Journal of Qualitative Studies on Health and Well-being, 1*(1), 20–26.

Morse, J. M. (1991). Negotiating commitment and involvement in the patient–nurse relationship. *Journal of Advanced Nursing, 16,* 455–468.

Morse, J. M. (1992). Comfort: The refocusing of nursing care. *Clinical Nursing Research, 1,* 91–113.

Morse, J. M. (1997). Responding to threats to integrity of self. *Advances in Nursing Science, 19*(4), 21–36.

Morse, J. M. (2000a). Responding to the cues of suffering. *Health Care for Women International, 21,* 1–9.

Morse, J. M. (2000b). On comfort and comforting. *American Journal of Nursing, 100*(9), 34–38.

Morse, J. M. (2001). Toward a praxis theory of suffering. *Advances in Nursing Science, 24*(1), 47–59.

Morse, J. M. (2005). Creating a qualitatively-derived theory of suffering. In U. Zeitler (Ed.), *Clinical practice and development in nursing* (pp. 83–91). Aarhus, Denmark: Center for Innovation in Nurse Training.

Morse, J. M., Beres, M., Spiers, J., Mayan, M., & Olson, K. (2003). Identifying signals of suffering by linking verbal and facial cues. *Qualitative Health Research, 13*(8), 1063–1077.

Morse, J. M., & Carter, B. (1996). The essence of enduring and the expression of suffering: The reformulation of self. *Scholarly Inquiry for Nursing Practice, 10*(1), 43–60.

Morse, J. M., Havens, G., DeLuca, A., & Wilson, S. (1997). The comforting interaction: Developing a model of nurse–patient relationship. *Scholarly Inquiry for Nursing Practice, 11*(4), 321–343.

Morse, J. M., & Johnson, J. L. (Eds.). (1991). *The illness experience: Dimensions of suffering.* Newbury Park, CA: Sage.

Morse, J. M., & Mitcham, C. (1997). Compathy: The contagion of physical distress. *Journal of Advanced Nursing, 26,* 649–657.

Morse, J. M., & Mitcham, C. (1998). The experience of agonizing pain and signals of disembodiment. *Journal of Psychosomatic Research, 44*(6), 667–680.

Morse, J. M., Mitcham, C., & van der Steen, V. (1998). Compathy or physical empathy: Implications for the caregiver relationship. *Journal of Medical Humanities, 19*(1), 51–65.

Morse, J. M., & O'Brien, B. (1995). Preserving self: From victim, to patient, to disabled person. *Journal of Advanced Nursing, 21,* 886–896.

Morse, J. M., & Penrod, J. (1999). Linking concepts of enduring, suffering, and hope. *Image: Journal of Nursing Scholarship, 31*(2), 145–150.

Morse, J. M., Penrod, J., Kassab, C., & Dellasega, C. (2000). Evaluating the efficiency and effectiveness of approaches to nasogastric tube insertion during trauma care. *American Journal of Critical Care, 9*(5), 325–333.

Morse, J. M., & Pooler, C. (2002). Patient–family–nurse interactions in the trauma resuscitation room. *American Journal of Critical Care, 11*(3), 240–249.

Morse, J. M., & Proctor, A. (1998). Maintaining patient endurance: The comfort work of trauma nurses. *Clinical Nursing Research, 7*(3), 250–274.

Morse, J. M., Solberg, S., & Edwards, J. (1993). Caregiver–infant interaction: Comforting the postoperative infant. *Scandinavian Journal of Caring Sciences, 7,* 105–111.

Olson K., Morse, J. M., Smith, J., Mayan, M., & Hammond, D. (2000–2001). Linking trajectories of illness and dying. *Omega, 42*(4), 293–308.

Penrod, J., Morse, J. M., & Wilson, S. (1999). Comforting strategies used during nasogastric tube insertion. *Journal of Clinical Nursing, 8,* 31–38.

Proctor, A., Morse, J. M., & Khonsari, E. S. (1996). Sounds of comfort in the trauma center: How nurses talk to patients in pain. *Social Sciences & Medicine, 42,* 1669–1680.

Sasano, P., & Morse, J. (2006). *What is a patient's comfort level? Defining a nursing concept.* Unpublished paper, University of Alberta, Canada.

Solberg, S., & Morse, J. M. (1991). The comforting behaviors of caregivers toward distressed post-operative neonates. *Issues in Comprehensive Pediatric Nursing, 14*(2), 77–92.

# Reference List for Table 23-1

1. Morse, J. M. (1983). An ethnoscientific analysis of comfort: A preliminary investigation. *Nursing Papers/Perspectives in Nursing, 15*(1), 6–19.

2. Johnson, J. L., & Morse, J. M. (1990). Regaining control: The process of adjustment following myocardial infarction. *Heart and Lung, 19*(2), 126–135.

3. Wilson, S., & Morse, J. M. (1991). Living with a wife undergoing chemotherapy: Perceptions of the husband. *Image: Journal of Nursing Scholarship, 23*(2), 78–84.

4. Thomas, A., & Morse, J. M. (1991). Managing urinary incontinence. *Journal of Gerontological Nursing, 17*(6), 9–14.

5. Côté, J. J., Morse, J. M., & James, S. G. (1991). The pain experience of the post-operative newborn. *Journal of Advanced Nursing, 16,* 378–387.

6. Morse, J. M. (1991). Negotiating commitment and involvement in the patient–nurse relationship. *Journal of Advanced Nursing, 16,* 455–468.

7. Solberg, S., & Morse, J. M. (1991). The comforting behaviors of caregivers toward distressed post-operative neonates. *Issues in Comprehensive Pediatric Nursing, 14*(2), 77–92.

8. Morse, J. M. (1991). The structure and function of gift-giving in the patient–nurse relationship. *Western Journal of Nursing Research, 13,* 597–615.

9. Solberg, S., & Morse, J. M. (1991). The comforting behaviors of caregivers toward distressed post-operative neonates. *Issues in Comprehensive Pediatric Nursing, 14*(2), 77–92.

10. Morse, J. M., & Johnson, J. L. (Eds.). (1991). *The illness experience: Dimensions of suffering.* Newbury Park, CA: Sage.

11. Morse, J. M., Bottorff, J., Neander, W., & Solberg, S. (1991). Comparative analysis of the conceptualizations and theories of caring. *Image: Journal of Nursing Scholarship, 23*(2), 119–126.

12. Morse, J. M. (1992). Comfort: The refocusing of nursing care. *Clinical Nursing Research, 1,* 91–113.

13. Estabrooks, C., & Morse, J. M. (1992). Toward a theory of touch: The touching process and acquiring a touching style. *Journal of Advanced Nursing, 17*, 448–456.

14. Morse, J. M., Bottorff, J., Anderson, G., O'Brien, B., & Solberg, S. (1992). Beyond empathy: Expanding expressions of caring. *Journal of Advanced Nursing, 17*, 809–821.

15. Morse, J. M., Anderson, G., Bottorff, J., Yonge, O., O'Brien, B., Solberg, S., & McIlveen, K. (1992). Exploring empathy: A conceptual fit for nursing practice? *Image: Journal of Nursing Scholarship, 24*(4), 274–280.

16. Morse, J. M., Solberg, S., & Edwards, J. (1993). Caregiver–infant interaction: Comforting the postoperative infant. *Scandinavian Journal of Caring Sciences, 7*, 105–111.

17. Laskiwski, S., & Morse, J. M. (1993). The spinal cord injured patient: The modification of hope and expressions of despair. *Canadian Journal of Rehabilitation, 6*(3), 143–153.

18. Morse, J. M., Solberg, S., & Edwards, J. (1993). Caregiver–infant interaction: Comforting the postoperative infant. *Scandinavian Journal of Caring Sciences, 7*, 105–111.

19. Morse, J. M., Bottorff, J. L., & Hutchinson, S. (1994). The phenomenology of comfort. *Journal of Advanced Nursing, 20*, 189–195.

20. Siegl, D., & Morse, J. M. (1994). Tolerating reality: The experiences of parents with HIV positive sons. *Social Science & Medicine, 38*, 959–971.

21. Bottorff, J. L., & Morse, J. M. (1994). Identifying types of attending: Patterns of nurses' work. *Image: Journal of Nursing Scholarship, 26*(1), 53–60.

22. Morse, J. M., Bottorff, J. L., & Hutchinson, S. (1994). The phenomenology of comfort. *Journal of Advanced Nursing, 20*, 189–195.

23. Morse, J. M., Miles, M. W., Clark, D. A., & Doberneck, B. M. (1994). Sensing patient needs: Exploring concepts of nursing insight and receptivity used in nursing assessment. *Scholarly Inquiry for Nursing Practice, 8*(3), 233–254.

24. Morse, J. M., Bottorff, J. L., & Hutchinson, S. (1995). The paradox of comfort. *Nursing Research, 44*(1), 14–19.

25. Applegate, M., & Morse, J. M. (1994). Personal privacy and interaction patterns in a nursing home. *Journal of Aging Studies, 8*(4), 413–434.

26. McIlveen, K. M., & Morse, J. M. (1995). The role of comfort in nursing care: 1900–1980. *Clinical Nursing Research, 4*(2), 127–148.

27. Morse, J. M., & Carter, B. J. (1995). Strategies of enduring and the suffering of loss: Modes of comfort used by a resilient survivor. *Holistic Nursing Practice, 9*(3), 33–58. Reprinted in Danish: N. Gress (Ed.), *Klinisk Sygrpleje, bd 1,11, og 111, 2000.*

28. Morse, J. M., & O'Brien, B. (1995). Preserving self: From victim, to patient, to disabled person. *Journal of Advanced Nursing, 21*, 886–896. DOI:10.1046/j.1365-2648.1995.21050886.x

29. Miles, M., & Morse, J. M. (1995). Utilizing the concepts of transference and countertransference in the consultation process. *Journal of the American Psychiatric Nurses Association, 1*(2), 42–47.

30. Hyland, L., & Morse, J. M. (1995). Orchestrating comfort: The role of funeral directors. *Death Studies, 19*, 453–474.

31. Hupcey, J. E., & Morse, J. M. (1995). Family and social support: Application to the critically ill patient. *Journal of Family Nursing, 1*(3), 257–280.

32. Morse, J. M., & Doberneck, B. M. (1995). Delineating the concept of hope. *Image: Journal of Nursing Scholarship, 27*(4), 277–285.

33. Dewar, A., & Morse, J. M. (1995). Unbearable incidents: Failure to endure the experience of illness. *Journal of Advanced Nursing, 22*(5), 957–964.

34. Proctor, A., Morse, J. M., & Khonsari, E. S. (1996). Sounds of comfort in the trauma center: How nurses talk to patients in pain. *Social Sciences & Medicine, 42*, 1669–1680.

35. Hogan, N., Morse, J. M., & Tasón, M. C. (1996). Toward an experiential theory of bereavement. *Omega, 33*(1), 43–65.

36. Morse, J. M., & Carter, B. (1996). The essence of enduring and the expression of suffering: The reformulation of self. *Scholarly Inquiry for Nursing Practice, 10*(1), 43–60.

37. Morse, J. M., & Mitcham, C. (1997). Compathy: The contagion of physical distress. *Journal of Advanced Nursing, 26,* 649–657.

38. Morse, J. M. (1997). Responding to threats to integrity of self. *Advances in Nursing Science, 19*(4), 21–36.

39. Penrod, J., & Morse, J. M. (1997). Strategies for assessing and fostering hope: The Hope Assessment Guide. *Oncology Nurses Forum, 24*(6), 1055–1063.

40. Morse, J. M., & Mitcham, C. (1998). The experience of agonizing pain and signals of disembodiment. *Journal of Psychosomatic Research, 44*(6), 667–680.

41. Penrod, J., Morse, J. M., & Wilson, S. (1999). Comforting strategies used during nasogastric tube insertion. *Journal of Clinical Nursing, 8,* 31–38.

42. Morse, J. M., Havens, G., DeLuca, A., & Wilson, S. (1997). The comforting interaction: Developing a model of nurse–patient relationship. *Scholarly Inquiry for Nursing Practice, 11*(4), 321–343.

43. Morse, J. M., Mitcham, C., & van der Steen, V. (1998). Compathy or physical empathy: Implications for the caregiver relationship. *Journal of Medical Humanities, 19*(1), 51–65.

44. Wilson, S., Morse, J. M., & Penrod, J. (1998). Developing reciprocal trust in the caregiving relationship. *Qualitative Health Research, 8,* 446–465.

45. Morse, J. M., & Proctor, A. (1998). Maintaining patient endurance: The comfort work of trauma nurses. *Clinical Nursing Research, 7*(3), 250–274.

46. Morse, J. M. (2000). On comfort and comforting. *American Journal of Nursing, 100*(9), 34–38.

47. Wilson, S., Morse, J. M., & Penrod, J. (1998). Absolute involvement: The experience of mothers of ventilator-dependent children. *Health & Social Care, 6*(4), 224–233.

48. Hupcey, J. E., Penrod, J., & Morse, J. M. (2000). Establishing and maintaining trust during acute care hospitalizations. *Scholarly Inquiry for Nursing Practice: An International Journal, 14*(3), 227–242.

49. Morse, J. M. (2000). Responding to the cues of suffering. *Health Care for Women International, 21,* 1–9.

50. Morse, J. M., & Penrod, J. (1999). Linking concepts of enduring, suffering, and hope. *Image: Journal of Nursing Scholarship, 31*(2), 145–150.

51. Morse, J. M., Penrod, J., Kassab, C., & Dellasega, C. (2000). Evaluating the efficiency and effectiveness of approaches to nasogastric tube insertion during trauma care. *American Journal of Critical Care, 9*(5), 325–333.

52. Morse, J. M., Wilson, S., & Penrod, J. (2000). Mothers and their disabled children: Refining the concept of normalization. *Health Care for Women International, 21*(8), 659–676.

53. Olson, K., Morse, J. M., Smith, J., Mayan, M., & Hammond, D. (2000–2001). Linking trajectories of illness and dying. *Omega, 42*(4), 293–308.

54. Morse, J. M. (2001). Toward a praxis theory of suffering. *Advances in Nursing Science, 24*(1), 47–59. [Italian: Verso una teoria della prassi della sofferenza, (traduzione di Luca Mori). *Salute e Società, 1,* a cura di Enzo Giorgo e Willem Tousijn, FrancoAngeli, 2003, pp. 169–185; Commentary: Mori, L. l'osserfvzione della sofferenza nel lavoro di Janice Morse, pp. 186–189].

55. Hupcey, J., Penrod, J., Morse, J., & Mitcham, C. (2001). An exploration and advancement of the concept of trust. *Journal of Advanced Nursing, 36*(2), 282–293.

56. Morse, J. M., & Pooler, C. (2002). Patient–family–nurse interactions in the trauma-resuscitation room. *American Journal of Critical Care, 11*(3), 240–249.

57. Morse, J. M., Beres, M., Spiers, J., Mayan, M., & Olson, K. (2003). Identifying signals of suffering by linking verbal and facial cues. *Qualitative Health Research, 13*(8), 1063–1077.

58. Mayan, M., Morse, J. M., & Eldershaw, L. P. (2006). Developing the concept of self-reformulation. *QHW: International Journal of Qualitative Studies on Health and Well-being, 1*(1), 20–26.

59. Weaver, K., Morse, J. M., & Mitcham, C. (2008). Ethical sensitivity in practice: Concept analysis. *Journal of Advanced Nursing, 62*(5), 607–618.

60. Bergstrom, L., Richards, L., Proctor, A., Bohrer-Avila, L., Morse, J., & Roberts, J. (2009). Birth talk in second stage labor. *Qualitative Health Research, 19*, 954–964.

61. Bergstrom, L., Richards, L., Morse, J., & Roberts, J. (2009). How caregivers manage pain and distress in second stage labor. *Midwifery, 55*(1), 38–45.

62. Morse, J. M., Konrad, S. J., Pooler, C., & Mott, R. (Submitted). Awaiting the diagnosis of breast cancer: Patterns of emotional responses.

63. Morse, J. M., Konrad, S. J., Pooler, C., & Mott, R. (Submitted). The release from enduring: Receiving the news your breast biopsy is negative.

# PART 5

# Tools for Integrating and Disseminating Knowledge in Advanced Nursing Practice

# Theory Testing and Theory Evaluation

*Jacqueline Fawcett*

## Introduction

The focus of this chapter is the science and art of theory development and evaluation. It begins with a definition of theory and a description of the process of theory development, and then continues with a discussion of the critical thinking that is required for the evaluation of theories. The emphasis in this chapter is theory development and evaluation activities that are required for advanced nursing practice. The content of this chapter is especially relevant to two essentials for doctor of nursing practice programs: *Essential I, Scientific Underpinnings for Practice*, and *Essential III, Clinical Scholarship and Analytical Methods for Evidence-Based Practice*.

## The Science and Art of Theory Development

The term *theory* is used to refer to diverse works, ranging from very abstract and general conceptual models to less abstract and general grand theories, to relatively concrete and specific middle-range theories, to very concrete and specific narrow-range, situation-specific theories. Despite the lack of consensus about the meaning of theory, King and Fawcett (1997) found considerable agreement about the existence of levels of abstraction for theoretical work. In this chapter, the

Portions of this chapter are adapted from Fawcett, J., & Garity, J. (2009). *Evaluating research for evidence-based nursing practice*. Philadelphia, PA: F. A. Davis. Used with permission.

term refers to middle-range theories. The term *conceptual model* refers to the very abstract and general work from which theories are derived.

## Theories

A theory is made up of concepts and propositions about a phenomenon. A *concept* is a word or phrase that captures the essence of something, such as functional status or mood. It may have one or more dimensions. An example of a single-dimensional concept is physical energy. An example of a multidimensional concept is functional status; the dimensions in this case include family care activities, household activities, social activities, community activities, personal care activities, and occupational activities (Tulman & Fawcett, 2007).

A *proposition* is a statement about one or more concepts. A proposition about one concept is a definition or a description of the concept; functional status, for example, can be defined as the performance of the usual activities of daily living. A proposition about two or more concepts states an association between the concepts, including the relationship between the concepts or the effect of one concept on one or more other concepts. For example, the following statement outlines the relationship between two concepts: "Functional status is related to mood." An example of a statement about the effect of a concept on another concept typically involves the effect of some intervention on some outcomes, such as: "An exercise intervention improves functional status and mood."

Nursing theories usually focus on experiences of health conditions and health-related events. Examples of health conditions include such medical diagnoses as cancer, multiple sclerosis, and diabetes. Examples of health-related events include pregnancy, childbirth, the postpartum period, and aging. The health condition or health event of interest provides a context for a theory. For example, the concepts of exercise intervention, functional status, and mood and the propositions about those concepts could make up a theory about the effects of an exercise intervention on the functional status and mood of women with breast cancer. Alternatively, the concepts of functional status and mood might make up a theory about the relationship between functional status and mood during the postpartum period.

## Types of Theories

Three types of theories are distinguished: descriptive, explanatory, and predictive. *Descriptive theories* simply describe some phenomenon. They typically comprise one concept and one proposition that is a definition or description of the concept. An example of a descriptive theory is the theory of functional status. In this case, the theory concept is functional status. The theory proposition asserts that functional status is a multidimensional concept that is defined as the performance of usual family care activities, household activities, social activities, community activities, personal care activities, and occupational activities (Tulman & Fawcett, 2007).

*Explanatory theories* specify how concepts are related to one another; they provide explanations for phenomena. They consist of two or more concepts, the propositions that are definitions or descriptions of each concept, and the propositions that specify the relationship(s) between the concepts. An example is the theory of chronic pain (Tsai, Tak, Moore, & Palencia, 2003). In this case, the theory concepts are chronic pain, physical disability, social support, age, gender, perceived daily stress, and depression. The propositions are definitions of each concept:

- Chronic pain is defined as the frequency and severity of pain (Tsai et al., 2003).
- Physical disability is defined as the frequency and extent of mobility, walking, bending, and hand and finger function (Tsai et al., 2003).
- Social support is defined as "perceived levels of social support . . . [including] (a) provision of attachment/intimacy, (b) social integration, (c) opportunity for nurturant behavior, (d) reassurance of worth, and (e) availability of informational, emotional, and material help" (Tsai et al., 2003, p. 162).
- Age is defined as age in years (Tsai et al., 2003).
- Gender is defined as male or female (Tsai et al., 2003).
- Perceived daily stress is defined as "the degree to which older persons experience daily stress from irritating, frustrating, or repeated occurrences in their lives" (Tsai et al., 2003, p. 162).
- Depression is defined as the frequency of depressed mood symptoms within the past week (Tsai et al., 2003).

The theory proposition that specifies the relationship between the concepts is as follows: "Chronic pain, physical disability, social support, age, and gender are related to perceived daily stress, which is related to depression."

*Predictive theories* specify how a concept affects one or more other concepts. They are made up of two or more concepts, the propositions that are definitions or descriptions of each concept, and the propositions that specify the effect(s) of one concept on one or more other concepts. An example is the theory about the effects of cancer support groups with coaching on symptom distress, emotional distress, functional status, and the quality of the cancer patient's relationship with a significant other (Samarel, Fawcett, & Tulman, 1997). In this case, the theory concepts are the cancer support group, symptom distress, emotional distress, functional status, and the quality of the relationship with a significant other. The propositions that are definitions of each concept are as follows:

- Cancer support group is defined as a "professionally led, structured 2-hr [cancer support group]" (Samarel et al., 1997, p. 18). The experimental treatment cancer support group included the woman's significant other, who served as a coach. One control treatment was a cancer support group that did not include coaches. The second control treatment was no support group.

- Symptom distress is defined as "the amount of physical distress or unpleasant body sensation experienced during treatment for breast cancer" (Samarel et al., 1997, p. 20).
- Emotional distress is defined as "the amount of psychological, or affective distress experienced during treatment for breast cancer" (Samarel et al., 1997, p. 20).
- Functional status is defined as "the extent to which usual household, family, social and community, personal care, and occupational activities were continued following the diagnosis of cancer" (Samarel et al., 1997, p. 21).
- The quality of the relationship with a significant other is defined as an individual's "perception of changes since diagnosis in the relationship with . . . an identified significant other . . . with regard to satisfaction, communication, trust, sensitivity, openness, and understanding" (Samarel et al., 1997, p. 21).

The theory proposition that specifies effects is as follows: "Women with breast cancer who participated in [a cancer support group with coaching] would have less symptom distress, less emotional distress, greater functional status, and a higher quality of relationship with a significant other . . . than women who participated in [a cancer support group without coaching] and women [who did not participate in any support group]" (Samarel et al., 1997, p. 17).

## Empirical Indicators and Other Empirical Methods

Most theory concepts and propositions cannot be directly observed or measured. Instead, each concept must be connected to an *empirical indicator*, which serves as a real-world proxy for a concept. Empirical indicators that are particularly useful for advanced nursing practice are assessment tools and intervention protocols. *Assessment tools* include various types of questionnaires, such as checklists and rating scales, that comprise one or more items. For example, functional status can be measured by a multiple-item checklist of activities of daily living performed during a particular period of time, a multiple-item rating scale such as the Comprehensive Inventory of Functioning—Cancer (Tulman & Fawcett, 2007), or a one-item rating scale that asks the patient to indicate, on a scale of 0 to 10, the extent to which he or she is performing the usual activities of daily living. One-item assessment tools are particularly useful in advanced nursing practice because they do not impose a burden on the patient, such as may occur when a tool with many items is used. One-item assessment tools also are useful because they do not impose an undue burden on the advanced practice nurse, such as may occur with use of a multi-item tool that requires calculation of a score.

*Intervention protocols* are explanations of procedures that are administered to or engaged in by patients; they are analogous to the experimental and control treatments used in experimental research and to the procedures included in clinical guidelines or a hospital procedure manual. The explanation for all procedures used to conduct a cancer support group is an example (Samarel et al., 1997; Samarel, Tulman, & Fawcett, 2002). Other empirical methods that are part of nursing practice and research include the number of times and the ways in which the assessment tool and intervention protocol are applied (the research design and data collection procedures), the number of patients who are assessed and receive the intervention (the sample of research participants), and the ways in which the results of the assessment and outcomes of the interventions are analyzed for quality improvement initiatives (the data analysis techniques).

## Conceptual Models

Theories are developed through a melding of science and art in the form of creative conversion of ideas stemming from provocative facts (Levine, 1966) observed in practice and in the literature. These facts are noticed because they fit with the observer's frame of reference about nursing, which also is called a *conceptual model* of nursing. Among the best-known conceptual models are Levine's conservation model, Neuman's systems model, Orem's self-care model, and Roy's adaptation model. Overviews of these and other conceptual models of nursing can be found in Appendix N-1 of *Taber's Cyclopedic Medical Dictionary* (Fawcett, 2009). A comprehensive analysis and evaluation of each of these and other conceptual models of nursing can be found in Fawcett and DeSanto-Madeya's book, *Contemporary Nursing Knowledge: Analysis and Evaluation of Nursing Models and Theories* (2013).

Each conceptual model of nursing is made up of concepts and propositions that are more abstract and general than those of a theory. Examples of concepts from Roy's adaptation model include stimuli and adaptation. An example of a proposition that defines a concept is as follows: Adaptation is defined as "The process and outcome whereby thinking and feeling people, as individuals and in groups, use conscious awareness and choice to create human and environment integration" (Roy, 2009, p. 26). An example of a proposition that links the concepts of stimuli and adaptation is as follows: Stimuli are related to the modes of adaptation, which are physiological, self-concept, role function, and interdependence (Fawcett, 2003).

## Conceptual–Theoretical–Empirical Structures for Theory Development

*Theory development* involves specification of a conceptual–theoretical–empirical (C-T-E) structure made up of three components:

1. A conceptual model
2. A theory
3. Empirical indicators and other empirical methods

Theory development is the product of research, which itself is a systematic process of inquiry (Fawcett & Garity, 2009). Thus, every study is explicitly or implicitly designed to develop a theory. Although the conduct of research typically is thought of as a rigorous scientific process, it is also a creative endeavor involving an appreciation of the beauty of logical reasoning and the "aha" moments that come when developing elegant C-T-E structures, designing studies, and interpreting data.

**TABLE 24–1    Theory-Generating and Theory-Testing Research: Types of Theories and Research Designs**

| Type of Research | Type of Theory | Type of Research Design |
|---|---|---|
| Theory-generating research | Descriptive theories | Descriptive research |
| Theory-testing research | Descriptive theories | Descriptive research |
| | Explanatory theories | Correlational research |
| | Predictive theories | Experimental research |

*Source:* Adapted from: Fawcett, J., & Garity, J. (2009). *Evaluating research for evidence-based nursing practice.* Philadelphia, PA: F. A. Davis, p. 27. Used with permission.

## Conceptual–Theoretical–Empirical Structures for Theory Generation

Theory development may involve inductive reasoning from specific observations of a phenomenon to a general concept and one or more propositions about the concept. This type of theory development is called *theory generation*. Theory generation typically is accomplished by conducting descriptive research, which may be qualitative or quantitative. The product of the descriptive research is descriptive theories (see **Table 24–1**).

As can be seen in **Figure 24–1**, the C-T-E structure for theory generation proceeds from the conceptual model to the empirical indicators and other empirical methods to the concepts and propositions of a new theory. **Figure 24–2** shows an example of a C-T-E structure for theory generation. This example was constructed from the report of a study designed to generate a theory of living with multiple sclerosis (Gagliardi, Frederickson, & Shanley, 2002). The authors' theory-generating research was guided by Roy's adaptation model; the empirical indicators were interview guides. The Roy model concept of modes of adaptation was used to guide the analysis of data collected by interviews of people with multiple sclerosis. Thus, each of the five themes identified in the interview data—"We're not completely the same," "Let me tell you about my feelings," "How I view my future," "How I see work," and "Let me tell you about my life"—was

**FIGURE 24–1    Conceptual-Theoretical-Empirical Structure for Theory-Generation: From conceptual model to empirical indicators to theory.**

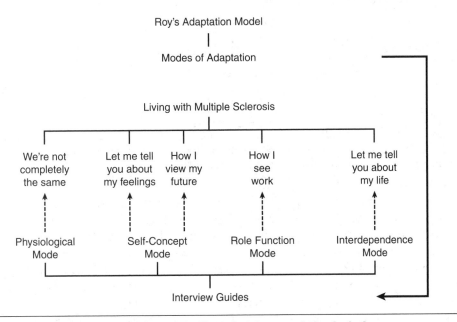

**FIGURE 24–2    C-T-E structure for Gagliardi, Frederickson, and Shanley's theory-generating study.**

linked to one of the modes of adaptation: physiological, self-concept, role function, or interdependence. The themes are considered the dimensions of the theory concept, living with multiple sclerosis.

## Creating Conceptual–Theoretical–Empirical Structures for Theory Generation

Advanced practice nurses can create C-T-E structures for their own studies designed to generate a new theory, or they can prepare a diagram of the C-T-E structure for an existing study. The C-T-E structure begins with the identification of the conceptual model concept that guides the selection of the empirical indicator used to collect data. This structure is completed when the theory concept and any concept dimensions are identified (see Figure 24–1 and Figure 24–2).

## Conceptual–Theoretical–Empirical Structures for Theory Testing

Theory development also may involve deductive reasoning from one or more general concepts and propositions to a specific set of concepts and propositions. This type of theory development is called *theory testing*. Theory testing typically is accomplished by means of the conduct of descriptive research, correlational research, or experimental research. The product of theory-testing descriptive research is a descriptive theory, the product of correlational research is an explanatory theory, and the product of experimental research is a predictive theory (see Table 24–1).

Conceptual Model

Theory

Empirical Indicators

**FIGURE 24–3    Conceptual–Theoretical–Empirical structure for theory-testing: From conceptual model to theory to empirical indicators.**

As can be seen in **Figure 24–3**, theory testing proceeds from the conceptual model to the theory that is to be tested to the empirical indicators and other empirical methods. **Figure 24–4** shows an example of a C-T-E structure for theory testing. This example was constructed from the report of a study designed to test a theory about the effects of a cancer exercise program on fatigue, physical function, and mood experienced by patients with various types of cancer (Hanna, Avila, Meteer, Nicholas, & Kaminsky, 2008). The authors' research was guided by Levine's conservation model. As can be seen in Figure 24–4, the conservation model concept of therapeutic intervention was linked with the theory concept of cancer exercise program, which was implemented by means of the empirical indicator that specified the precise intervention protocol. Additionally, the conservation model concepts of therapeutic intervention, conservation of energy, structural integrity, personal integrity, and social integrity were linked to the theory concepts of fatigue, physical function, and mood, respectively. The empirical indicator used to measure fatigue was the Piper Fatigue Scale. The empirical indicator for

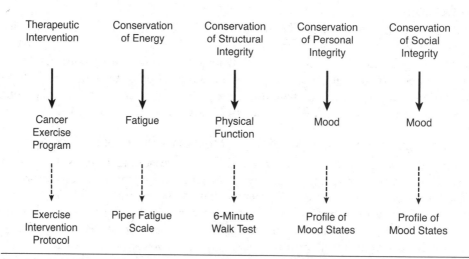

**FIGURE 24–4    C-T-E structure for Hanna, Avila, Meteer, Nicholas, and Kaminsky's theory-testing study.**

physical function was the 6-minute walk test. The empirical indicator for mood was the Profile of Mood States.

## Creating Conceptual–Theoretical–Empirical Structures for Theory Testing

Advanced practice nurses can create C-T-E structures for their own studies designed to test an existing theory, or they can prepare a diagram of the C-T-E structure for an existing study. The most important aspect of creating C-T-E structures for theory testing is the linkage of a conceptual model to a theory. Three approaches have been identified.

The first approach is the selection of the conceptual model of nursing and the direct derivation of a theory from that conceptual model. For example, two theories of family health have been directly derived from King's conceptual system (Doornbos, 1995, 2000; Wicks, 1995, 1997). This approach ensures a logical linkage between the conceptual model and the theory. The logic is ensured because the philosophical assumptions undergirding the conceptual model and the theory are the same.

The second approach is to select a conceptual model of nursing and then link an existing nursing theory to that conceptual model. For example, a researcher might want to link the nursing theory of uncertainty in illness (Mishel, 1990) to Roy's adaptation model. This approach is problematic in that the philosophical assumptions undergirding the conceptual model of nursing and the philosophical assumptions undergirding the conceptual model from which the theory of uncertainty in illness was derived may not be logically congruent. Logical congruence is evident only if the philosophical assumptions undergirding both conceptual models are the same.

The third approach is to select a conceptual model of nursing and then link an existing theory borrowed from another discipline to that conceptual model. For example, the theory of planned behavior (Ajzen, 1991), taken from the discipline of social psychology, has been linked to Neuman's systems model and with Orem's self-care framework (Villarruel, Bishop, Simpson, Jemmott, & Fawcett, 2001). Like the second approach, this approach can be problematic in that the philosophical assumptions undergirding the conceptual model of nursing and the philosophical assumptions undergirding the conceptual model from which the theory of planned behavior was derived may not be logically congruent. Logical congruence is evident only if the philosophical assumptions undergirding both conceptual models are the same.

Latham (2002) rejected the third approach on the grounds that it does not contribute to the advancement of the discipline of nursing. She declared:

> Grafting a particular borrowed theory onto a nursing conceptual model may be a questionable exercise. . . . Rather the emphasis could be placed on creating distinctive cognitive approaches with the parameters of nursing. . . . Nursing research will not advance knowledge if it continues to hang on the coattails of other disciplines. (p. 264)

The C-T-E structure for theory testing is completed when the theory concepts are linked to empirical indicators (see Figure 24–3 and Figure 24–4).

## Partnerships for Theory Development

Advanced practice nurses certainly may construct C-T-E structures and conduct research independently, but they may be more successful if they form partnerships with nurse researchers who are fully prepared to conduct research through research training from a doctor of philosophy or other research-intensive educational program. Such partnerships integrate the clinical expertise of the advanced practice nurse with the research expertise of the nurse researcher. An example of a successful partnership that brought together student nurses, staff nurses, advanced practice nurses, and nurse researchers is an international multisite study designed to test a theory of women's perceptions of and responses to cesarean birth that was guided by Roy's adaptation model (Fawcett et al., 2005; Fawsett et al., 2011).

# The Science and Art of Theory Evaluation

Many different sets of criteria for evaluating theories can be found in the nursing literature (e.g., Barnum, 1998; Duffy & Muhlenkamp, 1974; Fawcett, 2005; Fawcett & DeSanto-Madeya, 2013; George, 2002; Mariner-Tomey & Alligood, 2006; McEwen & Wills, 2007; Meleis, 2012; Parse, 2005). However, only one set of criteria includes the three components of C-T-E structures (Fawcett & Garity, 2009). That set of criteria is summarized in **Table 24–2**.

Evaluating C-T-E structures for theory generation and theory testing is a five-step process that requires thinking critically and making judgments about the extent to which the information about each component of the C-T-E structure satisfies a certain set of criteria. Critical thinking and making judgments is a primarily scientific endeavor grounded in the criteria, but it also involves the art of grasping the meaning of what is intended in the linkages among the C-T-E structural components and appreciating the beauty of the elegance of those linkages in a nonscientific, intuitive manner.

## Step 1: Evaluation of the Conceptual–Theoretical–Empirical Linkages

The first step in evaluation of C-T-E structures focuses on the conceptual model (C) component. The two criteria in this case are specification adequacy and linkage adequacy.

### Specification Adequacy

*Specification adequacy* refers to the amount of information about the conceptual model that is used to construct the C-T-E structure. It requires that the conceptual

**TABLE 24–2    Steps in the Evaluation of Conceptual–Theoretical–Empirical Structures**

| Steps | Criteria |
|---|---|
| 1. Evaluation of the conceptual–theoretical–empirical linkages | *Specification adequacy* is evident.<br>• Refers to the amount of information about the conceptual model.<br>  ◆ The conceptual model is explicitly identified.<br>  ◆ A clear and concise overview of the content of the conceptual model is given.<br><br>*Linkage adequacy* is evident.<br>• Refers to the clarity of the connections between the conceptual model, the theory, and the empirical indicators.<br>  ◆ The connections between the conceptual model, theory, and empirical indicators are explicit and complete. |
| 2. Evaluation of the theory | The theory is *significant*.<br>• Refers to the extent of social and theoretical importance of the theory.<br>  ◆ The theory should address a topic that is of practical importance to society.<br>  ◆ The theory should offer new insights about the topic.<br><br>The theory is *internally consistent*.<br>• Refers to the extent to which the theory is comprehensible.<br>  ◆ The concepts should be explicitly identified and clearly defined.<br>  ◆ The same term and same definition should always be used for each concept.<br><br>The theory is *parsimonious*.<br>• Refers to the extent to which the theory is stated as concisely as possible.<br>  ◆ The theory should be made up of as few concepts and propositions as necessary to convey its meaning.<br><br>The theory is *testable*.<br>• Refers to the extent to which the theory can be tested empirically.<br>  ◆ All concepts should be measurable. |

*(Continues)*

**TABLE 24-2    Steps in the Evaluation of Conceptual–Theoretical–Empirical Structures (*Continued*)**

| Steps | Criteria |
|---|---|
| 3. Evaluation of the empirical indicators | *Operational adequacy* is evident.<br>• Refers to the appropriateness of the empirical indicators.<br>   ♦ Empirical indicators yielding qualitative data should be dependable and credible.<br>   ♦ Empirical indicators yielding quantitative data should be reliable and valid measures of the theory concepts. |
| 4. Evaluation of research findings | The theory is found to be *empirically adequate* when tested.<br>• Refers to the extent to which the data agree with the theory.<br>   ♦ The concepts and propositions of the theory should be congruent with research findings. |
| 5. Evaluation of the utility and soundness of the conceptual model | The conceptual model is found to be *legitimate*.<br>• Refers to the extent to which the research supports the usefulness and soundness of the conceptual model.<br>   ♦ The conceptual model should be a useful guide for construction of theory-generating and/or theory-testing conceptual–theoretical–empirical structures.<br>   ♦ The content of the conceptual model is sound. |

*Source:* Adapted from: Fawcett, J., & Garity, J. (2009). *Evaluating research for evidence-based nursing practice*. Philadelphia, PA: F. A. Davis, pp. 51–53. Used with permission.

model be identified explicitly. It also requires that the content of the conceptual model that is relevant to the C-T-E structure be described clearly and concisely. An example of the content required is given in **Box 24–1**.

## Linkage Adequacy

*Linkage adequacy* refers to the clarity of the connections between the conceptual model, the theory, and the empirical indicators. It requires those connections to be stated explicitly and completely. An example of the content required is given in Box 24–1, and Figure 24–4 diagrams the complete C-T-E structure.

## Step 2: Evaluation of the Theory

The second step in evaluation of C-T-E structures focuses on the theory (T) component. The four criteria in this step are significance, internal consistency, parsimony, and testability.

## Box 24–1 Example of Narrative Content Required for the Criteria of Conceptual Model Specification Adequacy and Linkage Adequacy

### Specification Adequacy

The study was guided by Levine's conservation model. This conceptual model of nursing draws attention to individuals' needs for conservation of energy, structural integrity, personal integrity, and social integrity. As Levine (1988) explained:

> Conservation of energy refers to balancing energy output and energy input to avoid excessive fatigue, that is, adequate rest, nutrition, and exercise. Conservation of structural integrity refers to maintaining or restoring the structure of the body, that is, preventing physical breakdown and promoting healing. Conservation of personal integrity refers to maintenance or restoration of the patient's sense of identity, self-worth, and acknowledgement of uniqueness. Conservation of social integrity refers to the acknowledgment of the patient as a social being. (p. 227)

The conservation model includes two types of nursing interventions—therapeutic and supportive. Therapeutic nursing interventions are those nursing actions that have a positive influence on conservation of energy, structural integrity, personal integrity, and social integrity. Supportive nursing interventions are those actions used by nurses when energy, structural integrity, personal integrity, and social integrity cannot be conserved.

### Linkage Adequacy

As can be seen in Figure 24–4, therapeutic intervention was represented in this study by a cancer exercise program, which was implemented following a detailed protocol. Conservation of energy was represented by fatigue, which was measured by the Piper Fatigue Scale. Conservation of structural integrity was represented by physical function, which was measured by the 6-minute walk test. Conservation of personal integrity and conservation of social integrity were represented by mood, which was measured by the Profile of Mood States.

*Source:* Adapted from: Hanna, L. R., Avila, P. F., Meteer, J. D., Nicholas, D. R., & Kaminsky, L. A. (2008). The effects of a comprehensive exercise program on physical function, fatigue, and mood in patients with various types of cancer. *Oncology Nursing Forum, 35,* 461–469.

### Significance of the Theory

*Significance* refers to the extent to which the theory is socially important (social significance) and theoretically important (theoretical significance). It requires that the theory deal with a topic that society currently regards as practically important. It also requires that the theory offer new, compelling, and nontrivial insights into the topic. An example of narrative content that meets the criterion of significance is given in **Box 24–2**.

### Internal Consistency of the Theory

*Internal consistency* refers to the extent to which the concepts of the theory are comprehensible. It requires that the theory concepts be explicitly identified and clearly defined. It is also requires that the same terms be consistently used for the same concepts. For example, it is not appropriate to refer to the concept of mood as both "mood" and "emotion." An example of a narrative for internal consistency is given in **Box 24–3**.

---

**Box 24–2 Example of Narrative Content Required for the Criterion of Theory Significance**

#### Social Significance

*An estimated 1.4 million new cancer cases will be diagnosed in the United States in 2008. . . . All cancer treatments potentially have serious side effects.* (Hanna et al., 2008, p. 461)

#### Theoretical Significance

Side effects of cancer treatment "can include fatigue muscle loss, hair loss, nausea, pain, weakness, loss of appetite, depression, anxiety, sleep disruptions, and loss of ability to perform activities of daily living. . . . In the mid-1980s, studies emerged reporting exercise as an effective means of side effect management, particularly fatigue. . . . Some researchers have concluded the exercise currently offers the most promising nonpharmacologic treatment for [cancer-related fatigue] . . . Still, many unanswered questions remain, such as the ideal timing, intensity, and duration of exercise, particularly in patients actively receiving chemotherapy. . . . Research clearly has illustrated the usefulness of exercise in alleviation of the multiple symptoms of cancer and cancer treatment. None of the reported studies involved a comprehensive cancer exercise program achieving a significant improvement in physical function, fatigue, and mood in a mixed group of cancer diagnoses, staging, and treatment type. . . . The purpose of this study was to evaluate the effectiveness of a comprehensive exercise program using low-to-moderate intensity aerobic and resistance exercise for patients with various types of cancer on physical function, fatigue, and mood" (Hanna et al., 2008, pp. 461–462).

## Box 24–3 Example of Narrative Content Required for the Criterion of Theory Internal Consistency

The concepts of Hanna et al.'s (2008) theory are the cancer exercise program, fatigue, physical function, and mood.

- The cancer exercise program is defined as "a comprehensive program based on three key elements: exercise, education, and support" (Hanna et al., 2008, p. 464).
- Fatigue is defined as a multidimensional, complex concept that reflects the body's attempt to heal and as a symptom of adaptation (Hanna et al., 2008).
- Physical function is defined as "the distance walked in six minutes" (Hanna et al., 2008, p. 463).
- Mood is defined as feelings of "tension, anger, fatigue, depression, confusion, and vigor" (Hanna et al., 2008, p. 464).

## Parsimony of the Theory

*Parsimony* refers to the extent to which content of the theory is stated as concisely as possible. It requires that the theory be made up of as few concepts and propositions as necessary to clearly convey the meaning of each concept and proposition. An example of parsimony is evident in Figure 24–4. Hanna et al.'s (2008) review of the literature about the side effects of cancer and cancer treatment and the effects of exercise on side effects, for example, led these researchers to identify a parsimonious set of concepts that they regarded as plausible outcomes of a cancer exercise program—namely, fatigue, physical function, and mood. Furthermore, propositions that specified the definition of each concept and propositions that specified effects of the cancer exercise program on fatigue, physical function, and mood were stated concisely.

## Testability of the Theory

*Testability* refers to the extent to which the theory can be empirically tested. Each concept of the theory must be empirically measurable, which is accomplished when each concept is explicitly linked to an empirical indicator. Figure 24–4 provides an example of the linkage of theory concepts and empirical indicators; the narrative supporting testability is evident in the linkage adequacy section of Box 24–1, in which the theory concepts are explicitly linked to their respective empirical indicator.

## Step 3: Evaluation of the Empirical Research Methods

The third step in the evaluation of C-T-E structures research focuses on the empirical indicators and other empirical methods. The criterion in this step is operational adequacy.

## Box 24–4 Example of Narrative Content Required for the Criterion of Operational Adequacy

### Operational Adequacy of an Empirical Indicator Yielding Qualitative Data

Word data from interview guides were analyzed using content analysis. "Credibility of the data analysis was established by continuously confirming results until they accounted for all participants' responses. . . . To help reduce bias, portions of the logs and analytic memos were coded by an external auditor and compared with the first author's codes. Differences were explored for clarification. . . . The external auditor and first author achieved 95% agreement on the codes and themes. Participants also helped to clarify, confirm, and disconfirm findings" (Gagliardi et al., 2002, p. 232).

### Operational Adequacy of an Empirical Indicator Yielding Quantitative Data

The Profile of Mood States is regarded as a reliable and valid measure of mood. Investigators have reported "good reliability and validity data. Internal consistency coefficients across the five moods ranged from 0.84–0.95 in two different validation studies, and the test–retest reliability coefficients ranged from 0.65–0.74 for the five moods" (Hanna et al., 2008, p. 464).

*Operational adequacy* refers to the appropriateness of the empirical indicators as measures of the theory concepts. When the empirical indicator used to measure a theory concept yields qualitative data—that is, data that are words—it should be dependable and credible. When the empirical indicator used to measure a theory concept yields quantitative data—that is, data that are numbers—it should be reliable and valid. Examples of the narrative content needed to meet the criterion of operational adequacy for empirical indicators yielding qualitative and quantitative data are given in **Box 24–4**. Operational adequacy also refers to the appropriateness of the research design, the sample, the data collection procedures, the procedures used to protect research participants, and the data analysis techniques (Fawcett & Garity, 2009).

## Step 4: Evaluation of the Research Findings

The fourth step in evaluation of C-T-E structures again focuses on the theory (T) component. The criterion in this step is empirical adequacy.

*Empirical adequacy* refers to the extent to which the data from a study designed to generate or test the theory agree with the theory concepts and propositions. If the data are not completely congruent with theory concepts and propositions, the theory cannot be regarded as empirically adequate. Such a result could mean that the theory is more or less parsimonious than initially proposed. Alternatively, such a result could mean that the theory has no merit and should be discarded. An example of an empirically adequate theory is Hanna et al.'s (2008) theory of the effects of a cancer exercise program on fatigue, physical function, and mood. Analysis of the data from their theory-testing pretest, post-test quasi-experimental study indicated that—as hypothesized—the cancer exercise program resulted in decreased fatigue, increased physical function, and more positive mood.

## Step 5: Evaluation of the Utility and Soundness of the Conceptual Model

The fifth step in evaluation of C-T-E structures focuses on the conceptual model (C) component. The criterion in this step is legitimacy.

*Legitimacy* refers to the extent to which research findings support the usefulness of the conceptual model as a guide for construction of C-T-E structures for theory generation and theory testing, as well as the soundness of its content. The research findings cannot reveal any major flaws in the conceptual model concepts and propositions. Discovery of any flaws indicates that revisions in the content of the conceptual model are required or that the conceptual model should be discarded. Examples of narratives addressing legitimacy of a conceptual model appear in **Box 24–5**.

---

### Box 24–5 Example of Narrative Content for the Criterion of Legitimacy

#### Example from a Theory-Generating Study

"Collectively, the five themes identified in the data [see Figure 24–2] clearly reflect Roy's (1983) conceptualization of adaptation as "a process involving a holistic functioning of the person using his/her potential to affect health positively" (p. 266). . . . The Roy adaptation model (Roy & Andrews, 1999) directs nurses to assess behaviors in each mode of adaptation—physiological, self-concept, role function, and interdependence. The data from this study support the need for such a comprehensive assessment of each individual with MS" (Gagliardi et al., 2002, p. 235).

#### Example from a Theory-Testing Study

"Per Levine's Conservation Model, the present study emphasizes the need to use exercise to offset [cancer-related fatigue]. . . . The study results aligned with Levine's [conceptual model], validating favorable patient responses when incorporating exercise to treat fatigue" (Hanna et al., 2008, p. 467).

---

# Conclusion

This chapter's focus is on the C-T-E structures that need to be constructed for systematic theory generation and theory testing. The chapter also presented a discussion of criteria used to evaluate C-T-E structures. These go beyond the norm for theory evaluation theories by including criteria to evaluate conceptual models and empirical indicators.

# References

Ajzen, I. (1991). The theory of planned behavior. *Organizational Behavior and Human Decision Processes, 50,* 179–211.

Barnum, B. J. S. (1998). *Nursing theory: Analysis, application, evaluation* (5th ed.). Philadelphia, PA: Lippincott.

Doornbos, M. M. (1995). Using King's systems framework to explore family health in the families of the young chronically mentally ill. In M. A. Frey & C. L. Sieloff (Eds.), *Advancing King's systems framework and theory of nursing* (pp. 192–205). Thousand Oaks, CA: Sage.

Doornbos, M. M. (2000). King's systems framework and family health: The derivation and testing of a theory. *Journal of Theory Construction and Testing, 4,* 20–26.

Duffy, M., & Muhlenkamp, A. F. (1974). A framework for theory analysis. *Nursing Outlook, 22,* 570–574.

Fawcett, J. (2003). The Roy adaptation model: A program of nursing research. *Japanese Journal of Nursing Research, 36*(1), 67–73.

Fawcett, J. (2005). Criteria for evaluation of theory. *Nursing Science Quarterly, 18,* 131–135.

Fawcett, J. (2009). Appendix N-1: Conceptual models and theories of nursing. In D. Venes (Ed.), *Taber's cyclopedic medical dictionary* (21st ed., pp. 2646–2677). Philadelphia, PA: F. A. Davis.

Fawcett, J., Aber, C., Haussler, S., Weiss, M., Myers, S. T., Hall, J. L., . . . Silva, V. (2011). Women's perceptions of caesarean birth: A Roy international study. *Nursing Science Quarterly, 24,* 352–362.

Fawcett, J., Aber, C., Weiss, M., Haussler, S., Myers, S. T., King, C., . . . & Silva, V. (2005). Adaptation to cesarean birth: Implementation of an international multisite study. *Nursing Science Quarterly, 18,* 204–210.

Fawcett, J., & DeSanto-Madeya, S. (2013). *Contemporary nursing knowledge: Analysis and evaluation of nursing models and theories* (3rd ed.). Philadelphia, PA: F. A. Davis.

Fawcett, J., & Garity, J. (2009). *Evaluating research for evidence-based nursing practice.* Philadelphia, PA: F. A. Davis.

Gagliardi, B. A., Frederickson, K., & Shanley, D. A. (2002). Living with multiple sclerosis: A Roy adaptation model-based study. *Nursing Science Quarterly, 15,* 230–236.

George, J. B. (Ed.). (2002). *Nursing theories: The base for professional nursing practice* (5th ed.). Upper Saddle River, NJ: Prentice Hall.

Hanna, L. R., Avila, P. F., Meteer, J. D., Nicholas, D. R., & Kaminsky, L. A. (2008). The effects of a comprehensive exercise program on physical function, fatigue, and mood in patients with various types of cancer. *Oncology Nursing Forum, 35,* 461–469.

King, I. M., & Fawcett, J. (1997). *The language of nursing theory and metatheory.* Indianapolis, IN: Sigma Theta Tau International Center Nursing Press.

Latham, L. (2002). Letter to the editor. *Nursing Science Quarterly, 15*, 264.

Levine, M. E. (1966). Trophicognosis: An alternative to nursing diagnosis. In *American Nurses Association Regional Clinical Conference* (Vol. 2, pp. 55–70). New York, NY: American Nurses Association.

Levine, M. E. (1988). Myra Levine. In T. M. Schorr & A. Zimmerman (Eds.), *Making choices, taking chances: Nurse leaders tell their stories* (pp. 215–228). St. Louis, MO: Mosby.

Mariner-Tomey, A., & Alligood, M. R. (2006). *Nursing theorists and their work* (6th ed.). St. Louis, MO: Mosby Elsevier.

McEwen, M., & Wills, E. M. (2007). *Theoretical basis for nursing* (2nd ed.) Philadelphia, PA: Lippincott Williams & Wilkins.

Meleis, A. I. (2012). *Theoretical nursing: Development and progress* (5th ed.). Philadelphia, PA: Wolters Kluwer/Lippincott Williams & Wilkins.

Mishel, M. H. (1990). Reconceptualization of the uncertainty in illness theory. *Image: Journal of Nursing Scholarship, 22*, 256–262.

Parse, R. R. (2005). Fawcett's criteria for evaluation of theory with a comparison of Fawcett's and Parse's approaches. *Nursing Science Quarterly, 18*, 135–137.

Roy, C. (1983). The expectant family. Analysis and application of the Roy Adaptation Model. In I. W. Clements & F. B. Roberts (Eds.), *Family health: A theoretical approach to nursing care* (pp. 298–303). New York, NY: Wiley.

Roy, C. (2009). *The Roy adaptation model* (3rd ed.). Upper Saddle River, NJ: Pearson Prentice Hall.

Roy, C., & Andrews, H. (1999). *The Roy adaptation model* (2nd ed.). Upper Saddle River, NJ: Pearson Prentice Hall.

Samarel, N., Fawcett, J., & Tulman, L. (1997). Effects of support groups with coaching on adaptation to early stage breast cancer. *Research in Nursing and Health, 20*, 15–26.

Samarel, N., Tulman, L., & Fawcett, J. (2002). Effects of two types of social support and education on adaptation to early stage breast cancer. *Research in Nursing and Health, 25*, 459–470.

Tsai, P. F., Tak, S., Moore, C., & Palencia, I. (2003). Testing a theory of chronic pain. *Journal of Advanced Nursing, 43*, 158–169.

Tulman, L., & Fawcett, J. (2007). Development of the Comprehensive Inventory of Functioning—Cancer. *Cancer Nursing, 30*, 205–212.

Villarruel, A. M., Bishop, T. L., Simpson, E. M., Jemmott, L. S., & Fawcett, J. (2001). Borrowed theories, shared theories, and the advancement of nursing knowledge. *Nursing Science Quarterly, 14*, 158–163.

Wicks, M. N. (1995). Family health as derived from King's framework. In M. A. Frey & C. L. Sieloff (Eds.), *Advancing King's systems framework and theory of nursing* (pp. 97–108). Thousand Oaks, CA: Sage.

Wicks, M. N. (1997). A test of the Wicks family health model in families coping with chronic obstructive pulmonary disease. *Journal of Family Nursing, 3*, 189–212.

CHAPTER

# Using Theory in Evidence-Based Advanced Nursing Practice[*]

# 25

*Jacqueline Fawcett*

## Introduction

This chapter is focused on the use of theory as evidence in advanced nursing practice. It begins with a discussion of the equivalence of theory and evidence and a description of translational research, which is used to translate research findings into practical actions. The chapter continues with a presentation of the steps to follow and the criteria to be met to translate theories, in the form of research findings, into evidence-based best practices for advanced nursing practice. This chapter's content is especially relevant to three essentials for doctor of nursing practice programs: *Essential I, Scientific Underpinnings for Practice; Essential III, Clinical Scholarship and Analytical Methods for Evidence-Based Practice*; and *Essential VIII, Advanced Nursing Practice*.

## Theory and Evidence

Theories are typically thought of as formulations that are not relevant for practice, which is the source of the so-called *theory–practice gap*. Yet, "[n]othing is quite so practical as a good theory (Lewin, as cited in Van de Ven, 1989, p. 486). A central point of this chapter is that a theory does not *lead* to evidence but rather *is* the evidence. Thus, when we talk and write about evidence-based practice, we are actually talking and writing about theory-based practice. Accordingly, no gap

---

[*]Portions of this chapter are adapted from Fawcett, J., & Garity, J. (2009). *Evaluating research for evidence-based nursing practice*. Philadelphia, PA: F. A. Davis. Used with permission.

exists between theory and practice, as can be seen in the definition of evidence-based nursing practice given here: "Evidence-based nursing practice is the deliberate and critical use of theories about human beings' health-related experiences to guide [nursing] actions" (Fawcett & Garity, 2009, p. 8).

Of course, it is possible that no theory exists that can serve as evidence for a practical action. In this case, the evidence may be the tenacious beliefs of one or more individuals ("We always have done the procedure this way"), an authority ("The nurse manager said to do the procedure this way"; "The procedure manual [or textbook] said to do the procedure this way"), or common sense ("It seems reasonable to do the procedure this way") (Fawcett & Garity, 2009). Inasmuch as theory is regarded as the very best evidence, any nursing action that is not based on theory requires the generation of a new theory.

## Translational Research

Interest in translating theories into practical actions—such as assessment of health-related experiences and interventions used to promote positive responses to those experiences—has increased dramatically during the last several years in conjunction with an increased emphasis on evidence-based practice. *Translational research* is a research process used to determine which conditions, costs, and resources are required to progress from theory generation and theory testing to evidence-based practice. The goal of translational research is to decrease the time required for translation of theories into assessment tools and intervention protocols that will improve people's health-related quality of life.

## Types of Theories, Research, and Practice Tools

Five types of theories have been identified as what Carper (1978) and White (1995) referred to as the *fundamental patterns of knowing* in nursing: (1) empirical theories (the science of nursing), (2) aesthetic theories (the art of nursing), (3) ethical theories (the ethnics of nursing), (4) personal knowing theories (the interpersonal relationships of nursing), and (5) sociopolitical theories (the policies and politics of nursing). Collectively, the five types of theories constitute the evidence for nursing practice. The five types are integrated in nursing practice, although one type of theory may be more obvious than another in a given situation. For example, if an advanced practice nurse is caring for a patient who is hypo- or hyperglycemic, the best empirical theory about the most appropriate nursing intervention is applied. However, at the same time, the nurse will not neglect application of the other four types of theories.

Almost all contemporary discussions about evidence-based practice focus on empirical theories. Three primary types of empirical theories and research designs are (1) *descriptive theories* generated and tested by descriptive research, (2) *explanatory theories* tested by correlational research, and (3) *predictive theories* tested by experimental research. Most researchers and clinicians agree that

**TABLE 25–1    Types of Theories, Research Designs, and Practice Tools**

| Type of Theory | Type of Research Design | Type of Practice Tool |
| --- | --- | --- |
| Descriptive theories | Descriptive research | Assessment tools |
| Explanatory theories | Correlational research | Comprehensive assessment tools |
| Predictive theories | Experimental research | Intervention protocols |

predictive theories can be translated into intervention protocols. Nevertheless, few researchers or clinicians understand that descriptive and explanatory theories also have practical uses when translated into assessment tools.

Table 25–1 includes lists types of theories and research designs, as well as the types of practice tools that can be developed when research findings for each type of theory are translated for practice. As can be seen in the table, descriptive theories that are generated or tested by descriptive research can be translated into tools used to assess patients. An example is the assessment tool that DeSanto-Madeya (2006) included in her report of the generation of a descriptive theory of the experience of living with spinal cord injury. The Adaptation to Spinal Cord Assessment Tool, which is a semi-structured interview guide that also includes a one-item rating scale to measure adjustment to spinal cord injury, could be used to assess the physical, emotional, and role functioning of persons with spinal cord injuries, as well as their relationships with family and friends. Alternatively, the themes that make up the dimensions of the theory concept of the experience of living with a spinal cord injury could be translated into a more specific assessment tool. Each of the following themes, along with their descriptions, could, for example, be translated into a rating scale that would allow the nurse to assess the extent to which the patient has lived through each aspect of the experience of living with spinal cord injury:

- Looking for understanding of a life that is unknown
- Stumbling along an unlit path
- Being chained to the injury
- Viewing self though a stained glass window
- Moving forward in a new way of life
- Reaching normalcy
- Challenging the bonds of love (DeSanto-Madeya, 2006)

Explanatory theories that are tested by correlational research can be translated into comprehensive assessment tools. For example, a test of Dunn's (2005) explanatory theory of correlates of self-reported health revealed that the pain intensity, number of chronic health conditions, and depressive symptoms were related to self-reported health. This theory can be translated into a comprehensive assessment tool that includes one or more questions about each concept; alternatively, the research instruments used by Dunn could be evaluated for use as practice tools. **Box 25–1** is a summary of factors to take into account when considering the use of a research instrument as a practice tool.

## Box 25–1 Guidelines for Evaluating the Use of Research Instruments as Practice Tools

**What is the length of the research instrument?**

- Is the research instrument made up of one or many items?
  - ◆ Fewer items impose less burden on patients.
  - ◆ Fewer items also may impose less burden on the nurse when administering and scoring the tool and interpreting the patients' responses.

**What is the reading level of the research instrument?**

- No more than an 8th-grade reading level is recommended for use with patients.
- If the patient cannot read, can the instrument be administered orally by the nurse?

**Is the research instrument written in English or in the patient's native language?**

- If the instrument must be translated into the patient's native language, is the translation and back translation technique used? (See Varricchio, 2004.)
- If the instrument must be translated into the patient's native language, is cultural equivalence—including content equivalence, semantic equivalence, technical equivalence, criterion equivalence, and conceptual equivalence—documented? (See Cha, Kim, & Erlen, 2007, and Flaherty et al., 1988.)
  - ◆ *Content equivalence* refers to the relevance of each item to the culture of interest.
  - ◆ *Semantic equivalence* refers to the extent to which the connotative meaning of each item is the same in the original culture and the culture for which the instrument is being translated.
  - ◆ *Technical equivalence* refers to the extent to which the way the data were collected—such as interviews or survey questionnaires—is similar in each culture.
  - ◆ *Criterion equivalence* refers to the extent to which the interpretation of the data is similar across cultures.
  - ◆ *Conceptual equivalence* refers to the extent to which the researcher is able to measure the same middle-range theory concept in each culture.

**How easy are the research instrument items to complete?**

- Open-ended questions:
  - ◆ The patient has to write his or her response, or the nurse has to record the patient's response.
  - ◆ Example: How are you feeling physically?

*(Continues)*

- Visual analog scales:
  - ◆ The patient has to make a mark on a scale line. The scale line has to be 100 mm, and the nurse has to measure from one end of the line to the location of the patient's mark.
  - ◆ Example: Physically, I feel

    Dreadful ←——————————→ Great
- Rating scales:
  - ◆ The patient has to circle a number, or the nurse has to circle the number for the patient.
  - ◆ Example: On a scale of 1 to 10, where 1 = dreadful and 10 = great: Physically, I feel

    1  2  3  4  5  6  7  8  9  10

Predictive theories that are tested by experimental research can be translated into intervention protocols. For example, a test of the predictive theory of the effects of social support and education revealed that a combined individual telephone and in-person group social support and education intervention was just as effective as an individual telephone-only social support and education intervention in reducing mood disturbance and loneliness and improving the quality of a relationship with a significant other in women with early-stage breast cancer (Samarel, Tulman, & Fawcett, 2002). This theory could be translated into an individualized intervention for telephone-based social support and education using the detailed protocol given in Samarel et al.'s (2002) research report.

## Translating Theories into Practical Actions

Translation of theories into evidence-based assessment tools, intervention protocols, and any other practical actions follows a seven-step sequence. The seven steps identified in this chapter are adapted from the work of Melnyk, Fineout-Overholt, Stillwell, and Williamson (2010).

### First Step

The first step, which might seem obvious, is to identify a practice problem for which evidence is needed. This step requires an awareness of the problem and the possibility of a new way of assessing the problem or intervening to help people overcome it. Awareness may be catalyzed by something a patient experiences, an article in a nursing journal, a presentation at a workshop or conference, or a position statement from a government agency or professional society. An example of a problem is uncertainty about the effectiveness of cancer support groups for women with breast cancer as a way to reduce symptom and emotional distress, reduce interruptions in usual activities of daily living, and enhance relationships with family members.

## Second Step

The second step is to use the PICOT format to ask a question about the problem. This format takes into account the patient population (P), intervention or area of interest (I), group comparisons (C), the desired outcome (O), and time (T) (Melnyk et al., 2010).

- P: An example of a patient population is women with breast cancer who are or had been receiving chemotherapy in an outpatient clinic.
- I: An example of an intervention is a breast cancer support group.
- C: An example of group comparisons is receiving social support through a formal breast cancer support group versus receiving social support from a chemotherapy clinic nurse.
- O: An example of a desired outcome is enhanced adaptation, as manifested by minimal symptoms and emotional distress, minimal interruption in activities and daily living, and enhanced relationships with family members.
- T: An example of time is 13 months following the diagnosis of breast cancer.

## Third, Fourth, and Fifth Steps

The third, fourth, and fifth steps focus on the available evidence about the problem. The third step is a search of the published literature about the problem. Reference librarians at university, hospital, and public libraries can provide invaluable assistance with the search for relevant literature.

A scoping review of literature is recommended to determine the amount of literature available on the subject. As Hempel, Norman, Golder, Aguiar-Ibáñez, and Eastwood (2008) explained, "A scoping review, in contrast to a classic systematic review, formally documents the research that has been undertaken to date without providing detailed critical appraisal and synthesis of the individual studies" (p. 215). These authors pointed out that the primary outcome of a scoping review is determination of "whether enough [research] exists to conduct a full systematic review or identify research gaps in the existing literature" (p. 215). Davis, Drey, and Gould (2009) noted that a scoping review "provides a panoramic and intellectual overview of what is currently known and draws attention to areas where there are prominent knowledge gaps" (p. 1396). These authors concluded that the purpose of a scoping review is reconnaissance, which they explain "is generally synonymous with a [preliminary] investigation in which information is systematically gathered and examined in order to establish strengths and weaknesses" (p. 1396). Similarly, Bish, Kenny, Cert, and Nay (2012) explained, "[T]he goal is to scope a broad topic and include a wide range of study designs" (p. 412).

Literature reviews focus primarily on the theory component of conceptual–theoretical–empirical (C-T-E) structures, may include the empirical methods component (E), and should also include the conceptual model component (C). As Popper (1968) explained, "Theories are nets cast to catch what we call 'the world': to rationalize, to explain, and to master it. We endeavour to make the mesh ever finer and finer" (p. 59). Extrapolating from Popper's argument (1968), it can be said that the content of the conceptual model should be the net used to catch the relevant theory-generating and/or theory-testing research for the literature review. That is, the concepts and propositions of the conceptual model should be used to guide the search for and classification of the literature to be reviewed. Roy's adaptation model, for example, could be used as a search term.

Other search terms can be drawn from the PICOT format (Melnyk et al., 2010). For example, search terms drawn from the examples of the PICOT format given earlier in the discussion of the second step in translating theory into practical action might include the following: breast cancer, chemotherapy, social support, symptom distress, emotional distress, activities of daily living, and interpersonal relationships. The search can be narrowed when the conceptual model component (C) of the C-T-E structure being constructed is added.

The search terms also may include the type of article, such as a review article (including systematic reviews and state-of-the-science papers), practice guidelines, and best practices. More specifically, advanced practice nurses could take advantage of existing resources for evidence-based practice. Although most of these resources do not explicitly identify a conceptual model that guided the work or a theory that was generated or tested, they provide a summary of research findings, which advanced practice nurses will recognize as theories. Two especially useful resources are the practice guidelines available from the National Guideline Clearinghouse (http://www.guideline.gov/) and the best practices information sheets available from the Joanna Briggs Institute (JBI; http://www.joannabriggs.edu.au/). Practice guidelines are "systematically developed statements to assist health care practitioners' decisions about appropriate health care for specific clinical circumstances" (Wallin, 2005, pp. 248–249).

Best practices refer to "the organizational use of evidence to improve practice" (Driever, 2002, p. 593). These evidence-based practices include not only the actions required for assessment or intervention, but also specification of the most efficient and effective uses of human resources and equipment to attain the best possible patient outcomes. The JBI For example, Best Practice Information Sheets are available from the Joanna Briggs Institute (JBI; http://joannabriggs.org/Best%20Practice%20Information%20Sheets); these documents contain brief summaries of best practices gleaned from systematic reviews of research. Some of the many JBI Best Practice Information Sheets are listed here:

- Music as intervention in hospitals
- Strategies to reduce medication errors with reference to older adults
- Topical skin care in aged care facilities
- Effective dietary interventions for overweight and obese children
- Effectiveness of a pelvic floor muscle exercise program on urinary incontinence following childbirth
- Nurse-led cardiac clinics for adults with coronary artery disease

The fourth step in the process of translating theory into practical actions involves a critical evaluation of the literature. A realist review of literature is recommended as an efficient and effective approach to integrating the available literature that was identified in the scoping review. According to Pawson, Greenhalgh, Harvey, and Walshe (2005), a realist review "is a relatively new strategy for synthesizing research which has an explanatory rather than judgemental focus. [A realist review] seeks to unpack the mechanism of how complex programmes work (or why they fail) in particular contexts and settings" (p. 21). The conceptual and theoretical perspective(s) evident in the literature are of particular interest in a realist review. Indeed, Pawson et al. (2005) regard interventions (and other complex programs such as assessment tools) as theories that are derived from conceptual models. Elaborating on this point, these authors explained that healthcare programs "are always based on a hypothesis that postulates: if we deliver a programme in this way or we manage services like so, then this will bring about some improved outcome" (p. 22).

Realist reviews of the literature may involve appraisal and integration of theory-generating research, theory-testing research, or both. *Metasynthesis* and *metasummary* are techniques used to integrate theory-generating research (Finfgeld, 2003; Sandelowski, 2006; Sandelowski, Barroso, & Voils, 2007). *Meta-analysis* is a technique used to integrate theory-testing research (Rosenthal, 1991). *Critical interpretative synthesis* is a relatively new technique that is used to integrate both theory-generating and theory-testing research (Fleming, 2010).

A worksheet may be used to systematically record the research that is retrieved and the quality of each study. **Figure 25–1** shows an example of a worksheet. The quality of each study can be rated by using a levels-of-evidence schema; an example is given in **Box 25–2**. A different levels-of-evidence schema can be used to collectively evaluate all of the literature included in the review.

A schema that may be used to rate the overall level of evidence of an integrated review of literature, referred to as FAME (Feasibility, Appropriateness, Meaningfulness, Effectiveness, and Economic evidence, was developed by the JBI (http://joannabriggs.org/Levels%20of%20Evidence%20%20FAME). The highest level of evidence (Level 1) in each category of FAME comes from metasyntheses of research with consistent findings from experimental research. The lowest level of evidence (Level 4) in each category of FAME is expert opinion.

> Levels of evidence schemas usually include ratings for various types of research designs and even expert opinion, although the best ratings are typically assigned to integrated reviews of experimental research, especially RCTs [randomized controlled trials]. . . . [Furthermore,] levels of evidence [schemas] . . . ignore the different contributions of each type of research—descriptive, correlational, experimental—to practice [see Table 25–1]. (Fawcett & Garity, 2009, p. 268)

The fifth step in the translation of theory into practical actions is the use of the literature to inform all elements required for evidence-based practice—assessments and interventions, the context of care delivery, patient and family preferences, values,

| Citation Author(s)/ Year | Name of Conceptual Model | Name of Theory/ Concepts | Sample Size/ Characteristics | Instruments | Results | Effect Size (If Available) | Quality of the Study |
|---|---|---|---|---|---|---|---|
| | | | | | | | |
| | | | | | | | |
| | | | | | | | |
| | | | | | | | |
| | | | | | | | |
| | | | | | | | |
| | | | | | | | |
| | | | | | | | |
| | | | | | | | |
| | | | | | | | |
| | | | | | | | |
| | | | | | | | |
| | | | | | | | |
| | | | | | | | |

**FIGURE 25–1** Example of a literature review worksheet.

## Box 25–2  Example of a Levels-of-Evidence Schema to Rate Each Study Included in a Literature Review

**1++:** High-quality meta-analyses, systematic reviews of randomized controlled trials (RCTs), or RCTs with a very low risk of bias

**1+:** Well-conducted meta-analyses, systematic reviews of RCTs, or RCTs with a low risk of bias

**1−:** Meta-analyses, systematic reviews of RCTs, or RCTs with a high risk of bias

**2++:** High-quality systematic reviews of case control or cohort studies; high-quality case-control or cohort studies with a very low risk of confounding or bias and a high probability that the relationship is causal

**2+:** Well-conducted case-control or cohort studies with a low risk of confounding or bias and a moderate probability that the relationship is causal

**2−:** Case-control or cohort studies with a high risk of confounding or bias and a significant risk that the relationship is not causal

**3:** Nonanalytic studies (e.g., case reports, case series)

**4:** Expert opinion

*Source:* Scottish Intercollegiate Guidelines Network (SIGN). (2003, July). *Cutaneous melanoma: A national clinical guideline* (SIGN Publication No. 72), Edinburgh, Scotland: Author. Reprinted by permission.

and needs, and the nurse's expertise and clinical judgment (Driever, 2002; Fawcett, 2012; Pearson, Wiechula, Court, & Lockwood, 2007; Porter-O'Grady, 2006).

All five types of theories (empirical, aesthetic, ethical, personal knowing, sociopolitical) constitute the best evidence for assessments and interventions, although empirical theories tend to be the most obviously useful (Fawcett, 2012). Sociopolitical theories are the best evidence for the context of care delivery, which requires consideration of the policies and politics of the healthcare delivery system, including the extent to which healthcare resources are available and allocated for use by advanced practice nurses, in which the patient and nurse are located, such as the patient's home, a community health center, an outpatient clinic, an inpatient tertiary or rehabilitation hospital, or a long-term care facility.

Sociopolitical, aesthetic, and empirical theories provide the evidence for recognition of and accounting for patient and family preferences, values, and needs. These three types of theories sensitize the advanced practice nurse to consideration of the patient's and their family's culture, which has a major influence on the patient's and their family's health-related beliefs, values, and life ways (Leininger & McFarland, 2006) and on family dynamics regarding preferences for a particular approach to assessment and a specific intervention. These three types of theories also guide the nurse to consider the influence of social media (e.g., Facebook and Twitter) and public media (e.g., print and electronic news stories, advertisements, and television and radio talk shows) on patient and family preferences and values.

Aesthetic, ethical, personal knowing, and empirical theories are the evidence for the nurse's expertise and clinical judgment. Aesthetic theories guide the advanced practice nurse's understanding of the meaning of the individual patient's behavior and needs. Ethical theories are the guides to what the nurse should do in practice. Personal knowing theories undergird the nurse's understanding of how he or she expresses authentic caring with patients. Empirical theories tell the nurse what to expect when applying a particular assessment tool or intervention. The nurse's expertise and clinical judgment are the mechanisms by which all elements of evidence-based practice are integrated (Melnyk & Fineout-Overholt, 2011).

Although there is no magic formula for weighting, as Melnyk et al. (2010) noted, integration of all elements (assessments and interventions; context of care delivery; patient and family preferences, values, and needs; and the nurse's expertise and clinical judgment) and, we can add, all types of theories (empirical, aesthetic, ethical, personal knowing, sociopolitical), that need to be taken into account when considering implementing a new evidence-based practical action can be guided by the criterion of pragmatic adequacy of a theory. *Pragmatic adequacy* refers to the extent to which a theory serves as the evidence for practical actions, including assessment tools and interventional protocols. Theories that are judged to be pragmatically adequate are socially meaningful, compatible with a particular practice setting, feasible in the real world of practice, and consistent with patients' preferences for and expectations about care. In addition, for the purposes of this chapter, pragmatically adequate theories lead to actions that are within the legal scope of advanced nursing practice (Fawcett & Garity, 2009).

Evaluating the social meaningfulness of a theory requires consideration of the extent to which translation of the theory into a new assessment tool or intervention protocol would yield desired outcomes that are consistent with patient needs. Desired outcomes include comprehensive assessments of health-related experiences and positive effects of interventions, such as reduction in the incidence of physical or psychological symptom distress, and increased quality of life. Radwin, Washko, Suchy, and Tyman (2005, p. 93), for example, identified five desired outcomes of oncology nursing care:

1. Sense of well-being: "the patient's positive emotional state"
2. Trust: "the patient's confidence that care was appropriate and reliable and would be as successful as possible"
3. Fortitude: "the patient's strength and willingness to bear the effects of cancer treatments and the symptoms of the disease"

4. Optimism: "the patient's belief that he or she had made appropriate choices regarding treatment and the patient's feelings of hopefulness about treatment outcomes"
5. Authentic self-representation: "the patient's sense of genuine self-portrayal"

Social meaningfulness of qualitative theory-generating research depends on how confident the reader is that the new theory will be meaningful for practice and can be translated into a new assessment tool. The social meaningfulness of theory-testing research depends on both the statistical significance and the clinical significance of the research findings. Statistical significance is determined by the $p$ value. A caveat applies, however: "Statistical significance does not guarantee clinical significance and more to the point, the magnitude of the $p$ value (.05, .01, .001, .00029, or whatever) is no guide to clinical significance" (Slakter, Wu, & Suzuki-Slakter, 1991, p. 249).

Clinical significance is determined by the magnitude of the findings, which is calculated as an effect size. Effect sizes for different statistical tests can be classified as a small, medium, or large frequency of occurrence of a phenomenon, relationship between variables, or difference between groups (Cohen, 1992). Tulman and Fawcett (1996), for example, found small and medium effect sizes for the relationships between the concepts of their explanatory theory of biobehavioral correlates of functional status in women with breast cancer. Clinical significance also may take into account the cost-effectiveness of use of a new assessment tool or intervention (Leeman, Jackson, & Sandelowski, 2006). For example, Mock and colleagues (2004) pointed out that a home-based walking exercise intervention was "low-cost . . . and well received" by women receiving treatment for breast cancer (p. 475).

Evaluating the compatibility of the theory with a particular practice situation draws attention to the context of the situation and requires consideration of the demographic and health-related characteristics of the research participants and the setting in which the research took place. The theory that was generated or tested should be compatible with a particular practice specialty setting, a particular health condition, and particular ages or developmental phases of the people for whom the new assessment tool or intervention protocol is intended. Mock et al. (2004), for example, claimed that their predictive theory of the effects of a home-based walking exercise program on fatigue is "widely applicable . . . to many women with breast cancer" (p. 475).

Evaluating the feasibility of translating the theory into practical actions in a particular practice setting involves making clinical judgments about the complexity of implementing a new assessment tool or intervention protocol. Complexity is determined by considering the following factors:

- The type of training and the time needed to learn how to use the new practice tool or intervention protocol
- The number, type, and expertise of personnel required for all aspects of the design and implementation of the new practice tool or intervention protocol

- The number of contacts and amount of time for each contact required to use the new tool or to deliver and evaluate the new intervention
- The cost of in-service or other continuing education, salaries, and equipment

Feasibility also takes into consideration the willingness of those who control resources to utilize those resources. If they are not willing to surrender those resources to implement the new assessment tool or intervention protocol, the complexity of that practical action does not matter. However, it may be easier to convince whoever controls the resources to allocate them if the new assessment tool or intervention protocol has minimal cost and requires little training and a short time to learn how to use it, few personnel to implement it, and few contacts of short duration.

Furthermore, feasibility requires determining the willingness of nurses or other healthcare personnel to use a new tool or protocol. Making time to search and critically evaluate the literature and translate the theory that was generated or tested into a new assessment tool or intervention protocol can be especially difficult given the trend toward increasing patient acuity and the contemporary "fast-paced, high-risk [healthcare] environment" (Farrell, 2006, p. 119). Advanced practice nurses have to be leaders in fostering evidence-based practice. Advanced practice nurses can form partnerships with nurse researchers, who are fully prepared at the research doctoral level, to conduct research. An advanced practice nurse also can form a partnership with a nursing program or a nursing faculty member whose students have clinical experiences in the settings in which the advanced practice nurses work. The faculty member may be willing to develop a student assignment that focuses on a scoping review or even a realist review addressing a problem identified by the advanced practice nurse.

Evaluation of pragmatic adequacy also involves determining the extent to which the theory is consistent with patients' preferences for and expectations about care. For example, Mock et al. (2004) noted that implementation of their predictive theory about the effects of a home-based walking exercise program was "acceptable" to many women with breast cancer (p. 475). Their comment, coupled with their finding that almost three-fourths (72%) of the women in the experimental treatment group adhered to the walking exercise intervention, indicates that walking-type exercise was consistent with the women's preferences for and expectations about nursing care.

If the new assessment tool or intervention protocol is not consistent with patient preferences or expectations, either it should not be used or patients should be helped to change their preferences and expectations for care. Johnson's (1974) words of almost 40 years ago remain relevant today: "Current . . . practice is not entirely what it might become and [thus patients] might come to expect a different form of practice, given the opportunity to experience it" (p. 376). Suppose, for example, that a researcher found that listening to music the day before surgery reduced patients' anxiety on the morning of the surgery, and an advanced practice nurse decided to implement the music intervention as part of routine preoperative preparation. Some patients might be receptive to this intervention, whereas others might indicate that they did not want or expect to be asked to listen to music the day before their surgery. The advanced practice nurse would then have to explain the research results and the evidence base supporting the music intervention.

Evaluation of the pragmatic adequacy of a theory must also take into account whether the use of a particular assessment tool or intervention protocol is within the legal scope of advanced nursing practice. For example, prescribing medications has not always been included in the scope of advanced nursing practice.

The outcome of evaluation of pragmatic adequacy is a decision about translating the theory into a practical action. The decision tree shown in **Figure 25–2** illustrates the possible decisions. The decision can be a call for additional research ("what needs additional study"), advocacy of translating a theory into a new assessment tool or intervention protocol and adoption of the tool or protocol in advanced nursing practice ("what should be done"), a trial of a new tool or protocol in a practice setting ("what could be tried"), or discontinuation of a currently used tool or protocol or abandonment of a new tool or protocol ("what should not be done") (Fawcett & Garity, 2009).

Furthermore, as Fawcett and Garity (2009) explained:

> If the decision is to translate the theory into [a practical action]—What Should Be Done or What Could Be Tried—the how, when, and where of implementation of the new tool or protocol also need to be considered. How refers to the procedures to follow to actually use the tool or protocol. When refers to the time during an individual's experience in the healthcare system the tool or protocol is used, such as when the person initially seeks treatment, during the time that treatment is being received, or at the end of treatment. Where refers to the location in which the new tool or protocol will be used, such as in a hospital or at home. (p. 265)

**FIGURE 25–2    Decision tree for using a theory to guide practice.**
*Source:* Adapted from Fawcett, J., & Garity, J. (2009). *Evaluating Research for Evidence-Based Nursing Practice*. Philadelphia, PA: F. A. Davis, p. 265. Used with permission.

## Sixth Step

The sixth step in the process of translating theory into practical action involves evaluation of the innovative action, which occurs after the innovation has been implemented in practice. Evaluation may be done by means of a formal research project or through a healthcare organization's regular quality improvement or quality assurance program. An example of a formal research project is the evaluation of the Common Journey Breast Cancer Support Group, which is a breast cancer support group sponsored by a small community hospital in a rural New England state (Zeigler, Smith, & Fawcett, 2004). An example of a quality assurance program is a breast awareness project focused on breast examination, designed for nursing staff working with women with learning disabilities (Cowie & Fletcher, 1998).

## Seventh Step

The seventh step is dissemination of the results of the evaluation of the innovation. This means that the results of the evaluation of the innovation should be presented publicly—for example, at agency-based nursing rounds and at local, regional, national, and international conferences. In addition, they should be published, because the widest audience is made up of the readers of general and specialty journals. Presentations and publications are the necessary final step in translating theories into practical actions of evidence-based practice. As Melnyk et al. (2010) note, "Clinicians can achieve wonderful outcomes for their patients through [evidence-based practice], but they often fail to share their experiences with colleagues and their own or other healthcare organizations. This leads to needless duplication of effort, and perpetuates clinical approaches that are not evidence based" (p. 53).

## Conclusion

All nurses must have the skills needed for them to review current findings and evaluate if they are applicable for their setting (LaPierre, Ritchey, & Newhouse, 2004). The outcome of evaluating the applicability of research findings to a particular setting is a major element when nurses evaluate the pragmatic adequacy of a theory. The current emphasis on evidence-based nursing practice calls for advanced practice nurses to be leaders in evaluating the pragmatic adequacy of nursing theories and translating the theory, in the form of research findings, into evidence-based best practices. Advanced practice nurses also need to take the lead in helping all nurses understand that evidence-based practice is equivalent to theory-based practice.

## References

Bish, M., Kenny, A., Cert, G., & Nay, R. (2012). A scoping review identifying contemporary issues in rural nursing leadership. *Journal of Nursing Scholarship, 44,* 411–417.

Carper, B. A. (1978). Fundamental patterns of knowing in nursing. *Advances in Nursing Science, 1*(1), 13–23.

Cha, E. S., Kim, K. H., & Erlen, J. A. (2007). Translation of scales in cross-cultural research: Issues and techniques. *Journal of Advanced Nursing, 58*, 386–395.

Cohen, J. (1992). A power primer. *Psychological Bulletin, 112*, 135–159.

Cowie, M., & Fletcher, J. (1998). Breast awareness project for women with a learning disability. *British Journal of Nursing, 7*, 774–778.

Davis, K., Drey, N., & Gould, D. (2009). What are scoping studies? A review of the nursing literature. *International Journal of Nursing Studies, 46*, 1386–1400.

DeSanto-Madeya, S. (2006). A secondary analysis of the meaning of living with spinal cord injury using Roy's adaptation model. *Nursing Science Quarterly, 19*, 240–246.

Driever, M. J. (2002). Are evidence-based practice and best practice the same? *Western Journal of Nursing Research, 24*, 591–597.

Dunn, K. S. (2005). Predictors of self-reported health among older African-American central city adults. *Holistic Nursing Practice, 21*, 237–243.

Farrell, M. P. (2006). Living evidence: Translating research into practice. In K. Malloch & T. Porter-O'Grady (Eds.), *Introduction to evidence-based practice in nursing and health care* (pp. 107–123). Sudbury, MA: Jones and Bartlett.

Fawcett, J. (2012). Thoughts about evidence-based nursing practice. *Nursing Science Quarterly, 25*, 199–200.

Fawcett, J., & Garity, J. (2009). *Evaluating research for evidence-based nursing practice.* Philadelphia, PA: F. A. Davis.

Finfgeld, D. (2003). Metasynthesis: The state of the art—so far. *Qualitative Health Research, 13*, 893–904.

Flaherty, J. A., Gaviria, F. M., Pathak, D., Mitchell, T., Wintrob, R., Richman, J. A., & Birz, S. (1988). Developing instruments for cross-cultural psychiatric research. *Journal of Nervous and Mental Diseases, 176*, 257–263.

Fleming, K. (2010). Synthesis of quantitative and qualitative research: An example using critical interpretive synthesis. *Journal of Advanced Nursing, 66*, 201–207.

Hempel, S., Norman, G., Golder, S., Aguiar-Ibáñez, R., & Eastwood, A. (2008). Psychosocial interventions for non-professional carers of people with Parkinson's disease: A systematic scoping review. *Journal of Advanced Nursing, 64*, 214–228.

Johnson, D. E. (1974). Development of a theory: A requisite for nursing as a primary health profession. *Nursing Research, 23*(5), 372–377.

Lapierre, E., Ritchey, K., & Newhouse, R. (2004). Barriers to research use in PACU. *Journal of Perianesthesia Nursing, 19*(2), 78–83.

Leeman, J., Jackson, B., & Sandelowski, M. (2006). An evaluation of how well research reports facilitate the use of findings in practice. *Journal of Nursing Scholarship, 38*, 171–177.

Leininger, M. M., & McFarland, M. R. (2006). *Culture care diversity and universality: A worldwide nursing theory* (2nd ed.). Sudbury, MA: Jones and Bartlett.

Melnyk, B. M., & Fineout-Overholt, E. (2011). *Evidence-based practice in nursing and healthcare: A guide to best practice* (2nd ed.). Philadelphia, PA: Wolters Kluwer/Lippincott Williams & Wilkins.

Melnyk, B. M., Fineout-Overholt, E., Stillwell, S. B., & Williamson, K. M. (2010). The seven steps of evidence-based practice. *American Journal of Nursing, 110*(1), 51–53.

Mock, V., Frangakis, C., Davidson, N. E., Ropka, M. E., Pickett, M., Poniatowski, B., . . . McCorkle, R. (2004). Exercise manages fatigue during breast cancer treatment: A randomized controlled trial. *Psycho-Oncology, 14*, 464–477.

Pawson, R., Greenhalgh, T., Harvey, G., & Walshe, K. (2005). Realist review: A new method of systematic review designed for complex policy interventions. *Journal of Health Services Research and Policy, 10*(Suppl. 1), 21–34.

Pearson, A., Wiechula, R., Court, A., & Lockwood, C. (2007). A re-consideration of what constitutes "evidence" in the healthcare professions. *Nursing Science Quarterly, 20*, 85–88.

Popper, K. R. (1968). *The logic of scientific discovery.* New York, NY: Harper Torchbooks.

Porter-O'Grady, T. (2006). A new age for practice: Creating the framework for evidence. In K. Malloch & T. Porter-O'Grady (Eds.), *Introduction to evidence-based practice in nursing and health care* (pp. 1–29). Sudbury, MA: Jones and Bartlett.

Radwin, L. E., Washko, M., Suchy, K. A., & Tyman, K. (2005). Development and pilot testing of four desired health outcomes scales. *Oncology Nursing Forum, 32*, 92–96.

Rosenthal, R. (1991). *Meta-analytic procedures for social research* (rev. ed.). Newbury Park, CA: Sage.

Samarel, N., Tulman, L., & Fawcett, J. (2002). Effects of two types of social support and education on adaptation to early stage breast cancer. *Research in Nursing and Health, 25*, 459–470.

Sandelowski, M. (2006). "Meta-jeopardy": The crisis of representation in qualitative metasynthesis. *Nursing Outlook, 54*, 10–16.

Sandelowski, M., Barroso, J., & Voils, C. I. (2007). Using qualitative metasummary to synthesize qualitative and quantitative descriptive findings. *Research in Nursing and Health, 30*, 99–111.

Slakter, M. J., Wu, Y. W. B., & Suzuki-Slakter, N. S. (1991). *, **, and ***: Statistical nonsense at the .00000 level. *Nursing Research, 40*, 248–249.

Tulman, L., & Fawcett, J. (1996). Lessons learned from a pilot study of biobehavioral correlates of functional status in women with breast cancer. *Nursing Research, 45*, 356–358.

Van de Ven, A. H. (1989). Nothing is quite so practical as a good theory. *Academy of Management Review, 14*, 486–489.

Varricchio, C. G. (2004). Measurement issues concerning linguistic translations. In F. Frank-Stromborg & S. J. Olsen (Eds.), *Instruments for clinical health-care research* (3rd ed., pp. 56–64). Sudbury, MA: Jones and Bartlett.

Wallin, L. (2005). Clinical practice guidelines in nursing. *AWHONN Lifelines, 9*, 248–251.

White, J. (1995). Patterns of knowing: Review, critique, and update. *Advances in Nursing Science, 17*(4), 73–86.

Zeigler, L., Smith, P. A., & Fawcett, J. (2004). Breast cancer: Evaluation of the Common Journey Breast Cancer Support Group. *Journal of Clinical Nursing, 13*, 467–478.

# Index

Note: Page numbers followed by *b, f,* or *t* indicate material in boxes, figures, or tables, respectively.